THE LITTLE
BLACK BOOK
OF NEUROLOGY

Fifth
EDITION

THE LITTLE BLACK BOOK OF NEUROLOGY

Osama O. Zaidat, MD

Director, Interventional Neurology Program
Associate Professor of Neurology and Neurosurgery
Medical College of Wisconsin/Froedtert Hospital
Milwaukee, Wisconsin

Alan J. Lerner, MD

Associate Professor of Neurology
Case Western Reserve Universiy
School of Medicine;
Director, Memory and Aging Center
University Hospitals Health System
Cleveland, Ohio

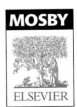

MOSBY
ELSEVIER

1600 John F. Kennedy Blvd.
Ste 1800
Philadelphia, PA 19103-2899

Notice

Neither the Publisher nor the Authors assume any responsibility for any loss or
injury and/or damage to persons or property arising out of or related to any use of
the material contained in this book. It is the responsibility of the treating practi-
tioner, relying on independent expertise and knowledge of the patient, to determine the best treatment and method of application for the patient.

The Publisher

Library of Congress Cataloging-in-Publication Data

The little black book of neurology. —5th ed. / Osama O. Zaidat, Alan J. Lerner.
     p. ; cm.
   Includes bibliographical references and index.
   ISBN 978-0-323-03950-5
1. Nervous system—Diseases—Handbooks, manuals, etc. 2. Neurology—
Handbooks, manuals, etc. I. Zaidat, Osama O. II. Lerner, Alan J.
   [DNLM: 1. Nervous System Diseases—Handbooks.   WL 39 L778 2008]
RC355.L58 2008
616.8—dc22   2007022809

Acquisitions Editor: Jim Merritt
Editorial Assistant: Greg Halbreich
Design Coordinator: Louis Forgione

ISBN-13: 978-0-323-03950-5

Working together to grow
libraries in developing countries

www.elsevier.com | www.bookaid.org | www.sabre.org

ELSEVIER   BOOK AID International   Sabre Foundation

Printed in the United States of America.

Last digit is the print number: 9   8   7   6   5   4   3   2

To

The soul of my father

Contributors

Nuhad E. AbouZeid, MD

Shahram Amina, MD

Eric M. Bershad, MD

Margo Block, MD

Robbie Buechler, MD, PhD, FAAN, FAASM

Jesse J. Corry, MD

Anh Dam, MD

Julia C. Durrant, MD

Matthew Eccher, MD

Eli Feen, MD

William B. Gallentine, MD

Catalina C. Ionita, MD

Prem A. Kandiah, MD

Bradley J. Kolls, MD, PhD

Wayne Wei-ku Lai, MD

Alan A. Lerner, MD

Fuhai Li, MD

Judah R. Lindenberg, MD

Marta Lopez-Vicente, MD

David L. McDonagh, MD

J. Douglas Miles, MD, PhD

Justin S. Moon, MD, MPH

Venkatesh Nagaraddi, MD

Eliza Cristina Olaru, MD

Santiago Ortega-Gutierrez, MD

Paul C. Peterson, MD, FACEP

Gautami K. Rao, MD

Jenice Robinson, MD

Sith Sathornsumetee, MD

Dharmen Shah, MD

William Stacey, MD, PhD

M. Badr Sultan, MD

Viktor Szeder, MD, PhD

Marshall Tolbert, MD, PhD

Jawad Tsay, MD

Osama O. Zaidat, MD, MS

Preface

The Little Black Book of Neurology has enjoyed a great reputation among health care providers for almost two decades; it has succeeded because it strived for simplicity, while being comprehensive and clinically relevant. This new edition, the fifth (LBBN-5e), retains the original concept of Dr. Robert Daroff of an easy-to-access guide, with topics arranged in alphabetical order and written by junior neurologists and residents.

In preparing for the fifth edition, we rethought the content and format. The concept of a comprehensive, authoritative book in a pocket format has run up against a bewildering explosion of new treatments, treatment algorithms, and evidence-based recommendations. Second, because of career moves, our focus has moved beyond the residency program at University Hospitals of Cleveland and Case Western Reserve University, which had provided authorship for previous editions.

The majority of the chapters have been updated or rewritten, with new tables and references added. At least one new suggested reading or reference of a landmark study or review article is provided at the end of most chapters, and we recommend that readers take note of those excellent references.

One major change is the provision of Neurologic Emergency and Therapeutic appendices at the back of the book. The Neurologic Emergency Appendix provides in short monograph, table, or algorithm format approaches to areas such as Acute Ischemic Stroke, Meningitis, Myasthenia Crisis, Headache, Hemorrhagic Stroke, Intracranial Pressure, Pain, Quadriplegia, Spinal Cord Injury, and Status Epilepticus. Topics covered in the Therapeutic Appendix include Dementia, Epilepsy, Headache, Insomnia, Multiple Sclerosis, Myasthenia Gravis, Pain Management, Parkinson's Disease, and Stroke.

We have also included the American Academy of Neurology (AAN) Guideline Summaries in a new appendix. These guidelines are important in our daily practice to provide better care of our patients and for Neurology Board Recertification. We conclude the appendices with a comprehensive scales index.

We hope the national breadth of this edition will provide perspective on many neurologic disorders that may not exist in an individual center. Authorship was a collaboration of adult and pediatric neurology, neuroradiology, and neurosurgery residents from three academic institutions across the United States: Case Western Reserve University, Cleveland, Ohio; Duke University, Durham, North Carolina; and Medical College of Wisconsin, Milwaukee, Wisconsin.

The new LBBN-5e is still the neurology pocket book that provides a concise, up-to-date, and easy-to-read practical overview of general neurology. This work will be very useful for neurologists, neurosurgeons, internists, family practitioners, physical medicine and rehabilitation staff, neuroradiologists, residents, medical students, nurses, physician assistants, and nurse practitioners, or any health care providers caring for neurologic patients. Our greatest satisfaction will be when the LBBN-5e is helpful in providing optimal patient care in the hands of health care providers.

I would like to thank our publisher, Elsevier, our managing editor, Jim Merritt, and his editorial assistant, Greg Halbreich, for their endless efforts and hard work to provide an excellent well-organized volume to our readers. Dr Alan Lerner has provided guidance through the formulation of this edition and contributed original text and practice recommendations.

I also would like to thank my wife, Sabreen Owais, and my kids, Bash, Kenan, and Tamim, for their patience with me during the long hours spent updating and editing the chapters.

Osama O. Zaidat
Milwaukee, Wisconsin

Contents

A

ABSCESS, BRAIN

Brain abscesses constitute less than 2% of intracranial masses and develop mainly in three clinical situations (15–20% are cryptogenic):

I. *Contiguous* spread (45–50% of all cases) via direct extension from local neighboring infection sites—frontal, ethmoid sinusitis or dental infection (frontal lobe abscess), middle ear or mastoid cell infection (temporal lobe and cerebellar abscess), spread by local osteomyelitis or by septic thrombophlebitis of emissary vein.

II. *Hematogenous* spread from distant sites of infection (25%), usually multiple and multiloculated in the middle cerebral artery distribution. Common sources of metastatic brain abscesses are chronic infection of lungs or pleura (bronchiectasis, empyema, lung abscess), congenital heart malformations with right-to-left shunts (oral bacterial flora after dental procedures), or bacterial endocarditis, or hepatic abscesses.

III. *Penetrating head injury or neurosurgical procedures* (10%)—compound depressed skull fractures, basal skull fractures with CSF fistulae/leak, and previous craniotomy can cause brain abscess formation, sometimes months or years after the acute event. Postneurosurgical abscesses occur, especially when surgery involves paranasal air sinuses.

Pathogens isolated from abscesses are related to the site of origin, as follows (organisms are listed in order of significance; many abscesses are polymicrobial):

I. Middle ear infection: streptococci (aerobic and anaerobic), *Bacteroides fragilis*, and Enterobacteriaceae (*Proteus*).

II. Sinusitis: same as middle ear infections, plus *Staphylococcus aureus*, *Haemophilus* species, and mucormycosis (also seen with orbital cellulitis).

III. Penetrating head trauma: *S. aureus*, streptococci, Enterobacteriaceae, and *Clostridium* species.

IV. AIDS/immunocompromised: *Toxoplasma, Mycobacterium, Listeria* species infection, although fungal abscesses may also occur.

CLINICAL FEATURES

Clinical features usually resemble those of other space-occupying lesions (focal signs, seizures in 25–35% of patients) with most symptoms related to increased intracranial pressure (ICP) (headache, nausea, vomiting, lethargy, and stupor). Fever occurs in only 50% of cases.

HISTOPATHOLOGIC STAGES

Days 1 to 3: Early cerebritis produces a local inflammatory response (usually within white matter or at the gray-white matter junction) around a necrotic center.

Days 4 to 9: Late cerebritis is characterized by increased necrosis and inflammation, with initial fibroblastic formation of the collagen capsule.

Days 10 to 13: Early encapsulation stage shows further development of the collagen capsule, which is typically thinner on the less vascular ventricular side.

Days 14 and later: Late capsular stage shows five distinct histologic layers—the necrotic center, inflammatory cells and fibroblasts, collagen capsule, neovascular layer, and surrounding reactive gliosis and edema.

WORKUP

I. Blood cultures should be drawn (positive in 15% of cases) and empiric parenteral antibiotic therapy must be initiated before CT scan or MRI.

II. CT scans correlate well with the histopathologic stages. In the cerebritis stage, CT without contrast shows the necrotic center as a hypodensity. Ring enhancement begins in the later stages of cerebritis. In capsular stages the capsule becomes visible on CT without contrast as a faint hyperdense ring that produces ring-enhancing lesion with contrast, which is thinner on the ventricular side.

III. MRI appearance is bright on diffusion-weighted images (DWI): T_1 delineates the abscess capsule as hyper/isointense and hypointense center and surrounding edema; T_2 demonstrates the hyperintense edema and center and hypointense capsule, enhances with gadolinium.

IV. MR spectroscopy can differentiate between abscess, necrotizing tumor, or granuloma. The main finding of MRS in abscesses is elevation of metabolites of bacterial origin, including acetate, lactate, succinate, and amino acids versus necrotic brain tumors with elevated choline and decreased *N*-acetylaspartate (NAA). The MRS pattern may monitor effectiveness of medical treatment of a brain abscess, showing a decline of the metabolites after a positive response to therapy.

V. EEG abnormalities include focal slowing, seizure activity, and sometimes evidence of diffuse encephalopathy. These findings are nonspecific and rarely of value in confirming the diagnosis.

If brain abscess is suspected, lumbar puncture should not be performed because organisms have a poor yield and the risk of herniation is greater with abscess than with other mass lesions. Angiogram, if performed, will show avascular mass and luxury perfusion.

TREATMENT

A combination of broad-spectrum antimicrobials, neurosurgical drainage or excision, and eradication of the primary infectious focus is indicated. If CT shows only cerebritis or abscess less than 2.5 cm and the patient is neurologically stable, antibiotics without surgery may suffice. Neurologic deterioration usually mandates surgery. Empiric antibiotics should be given based on the route of infection and adjusted based on the cultures. When the cause is unknown, the patient should receive a third- or fourth-generation cephalosporin, for example, ceftazidime 2 g IV q 8 hr (or ceftriaxone

2 g IV q 12 hr), penicillin (PCN) G 5 MU IV q 6 hr, and metronidazole 500 mg IV q 6 hr. For paranasal sinus sources administer PCN and metronidazole. In treatment of posttraumatic cases, nafcillin 2 g IV q 2 hr (or vancomycin 1 g IV q 12 hr) and a third-generation cephalosporin such as ceftazidime 2 g IV q 8 hr. Treatment should be given for 6 to 8 weeks, often followed by additional 2 to 6 months of oral therapy or until the resolution of neuroimaging findings. In patients who are positive for HIV, coverage should be added for toxoplasmosis with pyrimethamine plus sulfadiazine or clindamycin. Mucormycosis is treated with amphotericin B. Antiepileptic drugs may be given for up to 3 months. Routine corticosteroid administration is controversial and should be used only when mental status is significantly depressed and substantial mass effect can be demonstrated on imaging.

PROGNOSIS
Mortality rates range from 5% to 30%. Poor prognosis is associated with very young or old age; anaerobic pathogens; large, multiple, deep, cerebellar, or multiloculated abscesses; acute clinical presentation with stupor/coma; rupture into ventricle or subarachnoid space; concomitant pulmonary infection or sepsis; and specific organisms (i.e., *Aspergillus* and *Pseudomonas* species).

REFERENCES
Greenberg MS: *Handbook of neurosurgery*, ed 5, Lakeland, FL, Greenberg Graphics, 2001.

Infection in Neurosurgery Working Party of the British Society for Antimicrobial Therapy: *Br J Neurosurg* 14:525, 2000.

Karampekios et al: Cerebral infections. *Eur Radiol* 15(3):485–493, 2005.

ABSCESS, EPIDURAL

Spinal epidural abscesses most commonly spread via a hematogenous route. Risk factors include intravenous drug abuse, diabetes, alcoholism, and chronic renal failure.

CLINICAL FEATURES
Spinal and radicular pain that progresses to weakness over hours to days. Back pain, fever, spine tenderness, progressive myelopathy with bowel/bladder disturbance, and weakness progressing rapidly to para- and quadriplegia may occur.

PATHOGENS
Staphylococcus and gram-negative organisms.

PATHOPHYSIOLOGY OF SPINAL CORD DYSFUNCTION
Features consist of mechanical compression, vascular mechanisms leading to venous thrombosis, and infectious spread (myelitis) by direct extension. If epidural abscess is suspected, *emergency imaging* is indicated.

A

ABSCESS, EPIDURAL

TREATMENT

Adequate surgical drainage and broad-spectrum antibiotic coverage with third-generation cephalosporin and aminoglycosides such as ceftriaxone 2 gm IV q 12 h and tobramycin 3 mg IV q 24 h.

PROGNOSIS

Prognosis is poor; mortality rate can be as high as 25% of cases. Patients who are paralyzed before surgery rarely improve.

REFERENCE

Greenberg MS: *Handbook of neurosurgery*, ed 5, Lakeland, FL, Greenberg Graphics, 2001.

ACALCULIA

This acquired impairment of arithmetic calculations may be disabling for a patient by interfering with basic daily activities such as shopping, balancing a checkbook, or calculating a restaurant tip. The ability to perform mathematical calculations requires not only an arithmetic brain center but also the cognitive functions of attention, language processing (receptive and expressive), and spatial orientation.

Acalculia may be classified as one of the following: (1) *aphasic*, an inability to read or write numbers, usually occurring with left posterior parietal lesions; (2) *spatial*, a mental misalignment of numbers that usually occurs with right posterior hemispheric lesions; or (3) *anarithmetria* or *dyscalculia*, a primary loss of ability to perform mathematical operations, associated with left inferior parietal lobule and angular gyrus lesions.

Acalculia usually is observed as part of Gerstmann's syndrome of acalculia, agraphia, right-left disorientation, and finger agnosia, but more rarely it may be an isolated problem. The differential diagnosis of acalculia includes focal structural lesions, as seen in stroke, tumor, trauma, or abscess, or may be part of global brain dysfunction such as with encephalopathy or dementia.

ACID-BASE DISTURBANCES

RESPIRATORY ALKALOSIS

This condition is frequently observed in patients with bronchial asthma, hepatic cirrhosis, salicylate intoxication, hypoxia, sepsis, pneumonia, and acute anxiety (hyperventilation syndrome). Acute respiratory alkalosis constricts the cerebral arterioles and decreases the cerebral blood flow. Confusion accompanied by a slow EEG may develop.

More severe alkalosis (pH 7.52 to 7.65) in patients with respiratory insufficiency and hypoxia may result in a symptom complex of hypotension, seizures, asterixis, myoclonus, and coma. Other neurologic manifestations of milder respiratory alkalosis include paresthesias, dizziness, cramps as a result of coexistent tetany, hyperreflexia, and muscle weakness.

RESPIRATORY ACIDOSIS

Acute respiratory acidosis is a condition of low pH and high PCO_2, occurring as a result of impairment of the rate of alveolar ventilation. Lethargy and confusion occur as the PCO_2 rises above 55 mm Hg. Seizures, stupor, or coma may occur with levels greater than 70 mm Hg. The serum bicarbonate level is either normal or high, depending on how rapidly the respiratory failure developed.

Neurologic manifestations resulting from cerebral vasodilation include headache, increased intracranial pressure, and papilledema. Hyperreflexia or hyporeflexia and myoclonus may also occur. Causes of acute respiratory acidosis include sedative drugs, brainstem injury, neuromuscular disorders, chest injury, airway obstruction, and acute pulmonary disease.

Chronic respiratory acidosis generally occurs in patients with chronic bronchitis, emphysema, extreme kyphoscoliosis, or extreme obesity (pickwickian syndrome). It is most often symptomatic with acute exacerbations of disease. Compensatory polycythemia often results from chronic hypercapneic states. Hypoventilation or pickwickian syndrome may manifest as excessive daytime somnolence.

Therapy involves ventilatory support and treating the underlying disorder. The possibility of sedative or narcotic drug ingestion must be suspected in otherwise healthy patients who suddenly develop acute respiratory depression.

METABOLIC ALKALOSIS

Metabolic alkalosis may result from either excessive ingestion of base or excessive loss of acid. Delirium and stupor owing to this condition are rarely severe. Severe metabolic alkalosis produces a blunted, confused state rather than stupor or coma and may result in cardiac arrhythmias and severe compensatory hypoventilation.

Neurologic manifestations include paresthesias, cramps (due to tetany), muscle weakness (due to associated hypokalemia), and hyporeflexia. Causes of hypokalemic metabolic alkalosis include Cushing syndrome, vomiting or gastric drainage, diuretic therapy, and primary aldosteronism. Treatment depends on the underlying cause.

METABOLIC ACIDOSIS

Metabolic acidosis occurs when a decrease in plasma bicarbonate level lowers pH. Cardinal features are hyperventilation and, when severe, Kussmaul's respirations. In chronic metabolic acidosis, hyperventilation may be difficult to detect on clinical examination. The presence of neurologic symptoms depends on various factors, including the type of systemic metabolic defect, whether the fall in systemic pH affects the pH of the brain and CSF, the rate at which acidosis develops, and the specific anion causing the metabolic disorder. All forms of metabolic acidosis produce hyperpnea as the first neurologic symptom. Other manifestations include lethargy, drowsiness, confusion, and mild, diffuse skeletal muscle hypertonus. Extensor plantar responses occur at a later stage. Stupor, coma, or seizures generally develop only preterminally.

The most common causes of metabolic acidosis sufficient to produce coma and hyperpnea include uremia, diabetes, lactic acidosis, and ingestion of acidic poisons. Ketoacidosis occasionally develops in severe alcoholics after prolonged drinking episodes. In diabetics treated with oral hypoglycemic agents, lactic acidosis and diabetic ketoacidosis must be considered.

Because metabolic acidosis is a manifestation of a variety of different diseases, the treatment varies depending on the underlying process and on the acuteness and severity of the acidosis.

REFERENCES

Layzer RB: *Neuromuscular manifestations of systemic disease*, Philadelphia, FA Davis, 1985.

Plum F, Posner JB: *The diagnosis of stupor and coma*, ed 3, Philadelphia, FA Davis, 1982.

AGNOSIA

This rare condition is characterized by impaired recognition of objects, people, and sounds despite intact primary visual, auditory, and tactile senses. An agnosic patient will be able to sense the presence of an object, but will not be able to apply meaning to the previously recognized object and thus fails to recognize it. Agnosia is seen in a variety of neurologic insults including stroke, tumor, neurodegenerative conditions, and trauma. It is important to demonstrate intact vision, hearing, and sensation modalities before diagnosing agnosia. It is also important to rule out anomic aphasia prior to diagnosing any visual agnosia. In both visual agnosia and anomic aphasia, a patient will not be able to name an object. However, a patient with anomic aphasia will recognize the object.

There are three forms of agnosia:

I. *Visual agnosia* refers to inability to visually recognize familiar objects. There are two main forms of visual agnosia.
   A. The *apperceptive* type is a deficit of visual processing in which abnormal visual percepts are formed and may occur after *bilateral injury to the primary visual cortex*. Patients are unable to copy or match visually presented items.
   B. The *associative* type occurs when the deficit occurs after percept formation but before meaning has been associated. Patients may be able to copy objects, but will not recognize them. The majority of these patients have associated achromatopsia.

Object agnosia (inability to recognize objects), *prosopagnosia* (loss of recognition of specific members of a generic group; distinguishing and recognizing faces, cars, houses, etc.), and achromatopsia (inability to perceive color) are associative visual agnosias occurring with *bilateral occipito-temporal lesions*. *Simultanagnosia* is a visual agnosia in which the patient will be able to recognize individual parts of an object or single objects but not a scene as whole. This is seen as part of *Balint's* syndrome of simultanagnosia, optic ataxia and ocular motor apraxia usually due to bilateral occipito-parietal lesions.

The image in Figure 1 may be used to detect simultanagnosia. A patient is presented with the image and asked to describe the scene. A normal patient will be able to describe the actions occurring in the scene; however, a patient with simultanagnosia may be able to recognize a few individual objects, but not their relationship to each other.

II. *Auditory agnosia* refers to an inability to recognize sounds that cannot be attributed to a hearing defect. It may be restricted to nonspeech sounds (selective auditory agnosia) or speech sounds (pure word deafness), or may involve both (generalized auditory agnosia). Thus, a patient may be able to hear a bird chirping, but not recognize that the sound is originating from a bird.

III. *Tactile agnosia* refers to the inability to recognize objects by the tactile sense, despite intact primary sensation sense (light touch, temperature, pinprick, etc.). The patient usually can visually recognize the object. *Astereognosis*, an inability to recognize objects placed in the hand, is not well characterized due to the difficulty of separating it from primary sensory loss.

There is also a rare agnosia called *anosagnosia* that refers to a denial of illness. This may be seen as part of a neglect syndrome with right hemispheric damage. The patient may not recognize a body part, such as an arm, as belonging to self.

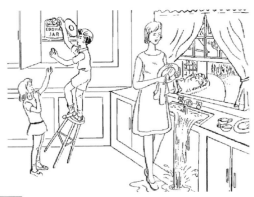

FIGURE 1

Simultagnosia test. Simultagnosia is characterized by the inability to recognize two or more things at the same time.

AGRAPHIA

The acquired inability to write, "aphasia of writing," occurs in five clinical forms:

I. *Pure agraphia* (no other language abnormality present) is seen with lesions of the *second frontal convolution* (Exner's area), *superior parietal lobule*, and the *posterior sylvian region*.

II. *Aphasic agraphia* is the writing disturbance of aphasics that usually resembles their spoken speech.

III. *Agraphia with alexia* is produced by a dominant angular gyrus lesion.

IV. *Apractic agraphia*, in which production of letters and words is abnormal, usually occurs with a dominant superior parietal lobule lesion.

V. *Spatial agraphia* with abnormalities of spacing letters and maintaining a horizontal line is usually produced by nondominant parietal lesions.

Neuropsychologists have defined two systems of writing. The *phonological system* decodes speech sounds (phonemes) into letters. In phonological agraphia, produced by lesions of supramarginal gyrus or the insula medial to it, the patient is unable to spell nonsense words but is capable of spelling familiar words. The *lexical system* retrieves visual word images when spelling. Lexical agraphia is marked by errors in spelling irregular words, but these errors are phonologically correct (rough spelled as ruf). Lexical agraphia occurs with lesions at the junction of the posterior angular gyrus and parieto-occipital lobule.

REFERENCES

Heilman KM, Valenstein E: *Clinical neuropsychology*, New York, Oxford University Press, 1993.

Mesulam MM: *Principles of behavioral and cognitive neurology*, New York, Oxford University Press, 2000.

AIDS

DEFINITION

Acquired immunodeficiency syndrome is caused by the human immunodeficiency virus (HIV), a retrovirus. Neurologic manifestations can occur at any level of the neuraxis at any stage of infection and can be a result of direct HIV infection, HIV-induced immune dysregulation, opportunistic infections, or pharmacologic therapy for the disease and its complications. Specific syndromes tend to occur more frequently during particular phases of HIV infection (but can appear at almost any point during the course) and virtually all have been described as the initial presenting feature of HIV infection. Coexistent systemic infections are common and should be specifically sought and treated concomitantly. The standard method for diagnosing HIV infection is measurement of antibody by ELISA followed by Western blot for confirmation of ELISA-positive samples. Prior to host antibody response ("window period") HIV antigen tests (e.g., p24 protein antigen) and nucleic acid (RNA, proviral DNA) tests are more sensitive. Rate of disease progression is directly related to HIV RNA levels (viral load).

MAJOR HIV-ASSOCIATED CNS DISORDERS CLASSIFIED BY NEUROANATOMIC LOCALIZATION

Meninges
 I. Aseptic HIV meningitis
 II. Cryptococcal meningitis
 III. Tuberculous meningitis
 IV. Syphilitic meningitis
 V. *Listeria monocytogenes* meningitis
 VI. Lymphomatous meningitis

Brain (Predominantly Nonfocal)
 I. HIV-associated dementia (HAD)
 II. HIV-associated minor cognitive dysfunction (MCMD)
 III. *Toxoplasma* encephalitis
 IV. Cytomegalovirus (CMV) encephalitis
 V. *Aspergillus* encephalitis
 VI. Herpes encephalitis
 VII. Metabolic encephalopathy (alone or concomitantly)

Brain (Predominantly Focal)
 I. Cerebral toxoplasmosis
 II. Primary CNS lymphoma (PCNSL)
 III. Progressive multifocal encephalopathy (PML)
 IV. Cryptococcoma
 V. Tuberculoma
 VI. Varicella-zoster virus (VZV) encephalitis
 VII. Stroke

Spinal Cord
 I. Vacuolar myelopathy (VM)
 II. Cytomegalovirus (CMV) myeloradiculopathy
 III. VZV myelitis
 IV. Spinal epidural or intradural lymphoma (metastatic)
 V. HTLV-1-associated myelopathy

CLASSIFICATION OF HIV-ASSOCIATED NEUROMUSCULAR DISORDERS

Peripheral Neuropathies
 I. Early stages (immune dysregulation)
　　A. Acute inflammatory demyelinating polyneuropathy (AIDP)
　　B. Chronic inflammatory demyelinating polyneuropathy (CIDP)
　　C. Vasculitic myelopathy
　　D. Brachial plexopathy
　　E. Lumbosacral plexopathy
　　F. Cranial mononeuropathy
　　G. Multiple mononeuropathies

II. Mid- and late stages (HIV-replication driven)
  A. Distal sensory polyneuropathy
  B. Autonomic neuropathy
III. Late stages (opportunistic infection, malignancy)
  A. CMV polyradiculomyelitis
  B. Syphilitic polyradiculomyelitis
  C. Tuberculous polyradiculomyelitis
  D. Lymphomatous polyradiculopathy
  E. Zoster ganglionitis
  F. CMV mononeuritis multiplex
  G. Nutritional neuropathy (vitamins B_{12}, B_6)
  H. AIDS-cachexia neuropathy
  I. ALS-like motor neuropathy
IV. All stages (toxic neuropathy)
  A. Nucleoside reverse transcriptase inhibitors (ddl, ddC, d_4T)
  B. Other drugs (vincristine, INH, ethambutol, thalidomide)

Myopathies
  I. Polymyositis
  II. Pyomyositis
  III. Inclusion body myositis
  IV. Toxic (zidovudine) myopathy
  V. AIDS-cachexia myopathy

NEUROLOGIC EVENTS IN HIV INFECTION
Early HIV Infection
Initial HIV infection usually manifests as a nonspecific viral syndrome of fever, arthralgias, myalgias, and malaise lasting several days. Formed antibodies to HIV proteins take 6 months to appear. Prior to seroconversion, standard anti-HIV antibody assays are negative, and diagnosis can be made only by means of Western blot assay for viral antigen. Several syndromes can be associated with this early phase of infection, and their association with HIV may be discerned only if Western blot is obtained.
  I. HIV meningoencephalitis—a viral meningitis can accompany the syndrome of initial infection. In a few patients, this affects the brain parenchyma as well, resulting in a self-limited encephalopathy.
  II. Transverse myelitis rarely accompanies acute HIV infection.
  III. Acute inflammatory demyelinating polyneuropathy can occur upon or shortly after initial infection. It may be differentiated from Guillain-Barré syndrome (GBS) (also known as acute inflammatory demyelinating polyneuropathy [AIDP]) by the presence of CSF pleocytosis. Course and treatment are similar to those for idiopathic GBS.
  IV. Sensory ganglioneuropathy.
  V. Brachial plexitis.
  VI. Rhabdomyolysis can accompany initial infection. Steroids can be beneficial.

Midstage HIV Infection (CD4 Count 200 to 500/μL)

I. HIV meningitis can recur at any point and may remain asymptomatic. The resulting elevated CSF protein and pleocytosis significantly complicates workup for other infections.

II. CIDP is the chronic form of AIDP. Patients can benefit from intravenous immunoglobulin or plasmapheresis.

III. Mononeuritis multiplex, when apparent in early or midstage HIV infection, is often self-limited.

IV. Nucleoside antiviral polyneuropathy—didanosine, zalcitabine, and stavudine can all cause a dysesthetic sensory neuropathy, especially at higher doses. Often of subacute onset over weeks, it gradually improves after change of offending agent; both features help to distinguish this from HIV-related distal sensory neuropathy.

V. Inflammatory myopathy presents as proximal muscle weakness and sometimes myalgia. Biopsy shows inflammation. Steroids are beneficial, if immune status permits.

VI. Zidovudine (AZT) myopathy occurs because AZT is a mitochondrial toxin. Presentation is similar to inflammatory myopathy. Biopsy suggests mitochondrial dysfunction but may show inflammation as well. Clinical improvement after AZT withdrawal is the best means of diagnosis.

Late HIV Infection (CD4 Count >200/μL)

I. Focal brain lesions

A. Cerebral toxoplasmosis—caused by intracerebral reactivation of infection with the parasite *Toxoplasma gondii*, this syndrome is usually manifested in fever, headache, confusion, seizures, and focal neurologic signs, although any or all of these can be lacking. Neuroimaging typically reveals multiple ring-enhancing lesions. Antibiotics are usually quite effective.

B. Primary CNS lymphoma (PCNSL) occurs in 2% of AIDS patients. PCNSL is the second most common cause of ring-enhancing lesions on CT/MRI and is usually unifocal. It can be distinguished from *T. gondii* by single-photon emission CT (SPECT) or positron emission tomography (PET). Any patient with ring-enhancing lesions that are atypical for toxoplasmosis or do not respond to several weeks of anti-*Toxoplasma* therapy must undergo biopsy. Mean survival is 1 month from diagnosis without whole-brain radiotherapy and 4 to 6 months with it.

C. Progressive multifocal leukoencephalopathy (PML) results from reactivation of JC virus, an infection generally of no consequence to the immunocompetent. Reactivation in oligodendroglia leads to demyelinating white matter disease, focal neurologic deficits, and non–ring-enhancing white matter lesions on scan. Mean survival is 2 to 4 months. Ten percent of patients have enhancing lesions, which may be associated with increased survival. No specific therapy is known, although occasional patients have responded to treatment with cytarabine or cidofovir.

D. Stroke is not a complication of HIV per se, but 4% of AIDS patients have a symptomatic stroke during their lives. Ischemic stroke may be caused by AIDS-related bacterial endocarditis, viral-associated vasculitis, or perivascular infection, or it may be a result of more traditional risk factors such as hypertension and hyperlipidemia; intracranial hemorrhage can complicate PCNSL, metastatic Kaposi sarcoma, or (rarely) toxoplasmosis.

E. Focal brain lesions in AIDS patients can be due to any of the abovementioned, plus cysticercosis, fungal abscess (due to *Candida* infection, *Aspergillus* infection, mucormycosis, coccidioidomycosis, etc.), bacterial abscess (caused by mycobacteria, *T. pallidum*, *Nocardia*, *Listeria*, etc.), or other tumors (glioma, Kaposi sarcoma, other metastases). The usual approach in a patient with typical imaging findings such as a ring-enhancing lesion and positive toxoplasma serologic test is to treat empirically for toxoplasmosis and proceed to biopsy if repeat scan shows no improvement. Those with negative serologic findings or atypical scan should undergo biopsy immediately.

II. Cryptococcal meningitis develops in 10%. It often presents as a combination of cognitive impairment, personality change, lethargy, cranial neuropathies, and increased intracranial pressure, with or without typical signs and symptoms of meningismus. Fungal CSF culture is the gold standard, but results take weeks; CSF cryptococcal antigen is rapid and highly sensitive and specific. India ink smear is also rapid and increases sensitivity. Initial treatment should be amphotericin B with flucytosine. Unfortunately, response can be as low as 40%, and recurrence is common; however, in those surviving the initial infection, long-term suppression with daily fluconazole can be effective.

III. Syphilitic meningitis and meningovasculitis frequently complicate HIV infection, because *T. pallidum* shares some risk factors with HIV. Findings include meningismus, cranial neuropathies, and with chronic infections, classic tertiary syphilis. Diagnosis depends on a combination of serologic testing and clinical suspicion. Treatment is with penicillin.

IV. Tuberculous meningitis is more common in AIDS patients than in the nonimmunosuppressed. Tuberculomas may also rarely occur. CSF PCR can complement culture.

V. HIV encephalopathy (AIDS dementia complex, HIV-associated dementia) is a subcortical dementia of unclear pathogenesis characterized by cognitive slowing, emotional blunting, and motor impairment. Prevalence estimates vary widely (5–60%); in the pediatric population, the prevalence is much higher (90%). Workup consists of ruling out treatable infections (cryptococcus, syphilis, CMV encephalitis) and medical conditions (hypothyroidism, vitamin B_{12} deficiency). No specific treatment beyond antiviral therapy is known.

VI. Vacuolar myelopathy is present in up to 55% on autopsy but symptomatic in far fewer. It is of uncertain pathogenesis, and pathologic findings include vacuolization in the dorsal and lateral columns of the spinal cord. Symptoms, which develop late, include constipation, urinary disturbances, ataxia, and spastic paraparesis. There is no treatment. The process is painless and slowly progressive; pain or rapid progression should prompt evaluation for other causes, such as viral myelitis, metastatic cord compression, or epidural abscess. Other subacute myelopathies sometimes associated with AIDS include syphilis and vitamin B_{12} deficiency.

VII. Mononeuritis multiplex in late HIV infection is often due to CMV and benefits from ganciclovir. CMV can also cause encephalitis, meningitis, retinitis, myelitis, or polyradiculitis. CSF PCR for central nervous system CMV infections has approximately 90% sensitivity.

VIII. Varicella-zoster virus (VZV) can cause encephalitis, Ramsay-Hunt syndrome, myelitis, vasculitis, and segmental zoster rashes (shingles). Herpes simplex virus (HSV) can cause encephalitis or myelitis. Both HSV and VZV are treated with acyclovir.

IX. Distal symmetrical polyneuropathy is an axonal, predominantly sensory neuropathy with impairment of all sensory modalities, often with paresthesias, which can be painful. Tricyclic antidepressants and anticonvulsants can help dysesthetic symptoms, but some patients may require opiates. Capsaicin may also help.

All Stages

I. HIV-related meningitis: aseptic (acute or recurrent) or chronic
II. Asymptomatic CSF abnormalities: elevated protein, lymphocytic pleocytosis, normal glucose
III. Nucleoside neuropathy and zidovudine myopathy
IV. Inflammatory myopathy

FOR MORE INFORMATION

www.cdcnpin.org (epidemiologic data)
www.cc.nih.gov/phar/hiv-mgt. (consensus panel reports on treatment of HIV infection)

REFERENCES

AAN Quality Standards Subcommittee: *Neurology*, 50:21–26, 1997.
Berger JR, Major EO: *Semin Neurol* 19:193–200,1999.
Bradley WG, Daroff RB, et al: *Neurology in clinical practice*, ed 4, Philadelphia, Butterworth-Heinemann, 2004.

ALCOHOL

Neurologic effects of alcohol are due to a combination of its direct neurotoxic effects, its metabolites, nutritional factors, and genetic predisposition. Neurologic complications associated with alcohol abuse can be conceptually divided into the following five categories (Table 1):

TABLE 1	
NEUROLOGIC COMPLICATIONS ASSOCIATED WITH ALCOHOL ABUSE	
Causes	Complications
Direct effects of alcohol	Acute intoxication
	Fetal alcohol syndrome
Alcohol withdrawal	Delirium tremens
	Seizure
Nutritional deficiency	Wernicke's encephalopathy
	Korsakoff's syndrome
Other related syndromes	Cerebellar degeneration
	Peripheral neuropathy
	Optic neuropathy
	Myopathy
Disease of uncertain pathogenesis	Central pontine myelinolysis
	Marchiafava-Bignami disease
	Cortical atrophy

I. *Intoxication with alcohol* correlates roughly with blood concentrations. Cognitive dysfunction tends to occur early, and cerebellar, autonomic, and vestibular symptoms tend to occur at higher blood levels. Positional vertigo may result from alcohol diffusing into the cupula when the recumbent position is assumed. As the alcohol concentration rises to a certain level, the intoxication is greater than when it falls to the same level. Blackouts are periods of amnesia, usually during binge drinking, and occur in persons with and without alcohol dependence.

II. *Withdrawal syndromes* in individuals with alcohol dependency result from either decreased intake or abrupt cessation of drinking. The syndromes may be early or late. Most common are the early symptoms, which begin 12 to 24 hours after decreased intake. Tremulousness is common and may be accompanied by nausea, vomiting, insomnia, and hallucinations (visual, tactile, or auditory). Treatment consists of benzodiazepines. Auditory hallucinations may persist, necessitating the use of neuroleptics.

Withdrawal seizures are always generalized tonic-clonic and begin within the first 24 hours but may occur after several days. Focal seizures should not be attributed to alcohol withdrawal and should warrant further investigation including CT of head to rule out any structural abnormality.

Treatment of withdrawal seizures is controversial because they are usually self-limited. Initial loading with phenytoin and slowly tapering off after several days is one approach. Thiamine is routinely given and hypomagnesemia, if present, is treated.

Delirium tremens are a serious complication and have a peak incidence 72 to 96 hours after decreased alcohol intake. Severe confusion, agitation, vivid hallucinations, tremors, and increased autonomic activity (tachycardia, fever, sweating, and orthostatic hypotension) are characteristic. These symptoms can last 1 to 3 days and can be fatal (~10%). Treatment consists of sedation with benzodiazepines, hydration with IV fluids, and administration of thiamine, multivitamins, and magnesium (if indicated). Autonomic hyperactivity should be treated aggressively if present.

III. *Wernicke-Korsakoff's syndrome* is the most common deficiency syndrome due to chronic alcoholism. Wernicke's syndrome, which is reversible, represents the acute phase and classically has the triad of *encephalopathy, ataxia*, and *ocular motor disturbance* (nystagmus, ophthalmoplegia, and gaze palsy). However, a complete triad of signs is often not present. Atrophy of the mammillary bodies is common.

Korsakoff's syndrome, which is irreversible, is a more chronic condition and includes anterograde amnesia (the inability to incorporate ongoing experience into memory) leading to confabulation. Both syndromes are attributed to thiamine deficiency and can also be seen in nonalcoholic malnutrition states, although much less commonly.

Treatment consists of thiamine, 100 mg/day for 3 days parenterally, followed by oral thiamine indefinitely. IV glucose should never be given without thiamine to a chronic alcoholic because of the risk of precipitating Wernicke's encephalopathy. As with most alcohol-related syndromes, supplemental vitamins and magnesium may be beneficial.

IV. *Other alcohol-related syndromes* include cerebellar degeneration, peripheral neuropathy, optic neuropathy, and myopathy.

Cerebellar degeneration invariably involves the anterior and superior cerebellar vermis and paravermian regions with resultant truncal and gait ataxia. Limb ataxia, if present, is much milder than truncal ataxia and more severe in the legs than in the arms.

Peripheral neuropathy, which can involve both sensory and motor nerves, is usually heralded by complaints of numb, burning feet involving distal limbs symmetrically. Minor motor signs may evolve. Pathogenesis seems to involve both toxic alcohol effects as well as poor nutrition status. Abstinence from alcohol is paramount for treatment success.

Nutritional amblyopia (previously called tobacco-alcohol amblyopia) consists of gradual visual loss over a period of several weeks and is caused by selective lesion of the optic nerves secondary to poor nutrition and is not a direct toxic effect of alcohol. Treatment with a combination of adequate diet and B vitamins, despite the continuation of drinking and smoking, results in visual recovery.

Alcoholic myopathy is believed to be caused by the toxic effects of alcohol and improves with abstinence. It may occur as an acute necrotizing disorder with muscle pain and rhabdomyolysis, or as a more slowly progressive disease with proximal weakness. The combination of thiamine, multivitamins, and abstinence is the treatment of choice for these syndromes.

V. *Conditions of somewhat uncertain etiology* occurring in chronic alcoholics include central pontine myelinolysis, Marchiafava-Bignami syndrome, and cortical atrophy.

Central pontine myelinolysis is a rare cerebral white matter disorder, associated with basis pontis lesions with resultant progressive quadriparesis, horizontal gaze palsy, and obtundation leading to coma. It occurs with excessively rapid correction of hyponatremia.

Marchiafava-Bignami syndrome is a rare demyelinating disease of the corpus callosum and adjacent subcortical white matter, sometimes associated with excessive consumption of crude red wine. Patients can have cognitive impairment that resembles a frontal lobe or dementia syndrome, spasticity, dysarthria, and impaired gait. The CT scan appearance of "atrophy" or "parenchymal volume loss" is probably related to fluid shifts in the brain and may reverse with abstinence.

Alcoholics have an increased incidence of stroke related to a variety of factors, including rebound thrombocytosis, altered cerebral blood flow, and hyperlipidemia.

REFERENCES

Adams RD, Victor M: *Principles of neurology*, New York, McGraw-Hill, 1997.
Bradley WG, Daroff RB, et al: *Neurology in clinical practice*, ed 4, Philadelphia, Butterworth-Heinemann, 2004.

ALEXIA

The loss of a previously acquired reading ability occurs in three main forms:

I. *Alexia without agraphia (pure alexia)*. This form was described first by Dejerine in 1892. The patient loses the ability to read, but writing is intact. This is seen with left posterior cerebral artery infarct involving the medial left occipital lobe and splenium of the corpus callosum. Owing to dysfunction of the left occipital lobe, visual information must be processed by the intact right occipital lobe (Fig. 2). However, the visual information cannot pass from the right visual area to the left language centers because of infarction of the splenium. The patient will have associated right hemianopia and impaired color naming (achromatopsia).

II. *Alexia with agraphia*. The patient loses the ability to read or write. This is seen most often with mass lesion or *infarction* in the left middle cerebral artery distribution affecting the left inferior parietal lobule, especially the angular gyrus. The patient, in addition to having alexia with agraphia, may have the entire *Gerstmann's* syndrome of *agraphia, acalculia, left-right disorientation,* and *finger agnosia*. The patient may also have a right homonymous hemianopia or mild receptive (Wernicke's) aphasia as well.

III. *Aphasic alexia*. This form of alexia is secondary to underlying severe aphasia (language processing) including Broca's or Wernicke's aphasia. Depending on the subtype of aphasic alexia, different components of reading and language processing will be affected.

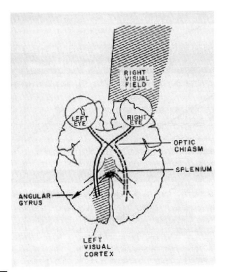

FIGURE 2
Left visual field.

REFERENCE
Bradley WG, Daroff RB, et al: *Neurology in clinical practice*, ed 4, Philadelphia, Butterworth-Heinemann, 2004.

AMAUROSIS FUGAX

Amaurosis fugax (AFx) or transient monocular blindness is a reversible loss of vision (partial or complete), classically from ischemia in the territory of central retinal or ophthalmic artery. Differential diagnosis includes "transient visual obscuration" resulting from increased intracranial pressure, arterial vasospasm, and ocular causes of transient visual loss. AFx has a short duration (seconds to minutes) and usually consists of negative symptoms (blackness or graying of the visual field) with an occasional positive phenomenon (scintillating scotomas or points of light). Funduscopic examination may show the cholesterol emboli (*Hollenhorst plaques*). Embolization from the internal carotid artery, aorta, or heart may be the cause (Table 2).

Treatment of classical AFx depends on the underlying cause. Aspirin and warfarin may be indicated, or endarterectomy may be necessary in cases of hemodynamically significant carotid artery stenosis. AFx due to vasospasm (i.e., particularly in young adults) may respond to calcium channel blockers nifedipine or verapamil.

TABLE 2

CAUSES OF TRANSIENT MONOCULAR BLINDNESS

I. Embolic
- A. Carotid embolism
- B. Cardiac and aortic embolism
- C. Embolism related to intravenous drug abuse

II. Hemodynamic
- A. Hypoperfusion
- B. Vasospasm
- C. Inflammatory arteritides such as temporal arteritis, Takayasu's syndrome, and polyarteritis nodosa
- D. Severe atherosclerotic occlusive disease of internal carotid or ophthalmic artery
- E. Carotid dissection
- F. Hypertensive crises

III. Ocular
- A. Anterior ischemic optic neuropathy
- B. Central retinal vein occlusion
- C. Intraocular causes such as hemorrhage, tumor, and glaucoma
- D. Drusen

IV. Neurologic disorders
- A. Disease of the vestibular or oculomotor system
- B. Optic neuritis (mainly demyelinating diseases)
- C. Optic nerve or optic chiasmal compression
- D. Increased intracranial pressure
- E. Migraine

V. Psychogenic

VI. Idiopathic

Adapted from Amaurosis Fugax Study Group: *Stroke* 21:201–208, 1990.

REFERENCES

Amaurosis Fugax Study Group: *Stroke* 21:201–208, 1990.
Winterkorn JM, Beckman RL: *J Neuroophthalmol* 15:209–211, 1995.

ANEURYSMAL SUBARACHNOID HEMORRHAGE

Incidence of aneurysmal subarachnoid hemorrhage (SAH) is about 2% to 3% and goes up to 6% to 9% in first-degree relatives and up to 15% in patients with polycystic kidney disease. Risk factors include female gender, smoking, cocaine drug abuse, and use of sympathomimetic drugs. The risk of rupture primarily depends on aneurysm size and location, with rupture associated with larger aneurysms, and posterior circulation.

CLINICAL PRESENTATION

The most common presentations of aneurysmal SAH are sudden, severe ("thunderclap") headache, stiff neck, photophobia, neurologic deficit, and altered mental status. Hunt and Hess (HH) grading is the most commonly used (I headache, II severe headache with cranial nerve palsy, III drowsiness with neurologic deficit, IV stupor, and V coma).

DIAGNOSIS

The diagnosis is made by CT scan demonstrating acute blood in the basal cisterns. An LP is indicated with a negative CT (3–5%) and a high clinical suspicion of SAH. Markedly elevated RBC count (>100,000 cells/mm^3), with no decrease in RBCs between tubes 1 and 4 is suggestive of SAH, although this may be secondary to a traumatic LP. Xanthochromia (yellow color) from RBC degradation in the CSF appears approximately 24 hours after aneurysm rupture. Conventional angiography remains the gold standard for identifying the aneurysm, although modern MRI and CT angiography may reliably detect aneurysms as small as 3 to 5 mm.

MANAGEMENT

All patients with aneurysmal SAH are admitted to the neurology ICU. Definitive treatment, either clip ligation or endovascular coiling, should occur at the earliest available opportunity *to avoid aneurysm rerupture*. The ISAT (International Subarachnoid Aneurysm Trial) study showed superiority for coiling in patients with SAH thought by surgeon and interventionalist to be suitable for either coiling or clipping (31% morbidity and mortality rates with clipping versus 24% with coiling). The risk of rebleeding is 4% to 6% in the initial 24 hours, then 1.5% per day for 14 days, 50% at 6 months, and stabilizing at 3% per year after 12 months. Indications for delayed treatment (i.e., on SAH days 10–14) may include subacute presentation (worse outcome associated with surgical clipping performed between SAH days 2 and 10) and poor clinical grade (HH grade 4, 5) at presentation (early treatment may not alter ultimate outcome). Nimodipine (40 mg PO q 6 hr for 21 days) may reduce morbidity risk from symptomatic vasospasm, although it may induce undesired hypotension. Euvolemia and normal blood pressure are maintained.

Vasospasm typically occurs between SAH days 3 and 10, with peak incidence at days 7 to 10. Neurologic deterioration necessitates a stat head CT to rule out ICH, hydrocephalus, or rehemorrhage; if none are present, vasospasm is assumed. Initial treatment is with "triple H therapy": hypertension (MAP >100), hypervolemia (CVP >8), hemodilution (HTC 28–30%). If there is no improvement, cerebral angiography with potential angioplasty or local intra-arterial papavarine or calcium channel blocker infusion is considered.

Treat other complications of SAH: Correct hyponatremia (cerebral salt wasting versus SIADH), dobutamine for neurogenic pulmonary edema, monitor cardiac abnormalities including myocardial infarction, vasopressin for diabetes insipidus, and external ventriculostomy or serial lumbar punctures for hydrocephalus.

OUTCOME

Outcome is poor; the 30-day mortality rate is 40% to 50% for those admitted to a hospital, and 15% die prior to reaching medical care.

Only one third of surviving patients return to their prerupture lifestyle, and one third remain moderately to severely disabled.

See also Endovascular Treatment of Cerebral Aneurysm.

REFERENCES

ISAT study. *Lancet* 361:431, 2003, and 366:809–817, 2005.
Kassel NF, Torner JC, Haley EC, et al: *J Neurosurg* 73:37–47, 1990.

ANGIOGRAPHY

Conventional cerebral angiography combines continuous fluoroscopy with injection of radiopaque contrast material directly into the arterial system of interest. This is done by advancing a catheter (usually through the femoral artery in the groin) into the aortic arch or selectively into the carotid or vertebrobasilar systems. Computerized digital subtraction techniques remove the bone density, improving visualization of the blood vessels. Angiography also provides evaluation of blood flow hemodynamics by following the movement/distribution of contrast agent through the blood vessels in real time. Indications for angiography include the evaluation of suspected vascular malformations, aneurysms, vasculopathies, stenotic or ulcerative vascular lesions, preoperative delineation of vascular anatomy and blood supply to tumors, and serving as a platform for endovascular procedures. Advances with high-resolution machines and 3D angiography technology and smaller catheter and less ionic contrast material made it more useful and safer.

The most common complication following angiography is a hematoma developing at the femoral arterial puncture site; this typically responds to local pressure. Uncommonly, a persistent arterial pseudoaneurysm develops, requiring ultrasound-guided thrombin injection. Acute stroke complicates less than 1% of procedures, with permanent neurologic deficit occurring in fewer than 0.5%. Elderly patients and those with preexisting carotid stenosis are at slightly higher risk. Allergic contrast reaction is rare, ranging from hives to anaphylaxis; a previous history of any contrast reaction obligates pretreatment with steroids. Patients with decreased renal function are at risk of developing contrast nephropathy; this risk may be reduced with adequate hydration before and after angiography, and pretreatment with *N*-acetylcysteine (Mucomyst) 600 mg PO q 12 hr 48 to 72 hours prior to angiography and sodium bicarbonate solution 1 hour before and 4 to 6 hours after.

Angiographic anatomy is depicted in Figures 3 and 4.

ANGIOMAS

Angiomas are congenital vascular lesions resulting from disordered embryogenesis. Histologic subtypes include the following (percentages refer to the frequency at autopsy): (1) *telangiectasias* (16%)—abnormal

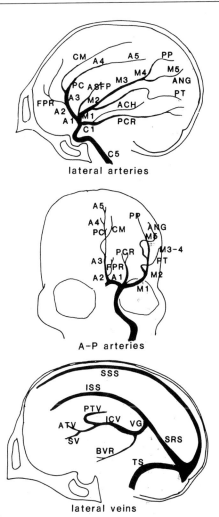

lateral arteries

A-P arteries

lateral veins

FIGURE 3

Internal carotid circulation. A_1–A, segments of anterior cerebral artery; ACH, anterior choroidal artery; ANG, angular artery; ASFP, ascending frontoparietal artery; ATV, anterior terminal vein; BVR, basal vein of Rosenthal; CM, callosomarginal artery; C_1–C_5, segments of internal carotid artery; FPR, frontopolar artery; ICV, internal cerebral vein; ISS, inferior sagittal sinus; M_1–M_5, segments of middle cerebral artery; PC, pericallosal artery; PCR, posterior cerebral artery; PP, posterior parietal artery; PTV, posterior terminal vein; SRS, straight sinus; SSS, superior sagittal sinus; SV, septal vein; TS, transverse sinus; VG, great cerebral vein of Galen.

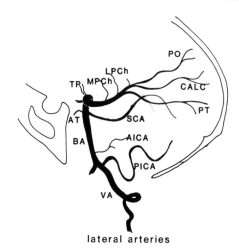

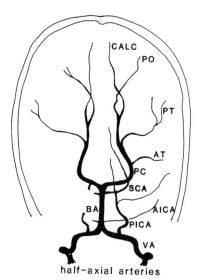

FIGURE 4

Vertebrobasilar circulation. AICA, anterior inferior cerebellar artery; AT, anterior temporal artery (branch of PC); BA, basilar artery; CALC, calcarine artery (branch of PC); LPCh, lateral posterior choroidal artery; MPCh, medial posterior choroidal artery; PC, posterior cerebral artery; PICA, posterior inferior cerebellar artery; PO, parieto-occipital artery (branch of PC); PT, posterior temporal artery (branch of PC); SCA, superior cerebellar artery; TP, thalamoperforate artery; VA, vertebral artery.

capillaries; (2) *venous angiomas* (59%)—anomalous veins; (3) *arteriovenous malformations* (AVMs) (14%)—clusters of abnormal vessels composed of arteries and veins without intervening capillaries; (4) *cavernous angiomas* (9%)—sinusoidal vessels without intervening neural tissue; and (5) *varices* (2%)—dilated veins. Angiomas are usually asymptomatic; symptoms usually are due to AVMs or cavernous angiomas. The most common intracranial locations are the cerebral hemispheres (75%) and basal ganglia (18%); posterior fossa angiomas are much less frequent (6%), occurring primarily in the pons; the spinal cord is a much rarer location (see Spinal Cord). Angiography detects most angiomas, with the notable exception of cavernous angiomas and telangiectasias. MRI is the preferred noninvasive neuroimaging modality.

AVMs are the most common symptomatic angioma; 80% to 90% are supratentorial. Clinical manifestations include hemorrhage (30% to 50%), seizures (approximately 30%), migraine-like headaches (20%), and gradually progressive focal neurologic deficits (10%). Hemorrhage occurs at a rate of 1% to 2% per year. Intraparenchymal hemorrhage occurs in two thirds of cases, subarachnoid hemorrhage in one third of cases. The short-term prognosis for patients with ruptured AVMs is better than that for patients with aneurysms, with lower rates of vasospasm (rare), death (10%), and rebleeding (6% in the first year, reverting to 1% to 2% subsequently). Recurrent hemorrhage is associated with higher rates of death and overall disability. The prognosis for patients with seizures alone is better than that after hemorrhage. Therapeutic modalities include surgical excision, embolization, and radiotherapy.

REFERENCES

Caplan LR: *Stroke: A clinical approach*, ed 2, Boston, Butterworth-Heinemann, 1993.
Mohr JP et al: In Barnett HJM et al (eds): *Stroke pathophysiology, diagnosis, and management*, ed 2, New York, Churchill Livingstone, 1992.

ANTIBODY TESTING IN NEUROMUSCULAR DISEASE

Immune-mediated neuromuscular disease is an important focus of diagnostic effort, as these disorders may respond to immunomodulatory therapy. In myasthenia gravis (MG) the pathogenic role of antibodies has been conclusively demonstrated. In many other conditions, however, associations with antibodies have been described, but the pathogenic role has not been fully demonstrated. The same antibody may be present in more than one condition, leading to poor specificity. In general, antibody testing should be performed to answer specific clinical questions. Table 3 summarizes some of the more established antibody associations.

MULTIFOCAL MOTOR NEUROPATHY

Multifocal motor neuropathy (MMN) is a rare, but important, treatable cause of neuropathy. It is more frequent in men than women, and presents

TABLE 3			
NEUROPATHY SYNDROMES ASSOCIATED WITH AUTOANTIBODIES			
Condition	Antigen	Antibody	% Positive
GANGLIOSIDE ANTIBODIES			
Multifocal motor neuropathy	GM1	Poly IgM	30–80
Distal lower motor neuron syndromes	GM1	Poly IgM	30–65
AMAN variant of Guillain-Barré syndrome	GM1, GD1a	Poly IgG, IgM	20–30
Miller-Fisher syndrome	GQ1b	Poly IgG	~95
GLYCOPROTEIN ANTIBODIES			
Monoclonal IgM to MAG	MAG	Mono IgM	50
RNA-BINDING PROTEIN ANTIBODIES			
Para-neoplastic sensory neuronopathy	Hu	IgG	>95
GLYCOSPHINGOLIPID ANTIBODIES			
Chronic sensory neuropathy	Sulfatide	Mono IgM	—
		Poly IgM, IgG	—
AMAN, acute motor axonal neuropathy; MAG, myelin-associated glycoprotein.			

between 20 and 50 years of age. Patients usually present with slowly progressive asymmetrical weakness in the distribution of named peripheral nerves with no sensory loss; early onset of diffuse weakness excludes the diagnosis of MMN. No spasticity, extensor plantar responses, clonus or pseudobulbar palsy should be present. Electrodiagnostic studies are crucial to the diagnosis of MMN. Typically, conduction block of motor nerves is found outside normal entrapment sites, along with normal sensory nerve responses. Criteria for the diagnosis of conduction block have been published by the American Association of Neuromuscular and Electrodiagnostic Medicine (AANEM). High titers of IgM antibody to GM1 and other glycolipids including asialo-GM1, GD1a, and GM2 may occur. Reported rates of anti-GM1 IgM range from 30% to 80%. This wide range has not been completely explained. Anti-GM1 antibodies also occur in other dysimmune neuropathies, as well as 5% of amyotrophic lateral sclerosis (ALS) patients. If anti-GM1 titers are very high (>1:6400), then specificity for MMN or a lower motor neuron syndrome is high, but levels this high occur in only 20% of MMN patients. The anti-GM1 antibodies role is not clear; hence diagnostic criteria for MMN published by the AANEM include no role for anti-GM1 antibodies. In practice, if MMN cannot be differentiated from motor neuron disease, a trial of intravenous gammaglobulin (IVIG) is appropriate, even if anti-GM1 antibodies are absent.

LOWER MOTOR NEURON SYNDROMES

Some patients present with clinical features of MMN, however, no conduction blocks are found on electrodiagnostic testing. These patients fall into a heterogeneous category of lower motor neuron syndromes (LMNS) that includes patients with primary lower motor neuron disease as well as some patients who may have a form of MMN. Anti-GM1 IgM antibodies are found in 30% to 65% of patients with a LMNS with distal asymmetrical weakness early in their course. In patients with a distal, asymmetrical onset of a LMNS with high anti-GM1 antibodies titers treatment with cyclophosphamide may be of benefit versus those who are antibody negative LMNS.

AMYOTROPHIC LATERAL SCLEROSIS
Although detectable serum levels of anti-GM1 have been reported in ALS, the titers are usually low compared to those with MMN. The frequency of a detectable positive anti-GM1 titer in ALS has been reported to be as high as 50%; however, one prospective series of ALS patients at a university center showed that none of the ALS patients had positive titers with a standard commercially available test. In the setting of classical ALS, there is no current utility for autoantibody testing.

GUILLAIN-BARRÉ SYNDROME
A high proportion of GBS patients, particularly those with *Campylobacter jejuni* infection, have a high titer of IgG and/or IgM antibodies to GM1. The presence of anti-GM1b antibodies appears to be associated with the acute motor axonal neuropathy (AMAN) form of GBS. There is some evidence that IgG antibodies are more linked to an axonal variant than are IgM antibodies. Other antibodies linked to the AMAN presentation of GBS are anti-GM1b, anti-GD1a, and anti-GalNAc-GD1a IgG antibodies. Similar antibody associations have been found in acute motor and sensory neuropathy (AMSAN) presentation as well, suggesting that AMAN and AMSAN are related entities. A consistent and useful association between the acute inflammatory demyelinating polyneuropathy (AIDP) presentation of GBS and specific anti-glycolipid antibodies has not been shown.

ANTI-GANGLIOSIDE GQ1b AND MILLER-FISHER SYNDROME
Miller-Fisher syndrome (MFS) is the most common variant of GBS. Clinically, it presents with a triad of ataxia, ophthalmoparesis, and areflexia. MFS overlaps clinically with GBS, and accounts for 5% to 10% of GBS cases. Although relatively uncommon, MFS provides a compelling example of a disorder in which ganglioside autoimmunity is believed to play a pathogenic role. Over 90% of patients with MFS have IgG antibodies to GQ1b, while these antibodies are absent in other conditions and in control populations. GQ1b is a ganglioside enriched in myelin and specifically present in the paranodal myelin of oculomotor, trochlear, and abducens nerves, but not the other cranial nerves. This finding appears to explain the ophthalmoplegia seen in MFS. GQ1b epitopes can be found on some strains of *C. jejuni*; the antecedent infection in some cases of MFS. IgG antibodies to GQ1b are also markers for GBS variants with acute ophthalmoplegia that do not meet full MFS criteria. Additionally, a case series of Bickerstaff's brainstem encephalitis, a condition that has overlap

with MFS clinically, showed that 60% of the group had anti-GQ1b IgG antibodies. Conversely, GBS patients without ophthalmoplegia are invariably anti-GQ1b negative. The high sensitivity and specificity of this antibody for MFS and ophthalmoplegic variants of GBS make this test clinically useful to rule out other causes of acute and subacute ophthalmoparesis.

ANTI-MYELIN-ASSOCIATED GLYCOPROTEIN AND ASSOCIATED NEUROPATHIES

Monoclonal gammopathy of undetermined significance (MGUS) is frequently associated with neuropathy, although the true prevalence is not well known. Approximately half of MGUS-associated neuropathies have IgM antibody activity directed against myelin-associated glycoprotein (MAG). IgM gammopathy with anti-MAG antibodies is not a frequent occurrence in a control population, and the presence of IgM anti-MAG is usually not an incidental finding. MAG is a membrane glycoprotein located in peripheral and central myelin.

The pathogenesis of the neuropathy is not well understood, but an animal model of anti-MAG neuropathy suggests that the antibodies are pathogenic and along with complement deposition mediate damage to the myelin sheath.

Anti-MAG neuropathy is the best characterized of the anti-nerve antibody syndromes. Typically, there is the insidious onset of sensory gait ataxia and progressive symmetrical ascending numbness with progression over months to years. Motor involvement is much less pronounced, and early on the clinical picture may resemble a *sensory neuronopathy*. Eventually, clinical motor involvement occurs in the majority of patients. Peripheral nerves may be thickened and palpable. EMG studies are crucial in diagnosing demyelinating peripheral neuropathy, as there is usually prolongation of distal latencies and dispersion of motor potentials, even when weakness is not evident. Sensory responses are frequently absent or attenuated. Spinal fluid often shows a protein of >100 mg/dL.

Compared with chronic inflammatory demyelinating polyneuropathy (CIDP) without IgM paraproteinemia, anti-MAG polyneuropathy is less responsive to steroids, plasmapheresis, and intravenous immunoglobulin (IVIG). Oral cyclophosphamide or intravenous cyclophosphamide with steroids may be effective.

ANTI-SULFATIDE ANTIBODIES AND SENSORIMOTOR NEUROPATHY

Polyneuropathies associated with serum IgM antisulfatide antibodies have been described. These neuropathies are usually more sensory than motor, with distal, symmetrical sensory loss. Pain is common. Tremor and gait ataxia have been reported. In patients with an associated M protein and a MGUS, EMG may show demyelination. In patients without an M protein EMG shows axonal loss. These antibodies also have been reported in patients with ALS. At this time there is no established diagnostic role for these antibodies in the routine evaluation of sensory or sensory-predominant peripheral neuropathy.

PARANEOPLASTIC NEUROMUSCULAR SYNDROMES

Many neurologic syndromes result from paraneoplastic causes (Table 4). This discussion is concerned with the neuromuscular syndromes only, although antibodies associated with non-neuromuscular syndromes are summarized in Table 4.

    I. *Paraneoplastic sensory neuronopathy* (PSN) is the classic paraneoplastic neuropathy. Presentation of neurologic symptoms classically precedes the tumor discovery by months. The neuropathy is painful, subacute in onset, often initially asymmetrical, and evolves into a complete loss of proprioception with prominent sensory ataxia and pseudoathetosis of the hands. Sensory neuronopathy has a limited differential diagnosis other than paraneoplastic causes that includes chemotherapy with platinum-containing agents, pyridoxine (vitamin B_6) intoxication, and Sjögren's syndrome. This condition is rare, but dramatic, affecting less than 1% of patients with small-cell lung carcinoma (SCLC) and rarely seen in other neoplasms. Anti-amphiphysin, anti-ANNA3, and anti-CV2 antibodies have also been associated, again usually with SCLC. Patients with anti-Hu may have more widespread disease that may include cerebellar degeneration and limbic or brainstem encephalitis (paraneoplastic encephalomyelitis/sensory neuronopathy [PEM/SN]). In the setting of a sensory neuronopathy, a positive anti-Hu is diagnostic of paraneoplastic etiology (specificity of 99% and a sensitivity of 82%) prompting a thorough evaluation for lung cancer. If no cancer is found, periodic screening should be performed, as cancer is eventually found in 80% to 90% of patients with anti-Hu. In general, recovery of sensation following treatment of the underlying cancer is poor, but the associated cancer is often limited and responds to treatment.

    II. *Sensorimotor polyneuropathy* may also be associated with anti-Hu or anti-CV2. The possibility of a paraneoplastic syndrome is often overlooked as patients with cancer may have multiple potential causes for a sensorimotor polyneuropathy.

  III. *Subacute autonomic neuropathy.* Paraneoplastic neuropathy may also present as a severe dysautonomia with anti-Hu antibodies.

  IV. *Lambert-Eaton myasthenic syndrome* (LEMS) is a presynaptic neuromuscular junction disorder associated with underlying cancer in about 60% of cases, usually SCLC but sometimes lymphoma. The syndrome presents with proximal leg weakness and less frequently arm weakness. Although progressive augmentation of muscle strength may occur initially with exercise, the dominant symptom is fatigable weakness, as in myasthenia gravis. Ocular symptoms are much less frequent than in myasthenia gravis, however. Characteristically EMG studies of LEMS show low motor CMAP amplitudes with an increment

A

ANTIBODY TESTING IN NEUROMUSCULAR DISEASE

TABLE 4

AUTOANTIBODIES IN NEUROLOGIC PARANEOPLASTIC SYNDROMES

Syndrome	Antibody for Diagnosis	Antibody for Paraneoplastic Etiology	Associated Cancer (Most Frequent)
Subacute sensory neuropathy		Anti-Hu	SCLC
		Anti-amphiphysin	SCLC
		ANNA-3	SCLC
		Anti-CRMP5/CV2	SCLC, thymoma
Sensory-motor peripheral neuropathy		Anti-Hu	SCLC
		Anti-amphiphysin	SCLC
		Anti-CRMP5/CV2	SCLC, thymoma
Stiff-man/person syndrome	Anti-GAD	Anti-amphiphysin	Breast
Myelitis		Anti-Hu	SCLC
Lambert-Eaton myasthenic syndrome	Anti-VGCC	Not available	SCLC
Myasthenia gravis	Anti-AchR, Anti-MUSK	Anti-titin	Thymoma
Dermatomyositis		Not available	Ovarian, lung, pancreas
Subacute cerebellar degeneration		Anti-Hu	SCLC
		Anti-PCA-2	SCLC
		ANNA-3	SCLC
		Anti-CRMP5/CV2	SCLC, thymoma

Syndrome	Antibody	Cancer
	Anti-Yo	Ovary, breast
	Anti-Ta/Ma2	Testis
	Anti-Ma	Multiple
	Anti-Ri	Breast
	Anti-Tr	Hodgkin's lymphoma
Opsoclonus/myoclonus (child)	Anti-Hu	Neuroblastoma
Opsoclonus/myoclonus (adult)	Anti-Ri	Breast
	Anti-Hu	SCLC
	Anti-Ma	Multiple
	Anti-Ta/Ma2	Testis
Limbic encephalitis	Anti-Hu	SCLC
	Anti-Ta/Ma2	Testicular
	ANNA-3	SCLC
	Anti-CRMP5/CV2	SCLC, thymoma
Retinopathy	Anti-recoverin, Anti-retinal	Lung
	Anti-Hu	SCLC
Extrapyramidal syndromes	Anti-Hu	SCLC
	Anti-Ta/Ma2	Testis
	Anti-Ma	Multiple
	Anti-CRMP5/CV2	SCLC, thymoma

ANTIBODY TESTING IN NEUROMUSCULAR DISEASE

A

in amplitude following brief exercise of greater than 100%. The prevalence of LEMS in patients with known SCLC is around 3%. Anti-voltage gated calcium channels are almost always present in LEMS, but do not differentiate between paraneoplastic and nonparaneoplastic causes. The presentation of LEMS may precede the diagnosis of the cancer by many months, and repeated screening is recommended.

V. *Myasthenia gravis* is considered elsewhere in this book.

VI. *Dermatomyositis* represents a paraneoplastic syndrome in approximately 30% of patients. Frequently associated tumors are ovarian, lung, pancreatic, stomach, colon, rectum, and non-Hodgkin's lymphoma. No serologic marker has been identified. *Polymyositis* is less frequently associated with a paraneoplastic form.

VII. *Stiff-man syndrome* is a rare condition characterized by chronic rigidity of axial musculature and spasms believed to arise from a functional deficit of GABA in the central nervous system. Antibodies to glutamic acid decarboxylase (anti-GAD) are present in serum and CSF in about 70% of patients. Stiff-man (stiff-person) syndrome is associated with other autoimmune conditions such as diabetes, autoimmune thyroiditis, pernicious anemia, and vitiligo. Epilepsy occurs in 10% of patients. In 5% of patients stiff-man syndrome is associated with cancer, particularly breast cancer. Anti-amphiphysin antibodies are found in the paraneoplastic stiff-man syndrome.

REFERENCES

AAEM: *Muscle Nerve* 8 (suppl):S225–229, 1999.

Katirji B et al, eds: *Neuromuscular disorders in clinical practice*, Boston, Butterworth-Heinemann, 2002.

Pourmand R: *Neurol Clin* 22:703–717, 2004.

Van den Berg L et al: *Muscle Nerve* 19:637–643, 1996.

Voltz R: *Lancet Neurol* 1:294–305, 2002.

Willison HJ, Yuki N: *Brain* 125:2591–2625, 2002.

ANTIDEPRESSANTS

Antidepressants encompass several groups of compounds, including tricyclic and tetracyclic compounds, selective serotonin reuptake inhibitors (SSRIs), and monoamine oxidase inhibitors. Table 5 summarizes the relative side effects of common antidepressants. Tricyclic antidepressants have notable anticholinergic side effects including blurred vision, dry mouth, constipation, urinary retention, memory dysfunction, and exacerbation of narrow-angle glaucoma. Patients with dementia and concomitant depression may worsen as a result of anticholinergic effects, whereas patients with Parkinson disease may improve. Patients with migraine or chronic pain may benefit from antidepressants with a relatively high affinity for serotonin receptors. Selective serotonin reuptake inhibitors (fluoxetine, sertraline, citalopram, and paroxetine) may cause headache. Choice of antidepressant must be based on assessment of the patient's

TABLE 5

FREQUENCY OF SIDE EFFECTS OF ANTIDEPRESSANT MEDICATIONS

Medication	Sedation	Agitation	Anti-cholinergic Effects*	Postural Hypotension	Gastrointestinal Upset	Sexual Dysfunction	Weight Gain	Weight Loss
Serotonin and norepinephrine reuptake inhibitors								
Tricyclics (tertiary amines)								
Amitriptyline	++++	0	++++	+++	+	+	++	0
Doxepin	++++	0	++++	+++	+	+	+	0
Imipramine	++++	0	++++	+++	+	+	+	0
Tricyclics (secondary amines)								
Desipramine	+++	0	+++	++	+	+	+	0
Nortriptyline	+++	0	+++	++	+	+	+	0
Bicyclic								
Venlafaxine	++	+	++	0	+++	++	0	+
Selective serotonin reuptake inhibitors								
Citalopram	0	0	+	0	++	+	+	+
Fluoxetine	+	++	+	0	++	++	+	+
Paroxetine	++	0	+	0	++	++	+	+
Sertraline	+	+	+	0	++	++	+	+
Serotonin antagonist								
Mirtazapine	+++	0	++	+	0	0	++	0
Norepinephrine and dopamine reuptake inhibitor								
Bupropion	+	++	++	0	++	0	+	++
Serotonin antagonists and reuptake inhibitors								
Nefazodone	++	0	++	+	+	0	0	0
Trazodone	++++	0	++	+	+	0	+	+

*Side effects may include dry mouth, dry eyes, blurred vision, constipation, urinary retention, tachycardia, or confusion.
0, none; +, minimal (>5% of patients); ++, low frequency (5–20%); +++, moderate frequency (21–40%); ++++, high frequency (greater than 40%).
Adapted from Whooley et al: *N Engl J Med* 2000.

A

ANTIDEPRESSANTS

TABLE 6

THE EFFECT OF BLOCKING OR STIMULATING CERTAIN CNS RECEPTORS

Receptor Type	Potential Side Effect
α^1 adrenergic receptor blocker	Orthostatic hypotension, reflex tachycardia
H1 histamine receptors blockers	Sedation, weight gain
M1 muscarine receptors blockers	Urinary retention, dry mouth, confusion, tachycardia
Serotonin 5-HT1 receptor stimulation	Antidepressant, anxiolytic effect, hypophagia
Serotonin 5-HT2 receptor stimulation	Sexual dysfunction, decreased libido or impotence, agitation, insomnia
Serotonin 5-HT3 receptor stimulation	Gastrointestinal side effects

clinical state, especially cardiac conduction and ability to tolerate orthostatic hypotension, as well as the specific drug's side effect profile. Suicide risk should be assessed in all depressed patients, because tricyclic antidepressant overdose is commonly fatal. There have been recent reports of increased suicide attempts in children taking an SSRI and new black-box warnings at this time are pending. Tables 6 and 7 summarize the side effects of blocking or stimulating certain CNS receptors and epileptogenicity of selected antidepressants.

REFERENCES

Sadock BJ, Sadock VA, Kaplan HL: *Kaplan and Sadock's comprehensive textbook of psychiatry,* ed 7, Philadelphia, Lippincott Williams & Wilkins, 2000.

Stimmel GL: In Herfindal ET, Gourley DR (eds): *Textbook of therapeutics,* ed 7, Baltimore, Williams & Wilkins, 2000.

APHASIA

Aphasia is the acquired disorder of previously intact language ability. As such, it is not interchangeable with failure of language development. Aphasic patients have disturbances of speech, writing, and reading. The great majority of patients with aphasia have left hemisphere lesions, although occasional patients have language dominance in the right hemisphere.

Benson and Geschwind developed the most widely used classification of aphasia. In this classification three aspects of language are used to classify aphasias (Tables 8 and 9).

I. *Fluency* refers to several features of spontaneous speech-rhythm, melody, articulation, and word production rate. Look for verbal (substitution of one word for another such as knife for spoon) and phonemic (substitution of incorrect sounds, such as "spork" for fork) paraphasic errors. Paraphasic errors (primarily in fluent aphasias) and naming abnormalities are the hallmark of aphasia.

II. *Comprehension* abilities vary from following midline commands (such as "stick out your tongue"), to performing multistep requests (such as "take

TABLE 7
EPILEPTOGENIC POTENTIAL OF ANTIDEPRESSANT DRUGS AND THEIR RECEPTOR SPECIFICATIONS

| Drug | Action on receptor: | | | | | | Seizures/epilepsy |
	H1	M1	NA	5-HT1	5-HT2	5-HT3	
Imipramine	–	–	+	+	+	+	0.1–4%, in overdose 3.8–8%
Paroxetine	0	0	0	+	+	+	Prolonged seizures during electroconvulsive therapy
							In overdose: no seizures in 15 patients with maximum dose 850 mg
Sertraline	0	0	0	+	+	+	Rare, secondary to SIADH
							In overdose: no seizures in 40 patients up to 8000 mg
Fluoxetine	0	0	0	+	+	+	<0.1%
Citalopram	0	0	0	+	+	+	No worsening of epilepsy in 16 patients. In overdose: 100–1.9 g 18%–49%
Reboxetine	0	0/–	+	0	0	0	0.13%
Venlafaxine	0	0	+	+	+	+	0.18%
Nefazodone	0	0	0	+	–	+	In overdose: seizures in dosages over 1 g then rare reports of convulsions
Mirtazapine	–	0	+	+	–	–	<0.1%

0, no or negligible effect; +, stimulation; –, blockade; H1, histamine; 5-HT1, 5-HT2, 5-HT3, serotonin receptors; M1, muscarine; NA, noradrenaline; SIADH, syndrome of inappropriate secretion of ADH.

A

APHASIA

TABLE 8

APHASIAS WITH DISORDERED REPETITION

Aphasia	Type of Speech	Comprehension*	Other Signs	Emotional State	Localization
Broca's	Nonfluent	+	Right hemiparesis worse in arm	Depressed	Lower posterior frontal
Wernicke's temporal	Fluent	−	Often none	Often euphoric and/or paranoid	Posterior superior
Conduction operculum	Fluent	+	Often none; cortical sensory loss in right arm	Depressed	Usually parietal
Global lesion	Nonfluent	−	Right hemiparesis worse in arm	Flat	Massive perisylvian

* +, relatively or fully intact; −, definitely impaired.
From Geschwind N: Used by permission of the Continuing Professional Education Center, Princeton, NJ.

TABLE 9

APHASIAS WITH INTACT REPETITION

Aphasia	Speech	Comprehension*	Localization
Transcortical motor	Nonfluent	+	Anterior to Broca's area or supplementary speech area
Transcortical sensory	Fluent	–	Surrounding Wernicke's area posteriorly
Transcortical mixed ("isolation syndrome")	Nonfluent	–	Both of the above
Anomic	Fluent	+	Lesion of angular gyrus or second temporal gyrus

* +, relatively or fully intact; –, definitely impaired.
From Geschwind N: Used by permission of the Continuing Professional Education Center, Princeton, NJ.

A

APHASIA

the paper in your left hand, fold it in half, and then put it on the floor"), to understanding relationships (as in "The lion was killed by the tiger. Which animal died?"), and to following more complex instructions.

III. *Repetition* of phrases may be impaired to various degrees; the most difficult phrases to repeat are those involving grammatical function or low frequency words (for instance, "The spy fled to Greece"). Additional testing of reading out loud, reading comprehension, and writing (to dictation or spontaneously) is useful.

Damage to the thalamus, caudate, putamen, and surrounding structures may produce aphasia (subcortical). Initial muteness improving to fluent or nonfluent hypophonic aphasia is common. Paraphasic errors in spontaneous speech, which disappear when the patient is asked to repeat phrases, and rapid resolution of deficits are hallmarks of these subcortical aphasias.

Other syndromes related to aphasia but involving only a single language modality include *aphemia* or pure word dumbness (inferior frontal lobe dominant hemisphere lesions), pure word deafness (lesions of the dominant superior temporal lobe or bilateral middle portion of the superior temporal gyrus), *alexia without agraphia* (left occipital lesions, including posterior corpus callosum), and *sign language aphasia* (deaf signers can become aphasic in American Sign Language or other sign languages with left hemispheric damage).

Lesion of the right hemisphere cortices may lead to difficulties with "*utterances*," which refers to the automaticity of the speech; "*discourse*," which refers to the skill with which one can organize narrative; and impaired "prosody," which refers to inflection, stress, and melody of speech.

The classification of aphasia is based on patients with stable deficits; the acutely ill patient may not be easily classified. Spontaneous recovery often occurs in the first month after onset and may continue for many months. Speech therapy individualized for the form of aphasia may be helpful in recovery of language function.

REFERENCES

Benson DF: In Heilman KH, Valenstein E (eds): *Clinical neuropsychology*, ed 3, New York, Oxford University Press, 1993.

Mesulam MM: *Principles of behavioral and cognitive neurology*, New York, Oxford University Press, 2000.

APRAXIA

Apraxia is the inability to perform a previously learned skilled movement in the presence of intact motor, sensory, coordination, and comprehension systems. *Ideomotor apraxia* is the inability to voluntarily complete an act in response to a verbal command. However, the same act can be performed spontaneously. It may involve buccofacial, limb, or truncal musculature. It is often associated with lesion in the left hemisphere and often complicates Broca's aphasia. A lesion in the arcuate fasciculus may result in bilateral apraxia and conduction aphasia. *Callosal apraxia* results from a lesion in the anterior corpus callosum and manifests as left-sided apraxia with intact right-sided praxis. *Limb-kinetic apraxia* refers to loss of fine skilled movement following a premotor lesion. The patient is often clumsy and slow in executing motor tasks. *Ideational apraxia* (apraxia for object use) is the inability to perform sequential movements to use common objects in a proper manner despite the retained ability in performing the individual movements. *Constructional apraxia* occurs in two thirds of patients with right parietal lobe lesions. The patient is unable to copy or spontaneously draw figures and construct or mentally manipulate three-dimensional structures. *Oculomotor apraxia* occurs as part of Balint's syndrome (bilateral occipito-parietal lesions), and *gait apraxia* is seen with frontal lesions and *dressing apraxia* with right parietal syndromes.

Testing for apraxia includes asking the patient to follow simple commands (such as "close your eyes" or "lick your lips"), to perform tasks with left and right extremities (for instance, comb hair, brush teeth, hammer a nail, or blow a kiss), and to use objects (as in lighting a match, or using the telephone). Patients with ideomotor apraxia are usually self-sufficient because they can manipulate objects correctly on their own, whereas patients with ideational apraxia are often unable to care for themselves.

REFERENCE

Devinsky O: *Behavioral neurology: 100 maxims,* St. Louis, Mosby, 1992.

ARNOLD-CHIARI MALFORMATIONS

Chiari malformation (named after pathologist Hans Chiari) is preferred for type I, and Arnold-Chiari malformation for type II.

PRESENTATION

Occipital headache (especially with straining and coughing), and lower cranial nerve palsies develop during adolescence or adulthood.

Type I: Cerebellar tonsils are herniated below foramen magnum (3 mm, mean of 13 mm versus normal mean of 1 mm); this type is associated with syringomyelia and bony deformities.

Type II: Cerebellar vermis, fourth ventricle, and medulla are displaced inferiorly and deformed; associated with spina bifida and lumbar meningomyelocele, polymicrogyria, heterotropias, syringomyelia, hydromyelia, enlargement of the foramen magnum, elongation of the cervical arches, platybasia, basilar invagination, assimilation of the atlas, and Klippel-Feil anomaly. Symptoms begin in infancy or early childhood, most commonly presenting as hydrocephalus or respiratory distress.

Type III: This type includes cervical spina bifida, cerebellar herniation through the defect, and a dystrophic posterior fossa; it is rarely compatible with postnatal life.

DIAGNOSIS
MRI shows tonsils below the foramen magnum and blockage of CSF flow; myelography and CT may also be indicated.

TREATMENT
New onset symptoms or deteriorating symptoms may be referred for decompressive surgery, which is better if done within 2 years of symptoms onset.

REFERENCES
Barkovich AJ: *Pediatric neuroimaging,* ed 3, Philadelphia, Lippincott Williams & Wilkins, 2000.

Bradley WG, Daroff RB, et al: *Neurology in clinical practice*, ed 4, Boston, Butterworth-Heinemann, 2003.

ARTERIOVENOUS MALFORMATION (See also CEREBRAL HEMORRHAGE)

DEFINITION
Cerebral AVM (cAVM) is a tangled bundle of abnormal vessels, with complex twists, linked by one or more fistulae. An important anatomic feature, also known as the *nidus*, is the lack of a capillary bed: arteries feeding the nidus are directly connected to the draining enlarged veins (shunting).

EPIDEMIOLOGY
cAVMs are assumed to arise during fetal development with increase in size and complexity over time (rarely familial). It is a rare disease (1–2 per 100,000 persons annually).

CLINICAL FEATURES
This defect presents in the third decade of life. cAVM may present with headache, seizure, or focal neurologic deficit or may be an incidental

ARTERIOVENOUS MALFORMATION

finding on head CT or MRI. Most common presentation is cerebral hemorrhage (ICH) in 50% of the cases, although cAVM accounts for 2% of all hemorrhagic stroke. *Risk of bleeding from cAVM* depends on deep location of the nidus, deep versus cortical feeders, and deep draining vein versus cortical. Age, vascular anatomy, size, location, and history of prior rupture affect the future risk of rupture. The risk of rebleed is 2% to 4% per year and is highest in the first year after ICH (18%). Associated aneurysm is seen in 10% to 23% of the cases.

PROGNOSIS
Mortality rate from ICH varies and averages around 5%.

DIAGNOSIS
CTOH shows mixed heterogeneous flow void signals with dilated veins. MRI (Fig. 5A) can detect hemosiderin and old blood that may have been asymptomatic and associated with increased risk of rebleed. For anatomic characterization, the gold standard is the cerebral angiogram (Fig. 5B). CTA can be helpful. fMRI can be helpful in treatment planning.

TREATMENT
Endovascular embolization may be curative in 10% to 15% of patients. This is usually achieved by use of embolic agents, such as N-butylcyanoacrylate, polyvinyl alcohol particles, detachable coils, or onyx liquid polymer. The most common therapy is multimodal treatment with embolization followed by radiation or open surgical resection of the cAVM. Treatment of asymptomatic patients with small AVM is controversial. Classification to predict outcome from surgery (Spetzler-Martin classification) basically predicts worse surgical outcome from larger AVM

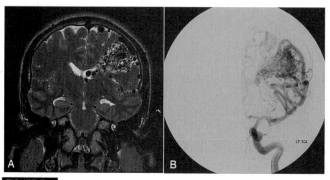

FIGURE 5
MRI (**A**) and angio (**B**) findings in cAVM with flow void signals of feeding arteries and draining veins on MRI and nidus appearance on angio and MRI.

nidus greater than 3 cm, with deep feeders and draining veins, and location in the dominant hemisphere.

REFERENCE
Stapf C, Mohr JP, Pile-Spellman J, et al: *Neurosurg Focus* 11(5):e1, 2001.

ASTERIXIS

DEFINITION
Asterixis, also known as "negative myoclonus," is a sudden loss of postural tone, usually manifesting as the inability to hold the wrists in forced dorsiflexion with arms extended.

PRESENTATION
Typically, sudden wrist flexion is followed by rapid correction to the original dorsiflexed position, resulting in a characteristic flapping tremor. The loss of postural tone can also be evident during tongue protrusion or forced eye closure.

Electrophysiologic studies reveal an electrically silent period on EMG corresponding to the lapse of posture, which can be preceded by EEG transients by 20 to 40 ms, suggesting a possible cortical generator of this phenomenon.

ETIOLOGY
Once thought to be pathognomonic of hepatic encephalopathy (hence the term "liver flap"), it can be seen in other toxic-metabolic conditions including uremia and drug intoxication. When asterixis is unilateral, however, ischemic or hemorrhagic cerebral lesions, especially in the thalamus, are the most common cause.

TREATMENT
Dopamine agonists or clonazepam at 0.1 to 0.3 mg PO bid may be tried if symptoms are persistent.

REFERENCE
Shibasaki H: In Jankovic JJ, Tolosa E (eds): *Parkinson's disease and movement disorders*, ed 4, Philadelphia, Lippincott Williams & Wilkins, 2002.

ATAXIA, SPINOCEREBELLAR DEGENERATION
Usually the hallmark of cerebellar dysfunction, ataxia is an abnormality of movement characterized by errors in rate, range, direction, timing, and force ("coordination") of motor activity. Patients report being clumsy, slow with movements, or unsteady when walking. Speech and vision may also become symptomatic. Elements of ataxia include:

I. *Asynergia*—decomposition of smooth movement into uncoordinated component parts.

II. *Dysmetria*—poorly controlled speed, force, or distance of movement; includes past-pointing, abnormal checking response, excessive rebound phenomenon.

III. *Dysdiadochokinesia*—impairment of rapid alternating movements.

Ataxia may involve limbs, trunk, eyes, or bulbar musculature and may be due to disease of the cerebellum, brainstem, spinal cord, or motor or sensory nerves. It results from defective timing of sequential contractions of agonist and antagonist muscles. Cerebellar hemispheric disease commonly produces limb ataxia, whereas midline cerebellar disease manifests as truncal and gait ataxia. Patients classically develop a broad-based gait to compensate for truncal instability. Owing to the double-crossing of the cerebellar pathways, ataxia is ipsilateral to cerebellar lesions.

Ataxia is frequently accompanied by other cerebellar findings:

I. *Tremor*, which classically becomes worse near the target

II. *Dysarthria*—slurring, aprosody, scanning

III. *Nystagmus*, which can produce blurring or vertigo

IV. *Saccadic dysmetria*—over/undershooting on saccades

Tremor in cerebellar disease may be an action or intention tremor (disease of dentate nucleus or superior cerebellar peduncle) or more coarse ("rubral tremor"). *Titubation*, a nodding-head tremor, is seen with midline cerebellar disease and may involve the trunk. *Ataxic speech* has abnormal variability of volume, rate, and phonation and may be slow and slurred or have alternating loudness and quietness. *Gait ataxia* may accompany vertigo in vestibular dysfunction. Impaired proprioception resulting from tabes dorsalis, hereditary disease, or dorsal root ganglionopathies may lead to *sensory ataxia* with impaired gait and presence of Romberg sign. This form of ataxia is distinct because it can produce ataxia without cerebellar disease. Worsening of the ataxia with eyes closed and absence of dysarthria and ocular symptoms suggest sensory rather than cerebellar involvement. Cerebellar ataxia normally persists despite visual clues.

ACUTE ONSET ATAXIA

This form often results from cerebellar hemorrhage or infarction. Hemorrhage is usually associated with headache. Multiple sclerosis, toxic disorders, and basilar migraine can also be acute causes. Viral cerebellitis causes an acute, reversible ataxia in children 2 to 10 years of age and is most common after chickenpox.

SUBACUTE ATAXIA

Hydrocephalus, foramen magnum compression, posterior fossa tumor, abscess, or parasitic infection in any age group can produce subacute ataxia. Other causes are infections (HIV, Creutzfeldt-Jakob disease, brainstem encephalitis), alcohol, vitamin deficiency (vitamin B_{12}, thiamine, vitamin E), celiac sprue (gliadin antibodies) and anti-GAD antibodies, drugs (antiepileptics, lithium, chemotherapy, solvents, metals [mercury, manganese, bismuth, thallium]), and paraneoplastic syndromes in association with bronchogenic or ovarian carcinoma.

ATAXIA WITH EPISODIC COURSE

Ataxia with episodic course may be encountered in the following conditions: multiple sclerosis, vertebrobasilar transient ischemic attacks, foramen magnum compression, intermittent obstruction of ventricular system due to colloid cyst and dominantly inherited, acetazolamide responsive episodic ataxia. In children, metabolic causes including inherited defects of the urea cycle, aminoaciduria, Leigh's disease, and mitochondrial encephalomyopathies should be considered.

ATAXIA WITH CHRONIC PROGRESSIVE COURSE

Chronic alcoholism with progressive cerebellar degeneration is common. Structural lesions such as posterior fossa tumors, foramen magnum compression, or hydrocephalus must be excluded first. Rarely, infectious agents such as chronic panencephalitis due to rubella in children can have a chronic progressive course. Multiple sclerosis occasionally manifests as chronic deterioration. Genetic diseases and other metabolic derangements can produce chronic ataxia as part of the clinical picture (see next section).

SPINOCEREBELLAR DEGENERATION

Spinocerebellar degeneration refers to a large group of disorders that produce ataxia as a primary symptom, often early in life (except for the dominant ataxias). Most are very rare. Autosomal recessive causes include Friedreich's ataxia, ataxia-telangiectasia, ataxia with isolated vitamin E deficiency, ataxia with oculomotor apraxia, abetalipoproteinemia, Unverricht-Lundborg disease, and others. Progressive ataxias are caused by leukodystrophies, xeroderma pigmentosum, coenzyme Q deficiency, vanishing white matter disease, GM2 gangliosidoses, Ramsay-Hunt syndrome, ceroid lipofuscinosis, sialidosis, sphingomyelin storage diseases, Wilson's disease, Leigh's disease, Refsum's disease, and hexosaminidase deficiency (Tay-Sachs). Mitochondrial diseases such as MELAS, MERRF, and Kearns-Sayre produce progressive ataxias along with many other typical symptoms. Abnormal metabolism such as disorders of urea metabolism, aminoacidurias (Hartnup's, branched chain), and various disorders of pyruvate/lactate metabolism can cause ataxia, sometimes intermittently. There is a large group of autosomal dominant ataxias that typically present after age 20 (see *spinocerebellar ataxia*).

Friedreich's ataxia is the most common type of spinocerebellar degeneration. It is caused by a triple nucleotide repeat (GAA) expansion at chromosome 9 that encodes the protein frataxin. Symptoms develop from 18 months to 24 years of age and consist of progressive limb and truncal ataxia, dysarthria, and areflexia in the lower extremities. Pyramidal signs and loss of position and vibration sense evolve gradually. There is degeneration of cranial nerves VIII, X, and XII, the cerebellar hemispheres

A

ATAXIA, SPINOCEREBELLAR DEGENERATION

and tracts, and large myelinated nerves throughout the body. Skeletal deformities (kyphoscoliosis and pes cavus) and cardiomyopathy are seen in more than two thirds of patients. Systemic involvement manifests by increased incidence of diabetes, blindness, and deafness. Ambulation is usually lost by age 25, and death frequently occurs in the fourth or fifth decade of life. Treatment is aimed at symptomatic management of the skeletal deformities, diabetes, and the cardiac disorders. *Early-onset cerebellar ataxia* with retained reflexes is often a variant with the frataxin mutation, but sometimes has unknown causes.

Ataxia-telangiectasia is characterized by progressive ataxia, neuropathy, choreoathetosis, areflexia, ocular telangiectasias (dilated capillaries in the conjunctiva), and frequent infections.

Ataxia sometimes occurs sporadically later in life with no identifiable cause. This condition is sometimes due to a degenerative condition known as olivopontocerebellar atrophy (OPCA). OPCA can progress to multisystem atrophy, which carries a very poor prognosis.

EVALUATION

Evaluation of a patient with progressive ataxia requires careful attention to disease progression, associated systemic and neurologic signs, and family history. Testing can include MRI, TSH, vitamin E, vitamin B_{12}, RPR, anti-GAD, gliadin antibody, paraneoplastic antibodies (Yo, Hu, Ri, Ta, Ma, CV2 antiglutamate), CSF (including cytology). In younger patients, specialized metabolic tests may be needed. DNA testing for most of the inherited disorders is available.

REFERENCES

http://www.emedicine.com/neuro/topic556.htm.
Evidente VG et al: *Mayo Clin Proc* 75:475–490, 2000.
Martin JB: *N Engl J Med* 340(25):1970–1980, 1999.
NICP Chapter 23.

ATHETOSIS (See also CHOREA)

Athetosis is an involuntary, slow, sinuous, irregular, writhing movement of any muscle group, usually most prominent in the distal extremities. It frequently coexists with other abnormal movements, particularly dystonia and chorea. Like those movements, athetosis is associated with lesions in the basal ganglia. EMG analysis reveals loss of reciprocation between agonists and antagonists. Common syndromes include posthemiplegic athetosis, generalized athetosis ("double athetosis" seen in cerebral palsy and postkernicterus), and drug-induced athetosis (e.g., levodopa-induced dyskinesias). Athetosis may be seen in many inherited metabolic diseases such as Huntington disease, Wilson disease, Lesch-Nyhan syndrome, glutaric acidemia, glyceric acidemia, sulfite oxidase deficiency, Niemann-Pick disease, familial calcification of the basal ganglia, and Hallervorden-Spatz disease.

ATTENTION-DEFICIT HYPERACTIVITY DISORDER

EPIDEMIOLOGY

Attention-deficit hyperactivity disorder (ADHD) is estimated to affect 3% to 5% of school age children. It is familial in 30% to 50% of cases, and is four to six times more common in boys. Comorbid conditions are frequent: 50% have obsessive-compulsive disorder (OCD), 30% to 50% have conduct disorders, 50% have oppositional defiant disorder, 15% to 20% have mood disorders, and 20% to 25% have anxiety disorders.

Although the underlying neurobiology is incompletely understood, it is generally felt that a hypodopaminergic state results in decreased activity of inhibitory areas of the prefrontal cortex, striatum, caudate, and thalamic nuclei leading to an inability of affected children to control their attention, impulses, and motor activity.

CLINICAL PRESENTATIONS

Table 10 lists clinical presentations of ADHD.

MANAGEMENT

I. Children and adolescents
   A. A combination of behavior management at home and school, targeted educational assistance, and medication therapy.
   B. Interdisciplinary team that includes patient, family, school officials, mental health professionals, and the physician
   C. Medications used most often include stimulants (methylphenidate, amphetamines, pemoline), atomoxetine (a serotonin and norepinephrine reuptake inhibitor), antidepressants (bupropion; rarely tricyclic antidepressants because of cardiac effects), α_2-adrenergic agents (clonidine, guanfacine). Stimulants are first-line drugs with a 70% to 90% response rate.
   D. The development of time-released medications (e.g., Concerta, Adderall XR) has helped with compliance and with preventing attention from waning due to short acting medication (Methylphenidate typically lasts about four hours) but also allows children to avoid the stigma of receiving medication from the school nurse.
   E. Side effects of stimulants include insomnia, anorexia, irritability, rebound phenomena, growth suppression, cardiovascular effects, potential for drug addiction, and an increase in seizure frequency. Some children may take drug holidays when attentional needs are relaxed, such as summer vacation.
   F. Children with strong family history of tics or Tourette's disorder should be referred to a specialist prior to initiating therapy as both conditions may be precipitated prematurely by stimulant use. Pemoline can be used with substance-abusing patients but is associated with acute liver failure. Nonstimulants are used in

---

TABLE 10

DSM-IV DIAGNOSTIC CRITERIA FOR ATTENTION-DEFICIT
HYPERACTIVITY DISORDER

DIAGNOSTIC CRITERIA

1. Onset before age 7 years
2. Some impairment in two or more settings (e.g., school and home)
3. Clinically significant impairment in social, academic, or occupational functioning
4. Absence of pervasive developmental or other mental disorder
5. *Either* six or more symptoms of inattention *or* six or more symptoms of hyperactivity-impulsivity, for at least 6 months, that are maladaptive and inconsistent with developmental level

SYMPTOMS OF INATTENTION

1. Failure of close attention to details
2. Has difficulty sustaining attention in tasks
3. Often does not listen when spoken to directly
4. Often does not follow through on instructions or fails to finish tasks
5. Has difficulty organizing tasks or activities
6. Often loses things necessary for tasks
7. Is easily distracted by extraneous stimuli
8. Is often forgetful in daily activities

SYMPTOMS OF IMPULSIVITY

1. Often blurts outs answers before questions are completed
2. Often has difficulty awaiting turn
3. Often interrupts or intrudes on others

SYMPTOMS OF HYPERACTIVITY

1. Often fidgets with limbs or squirms in seat
2. Often leaves seat in classroom or other places where sitting is expected
3. Often runs or climbs excessively
4. Has difficulty playing quietly
5. Is often "on the go" or often acts as if "driven by a motor"
6. Often talks excessively

SUBTYPES

1. *Combined*: six or more symptoms are from inattentive list, and six or more symptoms are from hyperactive-impulsive lists
2. *Predominantly inattentive subtype*: the six symptoms are from the inattentive group
3. *Predominantly hyperactive-impulsive subtype:* the six symptoms are from the hyperactive-impulsive lists

From American Psychiatric Association: Diagnostic and statistical manual of mental disorders, ed 4,. Washington, DC, APA, 1994.

---

children who fail to respond to or cannot tolerate the stimulants and in those with significant comorbid conditions such as anxiety, depression, tics, aggression, or substance abuse.

II. Adults
   A. ADHD is being increasingly recognized in adulthood, but the diagnosis requires obligate onset in childhood, even if it was not diagnosed as such. The presentation is similar, but they are often of the primarily inattentive subtype.

B. Thirty percent of ADHD patients diagnosed in childhood will outgrow their symptoms, 40% will continue to display significant symptoms often accompanied by depression and anxiety, and 30% will decline with development of additional psychopathology such as alcoholism, substance abuse, or antisocial personality disorders. About 60% will continue with symptoms into adulthood where it may impact social or occupational functioning.

C. Many patients may discontinue medication in early adulthood, only to find that tasks such as college coursework or job-related functions are difficult because of lack of ability to organize and attend to details.

D. Differential diagnosis includes adult onset attentional disorders (e.g., dementia, focal lesions, medication effects), substance abuse, and mood disorders

E. Treatment for adults is similar to that for children. Note that stimulants often are dosed by weight, so that higher dosages may be required for efficacy.

REFERENCE
Rapply MD: *N Engl J Med* 352(2):165–173, 2005.

AUTISM

Normal early milestones are followed by regression at age 1 to 3 years characterized by abnormal language (parrotlike and echolalic), social dysfunction (aloof, passive, or odd), and restricted range of behaviors, interests, or activities (repetitive, stereotyped movements or idiot savant). One third of patients with autism develop epilepsy. *Diagnostic evaluation* should include formal audiologic assessment and EEG. Imaging is rarely indicated. *Treatment* consists of special education and behavior modification programs and medications targeted at specific behaviors.

I. Autistic spectrum
  A. *Asperger syndrome:* flat affect, insensitive to social cues, obsessively indulged special interests, need for sameness, unable to communicate effectively, though language skills develop normally
  B. *Pervasive developmental disorder:* onset after 30 months of age; impaired social skills, anxious, resistant to change, odd mannerisms and speech, and occasionally self-mutilation

II. Syndromes with prominent autistic features
  A. *Fragile X syndrome:* most common cause of mental retardation; dysmorphic faces, macro-orchidism after puberty, hyperactive; one third of female heterozygotes are mildly retarded.
  B. *Angelman's syndrome* ("happy puppet" syndrome): maternal 15q deletion; infantile feeding problems, severe retardation, microcephaly, autism, jerky puppetlike ataxia, paroxysmal laughter, protruding tongue. By contrast, *Prader-Willi syndrome* (paternal 15q

deletion) presents with hypotonia at birth; dysmorphism, mental retardation; and later, hyperphagia, hypogonadism, pickwickian syndrome.
  C. *Rett's syndrome:* girls develop normally until 6 to 12 months of age; thereafter, regression with acquired microcephaly, ataxia, and autistic-like behavior; repetitive hand-wringing or hand-wetting movements; irregular breathing.
  D. *Others:* tuberous sclerosis; hypomelanosis of Ito.

REFERENCES

Gillberg C: *Curr Opin Neurol* 11:109–114, 1998.
Menkes JH: *Textbook of child neurology*, Baltimore, Williams & Wilkins, 1995.

AUTONOMIC DYSFUNCTION

CLASSIFICATION

Disorders marked by autonomic dysfunction are given in Table 11. Progressive autonomic failure can occur either as an isolated syndrome of orthostatic hypotension or in association with spinocerebellar or parkinsonian features in the syndromes collectively referred to as multiple-system atrophy (MSA). Autonomic dysreflexia occurs in the context of spinal cord lesions *above the T6 level*. This is mediated by an interruption in the brain's ability to dilate the splanchnic vascular bed and manifests as a marked rise in blood pressure along with headache, goose flesh, diaphoresis, flushing, or chills; it affects half to three quarters of this population. Acute pandysautonomia may occur as a variant of Guillain-Barré syndrome or may complicate more typical cases of Guillain-Barré syndrome. A number of hereditary acquired or peripheral small fiber neuropathies can have autonomic features.

DIAGNOSIS

Autonomic dysfunction is suspected in the presence of orthostatic hypotension or other derangement of cardiovascular regulation, loss of sweating, bladder or bowel dysfunction, impotence, or pupillary abnormalities. The following screening tests can be performed at the bedside:
  I. *Orthostatic blood pressure and heart rate.* An estimate is made of the time typically required to produce symptoms on standing. After 20 minutes of inactivity, baseline supine heart rate and blood pressure are recorded. The standing measurements are taken at 3 minutes or after the estimated time interval that takes the patient to become symptomatic. The cuff on the arm is kept at the level of the heart at all times. *Orthostatic hypotension is defined as a reduction in SBP of at least 20 mm Hg or reduction in DBP of at least 10 mm Hg within 3 minutes of standing.* HR normally increases by 11 to 29 beats/minute immediately on standing. If the patient has had ECG leads placed prior to testing, the ratio between the longest R-R interval (slowest rate),

TABLE 11

CLASSIFICATION OF AUTONOMIC DISORDERS

I. Diseases affecting the central nervous system
   A. Progressive autonomic failure (PAF), idiopathic orthostatic hypotension
      1. Pure PAF
      2. PAF with multiple-system atrophy (Shy-Drager syndrome)
         a. With parkinsonian features
         b. With spinocerebellar degeneration
   B. Parkinson's disease
   C. Spinal cord lesions
   D. Wernicke's encephalopathy
   E. Miscellaneous diseases
      1. Cerebrovascular disease
      2. Brainstem tumors
      3. Multiple sclerosis
      4. Adie's syndrome
      5. Tabes dorsalis
II. Diseases affecting the peripheral autonomic nervous system
   A. Disorders with no associated sensory-motor peripheral neuropathy
      1. Acute and subacute autonomic neuropathy
         a. Pandysautonomia
         b. Cholinergic dysautonomia
      2. Botulism
   B. Diseases associated with sensory-motor peripheral neuropathy in which autonomic dysfunction is clinically important
      1. Diabetes
      2. Amyloidosis
      3. Guillain-Barré syndrome
      4. Acute intermittent porphyria
      5. Familial dysautonomia (Riley-Day syndrome: HMSN III [hereditary motor-sensory neuropathy])
      6. Chronic sensory and autonomic neuropathy
   C. Disorders in which autonomic dysfunction is usually clinically unimportant
      1. Alcohol-induced neuropathy
      2. Toxic neuropathies (caused by vincristine sulfate, acrylamide, heavy metals, perhexiline maleate, or organic solvents)
      3. HMSNs I, II and V
      4. Malignancy
      5. Vitamin B_{12} deficiency
      6. Rheumatoid arthritis
      7. Chronic renal failure
      8. Systemic lupus erythematosus
      9. Mixed connective tissue disease
      10. Fabry's disease
      11. Chronic inflammatory neuropathy

Adapted from McLeod JG, Tuck RR: *Ann Neurol* 21:419–430, 1987.

A

AUTONOMIC DYSFUNCTION

which occurs about 30 beats after standing, divided by the shortest R-R interval, which occurs at about 15 beats, is called the 30:15 ratio. Normal 30:15 ratio is above 1.04 with slight age-related variation. *Orthostatic BP assesses sympathetic adrenergic efferents, and the heart rate tests assess parasympathetic cholinergic (cardiovagal) efferents*; both assess baroreceptor and CN IX and X integrity.

II. *Respiratory-HR variation*. The patient breathes deeply at 6 breaths/minute, and the times of inspiration and expiration are noted on the ECG tracing. HR difference between inspiration and expiration of less than 10 beats/minute or an expiration-to-inspiration ratio of R-R intervals of less than 1:2 is abnormal in individuals under age 40. Normally the HR increases during inspiration (respiratory sinus arrhythmia) due to decreased cardiovagal activity. This is the single best cardiovagal test, though the effect decreases with advancing age.

III. *Tests of pupillary function*. Installation of dilute 0.1% epinephrine into the conjunctival sac has no effect on normal pupil but dilates a pupil with postganglionic sympathetic innervation lesion; this reaction is due to denervation supersensitivity. Likewise, dilute 0.125% pilocarpine causes little or no constriction in normal pupils but causes miosis if abnormal parasympathetic innervation is present. Pharmacologic tests are distorted by corneal trauma (e.g., contact lenses, corneal reflex testing) within 24 hours of the eye drops.

IV. *Other tests*. More extensive autonomic testing includes measurement of plasma norepinephrine levels and determination of denervation supersensitivity, Valsalva maneuver and tilt-table testing, baroreflex sensitivity testing, thermal sweat testing, and skin blood flow measurements.

TREATMENT

Management of orthostatic hypotension begins with supportive measures:

I. Avoid or optimize drugs that cause orthostasis (e.g., diuretics, antihypertensives, and psychotropic agents).

II. Avoid sudden standing, straining during urination or defecation, excessive heat, large meals, and alcohol. Elevation of the head of the bed reduces nocturnal volume loss and is recommended, as is increased salt intake unless there is congestive heart failure.

III. Waist-high elastic garments may be helpful but are cumbersome.

IV. Drinking coffee after large meals may help reduce postprandial hypotension.

PHARMACOLOGIC THERAPY

I. Fludrocortisone—Start at 0.1 mg/day and increase by 0.1 mg every 3 to 4 days until symptoms are controlled or maximum dosage of 1 mg/day is reached. Complications: supine hypertension, peripheral edema, hypokalemia, and congestive heart failure.

II. Midodrine—Start at 10 mg tid.
III. Pseudophedrine—Give 30 mg qid.

REFERENCES

Grubb BP: *Am J Cardiol* 84(8A):3Q–9Q, 1999.
Ravits JM: *Muscle Nerve* 20(8):919–937, 1997.

B

BALINT'S SYNDROME

Described in 1909 by Reszö Bálint, this syndrome consists of a rare triad of simultagnosia, optic apraxia, and ocular ataxia.
 I. *Simultagnosia* refers to the inability to see the totality of a scene, despite being able to see the individual characteristics of the whole. A diagram showing a familiar scene with people and objects (also used as part of the NIH stroke scale) can be used to test for simultagnosia (see Figure 1). A normal patient will be able to describe actions of the objects and people in relationship to each other. A patient with simultagnosia may only be able to describe parts of the scene or only parts of objects, but not their relationships to each other.
 II. *Optic apraxia*, described originally as "psychic paralysis of gaze," refers to an inability to shift gaze voluntarily to objects of interest despite unrestricted eye movements.
III. *Ocular ataxia* refers to difficulty reaching objects under visual guidance despite normal limb strength and intact joint position sense.
 Traditionally, Balint's syndrome is thought to be due to *bilateral occipitoparietal* lesions. However, a comprehensive review suggests that not all cases reported originated from same anatomic substrates. For example, bifrontal lesions resulting in attentional impairment or right hemispheric lesions producing a neglect syndrome may in part mimic Balint's syndrome.
 The etiology for Balint's syndrome may include stroke, tumors, trauma, neurodegenerative diseases such as Creutzfeldt-Jakob or Alzheimer's disease, and HIV infection.

REFERENCE

Rizzo M, Vecera SP: *J Neurol Neurosurg Psychiatry* 72:162–178, 2002.

BENZODIAZEPINES

Benzodiazepines are used in the treatment of anxiety, insomnia, epilepsy, vertigo, and certain movement disorders. They are also used in the management of ethanol withdrawal. Prolonged use of any drug in this class may cause physical dependence, particularly in patients with a history of alcohol or substance abuse. Therefore, only the lowest effective doses should be used for the shortest possible period. Side effects include sedation, suppression of REM sleep, amnesia, agitation, and gait disorder. Withdrawal symptoms may occur after 4 to 6 weeks of use and include flulike symptoms, insomnia, irritability, seizures, nausea, headache, tremor, and muscle cramps. In those at risk for withdrawal, the dose should be tapered over several weeks. Acute intoxication with depressed mental status may be reversed with the benzodiazepine receptor antagonist flumazenil, starting at 0.2 mg IV over 30 seconds. Failure to respond to a total dose of 5 mg makes it unlikely that sedation is due to benzodiazepines.

BLADDER

Normal bladder function is controlled by bladder stretch receptors (generating sympathetic input to the spinal cord), the bladder wall detrusor muscle (activated by parasympathetic outflow), the internal sphincter (smooth muscle), and the external sphincter (striated muscle under voluntary control). Neural control is mediated by cerebral hemispheric centers (orbitofrontal cortex), the pontine micturition center, the sacral micturition center, and the hypogastric, pelvic, and pudendal nerves (Fig. 6).

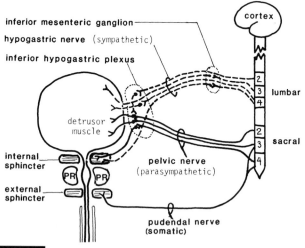

FIGURE 6

Neuroanatomy of bladder control.

These centers and nerves work together to achieve (1) storage of urine without leaking; (2) adequate perception of increased intravesical pressure; (3) release of cortical inhibition of emptying in appropriate circumstances; (4) proper synergy of urinary tract muscular structures; and (5) complete bladder emptying.

Disorders of bladder control can be caused by local factors (such as previous childbirth, pelvic surgery, or urinary tract infection) or disorders of the upper or lower motor neuron (Table 12).

Detrusor hyperreflexia resulting from *cerebral cortical dysfunction* is a deficit of normal inhibitory mechanisms in which the micturition reflex itself is intact, and the lesion is above the pontine micturition center. Symptoms include frequency, urgency, and urge incontinence. Common neurologic disorders leading to uninhibited bladder contraction include *stroke, mass lesion, and hydrocephalus.*

Bladder dyssynergia due to *suprasacral spinal cord lesions* leads to loss of detrusor-sphincter coordination. Simultaneous contraction of detrusor and sphincter can lead to increased intravesical pressures and upper urinary tract damage. *Multiple sclerosis, spinal cord tumor or trauma, vascular malformation, and herniated intervertebral disk are common causes.*

Detrusor areflexia is due to lesions of the *sacral micturition center* or its connections to the bladder. Sphincter function is preserved but detrusor contraction is not activated, commonly resulting in overflow incontinence. *Causes include myelopathy resulting from herniated disk or tumor and interruption of the reflex arc as a result of pelvic or pudendal nerve injury following trauma or operation.*

Autonomic dysreflexia occurs after spinal cord lesions above the region of major sympathetic outflow (T5 to L2). Splanchnic sympathetic outflow is no longer moderated by supraspinal centers, and bladder distention, catheterization, or other manipulation may cause an acute syndrome of severe hypertension, anxiety, diaphoresis, headache, and bradycardia. Prompt recognition and treatment (blood pressure control and treatment of local bladder problems) are essential.

Table 13 includes agents traditionally used in the pharmacologic management of upper and lower motor neuron bladder dysfunction. Tolterodine (Detrol) is a nonselective antimuscarinic agent which can be used for treatment of detrusor hyperreflexia (symptoms of frequency, urgency, urge incontinence). Its efficacy is equivalent to that of oxybutynin, and it offers the advantages of twice daily dosing and fewer anticholinergic side effects.

REFERENCES

Fowler CJ: *Brain* 122(Pt 7):1213–1231, 1999.
Madersbacher HG: *Curr Opin Urol* 9(4):303–307, 1999.
Millard R et al: *J Urol* 161:1551–1555, 1999.

TABLE 12
BLADDER DYSFUNCTION

	Upper Motor Neuron	Lower Motor Neuron
Characteristic Feature	Decreased capacity for storage	Decreased emptying ability
Cause	Injury to cerebral hemisphere or to spinal cord above T12 (trauma, multiple sclerosis, stroke, tumor)	1. Sensory: diabetes mellitus, tabes dorsalis 2. Motor: amyotrophic lateral sclerosis 3. Mixed sensory and motor: spinal dysraphism (meningomyelocele), tumor or trauma of lower cord, conus, or cauda
History	Urge incontinence with dry intervals Wet at night	Overflow incontinence Urinary retention Straining to void Wet or dry at night
Bulbocavernous Reflex	Present	Absent
Cystometrogram	Hyperreflexic bladder Small bladder capacity Small residual volumes Vesicoureteral reflux (and upper urinary tract damage) may occur at peak pressures.	Flaccid bladder Large bladder capacity Large residual volumes Vesicoureteral reflux and upper urinary tract damage can occur with persisting urinary retention.

TABLE 13

TREATMENT OF BLADDER DYSFUNCTION

Upper Motor Neuron	Lower Motor Neuron
Treatment goal: increase storage capacity	Increase bladder tone; avoid storage of large urinary volumes; promote bladder emptying
Treatment	

Oxybutynin (Ditropan) anticholinergic
Dose:
    Child: 2.5 mg PO bid–tid
    Adult: 5 mg PO tid–qid
	Bethanechol (Urecholine) cholinergic
	Dose:
	    Child: 5 mg/day, increase as below for adult
	    Adult: 2.5–10 mg SC tid–qid, or 5–50 mg PO tid–qid

Side effects: dry mouth, blurred vision	Contraindicated asthma, hyperthyroidism, coronary artery disease, ulcer disease

Propantheline bromide (Pro-Banthine) anticholinergic
Dose:
    Child: not currently approved for use (USA)
    Adult: 15–30 mg PO tid–qid
	Phenoxybenzamine (Dibenzyline) anti-adrenergic
	Dose:
	    Child: 0.3–0.5 mg/kg/day
	    Adult: 10–30 mg/day
	Side effects: retrograde ejaculation, drowsiness, orthostatic hypotension

Side effects: dry mouth, blurred vision	

Imipramine (Tofranil) mixed anticholinergic and adrenergic
Dose:
    Child: 1.5–2 mg/kg qid
    Adult: 25 mg PO qid
Side effects: dry mouth, blurred vision, constipation, tachycardia, sweating, fatigue, tremor	

Intermittent self-catheterization	Intermittent self-catheterization or Crédé maneuver

BOTULINUM TOXIN

One of the most potent toxins known to man, botulinum toxin first found its way into clinical use in 1981, when it was shown to be an effective treatment for strabismus. Since then, the clinical literature has exploded with new potential uses for this drug. To date, the FDA has given approval for its use in treatment of strabismus, cervical dystonia, *blepharospasm*, *hemifacial spasm*, axillary hyperhidrosis, and cosmetic treatment of frown lines.

Botulinum toxin is injected locally, at the site of the muscle whose action is to be inhibited. Onset of action is approximately 2 days after injection.

DURATION OF ACTION

The treatment should be effective for about 3 months, at which time the injections must be repeated.

ADVERSE REACTION

Adverse reactions depend on the site of injection. For treatment of blepharospasm, ptosis, dry eyes, and punctate keratitis are common side effects, whereas injection of neck muscles in treatment of cervical dystonia can result in dysphagia, upper respiratory infection, neck pain, and headache. Hypersensitivity reactions can occur.

MECHANISM OF ACTION

Once injected, botulinum toxin inhibits the release of acetylcholine from presynaptic neurons. It therefore affects not only the neuromuscular junction, but also cholinergic synapses in the autonomic nervous system.

Botulinum toxin resistance after repeated injections may be due to the formation of antibodies against the toxin. Development of neutralizing antibodies appears to be minimized when smaller doses of botulinum toxin are used, and when at least 2 to 3 months are allowed to elapse between doses.

Other potential uses for botulinum toxin include treatment of spasticity (e.g., in cerebral palsy, stroke, multiple sclerosis), headache, pain, dystonias, tics, stuttering, constipation, anal fissures, and other neurologic and non-neurologic ailments.

REFERENCES

Jankovic J: *J Neurol Neurosurg Psychiatry* 75:951–957, 2004.
Morton RE, Hankinson J, Nicholson J: *Arch Dis Child* 89:1133–1137, 2004.

BRACHIAL PLEXUS

The brachial plexus (Fig. 7) comprises the anastomoses derived from the anterior primary rami of vertebral segments C5 to T1. The plexus may be divided conceptually into the supraclavicular plexus (at the level of the nerve roots and trunks) and the infraclavicular plexus (at the level of the cords and terminal nerves). This distinction is useful clinically. Injuries to the supraclavicular plexus clinically resemble root injuries. Injuries to the infraclavicular plexus clinically resemble terminal nerve injuries. Causes and frequency of injury are also different between the two sites. Owing to its relative lack of protection, the supraclavicular plexus is more frequently damaged than the infraclavicular plexus.

ETIOLOGY

I. *Trauma* is the most common cause of damage to the supraclavicular plexus. The most severe traction injuries result in root avulsions, which usually result in severe pain and irreversible loss of function. Less severe traction injury may result in demyelination or axonal loss in either the upper or lower trunks. Chronic pressure on the shoulder may result in upper trunk injury (Pack palsy). Obstetric paralysis due to shoulder dystocia can damage either the *upper trunk (Erb's palsy)*

or the *lower trunk (Klumpke's palsy)*, but the upper trunk is more commonly injured.
II. Other causes of supraclavicular plexus injury include the burner syndrome, postmedian sternotomy lesions, true neurogenic thoracic outlet syndrome (TOS), classic postoperative paralysis, and neoplastic invasion. The *Pancoast syndrome* is a special case of neoplastic invasion, resulting from an apical lung tumor directly invading the lower trunk; in this case, the plexopathy may be the first sign of neoplasm. In general, however, patients with neoplastic invasion of the plexus are already known to have a malignancy.

CLINICAL PRESENTATION

Upper trunk lesions result in weakness of shoulder abduction, external rotation, forearm flexion and supination and variable amounts of triceps weakness. Sensory loss is variable and may involve the deltoid region, the external aspect of the upper arm, and the radial side of the forearm. Lower trunk lesions result in weakness of the intrinsic hand muscles, thenar muscles, long finger flexors, and finger extensors. Sensory loss may involve the medial arm, medial forearm, and the ulnar hand.

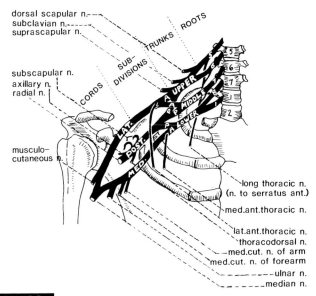

B

BRACHIAL PLEXUS

Brachial plexus. (From Haymaker W, Woodhall B: *Peripheral nerve injuries: Principles of diagnosis,* Philadelphia, WB Saunders, 1953.)

The *infraclavicular plexus* is less frequently injured. Traumatic injury to one of the cords may result from humeral head dislocation or axillary trauma, or penetrating injuries from gunshot or stab wound. Axillary artery cannulation or other perforation may result in medial brachial fascial compartment syndrome with symptoms typically involving predominantly the median nerve. Radiation-induced brachial plexopathy usually involves the infraclavicular plexus, most commonly after irradiation of the axillary lymph nodes in patients with breast cancer. Radiation-induced brachial plexopathy usually begins 12 to 20 months following radiation, but may begin years later. Typically symptoms of paresthesias and weakness initially occur in a lateral cord distribution and then spread gradually over years to involve the whole arm. Usually pain is not present, in direct contrast to neoplastic invasion of the plexus, which is typically very painful. *Needle EMG* may also be helpful in differentiating radiation-induced plexopathy from tumor infiltration. If present, myokymia (a spontaneous discharge pattern seen on needle EMG) is highly suggestive of radiation plexopathy. MRI of radiation-induced plexopathy typically shows diffuse thickening and enhancement without a mass.

Clinically, lateral cord lesions result in weakness of forearm flexion and pronation and wrist flexion with sensory loss in the radial forearm and the first three digits of the hand. Posterior cord lesions result in complete radial nerve palsies with additional weakness of shoulder abduction and adduction. Sensory loss involves the lateral arm, posterior arm and forearm, and the radial dorsal hand. Medial cord lesions result in a presentation that is almost identical to a lower trunk lesion, except that finger extensors are spared. Sensory loss again involves the medial arm, forearm, and ulnar hand.

Neuralgic amyotrophy (*Parsonage-Turner syndrome, idiopathic brachial plexitis*) is a relatively common disorder that is usually discussed with the brachial plexopathies; however, the actual site of pathology appears to be the terminal nerves. Typically shoulder pain develops suddenly, usually a few hours to a few weeks following an antecedent event such as illness or trauma. The shoulder pain is usually severe, and worsens at night, preventing sleep. The patient usually splints the extremity against the chest to avoid movement. Most frequently the pain begins to improve after 7 to 10 days. At this point the patient begins to notice weakness and muscle atrophy in the distribution of the affected nerves. The process may be bilateral. Neuralgic amyotrophy has a predilection to affect pure, or nearly pure, motor nerves. These include the anterior interosseous, posterior interosseous, long thoracic, suprascapular, and axillary nerves. The musculocutaneous nerve is less frequently affected. Prognosis for eventual recovery is usually good, although maximal motor recovery may require 2 to 3 years. Treatment consists of analgesia and physical therapy to prevent limitations of range of motion.

REFERENCE

Katirji B et al: *Neuromuscular disorders in clinical practice*, Boston, Butterworth-Heinemann, 2002.

BRAIN DEATH (See also COMA and TRANSCRANIAL ULTRASOUND WITH AAN GUIDELINES)

DEFINITION

Brain death is an irreversible loss of all clinical brain functions, including the brainstem. *Brain death is accepted as a definition of death in the United States*, although specific criteria for determining brain death and discontinuation of mechanical ventilation vary by state and institution. Historically, brain death as a clinical entity did not exist until the advent of mechanical ventilators, because brain dead patients cannot breathe spontaneously.

The triad of brain death is *coma, absence of brainstem reflexes*, and *apnea*. The American Academy of Neurology has published a practice parameter on the determination of brain death in adults in an effort to standardize the diagnosis.

B

BRAIN DEATH

CLINICAL CRITERIA OF BRAIN DEATH

I. Absolute prerequisites
 A. Clinical (e.g., by history or examination) or neuroimaging evidence shows a devastating, irreversible CNS injury that is compatible with brain death (i.e., could cause the irreversible loss of all clinical brain functions).
 B. Complicating conditions such as those due to metabolic or endocrine disturbances must be ruled out, and severe electrolyte disturbances or states of cardiovascular instability such as shock must be corrected.
 C. Drug intoxication such as that due to CNS depressants or neuromuscular-blocking drugs or poisoning must be excluded, because these conditions can mimic brain death and are potentially reversible. Any sedating agent must be stopped with level checked to confirm its clearance from the blood.
 D. Hypothermia (core body temperature < 32° C/90° F) must be corrected.
II. Required clinical features
 A. Once the foregoing prerequisites have been met, then, in the setting of a known, devastating brain injury which would be compatible with brain death, a single brain death examination including the following clinical features is sufficient. *However, it is generally recommended to perform the clinical examination for coma and brainstem function once and then repeat this examination together with the apnea test at least 6 hours later.* This will give time for the amelioration of the effect of any unsuspected drugs which may be unknowingly obscuring the clinical picture.
 B. Coma: there is no cerebral motor response to painful stimuli (e.g., withdrawal of extremities, posturing, or grimacing).

C. No brainstem functions (including reflexes) can be elicited.
   1. Pupils unreactive to light (midposition or dilated)
   2. Corneal reflexes absent
   3. Vestibular-ocular reflexes absent (No response to oculocephalic maneuvers and 50 mL ice water caloric stimuli in each ear.)
   4. Gag reflex absent (move endotracheal tube to elicit)
   5. No other brainstem reflexes (e.g., blink, ciliospinal, cough, snout)
D. Apnea testing
   1. Patients must have a core temperature of at least 36.5 °C (97 °F) and a systolic blood pressure of at least 90 mm Hg at the time of apnea testing.
   2. Patients must have a normal arterial Po_2 and Pco_2 (or at least a baseline Pco_2 in a given patient for patients whose baseline Pco_2 is higher than normal). Prior to starting the apnea test, patients should be preoxygenated with 100% Fio_2 for 10 to 30 minutes.
   3. When the patient is disconnected from the ventilator, 100% Fio_2 is supplied by a small catheter inserted through the endotracheal tube at 6 L/minute of oxygen. Care should be taken to avoid occluding the endotracheal tube with this catheter.
   4. After disconnection from the ventilator, the patient is observed for the absence of spontaneous respiration or respiratory effort during apneic oxygenation for 10 minutes. Blood gas levels are measured before the ventilator is disconnected and again at 5 and then 10 minutes after disconnecting the ventilator. The apnea test is consistent with brain death if the PCO_2 rises to 60 mm Hg or more or at least increases 20 mm Hg above the patient's baseline.

III. Confirmatory tests (optional testing)
   A. These confirmatory tests are not absolutely required in order to diagnose brain death except in infants. They may be used when, for example, the apnea test cannot be performed due to cardiovascular instability during apnea testing. In general, it is recommended to perform at least one confirmatory test.
   B. Isoelectric EEG. Technical standards have been published by the American Electroencephalographic society (see Guidelines in EEG in references).
   C. Brainstem auditory and somatosensory evoked potentials can provide additional evidence of absent brainstem functions.
   D. Absence of cerebral circulation may be demonstrated by cerebral arteriography, transcranial Doppler, or radioisotope angiography.

IV. Additional considerations
   A. Coordination of care with organ donation services varies according to state and institution.
   B. Deep tendon reflexes and other spinal reflexes may be present in brain dead patients. Families and caregivers of such patients often need counseling to reassure them that these reflexes do not reflect cerebral activity. In rare circumstances, quite elaborate movements

such as abdominal flexion mimicking an attempt to sit up have been described in brain dead patients.

REFERENCES

American Academy of Pediatrics Task Force on Brain Death in Children: *Pediatrics* 80:298–300, 1987.

Guidelines in EEG, pts. 1–7, *J Clin Neurophysiol* 3:131–168, 1986.

Quality Standards Subcommittee of the American Academy of Neurology: *Neurology* 45(5):1012–1014, 1995.

Ropper AH: *Neurology* 34:1089–1092, 1984.

Wijdicks EF: *N Engl J Med* 344(16):1215–1221, 2001.

BULBAR PALSY

"Bulbar" refers to the "bulb," an archaic term for the medulla. Bulbar palsy refers to the clinical picture of weakness or paralysis of muscles supplied by those cranial nerves which have motor nuclei in the medulla: IX, X, XI, and XII. The weakness may be due to lesions of the nuclei or nerves. Involved muscles include those of the pharynx, larynx, sternocleidomastoid, upper trapezius, and tongue.

CLINICAL PRESENTATION

Clinical features include dysarthria, hoarseness, nasal voice, dysphagia, palatal deviation, diminished gag reflex, or weakness of the sternocleidomastoid, upper trapezius, or tongue muscles. Atrophy and fasciculation may be present.

ETIOLOGY

Degenerative: motor neuron disease (e.g., progressive bulbar palsy)

Infections: meningitis, encephalitis, herpes zoster, poliomyelitis, diphtheria

Inflammatory: granulomatous disease, Brown-Vialetto-van Laere syndrome (also known as pontobulbar palsy with deafness), bone lesions (e.g., platybasia, Paget's disease), and postirradiation changes

Neoplastic: intra- and extramedullary posterior fossa tumors

Vascular: cerebrovascular lesions of the brainstem; ischemic stroke, AVM, and aneurysms (uncommon)

Trauma/congenital: syringobulbia

Bulbar palsy is also associated with syringomyelia.

Diseases that affect peripheral nerves in general, such as Guillain-Barré syndrome, may present with bulbar symptoms. Similarly, myasthenia gravis and other neuromuscular disorders must be considered in the differential diagnosis. Bulbar palsy must be differentiated from *pseudobulbar palsy*, which affects the pathways descending from the cortex to the cranial nerve motor nuclei.

REFERENCE

Albers JW et al: *Arch Neurol* 40(6):351–353, 1983.

C

CALORIC TESTING

Water that is colder or warmer than body temperature, when applied to the tympanic membrane, changes the firing rate of the ipsilateral vestibular nerve, causing ocular deviation and nystagmus. Cold water normally induces a slow ipsilateral deviation with contralateral "corrective" fast phases. Warm water induces a slow contralateral deviation and ipsilateral fast phases. Because the direction of nystagmus is conventionally described as that of the fast phase, the mnemonic COWS (cold opposite, warm same) indicates the direction of caloric nystagmus for cold and warm stimuli. Bilateral irrigation induces vertical nystagmus; the mnemonic CUWD (cold up, warm down) refers to the fast phases.

Caloric testing may be done qualitatively at the bedside or quantitatively in a laboratory. Quantitative caloric testing is used to evaluate vestibular function. Bedside caloric testing is used (1) to establish the integrity of the ocular motor system in patients with an apparent gaze paresis, and (2) to evaluate altered states of consciousness. Caloric stimulation may be used to elicit vestibular eye movements if oculocephalic maneuvers (see Vestibulo-ocular Reflex) have negative results or when a cervical injury is suspected.

Bedside caloric testing is performed after the external auditory canal has been examined, cerumen removed, and the patency of the tympanic membrane verified. The head is elevated 30 degrees from horizontal, aligning the lateral semicircular canal in the horizontal plane and maximizing lateral horizontal nystagmus. Water is gently injected with a syringe through a soft catheter inserted in the external auditory canal. Usually 1 mL of ice water is sufficient in alert patients and minimizes discomfort. Up to 100 mL of ice water can be used in unresponsive patients, and several minutes should be allowed for a response. Irrigation is repeated in the opposite ear after waiting at least 5 minutes for vestibular equilibration. Warm water (44°C) may also be used. Because of the risk of thermal injury, hot water should never be used.

Eye movements elicited by vestibular stimuli, whether with passive head rotation or caloric stimulation, may allow localization of lesions within the ocular motor system. Impaired movement of both eyes to one side occurs with lesions of the ipsilateral paramedian pontine reticular formation. Impaired abduction in one eye suggests a palsy of CN VI. Impaired adduction is seen in third-nerve palsies and in the eye ipsilateral to a medial longitudinal fasciculus lesion (internuclear ophthalmoplegia). Bilateral internuclear ophthalmoplegias cause, in addition to bilateral adduction weakness, impaired vertical vestibular eye movements. Eye deviation may occur in aberrant directions in patients with drug intoxication or structural disease of central vestibular connections.

As consciousness declines, the caloric stimulus-induced eye movements relate to the integrity of brainstem structures. Tonic eye deviation indicates integrity of brainstem function. Asymmetrical horizontal responses are interpreted as previously described and may give localizing information. Lack of any response may result from lesions of vestibulo-ocular reflex pathways in the medulla or pons, the eighth cranial nerve, or the labyrinth or from drug intoxications, such as those resulting from vestibular suppressants (barbiturates, phenytoin, tricyclic antidepressants, or major tranquilizers) and neuromuscular blockers. The presence of caloric-induced nystagmus in an unresponsive patient suggests a psychogenic etiology.

CARDIOPULMONARY ARREST (See also BRAIN DEATH, COMA)

Prediction of neurologic outcome following cardiopulmonary arrest requires serial evaluations and is a challenging task. Most patients with good outcome (independent self-care) emerge from coma within 24 to 48 hours. Conversely, coma duration greater than 48 hours has high likelihood of death or permanent neurologic deficit. Deterioration in level of consciousness is indicative of poor prognosis. Absence of the pupillary light reflex on initial examination, absence of motor responses at 1 day, failure to follow commands at 1 week, and bilaterally absent cortical somatosensory evoked potentials are all strong predictors of poor neurologic outcome.

Pre-arrest morbidity affects survival. Pre-existing pneumonia, hypotension, renal failure, cancer, and home-bound lifestyle are predictive of poor prognosis. *Arrest for longer than 15 minutes is associated with an in-hospital mortality rate of 95%.*

Therapeutic measures to improve neurologic outcomes, beyond cardiopulmonary resuscitation, are being aggressively pursued. Immediate treatment with induced *hypothermia* (32°C for 12–24 hours), following return of spontaneous circulation in comatose survivors of cardiac arrest, has been shown to be efficacious and is becoming the standard of care in many medical centers worldwide. (Table 14).

REFERENCE
Booth CM et al: *JAMA* 291:870–879, 2004.

CAROTID CAVERNOUS FISTULA

DEFINITION
A carotid cavernous fistula (CCF) is a communication between the carotid artery or its branches and the cavernous sinus.

C

CAROTID CAVERNOUS FISTULA

TABLE 14

NEUROLOGIC SIGNS AND NEUROLOGIC PROGNOSIS AFTER
CARDIOPULMONARY ARREST

Physical Finding	Overall Likelihood Ratio of Poor Neurologic Outcome (95% CI)	
	Positive	Negative
At time of Coma		
Absent withdrawal to pain	1.7 (0.7–4.2)	0.4 (0.1–1.1)
At 24 Hours		
Absent withdrawal to pain	4.7 (2.2–9.8)	0.2 (0.1–0.6)
Absent pupil reflex	10.2 (1.8–48.6)	0.8 (0.4–1.4)
Absent motor response	4.9 (1.6–13)	0.6 (0.3–1.3)
Absent corneal reflex	12.9 (2.0–68.7)	0.6 (0.2–1.9)
At 72 Hours		
Absent pupil reflex	3.4 (0.5–23.6)	0.9 (0.4–2.1)
Absent motor response	9.2 (2.1–49.4)	0.7 (0.3–1.3)
Seizure or myoclonus	1.4 (0.5–3.9)	0.8 (0.3–2.1)

CLINICAL FEATURES

Dandy's clinical triad of pulsatile exophthalmos, chemosis, and orbital pain is common. Proptosis occurs in 90% of patients, and pain is the common presentation. Double vision may occur in less than 50% of patients, and cranial nerve (CN V, IV, III, and VI) palsies may be found. Venous hypertension intracranially ipsilateral to the side of the CCF may occur and may result in intracranial or subarachnoid hemorrhages. Massive epistaxis to such an extent that it can be life-threatening may also occur in 1% to 2% of cases.

CCF can be classified as spontaneous or traumatic according to the cause, or slow versus high flow rate according to the angiographic appearance. Barrow classification of CCF indicates four angiographic types:
Type A: direct fistula from internal carotid artery (ICA) to cavernous sinus (CS), communication usually high flow rate
Type B: supplied by only dural branches of the ICA
Type C: supplied by only dural branches of the external carotid arteries
Type D (most common type): supplied by dural branches of both internal and external carotid arteries, unilaterally or bilaterally

DIAGNOSIS

CTA, MRA, or conventional angiography (see Fig. 8) are used for diagnosis. Slow fistula is best diagnosed with selective conventional angiography.

TREATMENT

Symptomatic high flow CCFs should be considered emergencies and can be vision- or life-threatening. Treatment is mainly endovascular via transfemoral approach or rarely via direct trans-cutaneous ophthalmic vein approach. Coiling with platinum coils or glue embolization or covered stent may be utilized.

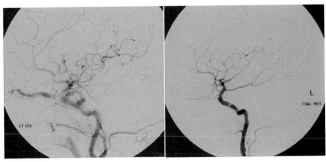

FIGURE 8

Pre- (*left*) and post- (*right*) treatment.

C

CAROTID STENOSIS

CAROTID STENOSIS (See also ISCHEMIA)

EPIDEMIOLOGY

As many as 20% to 30% of strokes are due to carotid artery disease. The *clinical presentation* is explained in the discussion of stroke under Ischemia. Briefly, stroke or transient ischemic attacks (TIAs) as confirmed by a neurologist have to be related to the territory of the stenosed artery to be symptomatic. Ophthalmic TIAs and amaurosis is a common presentation; anterior circulation MCA, ACA TIAs/minor or major strokes are common as well.

DIAGNOSIS

The gold standard is diagnostic cerebral angiogram, followed by good quality CTA and MRA, and finally carotid ultrasound (reliability in routine daily practice is not as good as has been shown in clinical studies).

TREATMENT

Approaches to therapy include surgery and stenting in appropriate settings, but medical therapy is a critical aspect of management of carotid artery disease. Best medical therapy for carotid stenosis has evolved into antiplatelet therapy, with aspirin 325 mg daily + ACE inhibitor + statin (regardless of lipid panel status). Newer antimetabolic syndrome agents are also on the way. Based on four randomized studies comparing carotid endarterectomy to aspirin in treating symptomatic carotid stenosis over 70% showed benefit most with an absolute risk reduction of 17% over 2 years with numbers needed to treat of 3 to 6, whereas in patients with asymptomatic carotid stenosis over 60%, the absolute risk reduction is 1% per annum (numbers needed to treat = 14 to 17). Surgeon morbidity is critical and is recommended to be below 3% (in asymptomatic patient) to show benefit.

Carotid angioplasty and stenting (CAS) is currently indicated for high-risk surgical patients; the most common indications are as follows:

I. Anatomic indication: infraclavicular lesions in the chest, high region at C2 and higher or at the angle of jaw or higher, tandem region in the intracranial inferior cerebellar artery with 50% or higher diameter stenosis

II. Prior radiation to the neck

III. Prior neck surgery and dissection

IV. Prior carotid endarterectomy (restenosis after old carotid endarterectomy is one of the most common indications for CAS)

V. Contralateral high-grade stenosis or occlusion

VI. Contralateral cranial nerve palsy and hoarseness from neck surgery

VII. Co-morbidities, coronary artery disease, congestive heart failure, ejection fraction < 30%, severe COPD, poorly controlled diabetes mellitus, end-stage renal disease

It definitely has to be done by a neuro-interventionalist well-trained and experienced in both cerebral angiograms and carotid stenting because recent studies have shown poor outcomes from poorly-trained physicians. The use of a distal embolic protection device is recommended.

REFERENCE

Barrett KM, Brott TG: *Neurol Clin* 24(4):681–695, 2006.

CARPAL TUNNEL SYNDROME

Carpal tunnel syndrome (CTS) occurs as a result of compression of the median nerve as it courses beneath the transverse carpal ligament. Incidence is 1:1000 population. Eighty-two percent of patients are over 40 years old, and 65% to 75% are women. Approximately half of the patients have bilateral symptoms. Acute CTS is commonly related to distal radius fracture; other causes include hemorrhage into the carpal tunnel (due to trauma or coagulopathy), burn, infections, and injection injuries. Chronic CTS is usually idiopathic or may be related to repetitive motion injury; other causes are anatomic (ganglion, neuroma, lipoma, and myeloma), neuropathic (diabetes, alcoholism, amyloidosis, and mucopolysaccharidoses), inflammatory (tenosynovitis, hypertrophic synovium, rheumatoid arthritis, gout, dermatomyositis, scleroderma, systemic lupus erythematosus), infection (tuberculosis), alteration of fluid balance (pregnancy, myxedema, obesity, long-term hemodialysis, congestive heart failure), acromegaly, and Paget's disease.

Patients characteristically complain of nocturnal numbness and paresthesias or burning pain in the median distribution (but may radiate to the forearm, elbow, or shoulder). Weakness and atrophy of the opponens pollicus, abductor pollicis brevis, and first two lumbricals and loss of two-point discrimination are late signs of long-term involvement. The symptoms are reproduced by tapping over the medial nerve at the carpal tunnel (*Tinel's sign*) or by maximum flexion of the wrist for 60 seconds (*Phalen's sign*), which has 75% to 88% sensitivity and 100% specificity. Also, inflating a sphygmomanometer to 150 mm Hg at the wrist for 30 seconds has a 100% specificity and 97% sensitivity. EMG studies show prolongation of distal median motor and sensory (more sensitive) latencies and a difference between the distal median and ulnar motor latencies. Fibrillation potentials are infrequent. Bilateral EMG and nerve conduction abnormalities are common, even in asymptomatic patients. Recently, sonography and MRI have been shown to help in establishing the diagnosis.

Differential diagnosis includes C6 or C7 radiculopathy, thoracic outlet syndrome, brachial plexopathy, peripheral polyneuropathy, sensory stroke, syringomyelia, and more proximal median neuropathies.

Treatment consists of avoiding activities that precipitate symptoms and wearing a wrist extension splint at night. Local steroid with or without lidocaine injections may provide limited relief. Indications for surgery are weakness, atrophy, or EMG evidence of denervation. Surgical treatment, which can be done by either open or endoscopic approach, is usually not necessary during pregnancy as symptoms resolve spontaneously.

REFERENCE
Sternbach G: *J Emerg Med* 17:519–523, 1999.

CATAMENIAL EPILEPSY

Catamenial epilepsy is vaguely defined as an increase in seizure frequency beginning immediately before or during menses.

One must take into consideration, however, that most published reports rely on self-reporting and patient perception. Prevalence reported from different studies ranges from 10% to 78%. Duncan and associates found that 78% of women claimed to have catamenial seizures, but only 12.5% fulfilled criteria. Herzog and associates described three patterns in 184 women with refractory temporal lobe epilepsy based on 1-month seizure and menstrual diary and midluteal progesterone levels:

1. Perimenstrual: Greater amount of seizures during days −3 to +3 compared with other phases.
2. Periovulatory: Greater than average daily seizure frequency during days 10 to 13.
3. Luteal: Greater during the ovulatory, midluteal, and menstrual phases.

To diagnose catamenial epilepsy ask the patient to keep a diary that tracks seizures in relation to menses; check progesterone level during seizures.

Treatment consists of antiepileptic drugs, acetazolamide, and hormonal therapy (be wary of giving progesterone to those interested in becoming pregnant).

REFERENCES
Duncan S, Read CL, Brodie MJ: *Epilepsia* 34:828–831, 1993.
Herzog AG, Klein P, Ransil BJ: *Epilepsia* 38:1082–1088, 1997.

C

CATAMENIAL EPILEPSY

CAUDA EQUINA AND CONUS MEDULLARIS

Clinical features of cauda equina and conus medullaris syndromes are summarized in Table 15.

TABLE 15

CLINICAL DIFFERENTIATION OF CAUDA EQUINA AND CONUS MEDULLARIS SYNDROMES

Feature	Conus Medullaris (Lower Sacral Cord)	Cauda Equina (Lumbosacral Roots)
Sensory deficit	Saddle distribution	Saddle distribution
	Bilateral, symmetrical	Asymmetrical
	Sensory dissociation present	Sensory dissociation absent
	Presents early	Presents relatively later
Pain	Uncommon	Prominent, early
	Relatively mild	Severe
	Bilateral, symmetrical	Asymmetrical
	Perineum and thighs	Radicular
Motor deficit	Symmetrical	Asymmetrical
	Mild	Moderate to severe
	Atrophy absent	Atrophy more prominent
Reflexes	Achilles reflex absent	Reflexes variably involved
	Patellar reflex normal	
Sphincter dysfunction	Early, severe	Late, less severe
	Absent anal and bulbocavernosus reflex	Reflex abnormalities less common
Sexual dysfunction	Erection and ejaculation impaired	Less common

Modified from DeJong RN: *The neurologic examination,* ed 4, New York, Harper & Row, 1979.

CEREBELLUM

I. Embryology
   A. Derived from rhombic lip
   B. Ten percent of brain volume, but contains more than half of all neurons in the brain
II. Cerebellar structure
   A. Layers
      1. Outer gray/molecular mantle (cortex; basket and stellate cells), Purkinje cells underneath in a single row
      2. Granular layer
      3. Internal white matter
      4. Intrinsic nuclei (provide cerebellar outflow; listed medial to lateral; see below for specific neuronal connections)
         a. Fastigial
         b. Interposed (globose and emboliform)
         c. Dentate

B. Fissures
   1. Primary fissure, located on the upper surface, divides the cerebellum into anterior and posterior lobes.
   2. Posterolateral fissure on the underside of the cerebellum separates the large posterior lobe from the small flocculonodular lobe.
   3. Shallower fissures subdivide the anterior and posterior lobes into several lobules from anterior to posterior: lingula, central, culmen, declive, folium, tuber, pyramis, uvula, tonsil, nodulus, and flocculus.
   4. Two longitudinal furrows, most prominent on the undersurface of the cerebellum's posterior lobe, separate three areas:
      a. Vermis, a thin midline longitudinal strip
      b. Left cerebellar hemisphere
      c. Right cerebellar hemisphere
C. Neuronal projections
   1. Vermis projects to fastigial nucleus—proximal muscle control
   2. Intermediate zone projects to interposed nuclei—distal muscular control
   3. Lateral zone projects to the dentate nucleus—connects to cerebral cortical projections
D. Cerebellar peduncles (Table 16)
   1. Inferior
   2. Middle
   3. Superior
III. Cellular organization of the cerebellum
   A. Molecular layer
      1. Axons of granular cells (known as parallel fibers)
      2. Interneurons
         a. Stellate cells
         b. Basket cells
   B. Purkinje cell layer (consists of Purkinje neurons that are arranged side by side in a single layer)
      1. Dendritic tree extends into molecular layer
      2. Axons project to intrinsic nuclei
         a. Only output of cerebellar cortex
         b. Inhibitory neurons
         c. Axons utilize GABA receptor
   C. Granular layer
      1. Vast numbers of densely packed small neurons, mostly small granule cells
      2. Cortical input; synapses with incoming fibers (Table 17)
IV. Functional divisions of the cerebellum (Fig. 9)
   A. Vestibulocerebellum
      1. Also called the archicerebellum
      2. Corresponds to the flocculonodular lobe

C

CEREBELLUM

TABLE 16

THE CEREBELLAR PEDUNCLES

Cerebellar Peduncle	Alternate Name	Source of Axons	Tract Name	Crosses	Termination
Inferior	Restiform body	Clark's column (C8–L3)	Dorsal spinocerebellar	Ipsilateral	Paleocerebellum and archicerebellum
		Accessory cuneate nucleus	Cuneocerebellar	Ipsilateral	
		Inferior olive	Olivocerebellar	Medulla	
		Vestibular nuclei and ganglion	Vestibulocerebellum	Ipsilateral	
		Purkinje cells		Ipsilateral	Vestibular nuclei
Middle	Brachium pontis	Pontine nuclei	Pontocerebellar	Pons	
Superior	Brachium conjunctivum	Deep cerebellar nuclei	Cerebellar efferents	Level of inferior colliculus	Red nucleus, thalamic nuclei (ventro-anterior and ventro-lateral)

TABLE 17

PRINCIPAL INPUT AND OUTPUT PATHWAYS OF CEREBELLUM

Functional Region	Anatomic Region	Principal Input	Deep Nucleus	Principal Destination	Functions
Vestibulocerebellum	Flocculonodular lobe	Vestibular labyrinth	Lateral vestibular	Medial systems: axial motor neurons	Axial control and vestibular reflexes
Spinocerebellum	Vermis	Vestibular labyrinth, proximal body parts, facial, visual, and auditory inputs to posterior lobe only	Fastigial	Medial systems: vestibular nucleus, reticular formation, and motor cortex	Axial and proximal motor control, ongoing execution of movement
	Intermediate part of hemisphere	Spinal afferents, distal body parts	Interposed	Lateral systems: red nucleus and distal motor cortex areas	Distal motor control, ongoing execution
Cerebrocerebellum	Lateral part of hemisphere	Cortical afferents	Dentate	Integration areas: red nucleus (parvocellular part) and premotor cortex (area 6)	Initiation, planning, and timing

CEREBELLUM

C

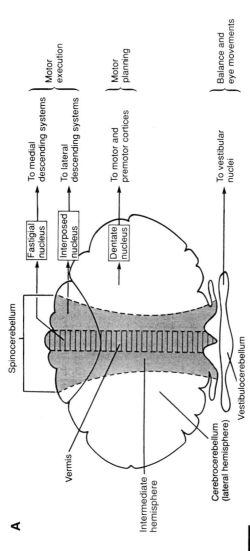

A

To medial descending systems
To lateral descending systems
} Motor execution

To motor and premotor cortices } Motor planning

To vestibular nuclei } Balance and eye movements

Fastigial nucleus
Interposed nucleus
Dentate nucleus

Spinocerebellum

Vermis

Intermediate hemisphere

Cerebrocerebellum (lateral hemisphere)

Vestibulocerebellum

FIGURE 9.

The cerebellum has three functional components (vestibulocerebellum, spinocerebellum, and cerebrocerebellum) with different outputs (**A**) and inputs (**B**). *cont'd*

B

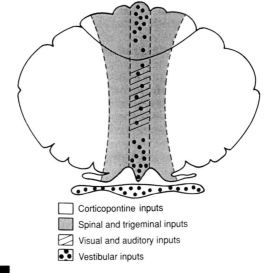

Corticopontine inputs

Spinal and trigeminal inputs

Visual and auditory inputs

Vestibular inputs

FIGURE 9
Cont'd

   3. Receives its input from the vestibular nuclei in the medulla and projects back to them
   4. Dominant afferents are semicircular canals and otolith
   5. These afferents are the only afferents that reach the cerebellar cortex directly
   6. Receives visual information from the lateral geniculate nucleus, superior colliculi, and striate cortex
   7. Output of the vestibulocerebellum: vestibular nuclei
B. Spinocerebellum
   1. Also called the paleocerebellum
   2. Extends rostrocaudally through the central part of both the anterior and posterior lobes and includes the vermis and the intermediate part of the hemispheres
   3. Fastigial nuclei
      a. Project bilaterally to the brainstem reticular formation and to the lateral vestibular nuclei, which give rise to fibers that descend to the spinal cord
      b. Crossed ascending projections reach the ventrolateral nucleus of thalamus
   4. Interposed nuclei
      a. Project to the contralateral magnocellular portion of the red nucleus in the brainstem via the superior cerebellar peduncle; many of these fibers continue to the ventral lateral nucleus of the thalamus

     b. The principal input is somatosensory information from the spinal cord through the topographically arranged spinocerebellar tracts

C. Neocerebellum
1. Also called the cerebrocerebellum
2. Lateral part of the cerebellar hemisphere
3. Receives input originating exclusively in pontine nuclei that relay information from the premotor, motor, and sensory cortices to the contralateral cerebellar hemisphere through the middle cerebellar peduncle
4. Output is via dentate nucleus via the superior cerebellar peduncle to the ventrolateral thalamus
5. The dentate nucleus also projects to the parvocellular component of the red nucleus, which is part of a complex feedback circuit that sends information back to the cerebellum, primarily through the ipsilateral inferior olivary nucleus
6. Lesions of the dentate nuclei or the overlying cortex produce four kinds of disturbances
    a. Delay in initiating and terminating movement
    b. Terminal tremor at the end of movement
    c. Disorders in the temporal coordination of movements involving multiple joints
    d. Disorders in the spatial coordination of hand and finger muscles

V. Signs and symptoms of cerebellar disease
A. Hypotonia
B. Ataxia
1. Dysmetria
2. Dysdiadochokinesia
3. Past-pointing
4. Classified by limb or affected function (e.g., gait ataxia)
C. Tremor (synonymous with limb ataxia; not a true tremor in the sense it is not a regular oscillation around a fixed point)
D. Cerebellar dysarthria: described as slow, scanning, irregular
E. Ocular dysmotility
1. Ocular dysmetria (overshooting on saccades analogous to limb ataxia)
2. Periodic alternating nystagmus with flocculonodular lesions

VI. Vascular blood supply of cerebellum
A. Posterior inferior cerebellar artery (PICA) is a branch of the vertebral artery or basilar artery, curves upward on the inferior surface of the cerebellum, and supplies the inferior cerebellar peduncle, ipsilateral portion of the inferior vermis (uvula and nodulus), cerebellar tonsil, and the inferior surface of the cerebellar hemisphere.
B. Anterior inferior cerebellar artery (AICA) arises from the basilar artery. It lies on the inferior surface of the cerebellum. Its branches supply the pyramids, tuber, flocculus, and parts of the inferior surface of the cerebellar hemisphere and the lower portion of the middle cerebellar

peduncle. Penetrating branches supply portions of the dentate nucleus and the surrounding white matter.

C. Superior cerebellar artery (SCA) arises near the distal segment of the basilar artery just below the terminal bifurcation into paired posterior cerebral arteries and lies on the superior surface of the cerebellum. It divides into medial and lateral branches. It supplies the superior surface of the cerebellar hemisphere, the ipsilateral portion of the superior vermis, most of the dentate nucleus, the upper portion of middle cerebellar peduncle, and the superior cerebellar peduncle.

VII. Cerebellar syndromes
  A. Rostral vermis syndrome (anterior lobe)
    1. Wide-based stance and gait
    2. Gait ataxia
    3. Limb ataxia may be mild or not present
    4. Hypotonia, nystagmus, and dysarthria (rare)
    5. Syndrome is seen in alcoholic patients. The pathologic changes in this condition affect the anterior and superior vermis; it may also be caused by vascular lesion, congenital malformation (Dandy-Walker malformation)
  B. The caudal vermis syndrome (flocculonodular and posterior lobe)
    1. Staggering gait
    2. Little or no limb ataxia
    3. Nystagmus (may have periodic alternating nystagmus)
    4. Seen with medulloblastoma, vascular lesions
  C. Hemispheric syndrome (posterior lobe, variably anterior lobe)
    1. Ipsilateral appendicular incoordination
    2. Causes: infarcts, neoplasms, and abscesses
  D. Pancerebellar syndrome
    1. Bilateral signs of cerebellar dysfunction affecting the trunk, limbs, and cranial musculature
    2. Causes: infectious and parainfectious processes, hypoglycemia, hyperthermia, paraneoplastic disorders, Creutzfeldt-Jakob disease, and other toxic-metabolic disorders

VIII. Syndromes of cerebellar infarction
  These syndromes account for 2% of all acute ischemic strokes and involve the following sites (in order of frequency): posterior inferior cerebellar artery (40%), superior cerebellar artery (35%), border zone infarcts (20%), and anterior inferior cerebellar artery (5%). SCA infarcts are more likely to produce mass effect and herniation; other types may also be accompanied with mass effect, depending on the size of the infarction.

C

CEREBELLUM

REFERENCES

Belden JR, Caplan LR et al: *Neurology* 53:1312–1318, 1999.

Brazis PW, Masdeu JC, Biller J, eds: *Localization in clinical neurology*, ed 3, Boston, Little Brown, 1996.

Carpenter MB: *Core text of neuroanatomy*, ed 4, Baltimore, Williams & Wilkins, 1991.

Kandel ER, Schwartz JH, Jessel TM: *Principles of neural science*, ed 3, Norwalk, CT, Appleton & Lange, 1991.

CEREBRAL ANEURYSMS

EPIDEMIOLOGY

Cerebral aneurysms occur in approximately 5% of the general population (9% in first-degree relatives). The ratio of ruptured to unruptured is approximately 1:1, although the number of incidentally discovered aneurysms may be increasing with the widespread use of MRI and CTA. Most are believed to be acquired, with only 2% occurring during childhood. An increased incidence of cerebral aneurysms is associated with various collagen synthesis disorders, such as Ehlers-Danlos syndrome, Marfan syndrome, autosomal dominant polycystic kidney disease (15%), α_1-antitrypsin deficiency, and neurofibromatosis type 1.

PATHOLOGY

Aneurysms occur along bends in the artery, or at arterial branch points, in direct line with the blood flow. *The underlying defect appears to be fragmentation of the internal elastic lamina and absent muscularis at the aneurysm neck*; the aneurysm wall is composed of a thin adventitia with or without an inner endothelium. Eighty-five percent occur in the anterior circulation, and 15% in the posterior circulation. They are evenly divided among midline, right, and left. The most common locations are the anterior or posterior communicating artery (25–30% each, depending on the study), middle cerebral artery (20%), and basilar artery (10%). Multiple aneurysms occur in 20%, usually at mirror locations.

CLINICAL PRESENTATION

The overall risk of aneurysm rupture is 0.5% to 1% per year. This risk is dependent on size, history of prior ruptured aneurysm, and location. The risk is 0.5% to 1% per year if less than 7 mm in diameter and 1% to 2% per year if greater than 7 mm in diameter; and the risk then increases with increasing size. Previous subarachnoid hemorrhage from another aneurysm is associated with 1% to 2% per year, regardless of size, and an 8- to 10-fold relative risk increase in posterior circulation and posterior communicating artery. Tobacco smoking is associated with a 3- to 10-fold increased risk of rupture, and is the only environmental factor definitively linked with rupture.

TREATMENT

Treatment involves a team approach with the neurologist, neuro-interventionalist, and neurosurgeon to consider potential aneurysm clipping versus endovascular coiling or observation.

REFERENCES

The International Study of Unruptured Intracranial Aneurysms Investigators: *N Engl J Med* 339:1725–1733, 1998.

International Subarachnoid Aneurysm Trial (ISAT) study group: *Lancet* 360:1267–1274, 2002 and 366:809–817, 2005.

Kassel NF, Torner JC, Haley EC et al: *J Neurosurg* 73:18–36, 1990.

CEREBRAL CORTEX

The cerebral cortex is a mantle of gray matter on the cerebral surface. Based on the difference in the number of cell layers, cerebral cortex can be divided into allocortex (three layers), mesocortex (three to six layers), and isocortex (six layers). The isocortex can then be divided into different areas (Brodmann's areas), based on cytoarchitectonics. Figure 10 shows Brodmann's areas in lateral and medial views.

CEREBRAL HEMORRHAGE, INTRACRANIAL HEMORRHAGE, SUBARACHNOID HEMORRHAGE

EPIDEMIOLOGY

Primary intracranial hemorrhage (ICH) accounts for 10% to 15% of all strokes. The annual incidence is 10 to 20 cases per 100,000 people with a prevalence of 37,000 to 52,000 cases per year in the United States. ICH is more common in persons older than 55 years of age, men, blacks, and Japanese. Chronic hypertension probably causes lipohyalinosis of the small intraparenchymal arteries, resulting in arteriolar wall weakness and subsequent rupture. *Location of hemorrhage* in order of frequency is as follows: putamen (35% to 50%), subcortical white matter (30%), cerebellum (15%), thalamus (10% to 15%), and pons (5% to 12%). The active bleeding usually lasts only a short time, and later clinical deterioration is most often ascribed to surrounding edema and ischemia, rather than continued hemorrhage.

ICH RISK FACTORS

Risk factors are hypertension, excessive use of alcohol, low serum cholesterol (<160 mg/dL), amphetamine and cocaine use, and genetic predilection (mutation of a subunit of factor XIII, β amyloid deposition in blood vessels, and presence of Σ_2 and Σ_4 alleles of apolipoprotein E).

CLINICAL FEATURES

The clinical presentation correlates with anatomic location, size, and degree of associated mass effect (Table 18). Headache is a frequent accompanying symptom.

Putamenal hemorrhage is associated with dense ipsilateral hemiplegia, hemianesthesia, and homonymous hemianopsia with aphasia or neglect (depending on which hemisphere is involved). There is also decreased level

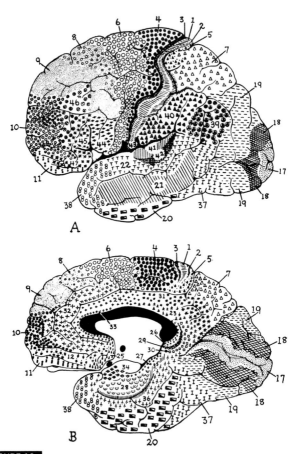

Brodmann's cytoarchitectural map of cerebral cortex, indicating major functional areas. **4**, Primary motor strip; **3, 1,** and **2**, sensory strip; **17**, primary visual cortex; **18** and **19**, visual association cortex; **8**, frontal eye fields; **6**, premotor cortex; **41** and **42**, auditory cortex; **5** and **7**, somaesthetic association cortex. Areas **13** to **16** (not shown) make up the insula. Labeling is from anterior to posterior. (From Carpenter MB: *Core text of neuroanatomy*, ed 4, Baltimore, 1991, Williams & Wilkins.)

of consciousness (disproportionate to the weakness), ipsilateral eye deviation, and normal pupils.

Thalamic hemorrhage produces dense contralateral hemisensory loss with variable hemiparesis, contralateral homonymous hemianopia, vertical or lateral-gaze palsies (including "wrong way" deviation), and occasionally, nystagmus.

TABLE 18

CLINICAL PRESENTATION OF INTRACRANIAL HEMORRHAGE

Location	Pupils	Eye Movements	Motor and Sensory Deficits	Other
Putaminal	Normal or dilated if herniation	Ipsilateral conjugate deviation	Contralateral hemiparesis or sensory loss	Decreased consciousness
Caudate	Ipsilaterally constricted	Conjugate deviation +/- ptosis	Transient hemiparesis	Headache, confusion
Thalamic	Small, poorly reactive	Upgaze palsy, lids retraction, medial and downward deviation	Mild hemiparesis, sensory loss	Aphasia, if left thalamus involved
Pontine	Constricted but reactive	Horizontal gaze palsy	Quadriplegia	Coma
Cerebellar	Ipsilateral slight constriction	Sixth nerve palsy, contr. Conjugate deviation	Ipsilateral limb ataxia, no hemiparesis	Gait ataxia

CEREBRAL HEMORRHAGE

C

Cerebellar hemorrhage is associated with severe occipital headache, sudden nausea and vomiting, and truncal ataxia. It is a potential neurosurgical emergency when brainstem compression is imminent or for lesions greater than 3 cm in diameter.

Pontine hemorrhage causes coma, pinpoint pupils (reactive to light), bilateral extensor posturing, impaired ocular motility, and caloric testing.

DIAGNOSIS

I. The size is estimated based on the CT findings using the simple volumetric formula: ABC/2 (A = width, B = length, C = height). Angiography may be necessary to exclude underlying vascular malformation or tumor.

MANAGEMENT

Immediate attention must be directed at the ABCs: airway, breathing, and circulation. Patients with a Glasgow coma score (GCS) of 8 or less or an impaired gag reflex need rapid sequence intubation. Sedation with short-acting drugs (propofol) prevents the intracranial pressure (ICP) spikes and allows frequent neurologic checks.

I. *Blood pressure* management is critical. Judicious lowering of the BP is indicated, although the exact BP and agents to use is controversial. Initial data seems to favor calcium channel blocker nicardipine at 3 to 5 mg/hour to keep systolic BP 140 to 160 mm Hg or mean arterial pressure (MAP) around 100 mm Hg to keep cerebral perfusion pressure (CPP) above 60 mm Hg. Other agents that are easily titratable with limited ICP changes are favored: labetalol, enalaprilat, and hydralazine. Chronic hypertension with autoregulation curve shifted to the right requires higher MAP.

II. *Adequate ventilation* and pulmonary/pharyngeal toilet must be maintained. Hyperventilation with induction of hypocapnia to keep Pco_2 30 mm Hg can also be used to decrease ICP.

III. *Antiedema agents* (osmotic diuretics, hypertonic saline, and steroids) may be used, but their efficacy is uncertain. This step is a temporary measure before the ultimate therapy to control ICP.

IV. *Intraventricular instillation of thrombolytic* agents to aid dissolution of mainly intraventricular clot remains controversial.

V. *Procoagulant* such as factor VII (rFVIIa) reduced the ICH mortality rate by 38% and improved outcome, with a slight increase in clotting complications. Third-phase clinical data are still pending.

VI. Neurosurgical evaluation should be obtained for superficially located cerebral hemorrhages and all cerebellar hemorrhages, for placing ICP monitors, EVD for obstructive hydrocephalus and IVH and possibility of intraventricular rtPA.

VII. *Other supportive measures:* Seizures generally occur within 72 hours of the ictus. Prophylactic use of anticonvulsant agents is reserved for patients with cortical involvement. Maintain adequate fluid and electrolyte balance. Raise the patient's head of the bed 30 degrees, barring contraindications due to spinal injury. Correct underlying coagulopathy. Prophylaxis for stress ulcer involves proton pump inhibitor, and for deep vein thrombosis (DVT) pneumatic sequential compression devices are needed. DVT is treated with placing a venous filter rather than anticoagulation.

PROGNOSIS AND COMPLICATIONS

Death from ICH is usually due to mass effect with herniation or brainstem compression and brainstem hemorrhages. Common ICH complications are *hematoma expansion* (20–40% within the first 24 hours, 26% within the first hour), intraventricular extension, and edema with shift, obstructive hydrocephalus, and increased ICP. ICH has the highest mortality rate of all strokes (23–58% at 6 months). *The main predictors of fatality are* (1) GCS at presentation; (2) hematoma volume; and (3) intraventricular extension. Mortality rate varies from 17% (GCS > 9 and hematoma volume < 30 mL) to 90% (GCS < 9 and hematoma volume > 60 mL). A survivor's long-term functional prognosis may be better than for infarction because there is more reversible injury.

Other causes of intraparenchymal hemorrhage (Table 19) include the following:

I. Trauma (accounts for up to 50% of nonhypertensive cerebral hemorrhage)
II. Ruptured AVM
III. Ruptured aneurysm with parenchymal extension
IV. Metastatic carcinoma, especially lung, choriocarcinoma, melanoma, and renal adenocarcinoma
V. Primary neoplasms (glioblastoma multiforme, pituitary adenoma)
VI. Embolic infarction with secondary hemorrhage (up to one third of embolic infarcts)
VII. Hematologic disorders, including leukemia, lymphoma, thrombocytopenic purpura, aplastic anemia, sickle cell anemia, hemophilia, hypoprothrombinemia, afibrinogenemia, and Waldenström's macroglobulinemia
VIII. Anticoagulant therapy
IX. Cerebral amyloid angiopathy. This usually presents as multiple, recurrent hemorrhages in the white matter or cortex, sparing deep gray matter (as opposed to hypertensive hemorrhages). Amyloid angiopathy may be the cause in 5% to 10% of sporadic intracerebral hemorrhage. It is associated with dementia in about 30% of cases; familial cases are associated with mutations in the amyloid precursor protein on chromosome 21 (Dutch and Icelandic forms). Attempts at surgical evacuation are usually futile because the vessels are very fragile, bleeding is very difficult to control, and there is a high incidence of recurrent hemorrhages.
X. Vasculopathies such as lupus, polyarteritis nodosa, and granulomatous arteritis

TABLE 19

CHARACTERISTICS OF SPONTANEOUS INTRACRANIAL HEMORRHAGE

Cause	Clinical History	Annual Recurrence Rate
Hypertension (HTN)	Longstanding uncontrolled HTN, middle-aged patients	< 2%
Amyloid angiopathy	Preexistent dementia, presents in sixth to eighth decades of life	21–31%
Intracranial aneurysm	Peak age for rupture 50 yr	50% within 6 months, 3% per year afterward for unsecured aneurysm
Arteriovenous malformation	Preexistent headaches, seizures, prior to 40 yr of age	2–4% without surgical correction
Cavernous angioma	Preexistent symptoms prior to 30 yr of age	0.5–1% initial, 4.5% afterward
Venous angioma	Broad range of age with a peak in the fourth decade	First rate of bleed 0.15%, recurrence rate undetermined
Brain tumors	Malignant astrocytomas, metastatic malignant melanoma, choriocarcinoma, renal cell carcinoma, thyroid cancer	1–15% overall estimate of bleeding
Drugs of abuse (cocaine, amphetamine, ecstasy)	Peak incidence in the third through fifth decades	Unknown

XI. Cortical vein thrombosis with secondary hemorrhage

XII. Drugs, including methamphetamine, amphetamine, pseudoephedrine, phenylpropanolamine, and cocaine

Subarachnoid hemorrhage occurs with an incidence of 15:100,000 with peak incidence at 55 to 60 years of age. The majority of cases are due to rupture of cerebral aneurysm or trauma (see Aneurysm for further discussion).

Subdural hemorrhage (SDH) may be acute or chronic. Acute SDH is usually due to trauma with tearing of bridging veins. There may be an initial loss of consciousness with regaining of consciousness (lucid interval) followed in several hours by progressive deterioration of mental status and headache. Lateralizing signs may be present. Diagnosis is based on clinical course, emergency CT (appears as hyperdensity over cortex), and if necessary, angiography. Treatment consists of neurosurgical evacuation and correction of underlying coagulopathies (if present). Dialysis patients and alcoholics are particularly prone to develop SDH.

Chronic SDH is less clearly related to trauma and may follow minor head trauma in the elderly and in patients on anticoagulants. Symptoms and signs resemble those in acute SDH but develop gradually over several days to months. Lateralizing signs are common. Mental status changes may suggest dementia. Diagnosis is as for acute SDH, although the lesion on CT is usually hypo- or isodense. Treatment is neurosurgical evacuation. The prognosis for survival and recovery in surgically treated patients is generally good, but the hemorrhage may recur.

Acute epidural hemorrhage results from skull fracture with laceration of the middle meningeal artery and vein. The clinical course is similar to acute SDH but is more rapidly progressive. Rapid herniation, respiratory depression, and death may ensue. The diagnosis is established emergently as for acute SDH. The CT appearance is a convex hyperdensity. This hemorrhage is a neurosurgical emergency and is treated by immediate evacuation.

REFERENCES

Bradley WG, Daroff RB, et al, eds: *Neurology in clinical practice*, ed 4, Boston, Butterworth-Heinemann, 2004.

Meyer S, Brun NC et al: *N Engl J Med* 352:777–785, 2005.

Suarez JI: *Critical care neurology and neurosurgery*, Totowa, NJ, Humana Press, 2004.

CEREBRAL PALSY

Static encephalopathy or cerebral palsy (CP) refers to a group of early-onset nonprogressive disorders of the CNS manifested by aberrant control of movement, tone, or posture.

Risk factors for development of CP:

I. Gestational age (prematurity and low birth weight)

II. Multiple gestation and transient hypothyroxinemia in premature infants

III. Intrauterine exposure to infection or inflammation (nine-fold increased risk for CP)

IV. Disorders of coagulation
V. Asphyxia (contributes 6% of spastic CP)
VI. Placental abnormalities leading to embolization to the fetal circulation, reaching cerebral circulation via the patent foramen ovale
VII. Maternal mental retardation. Interestingly, antenatal exposure to steroids may be protective and premature babies born to preeclamptic mothers have a lower risk of CP than babies born similarly premature for other indications.

Neurologic manifestations may include cognitive impairment, seizures, or impairments in vision (optic atrophy), hearing, or speech (pseudobulbar signs) in addition to the motor disability. The main categories are as follows:

I. *Spastic* form, which includes spastic *quadriplegia*, *diplegia*, or *hemiparesis* with unilateral hemispheric atrophy and thickening of the skull on the same side (*Davidoff-Dyke-Masson syndrome*)
II. *Dyskinetic* type consisting of chorea, choreoathetosis, or dystonia
III. *Ataxic* form
IV. *Hypotonic* or atonic variant
V. *Mixed* form

Diagnosis is usually made by exclusion. Imaging may be necessary to exclude remediable causes such as hydrocephalus.

Treatment includes the use of supportive care with physical therapy and orthosis. Surgical treatment involves tendon release and transfer. Medical treatment for the spastic type may be tried with dantrolene sodium or baclofen, for the ataxic type with gabapentin, and for the dyskinetic type with dopaminergic medications. Botulinum toxin may be used to treat dynamic equinus foot deformity due to spasticity in ambulant pediatric CP patients 2 years of age or older.

Prognosis depends on the severity of the disease; most of the hemiparetic patients tend to do well. Patients with seizure, mental retardation, or dyskinetic and ataxic types have less favorable outcomes.

REFERENCES
Carr LJ et al: *Arch Dis Child* 79:271–273, 1998.
Grice J: *Arch Dis Child* 80:300, 1999.
Nelson KB, Grether JK: *Curr Opin Pediatr* 11:487–491, 1999.

CEREBRAL SALT-WASTING SYNDROME

This syndrome is defined as hyponatremia in the setting of hypovolemia and renal sodium wasting. Some patients with hyponatremia do not have syndrome of inappropriate ADH secretion (SIADH) with resultant free water retention; instead, they have *inappropriate natriuresis*.

Primary cerebral tumors, carcinomatous meningitis, subarachnoid hemorrhage, and head trauma following intracranial surgery and pituitary surgery may cause this syndrome. The pathophysiology is considered to be either by alteration of atrial natriuretic peptide or of the neural input to the kidney. It is important to recognize this syndrome because the treatment is different from SIADH. Differentiation is done by careful assessment of volume status. If there is any doubt regarding the diagnosis, fluid restriction should be instituted. Then, if the natriuresis persists, cerebral salt-wasting should be suspected and treated appropriately. The syndrome responds to vigorous sodium and water replacement.

CEREBROSPINAL FLUID

FORMATION

Cerebrospinal fluid (CSF) is produced mainly by the choroid plexuses (95%) but also in the interstitial space and ependyma (5%). The rate of CSF formation is about 500 mL per day, and total CSF volume is 150 mL (50% intracranial, 50% spinal). Secretion is an energy-requiring process related to ion exchange (Na/K). Production is also dependent on the cytosolic enzyme carbonic anhydrase. Therefore, carbonic anhydrase inhibitors (e.g., acetazolamide) substantially reduce CSF formation. CSF is absorbed primarily by arachnoid villi extending into the dural venous sinuses. Normal CSF opening pressure during lumbar puncture (LP) should be less than 20 mm H_2O (Table 20).

APPEARANCE

Normal CSF is clear and colorless (specific gravity 1.007, pH 7.33 to 7.35); when cell counts reach approximately 200 WBC/mm^3 or 400 RBC/mm^3, it may become cloudy. Lower cell counts can be detected by observing for *Tyndall's effect*. This phenomenon refers to a sparkling quality of CSF when viewed in direct light and results from suspended particles scattering ambient light. *Viscous* CSF can result from large numbers of cryptococci within the CSF, secondary to their polysaccharide capsules.

TABLE 20

NORMAL VALUES FOR LUMBAR FLUID

Age	Protein mg/dL	Glucose mg/dL	Cell Count/mm^3	Lymph/PMN Ratio	Opening Pressure (mm CSF)
Preterm	115	50	9	40/60	
Term	90	52	8	40/60	80–100
Child	5–40	40–80	0–5		60–200
Adult	20–40	50–70	0–5	100/0	60–200
Ventricular	6–15				
Cervical	20–30				

IgG/albumin ratio (CSF IgG/Alb) upper limit: 0.27
IgG/albumin index (CSF IgG/Alb)/(serum IgG/Alb) upper limit: 0.60
Myelin basic protein upper limit: 4 ng/mL
Corrections
WBC: Reduce WBC by one cell for every 700 RBC (if hematocrit is normal)
or:
WBC (corr) = WBC(csf) − WBC(blood) × RBC(csf)/RBC(blood)
Protein: Subtract 1 mg/mL for every 1000 RBC

Clot or pellicle formation occurs with elevated proteins. *Froin's syndrome* refers to clot formation in the setting of complete spinal block and very high protein. CSF is perceived as grossly bloody with cell counts greater than 6000 RBC/mm^3, and at cell counts of more than 500, *xanthochromia* appears. Xanthochromia refers to the yellow, pink, or orange coloration of the CSF corresponding to the breakdown products of RBCs. Oxyhemoglobin released from RBCs can be detected within the supernatant fluid within 2 to 4 hours after the release of blood into the subarachnoid space; it reaches a maximum at about 36 hours and disappears in about 7 to 10 days. Supernatant fluid may, however, remain clear for up to 12 hours after a subarachnoid bleed. Differential diagnosis of xanthochromia includes hyperbilirubinemia, hyperproteinemia, hypercarotenemia, and drugs (rifampin).

CYTOLOGY

Cytologic analysis should be done soon after LP. Prompt refrigeration is necessary. Lymphocytes are the predominant leukocyte forms in normal CSF. An occasional granulocyte is seen in normal fluid and is not necessarily pathologic if the total WBC count is normal (0 to 3 cells/mm^3). A few or moderate numbers of granulocytes may occur following spinal anesthesia, myelography, or other intrathecal injections or with trauma, hemorrhage, or infarct in the absence of infection. No RBCs should be present in normal CSF. In a traumatic spinal tap, it is important to differentiate whether the WBCs are truly elevated or whether they are present in the same WBC/RBC ratio as in the peripheral blood. In a nonanemic patient, as an approximation, subtract 1 WBC for every 700 RBCs. *Fishman's formula* can be used for correction of WBC counts in the presence of significant anemia or peripheral leukocytosis. It estimates the WBC count in the CSF before the LP (actual WBC$_{CSF}$ = WBC$_{CSF}$ × RBC$_{CSF}$/RBC$_{blood}$). Detection of tumor cells is enhanced by collection of large volumes of CSF (20 mL), repeated CSF examination, and cisternal taps.

PROTEIN

Protein is a nonspecific indicator of disease. Normally, the blood-brain barrier keeps serum proteins out of the CSF (normal adult, 15 to 45 mg/dL). Many CNS diseases disrupt the barrier, allowing entrance of serum protein and consequently elevation of CSF protein (see Table 21). Increases greater than 500 mg/dL are rare and occur mainly in spinal block, meningitis, arachnoiditis, and subarachnoid hemorrhage (SAH). Metabolic conditions such as myxedema and diabetic neuropathy may cause an increase in protein levels. The major immunoglobulin in normal CSF is IgG. The IgG index and synthesis rate correct for serum IgG. Elevated levels may result from production within the CNS in various immune response disorders. Oligoclonal bands indicate the presence of an immune-mediated pathologic process such as multiple sclerosis and subacute sclerosing panencephalitis. Oligoclonal bands occur in 80% to 90% of patients with clinically definite

TABLE 21

CSF PROFILES IN VARIOUS DISEASES

Disease	Pressure	Cell Count/mm³	Protein (mg/dL)	Glucose (mg/dL)	Comments
Purulent meningitis	Increased (inc) in 90% 200–1500 mm H₂O	100–10,000 90%–95% PMN	Normal (Nl) to 2200	Decreased (dec)	
Aseptic meningitis	May be inc	10–1000 L + M (PMN early)	Nl to 400	Nl	
Fungal meningitis	Nl	Inc PMN + L + M	Nl or inc	Dec	Need to check india ink and cryptococcal antigen.
Tuberculous meningitis	Inc	50–500	100–1000	Dec	
Sarcoidosis	Nl or inc	10–100 L + M	50–200	Nl or dec	
Neoplastic meningitis	Nl or inc	0–500 PMN + L + M	Nl or inc	Nl or dec	Cytology may show atypical cells, and cell surface markers may be helpful
Subarachnoid hemorrhage	Inc	Nl or inc	Nl or inc	Nl or dec	Lysis of RBC begins after 2 to 4 hours. Xanthochromia is visible after 8 to 10 hours and may persist for weeks.
Herpes encephalitis	Nl	50–100 L + M	Nl	Nl	RBC and xanthochromia are often present (which distinguishes this disease from other viral meningitides).
Subacute sclerosing panencephalitis	Nl	Nl	Nl or inc	Nl	Gammaglobulins are markedly inc and may account for 50% of the total protein. Oligoclonal bands are present.

Cont'd

C

CEREBROSPINAL FLUID

TABLE 21

CSF PROFILES IN VARIOUS DISEASES—cont'd

Disease	Pressure	Cell Count/mm³	Protein (mg/dL)	Glucose (mg/dL)	Comments
Guillain-Barré syndrome	Nl	0–25 L + M	Nl or inc	Nl	Protein values peak between day 4 and day 18. Oligoclonal bands are often present.
Migraine	Nl or inc	5–15 L + M	Nl	Nl	A migrainous syndrome with WBC counts greater than 200/mm³ has been described.
Optic neuritis	Nl	Nl or inc Less than 25 L + M	Nl or inc	Nl	
Multiple sclerosis	Nl	Nl or inc Less than 25 L + M	Nl or inc	Nl	Oligoclonal bands, IgG/albumin index and ratio elevated, indicating intra-CNS antibody production. Myelin basic protein may increase with an exacerbation.
Acute disseminated encephalomyelitis	Nl or inc	5–150 L + M + PMN	Nl or inc	Nl	
Spinal block	Dec	Nl or inc	Markedly increased	Nl	Clotting (Froin's syndrome) occurs when the protein value is greater than 1000.
Seizure	Nl	Nl or inc Up to 25 L + M rarely PMN	Nl or inc	Nl	Pleocytosis is usually associated with prolonged or frequent seizures.

CNS Lyme disease	NI or inc	Inc L + M Up to 20% plasma cells	Inc	NI or dec	Oligoclonal bands, IgG/albumin index and ratio may be elevated, indicating intrathecal anti-*Borrelia* antibody production.
HIV and AIDS				
Encephalopathy	NI	NI	NI or inc	NI
Toxoplasmosis	NI or inc	Inc Positive *Toxoplasma* antibody	Inc	NI
Cryptococcosis	NI or inc	NI or inc Positive cryptococcal antigen	NI or inc	NI or dec
Polyneuropathy				
Distal, symmetrical	NI	NI	NI or inc	NI
Chronic inflammatory	NI or inc	Inc	Inc	NI

Inc, increased; L, leukocytes; M, macrophages; NI, normal; PMN, polymorphonuclear cells.

CEREBROSPINAL FLUID

C

multiple sclerosis. Myelin basic protein, a product of oligodendroglia, may be increased by any processes that result in myelin breakdown, such as stroke or anoxia; elevated levels are not a specific marker of demyelinating disease. Low CSF protein may occur with dural leaks and in benign intracranial hypertension. Protein in cisternal CSF is 50% of the lumbar value and is even lower (25%) within the lateral ventricles.

GLUCOSE

Glucose is derived from serum and is a reflection of the previous 4 hours of systemic glucose levels. Normal CSF to blood ratio is 0.6 with a usual value of 40 to 80 mg/dL. Simultaneous serum glucose level should be done. Hypoglycorrhachia occurs in bacterial, fungal, or tuberculosis meningitis, and inflammatory processes such as sarcoidosis, carcinomatous meningitis, and SAH. The mechanism of hypoglycorrhachia in meningeal disorders is related to an increase in anaerobic glycolysis in brain and spinal cord and, to a variable degree, PMNs as well as an inhibition of glucose entry from altered glucose membrane transport.

COMPLICATIONS OF LUMBAR PUNCTURE
Headache
Headache resulting from persistent dural CSF leak occurs in about 10% of LP procedures. Onset is 5 minutes to 4 days after LP. Pain is related to positioning and may be diminished or relieved when the head is raised. Post-LP headache usually resolves spontaneously, the majority within 1 week, but may persist up to several months. These headaches are more common in women and younger patients. The risk factors are related to needle size, the amount of CSF obtained, and placing the stylet back before removing the needle. Preventive measures include use of the smallest gauge needle, insertion of the needle bevel parallel to the dural fibers of the posterior longitudinal ligament, and the use of short bevel needles. Treatment of an established post-LP headache involves bed rest, adequate hydration (particularly if nausea and vomiting occur), and analgesics. Caffeine 300 to 500 mg PO and theophylline may be used. Intractable cases may be treated with epidural blood patching by injection of 10 mL of the patient's freshly drawn blood into the epidural space, where it can clot. It is curative in the majority of cases.

Brain Herniation
Brain herniation may occur immediately or up to 12 hours after an LP in patients with supratentorial mass lesions and midline shift or obstructing posterior fossa tumors.

Bleeding
Spinal subdural, epidural, and subarachnoid hemorrhage may occur in patients treated with anticoagulants or those with thrombocytopenia or bleeding diathesis.

Diplopia
Rare transient unilateral or bilateral abducens palsy can cause diplopia.

Others
Radicular irritation, meningitis, implantation of epidermoid tumor are also complications of LP.

LP Contraindications
Contraindications include infection over the site of entry, coagulopathy, presence of a known or suspected intracranial mass especially with midline shift, and noncommunicating hydrocephalus (always try to obtain CT before procedure). Elevated ICP as reflected by papilledema by itself is not an absolute contraindication to spinal tap because LP is actually used as a treatment in pseudotumor cerebri.

REFERENCES
Fishman RA: *Cerebrospinal fluid in diseases of the nervous system*, Philadelphia, WB Saunders, 1992.
Zaidat OO, Suarez JI: *JAMA* 283:1004, 2000.

CHANNELOPATHIES

DEFINITION AND PATHOPHYSIOLOGY
Ion channels consist of multiple subunits, each with very similar structure but different electrophysiologic characteristics. The differing neuronal expression and combination of these subunits into complexes gives rise to enormous diversity in the properties and distribution of ion channels, which is reflected in the variety of diseases that make up the neurologic channelopathies (Table 22). Disorders of ion channels (channelopathies) are increasingly being identified, making this a rapidly expanding area of neurology. Ion channel function may be controlled by changes in voltage (voltage gated), chemical interaction (ligand gated), or mechanical perturbation:

I. *Voltage-gated channelopathies* causing inherited muscle diseases include the *nondystrophic myotonias* and *familial periodic paralyses*. *Paramyotonia congenita* is due to mutation in the gene coding for the α_1 subunit of the sodium channel; *Thomsen's disease* (autosomal dominant myotonia congenita) and *Becker's disease* (autosomal recessive myotonia congenita) are allelic disorders associated with mutations in a gene coding for skeletal muscle chloride channel. *Familial hyperkalemic periodic paralysis* is due to mutations in the same sodium channel gene as that affected in *paramyotonia congenita*, while *familial hypokalemic periodic paralysis* results from mutations in the gene coding for the α_1 subunit of a skeletal muscle calcium channel.

The first demonstration that channelopathies could affect nerves as well as muscles came in 1995, when researchers discovered that *episodic ataxia type 1*, a rare autosomal dominant disease, results from

TABLE 22

CHANNELOPATHIES: MUSCLE AND NEURONAL DISEASES

Type of channel	Channel	Disease
	Muscle Diseases Related to Channelopathies	
VOLTAGE-GATED		
Na⁺ channels	α subunit of Na$_V$ 1.4 (skeletal muscle)	Hyper- and hypokalemic periodic paralysis
		Paramyotonia congenita and other myotonic disorders
K⁺ channels	α subunit of Kir2.1 inward rectifier (skeletal and smooth muscle)	Andersen's syndrome
		Hypokalemic periodic paralysis
	Accessory subunit MiRP2 (assembles with K$_V$ 3.4)	Hypokalemic periodic paralysis
Ca²⁺ channels	α subunit of Ca$_V$ 1.1 (skeletal muscle dihydropyridine-sensitive channel)	
		Malignant hyperthermia
	Ryanodine receptor (sarcoplasmic channel)	Malignant hyperthermia
		Central core disease
Cl⁻ channels	ClC1 (skeletal muscle chloride channel)	Myotonia congenita (dominant and recessive)
LIGAND-GATED		
Nicotinic Ach R	α₁ subunit (skeletal muscle)	Congenital myasthenic syndromes
	β₁ subunit (skeletal muscle)	Congenital myasthenic syndromes
	δ subunit (skeletal muscle)	Congenital myasthenic syndromes
	∈ subunit (skeletal muscle)	Congenital myasthenic syndromes

Neuronal Diseases Related to Channelopathies

VOLTAGE-GATED		
Na⁺ channels	α subunit of Na$_v$1.1 (somatic sodium channel)	Generalized epilepsy with complex febrile seizures
		Severe myoclonic epilepsy of infancy
	α subunit of Na$_v$1.2 (axonal sodium channel)	Generalized epilepsy with complex febrile seizures
	β₁ subunit of sodium channels	Generalized epilepsy with febrile seizures plus
K⁺ channels	α subunit of K$_v$ 1.1 (axonal/presynaptic delayed rectifier)	Episodic ataxia type 1
	M-type potassium channel subunit (with KCNQ3)	Benign familial neonatal convulsions
	M-type potassium channel subunit (with KCNQ2)	Benign familial neonatal convulsions
Ca²⁺ channels	α subunit of Ca$_v$ 2.1 (P/Q-type channel	Familial hemiplegic migraine
	in cerebellar neurons and presynaptic terminals)	
		Episodic ataxia type 2
		Spinocerebellar ataxia type 6
LIGAND-GATED		
Nicotinic ACh R	β₂ subunit of nicotinic receptors (with α₄)	Autosomal dominant nocturnal frontal lobe epilepsy
	α₄ subunit of nicotinic receptors (with β₂)	Autosomal dominant nocturnal frontal lobe epilepsy
Glycine receptors	α₁ subunit (spinal cord inhibitory synapses)	Familial hyperplexia
GABA$_A$ receptors	γ₂ subunit (brain inhibitory synapses)	Generalized epilepsy and complex febrile seizures
GLIAL		
Gap-junction proteins	Connexin 32 (paranodal myelin)	X-linked Charcot-Marie-Tooth disease

CHANNELOPATHIES

mutations in one of the potassium channel genes. The impairment of potassium channel function, which normally limits nerve excitability, results in the rippling of the muscles (myokymia) of the face and limbs seen in this disease. *Episodic ataxia type 2*, also autosomal dominant, is not associated with myokymia but responds dramatically to acetazolamide, an unexpected feature it shares with many channelopathies. The suspicion that it might be a channelopathy was confirmed when mutations in a gene coding for the α_1 subunit of a brain-specific calcium channel were found. Mutations in this same gene can also cause *familial hemiplegic migraine* and *spinocerebellar degeneration type 6*. It is unclear how different mutations of the same gene can give rise to such different phenotypes. In the case of *myotonia congenita* and *familial hyperexplexia*, point mutations in the same gene can result in either autosomal recessive or dominant inheritance.

II. *Ligand-gated channelopathies* that have recently been described include *familial startle disease*, which is due to mutations of the α_1 subunit of the glycine receptor, and *dominant nocturnal frontal lobe epilepsy*, which is due to mutations of the α_4 subunit of the nicotinic acetylcholine receptor. A gene for *familial paroxysmal choreoathetosis* has been mapped to a region of chromosome 1p where a cluster of potassium channel genes is located.

III. *Acquired channelopathies* are caused by toxins and autoimmune phenomena. The marine toxin ciguatoxin, which contaminates fish and shellfish, is a potent sodium channel blocker that causes a rapid onset of numbness, intense paresthesias and dysesthesia, and muscle weakness. Antibodies to peripheral nerve potassium channels may result in neuromyotonia (*Isaac's syndrome*). Lambert-Eaton myasthenia which is associated with small cell carcinoma of the lung in 60% of cases is caused by autoantibodies directed against a presynaptic calcium channel at the neuromuscular junction and against multiple calcium channels expressed by lung cancer cells. The abnormalities seen in Guillain-Barré syndrome, chronic inflammatory demyelinating polyneuropathy, and multiple sclerosis could also be explained by sodium channel dysfunction.

CLINICAL PRESENTATIONS

All these channelopathies have surprisingly similar clinical features. Typically, there are paroxysmal attacks of paralysis, myotonia, migraine, and ataxia precipitated by physiologic stressors. A channelopathy may cause an abnormal gain of function (such as myokymia, myotonia, and epilepsy) or an abnormal loss of function (such as weakness or numbness) depending upon whether loss of channel function leads to excessive membrane excitability or to membrane inexcitability.

TREATMENT

Many of the channelopathies respond predictably to membrane stabilizing drugs such as mexilitine and acetazolamide. The neuronal specificity of ion channels allows the potential for targeted drug therapy akin to the selective receptor agonists and antagonists currently available: 3,4-diaminopyridine, a potassium channel blocker, can relieve symptoms in patients with Lambert-Eaton syndrome and improves leg strength in patients with multiple sclerosis. Specific channel modulating drugs are currently being developed for migraine, chronic pain, and cardiac dysrhythmias and may be useful for neurologic channelopathies.

REFERENCES

Kullman MK, Hanna MG: *Lancet* 1:157–166, 2002.
Rose MR: *BMJ* 316:1104–1105, 1998.

C

CHEMOTHERAPY, NEUROLOGIC COMPLICATIONS

This section lists the neurotoxic signs caused by agents commonly used in patients with cancer.

I. Acute encephalopathy: corticosteroids, methotrexate (MTX), cis-platinum, vincristine, L-asparaginase, procarbazine, 5-FU (with levamisole), ara-C, nitrosoureas, cyclosporine, interleukin 2, ifosfamide/mesna, interferons, tamoxifen, VP-16 (high-dose), paclitaxel, OKT3

II. Chronic encephalopathy: MTX, BCNU (intra-arterial), ara-C, carmofur, fludarabine, thiotepa

III. Reversible posterior leukoencephalopathy: cisplatin, carboplatin, paclitaxel, melphalan (high dose), cytarabine, MTX, filgrastim, erythropoietin, cyclosporine, tacrolimus

IV. CNS demyelination: MTX, 5-FU (with levamisole), fludarabine (can induce promyelocytic leukemia, particularly in chronic lymphocytic leukemia patients), cladribine

V. Stroke/stroke-like/TIA: MTX, L-asparaginase, cisplatin (with 5-FU), interleukin 2

VI. Visual loss/other cranial neuropathy: tamoxifen, gallium nitrate, nitrosoureas (intra-arterial), cis-platinum, vincristine

VII. Cerebellar dysfunction/ataxia: ara-C, 5-FU, procarbazine, hexamethylmelamine, vincristine, cyclosporine A

VIII. Aseptic meningitis: IVIG, levamisole, monoclonal antibodies, metrizamide, OKT3, ara-C, MTX

IX. Seizures: MTX, VP-16 (high dose), OKT3 antibody, cis-platinum, vincristine, L-asparaginase, nitrogen mustard, BCNU, dacarbazine, PALA, mAmsa, busulfan (high dose), cyclosporine, ifosfamide, chlorambucil

X. Myelopathy: MTX (IT), ara-C (IT), thiotepa (IT), cyclosporine

XI. Peripheral neuropathy: cisplatin, carboplatin, oxaliplatin, hexamethylmelamine, procarbazine, 5-azacytidine, VP-16, VM-26, methyl-G, ara-C, paclitaxel, docetaxel, thalidomide, vinorelbine, suramin, mitotane, vincristine (subacute to chronic; almost 100%), cyclosporine, interferon-α, 5-FU, ifosfamide

XII. Myopathy: vincristine (subacute), cyclosporine, corticosteroids

REFERENCES

Dropcho EJ: *Semin Neurol* 24:419–426, 2004.

MacDonald DR: *Neurol Clin* 9(4):955–967, 1991.

Posner JB: *Neurologic complications of cancer*, ed 2, Philadelphia, FA Davis, 1995, pp 282–310.

CHILD NEUROLOGY, HISTORY, AND PHYSICAL EXAMINATION

I. History: acute or insidious, focal or generalized, progressive or static process? These questions are all helpful in generating a differential diagnosis.

   A. Birth history
      1. Prenatal—infections (especially TORCH), maternal complications (hypertension, bleeding, preterm labor), medications or toxin exposure (drugs, alcohol, tobacco).
      2. Perinatal—gestational age, birth weight, head circumference, mode and presentation of delivery, maternal medications during delivery, Apgar scores, complications of delivery, resuscitation.
      3. Postnatal—length of neonate's hospital stay, concomitant illnesses (jaundice, infection, seizures, IVH, respiratory problems/mechanical ventilation), newborn metabolic screen, hearing screen.

   B. Developmental history: gross motor, fine motor, speech, behavioral. These findings are very helpful in determining timing and progression of the underlying process. Remember to ask specifically about regression, to adjust for prematurity, and that girls typically achieve milestones earlier than boys (Figure 11 and Table 23 discuss developmental milestones and red flags). As the child ages, behavioral and academic history should also be obtained.

   C. Family history: seizures, dysmorphisms, ataxia, deafness, unexplained deaths or miscarriages, birth marks, mental retardation, developmental delay, learning and behavioral disorders, and psychiatric disorders. Be aware of ethnicity.

   D. Social history: ask about home, school, drugs, alcohol, sex, and abuse. When speaking to teenagers, parents should be out of the room.

II. General physical examination: Observation of the child during the interview is critical. In younger children, we would recommend performing as much of the examination as possible on the parent's lap. Save painful or irritating portions of the examination until the end.

   A. Measure weight, length, and head circumference and plot on the growth curves (Figs. 12 to 14). Average head circumference at birth is 35 cm, and average growth is 1 cm per month over the first year.

   B. Look for any dysmorphic features (low-set ears, epicanthal folds, colobomas, midline defects, abnormal body shape or structure, etc.). Evaluate head shape, palpate the fontanels and sutures, and auscultate for bruits. In neonates, look for external trauma such as cephalhematoma, subgaleal hematoma, or caput succedaneum.

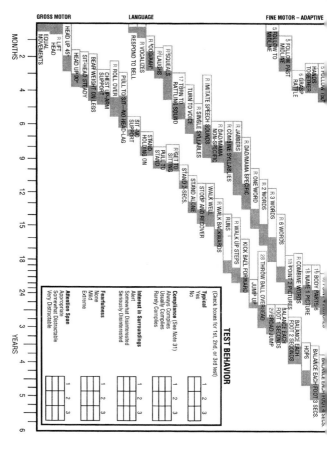

Dodds JB. The Denver Development Assessment (Denver II).

DIRECTIONS FOR ADMINISTRATION

1. Try to get child to smile by smiling, talking or waving. Do not touch him/her.
2. Child must stare at hand several seconds.
3. Parent may help guide toothbrush and put toothpaste on brush.
4. Child does not have to be able to tie shoes or button/zip in the back.
5. Move yarn slowly in an arc from one side to the other, about 8" above child's face.
6. Pass if child grasps rattle when it is touched to the backs or tips of fingers.
7. Pass if child tries to see where yarn went. Yarn should be dropped quickly from sight from tester's hand without arm movement.
8. Child must transfer cube from hand to hand without help of body, mouth, or table.
9. Pass if child picks up raisin with any part of thumb and finger.
10. Line can vary only 30 degrees or less from tester's line.
11. Make a fist with thumb pointing upward and wiggle only the thumb. Pass if child imitates and does not move any fingers other than the thumb.

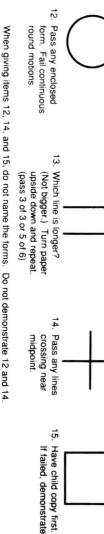

12. Pass any enclosed form. Fail continuous round motions.

13. Which line is longer? (Not bigger.) Turn paper upside down and repeat. (pass 3 of 3 or 5 of 6)

14. Pass any lines crossing near midpoint.

15. Have child copy first. If failed, demonstrate.

When giving items 12, 14, and 15, do not name the forms. Do not demonstrate 12 and 14.

16. When scoring, each pair (2 arms, 2 legs, etc.) counts as one part.
17. Place one cube in cup and shake gently near child's ear, but out of sight. Repeat for other ear.
18. Point to picture and have child name it. (No credit is given for sounds only.)

If less than 4 pictures are named correctly, have child point to picture as each is named by tester.

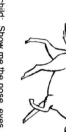
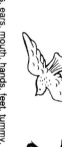
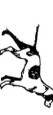
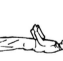

19. Using doll, tell child: Show me the nose, eyes, ears, mouth, hands, feet, tummy, hair. Pass 6 of 8.
20. Using pictures, ask child: Which one flies?... says meow?... talks?... barks?... gallops? Pass 2 of 5.
21. Ask child: What do you do when you are cold?... tired?... hungry? Pass 2 of 3, 3 of 3.
22. Ask child: What do you do with a cup? What is a chair used for? What is a pencil used for?
    Action words must be included in answers.
23. Pass if child correctly places **and** says how many blocks are on paper. (1, 5).
24. Tell child: Put block **on** table; **under** table; **in front of** me, **behind** me. Pass 4 of 4.
    (Do not help child by pointing, moving head or eyes.)
25. Ask child: What is a ball?... lake?... desk?... house?... banana?... curtain?... fence?... ceiling? Pass if defined in terms
    of use, shape, what it is made of, or general category (such as banana is fruit, not just yellow). Pass 5 of 8, 7 of 8.
26. Ask child: If a horse is big, a mouse is __? If fire is hot, ice is __? If the sun shines during the day, the moon shines
    during the __? Pass 2 of 3.
27. Child may use wall or rail only, not person. May not crawl.
28. Child must throw ball overhand 3 feet to within arm's reach of tester.
29. Child must perform standing broad jump over width of test sheet (8 1/2 inches).
30. Tell child to walk forward, ⟶⟶⟶➤ heel within 1 inch of toe. Tester may demonstrate.
    Child must walk 4 consecutive steps.
31. In the second year, half of normal children are non-compliant.

OBSERVATIONS:

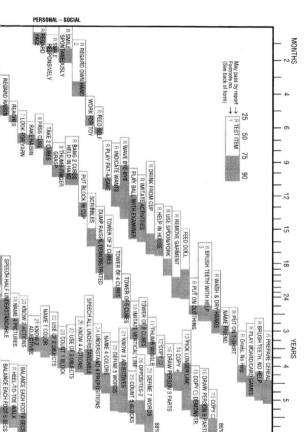

The Denver Development Assessment (Denver II). (From Frankenburg W, Colorado Medical School, 1990.)

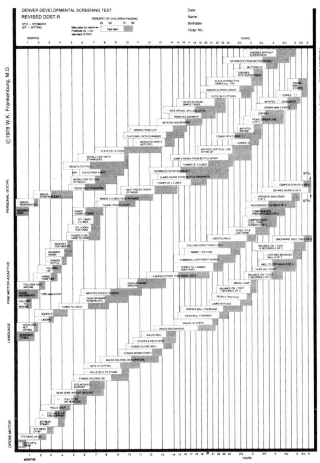

FIGURE 11

Denver Development Screening Test. (Courtesy of W. K. Frankenburg, MD.) *See foldout for second part of figure.*

C. Thorough ophthalmologic examination for cataracts, red reflex, chorioretinitis, optic nerve atrophy, papilledema, cherry red spot, retinitis pigmentosa, and retinal hemorrhages (often resulting from the birth process or trauma) should be performed.

D. Examine skin for any neurocutaneous stigmata; heart for signs of congestive heart failure or murmurs; abdomen for hepatosplenomegaly; back for scoliosis, sacral dimple, or hair tufts; and extremities for joint contractures or deformities.

TABLE 23

LANDMARK DEVELOPMENTAL MILESTONES

Age (Mo)	Gross Motor	Fine Motor	Language	Social
4	Rolls over	Moves arm in unison to grasp	Orients to voice	Enjoys looking around
6	Sits unsupported	Grasps with either hand, transfers	Babbles	Recognizes strangers
9	Crawls, pulls to stand	Pincer grasp, holds bottle	Understands "no"	Explores, plays pat-a-cake
12	Walks alone	Throws objects	Uses 2 words besides dada/mama	Imitates, comes when called
24	Walks up and down stairs alone	Turns single pages, removes clothes	Uses 2 word sentences; follows 2-step commands	Parallel play
36	Pedals tricycle	Dresses partially, draws a circle	Uses 3-word sentences, plurals	Group play, shares toys
48	Hops, skips	Buttons, catches ball	Knows colors, asks questions	Tells "tall tales"

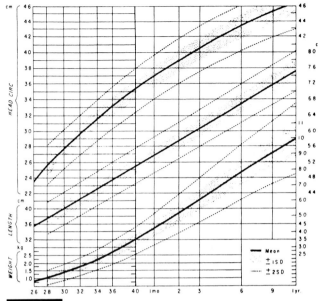

FIGURE 12

Fetal and infant norms: weight, length, and head circumference.

III. Neurologic examination: Examination needs to be adapted to the age of the child. Older children are typically quite cooperative and their examination is similar to that for an adult.

A. Mental status: be aware of feeding and nap cycles, which may affect the child's mental state.

B. Speech: developmental milestones (both receptive and expressive); *no words by 18 months is a red flag.*

C. Cranial nerves: pupillary light reflex present at 29 to 30 weeks; optokinetic nystagmus present at 36 weeks (lack of this response may be a sign of gross visual impairment); oculovestibular reflexes present at 30 weeks; spontaneous extraocular eye movement at 32 weeks; rooting reflex (sensory V) present at 34 weeks; suck reflex reflects a combination of CN V, IX, X, and XII function and is present at 34 weeks; assess tongue for atrophy/hypertrophy and fasciculations.

D. Motor: Observe resting posture, spontaneity and symmetry of movements. Much can be learned by just watching the child play. Tone depends on level of alertness and gestational age, and has a flexor progression in terms of gestational age (floppy at 28 weeks, strong flexor tone at term). Tone should be tested in both horizontal and vertical suspension as well as with traction from the supine position to assess head lag. Arching of the neck and back, scissoring of legs on

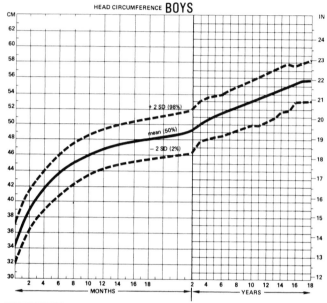

HEAD CIRCUMFERENCE BOYS

+ 2 SD (98%)

mean (50%)

− 2 SD (2%)

MONTHS — YEARS

Head circumference, boys. (From Nellhouse G: *Pediatrics* 41:106, 1968. Used by permission.)

vertical suspension, as well as fisting is indicative of increased tone. Hypotonic infants "slip through your fingers" at the shoulders, legs will flop apart in a frog-leg posture in supine position, and head will lag, as infant is pulled from supine to sitting by gentle arm traction. Formal manual muscle testing may be performed in older children.
E. Deep tendon reflexes are present at 33 weeks. Look for asymmetries. Cross-adductor reflex is normal until 1 year of age. Five to ten beats of ankle clonus is normal to 3 months.
F. Primitive reflexes (Table 24): Look for asymmetries, absence, or persistence. Occasionally these will be helpful in localization, but usually more useful for assessing general development.

REFERENCE

Swaimann, KF, Ashwal S: *Pediatric neurology: principles and practice*, ed 3, St. Louis, Mosby, 1999.

CHOREA

Chorea is involuntary, rapid, jerky, arrhythmic movements of muscle groups. It can involve the upper or lower extremities, trunk, neck, or face

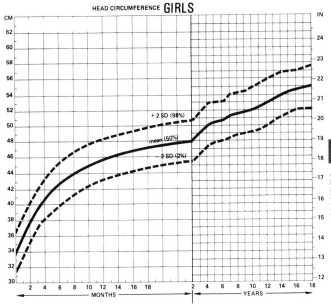

HEAD CIRCUMFERENCE GIRLS

FIGURE 14

Head circumference, girls. (From Nellhouse G: *Pediatrics* 41:106, 1968. Used by permission.)

and may be generalized, symmetrical, asymmetrical, or unilateral. Chorea is distinguished from other movement disorders by the random timing and distribution. The movements are often incorporated into deliberate movements by the patient that may camouflage the disorder. Grimacing and respiratory grunts may be manifestations.

Following are the most common causes of chorea:

I. Huntington's disease
II. Drug-induced (see later listing)
III. Systemic lupus erythematosus
IV. Polycythemia vera
V. Hyperthyroidism
VI. Pregnancy (chorea gravidarum) or oral contraceptive use
VII. Neuroacanthocytosis, a multisystem neurologic disease characterized by dementia, psychiatric disturbances, seizures, chorea, dystonia, tics, akinetic-rigid features, diminished deep tendon reflexes, muscle atrophy and weakness, and acanthocytes in peripheral blood

Other causes by group include the following:

TABLE 24
PRIMITIVE REFLEXES IN NEONATES AND INFANTS

Reflex	Response	Appears (Age)	Disappears (Age in mo)
Palmar grasp		28 wk	4–5
Moro reflex (drop baby's head suddenly in relation to trunk)	Opens hands, extends and abducts upper extremities and draws them together	28–32 wk	4–5
Gag		32 wk	Persists
Suck		34 wk	4
Tonic neck (rotate infant's head to the side while chest is maintained flat)	Arm and leg extend on side toward which face is rotated, flexion of limbs on opposite side; abnormal: asymmetric or obligatory and sustained pattern	34 wk	4
Reflex stepping (baby supported in upright position)		35 wk	5
Crossed adductor		35 wk	7
Plantar grasp		Birth	9–12
Extensor plantar response (Babinski)		Birth	10
Placing (dorsum of foot placed against edge of table)		1 day	Covered by voluntary action
Landau reflex (lift baby with one hand under its trunk, face downward)	Reflex extension of vertebral column → baby lifts head above horizontal	3 mo	24
Parachute response (suspend child horizontally about the waist, face down)	Arms extend and fingers spread	4–9 mo	Covered by voluntary action

I. Age-related
  A. Physiologic chorea of infancy
  B. Kernicterus
  C. Cerebral palsy
  D. Buccal-oral-lingual chorea of aging
  E. "Senile" chorea
II. Hereditary
  A. "Benign" familial (consider Huntington's disease)
  B. Amino acid, carbohydrate, and lipid disorders
  C. Lesch-Nyhan syndrome
  D. Wilson's disease
  E. Hallervorden-Spatz disease
  F. Ataxia-telangiectasia
  G. Tuberous sclerosis
  H. Sturge-Weber syndrome
  I. Myoclonic epilepsy
  J. Pelizaeus-Merzbacher disease
  K. Sickle-cell disease
  L. Leigh's disease
  M. Porphyria
  N. Paroxysmal kinesiogenic and dystonic choreas
  O. Familial basal ganglia calcification
  P. Olivopontocerebellar atrophy
III. Drug-induced and toxic
  A. Neuroleptics
  B. Antiparkinsonian agents: dopaminergic drugs, amantadine, anticholinergic agents
  C. Anticonvulsants: carbamazepine, phenytoin, phenobarbital
  D. Noradrenergic stimulants: amphetamine, methylphenidate, pemoline, aminophylline, theophylline, caffeine
  E. Anabolic steroids and oral contraceptives
  F. Opiates: methadone, heroin
  G. Others: antihistamines, lithium, tricyclics, isoniazid, reserpine, metoclopramide, digoxin, methyldopa, diazoxide, triazolam
  H. Toxins: ethanol intoxication and withdrawal, carbon monoxide, mercury, manganese, thallium, toluene
IV. Metabolic
  A. Hyponatremia and hypernatremia
  B. Hypocalcemia
  C. Hypomagnesemia
  D. Hypoglycemia and hyperglycemia
  E. Hypoparathyroidism
  F. Addison's disease
  G. Pregnancy
  H. Hepatic encephalopathy
  I. Renal failure
  J. Vitamin deficiencies: thiamine (beriberi), niacin (pellagra), vitamin B_{12}

C

CHOREA

V. Infectious or immunologic
   A. Sydenham's chorea (St. Vitus' dance), post-rheumatic fever
   B. Diphtheria, pertussis, typhoid fever, including postvaccinal
   C. Viral encephalitis
   D. Neurosyphilis
   E. Lyme disease
   F. Legionnaires' disease
   G. Sarcoidosis
   H. Systemic lupus erythematosus, Schönlein-Henoch purpura, Behçet's syndrome, periarteritis nodosa; antiphospholipid antibody syndrome
   I. Multiple sclerosis
VI. Cerebrovascular
   A. Basal ganglionic infarction or hemorrhage
   B. Arteriovenous malformation
   C. Migraine
VII. Miscellaneous
   A. Posttraumatic
   B. Brain tumors: primary, metastatic, lymphoma
   C. Epidural and subdural hematomas
   D. Electrical injury

REFERENCE

Joseph AB, Young RR, eds: *Movement disorders in neurology and neuropsychiatry*, Boston, Blackwell, 1992.

CHROMOSOMAL DISORDERS

Chromosomal abnormalities have been reported to occur in 4% to 34% of individuals with mental retardation. Diagnosis of these abnormalities is important in terms of defining prognosis, establishing risk of recurrence, avoiding further unnecessary testing, and providing families with an answer as to the cause of their child's problems. Significant advances in cytogenetics have substantially improved our diagnostic yield in the last decade. Current cytogenetic testing options include routine karyotyping (high-resolution chromosomal banding analysis), individual fluorescence in situ hybridization (FISH) assays, subtelomeric FISH assay, and comprehensive genomic hybridization (chromosomal microarray analysis). Indications for routine chromosomal analysis include mental retardation (MR) and developmental delay (DD), microcephaly, multiple congenital anomalies or dysmorphisms, sexual ambiguity, abnormal skin pigmentation, family history of mental retardation or miscarriages, or suspected genetic syndrome.

Specific guidelines regarding the type and resolution of chromosomal analysis required are still debated, but at minimum all cases of MR and DD without known cause deserve routine karyotyping. Further testing can be guided by clinical suspicion based on phenotypic findings characteristic of known syndromes (see later descriptions) via individual FISH (microdeletions, duplications, and subtelomeric rearrangements) or DNA analysis for specific gene abnormalities. If the patient does not fit any syndromic description and routine karyotyping is normal, comprehensive genomic hybridization may be of benefit. It encompasses all abnormalities that would be detected on routine chromosomal analysis and multiple individual FISH assays (all microdeletions, duplications, and telomeres), along with some single gene disorders.

I. Single gene disorders
   A. *Fragile X:* most common inherited cause of mental retardation (1 in 1500 males, 1 in 2000 females)
      Presentation: MR, long face with prominent chin, large ears, and macro-orchidism after puberty. Macrocephaly is frequently present. X-linked recessive inheritance, but some female carriers may have MR. DNA analysis shows an expanded number of CGG trinucleotide repeat in the *FMR-1 gene* on the X chromosome.
   B. *Rett syndrome:* 1 in 10,000 females
      Presentation: MR, language regression, loss of purposeful hand movement (replaced by stereotypical hand wringing), acquired microcephaly, seizures, and spastic diplegia. X-linked disorder caused by mutations (exons 1-4, 85%) or deletions (10%) in the *MECP2* gene. Phenotypic expression is quite variable, and occurrence has rarely been reported in males with MR. Both mutations and deletions are detectable with DNA analysis of the *MECP2* gene.

II. Trisomies
   A. *Trisomy 21 (Down syndrome):* 1 in 660 births; 94% of Down syndrome is secondary to trisomy 21, with the rest caused by either translocation (most commonly between chromosome 21 and chromosome 14) or mosaicism.
      Presentation: MR, hypotonia, infantile spasms, oblique palpebral fissures, median epicanthal fold, Brushfield spots (accumulation of fibrous tissue appearing as light colored spots encircling the periphery of the iris), low-set ears, thick protruding tongue, bilateral simian creases, short extremities and digits, heart anomalies, GI anomalies (duodenal atresia), and upper cervical spine malformation. In later life, these patients develop Alzheimer's disease with progressive cognitive decline with neuritic plaques and neurofibrillary tangles. They are also at risk for stroke in childhood due to congenital heart disease. Seizures are also common in later adult life.
   B. *Trisomy 13:* 1 in 5000 births
      Presentation: Severe MR, microcephaly, microphthalmos, holoprosencephaly, median facial anomilies, low-set dysplastic ears, polydactyly, cutis aplasia, "rocker bottom feet," and congenital heart disease.
   C. *Trisomy 18* (Edward syndrome): 1 in 4500 births

Presentation: Severe MR, brain grossly and microscopically normal in 50%, long narrow skull, low-set dysplastic ears, second finger overlies third, thumb distally implanted and retroflexible, heart anomalies, polycystic kidneys.

III. Subtelomeric rearrangements: Approximately 6% to 7% of patients with moderate MR have a subtelomeric chromosomal abnormality. Abnormalities are detected on telomeric FISH assay.

Presentation: Intrauterine growth retardation, postnatal failure to thrive or overgrowth, two or more facial dysmorphic features, one or more nonfacial dysmorphic features or congenital anomalies, and family history of MR.

IV. Microdeletion syndromes

A. DiGeorge (DG)/velocardiofacial (VCF) syndrome

Presentation: Mild to moderate MR, cardiac defects (conotruncal), thymic aplasia/hypoplasia, and hypocalcemia. VCF syndrome has MR, with cleft palate, cardiac defects, hypotonia, dysmorphic facies, short stature, and velopharyngeal incompetence. Significant overlap occurs between these two syndromes, as well as extreme phenotypic variability. Both syndromes are associated with 22q11.2 deletion (95%), and are detected by FISH analysis. DG syndrome has also been associated with a second deletion of 10p13p14.

B. Prader-Willi syndrome (PWS)

Presentation: MR, infantile hypotonia and failure to thrive, short stature, small hands and feet, micropenis and cryptorchidism, childhood onset obesity secondary to hyperphagia, blond hair, blue eyes, fair skin, and almond-shaped palpebral fissures. About 70% of cases are secondary to a paternal deletion in the 15q11-q13 chromosome, which may be detected using FISH analysis. Other chromosomal abnormalities associated with PWS include maternal uniparental disomy of chromosome 15 (25%) and nonexpression of the paternal genes on the same chromosome (2%). Neither of these abnormalities is detected by FISH; thus, it is recommended that when PWS is suspected, testing via DNA methylation be performed. This will detect all of the previously mentioned abnormalities.

C. Angelman syndrome (AS)

Presentation: Severe MR, microbrachycephaly, large mouth, prognathia "puppet-like" ataxic gait, absent speech, seizures, and paroxysms of laughter. About 70% of cases are due to a maternal deletion in the 15q11-q13 chromosome which may be detected using FISH analysis. Other chromosomal abnormalities associated with AS include paternal uniparental disomy of chromosome 15 (3–5%), mutations in the *UBE3A* gene (5%), and nonexpression of the paternal genes on chromosome 15 (7–9%). None of these abnormalities is detected by FISH, and thus, it is recommended that when AS is suspected, testing via DNA methylation be performed; if negative, then further DNA sequence analysis for *UBE3A* mutations should be performed.

D. Smith-Magenis syndrome (SM)

Presentation: MR, brachycephaly with midface hypoplasia, self-abusive behavior. SM is associated with deletions on 17p11.2 detectable by FISH assay.

E. Williams syndrome

Presentation: MR, "elfin facies," blue eyes with stellate pattern iris, congenital heart disease (particularly supravavular aortic stenosis), intermittent hypercalcemia, loquacious personality, and hoarse voice; 90% are associated with deletions of the elastin gene on 7q11.23 detectable by FISH assay.

V. Sex chromosomal abnormalities

A. *XO (Turner syndrome)* (1 in 2000 females): Usually normal intelligence (but frequently problems with visuospatial skills), short stature, broad chest with widely spaced nipples, low posterior hairline, webbed neck, congenital lymphedema, cubitus valgus, ovarian dysgenesis.

B. *XXY (Klinefelter's syndrome)* (1 in 500 males): Mild MR, learning disabilities, language disorder, behavior disorders, intention tremor, tall with long limbs, hypogonadism with hypogenitalism, gynecomastia.

C. *XYY:* Borderline MR, learning disabilities, behavior disorders, tall stature.

D. *XXX:* MR without other specific findings.

REFERENCES

Battaglia A, Carney JC: *Am J Med Gen Part C* 117C:3–14, 2003.

Jones KL: *Smith's recognizable patterns of human malformation*, ed 5, Philadelphia, WB Saunders, 1997.

Online Mendelian Inheritance in Man, OMIM, McKusick-Nathans Institute for Genetic Medicine, Johns Hopkins University (Baltimore, MD) and National Center for Biotechnology Information, National Library of Medicine (Bethesda, MD), 2000. Accessed at http://www.ncbi.nlm.nih.gov/omim/.

COMA (See also BRAIN DEATH, CARDIOPULMONARY ARREST, and AAN GUIDELINE SUMMARIES APPENDIX)

Consciousness is the state of awareness of self and surroundings. Loss of awareness with concomitant defects in arousal constitutes coma or, when less pronounced, a state of lethargy, stupor, and obtundation. Coma is neither a unitary state nor an etiologic diagnosis. Its presence suggests specific dysfunction of both hemispheres or dysfunction of the brainstem reticular activating system, or both. The mechanism of dysfunction may be a structural lesion (supratentorial or subtentorial), a metabolic disturbance, or psychogenic.

Coma evaluation requires a detailed medical history and a general physical examination to establish potential causes. In addition to complete chemistry tests, blood cell count, and coagulation panels, blood gas levels (observe color and request CO level), toxicology screens (on blood, urine, and gastric contents), thyroid function tests, cortisol level, and cultures should be obtained at the time of initial evaluation of coma of unknown cause. Emergency management is outlined in Table 25.

TABLE 25

EMERGENCY MANAGEMENT OF COMA OF UNKNOWN CAUSE

1. Ensure oxygenation. Clear airway, suction, perform bag-valve-mask ventilation, and use intubation as needed. Immobilize cervical spine prior to neck extension until C-spine injury is excluded radiographically. Atropine, 1 mg IV, may prevent vagally mediated bradyarrhythmias during intubation.
2. Maintain circulation with fluids and pressors to keep mean arterial pressure above 100 mm Hg. Continuous ECG monitoring is necessary.
3. Thiamine, 100 mg IV, followed by glucose 25 g (50 mL D_{50}) IV, immediately after blood is drawn (large volume) for diagnostics.
4. Treat intracranial hypertension if suspected (see Intracranial Pressure).
5. Stop seizures when present (see Epilepsy).
6. Restore acid-base balance.
7. Treat drug overdose. For suspected narcotics give naloxone (Narcan) 0.4 mg IV, repeat as necessary if effective (short half-life) or in 5 min. For suspected anticholinergics (e.g., tricyclics), give physostigmine, 1 mg IV. For suspected benzodiazepine overdose, give flumazenil starting at 0.2 mg IV over 30 seconds. Failure to respond to a total dose of 5 mg makes it unlikely that coma is due to benzodiazepines.
8. Exclude intracranial masses by CT (uncontrasted).
9. Normalize body temperature.
10. Treat infection if suspected (see Meningitis).
11. Specific therapy should be instituted as soon as a diagnosis is established.

The neurologic examination is focused toward determining the pathophysiologic features by distinguishing the location and degree of CNS dysfunction, including the following.

I. Level of consciousness: Response to voice, shaking, or pain. Consider status epilepticus, akinetic mutism, vegetative state, locked-in (de-efferented) syndrome, and psychogenic states (see below).
II. Brainstem function
   A. Pupils: Light reflex tests for cranial nerves II and III (midbrain).
      1. Anisocoria: With Horner's syndrome, suggests hypothalamic or lateral medullary dysfunction; without Horner's syndrome, and if there are associated ocular motility deficits, consider transtentorial herniation.
      2. Miosis: Common in toxic or metabolic encephalopathy (preserved light reflex is a hallmark of metabolic coma) and central herniation with supratentorial mass lesion. Pinpoint, barely reactive pupils suggest acute pontine lesion or presence of opioids.
      3. Mydriasis: In association with absent light reflex and (sometimes) irregular pupils, suggests dorsal midbrain dysfunction. Beware of atropine or sympathomimetics commonly given during resuscitation.
      4. Fixed, midposition pupils suggest midbrain nuclear (third cranial nerve) dysfunction.

B. Eye movements: Assess conjugacy, gaze deviation or preference, nystagmus, and spontaneous movements. Oculocephalic responses and vestibulo-ocular testing with ice water evaluate brainstem connections of cranial nerves III, IV, VI, and VIII. Presence of nystagmus without ocular deviation to the irrigated ear on caloric testing suggests psychogenic coma, because it indicates integrity of brainstem and hemispheric pathways. Roving eye movements suggest an intact brainstem. Ocular bobbing and its variants suggest pontine lesions.

C. Corneal or sternutatory reflexes test cranial nerves V and VII (pons).

D. Gag (pharynx) or cough (larynx-trachea) reflexes test cranial nerves IX and X (medulla).

III. Breathing patterns

A. *Cheyne-Stokes respirations* consist of cyclically increasing, then decreasing respiratory depth and rate, separated by apneic phases. It results from the interaction of an increased ventilatory drive to Pco_2 and a decreased forebrain stimulus for respiration, when Pco_2 is decreased. It suggests bilateral cerebral hemispheric or diencephalic dysfunction but may be produced by any encephalopathic state. It is also common in severe congestive heart failure.

B. *Central neurogenic hyperventilation* is attributed to brainstem injury. *Tachypnea* is more common and is usually associated with hypocapnia and hypoxemia. It often resolves with correction of the metabolic abnormalities, whereas central neurogenic hyperventilation does not. Tachypnea with brainstem disease may be associated with neurogenic pulmonary edema.

C. *Apneustic breathing* consists of prolonged "jamming" of respiration in inspiratory and expiratory phases. Although rare, it is seen with dorsolateral pontine lesions at the level of the sensory trigeminal nucleus.

D. *Ataxic breathing* consists of generally slow, irregular respirations with variable amplitude and can progress rapidly to complete apnea. It is due to bilateral lesions of the reticular formation in the caudal dorsomedial medulla, where the respiratory rhythm is generated. Medullary compression, usually caused by acute lesions, may result in respiratory arrest, leading to cardiovascular collapse.

E. These breathing patterns may be a false localizing sign in cases of coexisting metabolic derangement. For example, metabolic acidosis and hypoxia cause reactive hyperventilation, simulating neurogenic hyperventilation.

IV. Sensorimotor function

A. Spontaneous activity. Assess for volitional movement, choreoathetosis, posturing (arms decorticate or flexor versus decerebrate or extensor), asterixis, myoclonus, and seizures.

B. Response to noxious stimuli (listed in order of increasing severity of coma). Lateralizing features of response should be noted.

1. Purposeful.
2. Flexion withdrawal.
3. Abnormal flexion (decorticate posturing): Usually slow, stereotyped flexion of arm, wrist, and fingers with shoulder adduction and variable leg extension.
4. Abnormal extension (decerebrate posturing): Extension of wrist and arm with adduction and internal rotation of shoulder; extension and internal rotation of leg with plantar flexion of foot.
5. No response.

C. Tone: Assess for flaccidity, rigidity, spasticity, clonus, and paratonia.
V. Tendon reflexes: Assess for asymmetry, increase, or decrease in response.

The Glasgow coma scale quantitates level of consciousness. It is easy to use and reliable, with low interobserver variability (Table 26). Because the scale does not assess brainstem reflexes, it does not communicate a complete neurologic assessment but is useful for rapid identification, reliable communication, serial quantitation, and aid in assessing prognosis, particularly when used in evaluation of posttraumatic coma.

CAUSES OF COMA

I. Accurate localization can identify likely causes of altered consciousness.
    A. Supratentorial lesion
        1. Subcortical destructive lesions
        2. Hemorrhage: epidural, subdural, subarachnoid, intracerebral; hypertensive, vascular malformation
        3. Infarction: thrombotic or embolic arterial occlusion, venous thrombosis
        4. Tumor: primary, metastatic

TABLE 26

GLASGOW COMA SCALE

Category	Response	Score*
Eye opening	Open spontaneously	4
	To verbal command	3
	To pain	2
	Do not open	1
Best motor response	Obeys to verbal command	6
	Localizes pain	5
	Flexion withdrawal	4
	Flexion-abnormal (decorticate)	3
	Extension-abnormal (decerebrate)	2
	No response	1
Best verbal response	Oriented and converses	5
	Disoriented and converses	4
	Verbalizes	3
	Vocalizes	2
	No response	1

* Total score ranges from 3 to 15.

       5. Abscess: intracerebral, subdural

       6. Closed head injury

  B. Infratentorial lesion

       1. Compressive: cerebellar hemorrhage, infarct, tumor, or abscess; posterior fossa subdural, extradural hemorrhages, basilar aneurysm

       2. Destructive: brainstem hemorrhage, infarction, tumor, demyelination, or abscess

  C. Diffuse brain dysfunction

       1. Intrinsic: encephalitis, progressive multifocal leukoencephalopathy, meningitis, concussion, ictal or postictal state, herniation

       2. Hypoxic or metabolic: anoxia, ischemia, nutritional (e.g., Wernicke's syndrome), hepatic encephalopathy, uremia, pulmonary disease

       3. Endocrine: nonketotic hyperglycemic hyperosmolar coma, ketoacidosis, disseminated intravascular coagulation, hypoglycemia, Addison's disease, myxedema, thyrotoxicosis, panhypopituitarism

       4. Toxic, drug-induced: amphetamines, cocaine, psychedelics, tricyclics, phenothiazines, lithium, benzodiazepines, methaqualone, glutethimide, barbiturates, alcohol, opiates, ibuprofen, aspirin

       5. Ionic and acid-base disorders: hypo-osmolarity or hyperosmolarity; hyponatremia or hypernatremia, hypocalcemia or hypercalcemia, hypophosphatemia, lactic acidosis, cerebral edema

       6. Hypothermia, hyperthermia

       7. Remote effects of cancer (paraneoplastic): limbic encephalitis, thalamic degeneration

  D. Psychogenic coma: conversion reaction, catatonic stupor, malingering

II. The clinical course may also suggest localization and cause.

  A. Supratentorial mass with diencephalic or brainstem compression

       1. Early focal cerebral dysfunction

       2. Rostral to caudal progression with signs referrable to one area at a time

       3. Asymmetrical motor signs

       4. Third-nerve palsy preceding coma (early herniation)

  B. Infratentorial mass or destruction

       1. Early brainstem dysfunction or sudden onset of coma with accompanying brainstem signs

       2. Vestibulo-ocular abnormalities present

       3. Cranial nerve palsies usually present

       4. Abnormal respirations common, appear early

  C. Metabolic causes

       1. Confusion and stupor precede motor signs

       2. Motor signs usually symmetrical

       3. Pupillary reactions usually preserved (except with certain drugs and toxins; see Pupil)

       4. Asterixis, myoclonus, tremor, and seizures are common

       5. Acid-base disturbance with hypoventilation or hyperventilation is common

C

COMA

D. Psychogenic unresponsiveness
1. Lids tightly closed
2. Pupils reactive or dilated (factitious mydriatics)
3. Oculocephalic responses highly variable; nystagmus and arousal occur with caloric stimuli
4. Motor tone normal or inconsistent
5. Breathing normal or rapid
6. Reflexes nonpathologic
7. Normal EEG

III. Other states may resemble coma.
A. Vegetative state: Subacute or chronic condition after severe brain injury characterized by wakefulness, sleep-wake cycles, and eye opening to auditory stimuli, without evidence of consistent cognitive function or response to stimuli. Blood pressure and respirations are maintained. Vegetative state may follow coma and persist for years (a duration longer than 1 month is called persistent vegetative state). About one third of patients eventually become more responsive (more common in traumatic than in hypoxic cases). May occur with forebrain, occipital, hippocampal, or diffuse cerebral or cerebellar destruction.
B. Akinetic mutism: Subacute or chronic condition characterized by seeming alertness, yet minimal vocalization or movement even with noxious stimuli. May occur with cingulate, limbic, corpus striatum, globus pallidus, thalamic, or reticular formation damage.
C. Locked-in syndrome: Intact consciousness plus quadriplegia and lower cranial nerve dysfunction. Voluntary vertical, and sometimes horizontal, eye movements are preserved. Usually occurs with ventral pontine infarcts, tumors, hemorrhages, or myelinolysis; ventral midbrain infarction; head injury; or severe neuromuscular disease. May be transient or chronic.

IV. Prognosis in coma, excluding traumatic and drug-related causes, is usually poor. Prediction is less reliable in cases of intoxications and trauma but more precise after cardiopulmonary arrest (see Cardiopulmonary Arrest). In general, the longer coma lasts, the lower the chance for regaining independent function (i.e., making a "good recovery").
A. Prediction: Data obtained from 500 patients, excluding known trauma or drug intoxication (Levy and associates, 1985).
1. At 6 hours after onset of coma, absence of any of the following was associated with less than 5% chance of good recovery:
a. Pupillary light reflex
b. Corneal reflexes
c. Oculocephalic reflexes
d. Vestibulo-ocular reflexes (calorics)
2. At 1 day after onset, none of the patients with absent corneal reflexes had satisfactory recovery.

3. At 3 days after onset, no patient with absence of any of the following had satisfactory recovery:
   a. Pupillary reflexes
   b. Corneal reflexes
   c. Motor function
4. Predictors of good outcome are less reliable than negative predictors.
   a. At 6 hours after onset, with moaning or better verbal response *plus* pupillary, corneal, *or* oculovestibular responses: 41% of patients had good recovery.
   b. At 1 day after onset, with inappropriate or better words *plus* any three of pupillary, corneal, oculovestibular, or motor responses: 67% had good recovery.
   c. At 3 days after onset, with inappropriate or better words *plus* corneal *and* motor responses: 74% had good recovery.
   d. At 7 days after onset, with eye opening to pain *plus* localizing motor response: 75% had good recovery.

B. Overall outcome (at 1 year):
   1. 16% of patients were back to independent life.
   2. 11% were severely disabled.
   3. 12% were in a vegetative state.
   4. 61% died without recovery.

REFERENCES

American Neurological Association committee on ethical affairs: *Ann Neurol* 33:386–390, 1993.

Levy D et al: *JAMA* 253:1420–1426, 1985.

Plum F, Posner JB: *The diagnosis of stupor and coma*, ed 3, Philadelphia, FA Davis, 1982.

COMPLEX REGIONAL PAIN SYNDROME (REFLEX SYMPATHETIC DYSTROPHY)

DEFINITION AND CLINICAL FEATURES

Complex regional pain syndrome (CRPS) is a disorder of the extremities, frequently following an injury or operation, which is characterized by pain, sensory, sudomotor and vasomotor disturbances, trophic changes, and impaired motor function (Table 27). Two types of CPRS have been identified. *CPRS type I* without definable nerve lesion represents the majority (90%) of clinical cases. In *CPRS type II*, a definable nerve lesion is present, limiting its responsiveness to treatment.

ETIOLOGY AND PATHOGENESIS

Causes include fracture (25–47%), soft tissue injury (40%), myocardial infarction (12%), stroke (12%), and occasionally no precipitating event is found (5–10%). Female-male ratio is 4:1. Proposed mechanisms include

TABLE 27

SIGNS AND SYMPTOMS OF COMPLEX REGIONAL PAIN SYNDROME

Region	Signs/Symptoms
Sensory	Spontaneous burning or stinging pain (80%) occurring with active or passive movements
	Pain spreads beyond initial site of injury
	Mechanical hyperesthesia (65%) e.g., clothes resting on skin
	Mechanical allodynia (74%)—pain with light touch or brushing
	Mechanical hyperalgesia (100%)—exaggerated response to pinprick
	Temperature allodynia—tested with cool or warm test tubes of water
	Extreme sensitivity to temperature changes
	In CRPS II, electrical sensation or shooting pain is common
	Hypoesthesia in affected nerve distribution with extreme allodynia; cold allodynia is also more common
	Foreign feeling of affected limb (30%)
Vasomotor	Asymmetry of color (66%) and temperature (56%)
	Sympathetic hypofunction—skin is red, hot and dry
	Sympathetic hyperfunction—skin is cold, blue, pale or mottled and sweaty
	Thermography may reveal a 1°C difference
Sudomotor and edema	Asymmetry in sweating (53%)
	Limb edema (80%)
	Smooth-handled instrument will glide more easily over sweaty area than a dry area
Motor	Decreased range of motion (70%)
	Weakness (56–77%)
	Tremor (9–20%) and myoclonus
	Exaggerated reflexes on affected side (40%)
	Focal dystonia (14%)
	Contractures and fibrosis if chronic in late stages
Trophic	Trophic changes in skin (20%), hair (9%), nails (9%)
	Osteoporosis on x-ray

trauma-related cytokine release, exaggerated neurogenic inflammation, sympathetically maintained pain, and cortical reorganization in response to chronic pain.

DIAGNOSIS

CRPS remains a clinical diagnosis. Diagnostic criteria for CPRS by the International Association for the Study of Pain (IASP) are listed here:

I. Preceding noxious event with (CPRS I) or without (CPRS II) an obvious nerve lesion

II. Continuing pain, allodynia, or hyperalgesia, not limited to a single nerve territory and disproportionate to the inciting event

III. Presence of edema, skin blood flow (temperature), or sudomotor (sweat) abnormality, motor symptoms, or trophic changes on the affected extremity

IV. Other diagnoses are excluded

Three stages of CRPS have been identified: Stage I (acute phase) includes pain, temperature changes, and hyperalgesia. Stage II (dystrophic phase) has worsening of stage I symptoms. Stage III (atrophic phase) usually includes irreversible tissue damage with thin skin, thickened fascia, muscle contracture, joint stiffness, diffuse osteoporosis, limb movement reduction, and allodynia.

The following tests support the diagnosis: Comparative x-ray examination may reveal spotty osteoporotic changes. Three-phase bone scan (scintigraphy) reveals tracer uptake in late images suggesting increased bone metabolism. MRI can exclude other causes (e.g., septic or inflammatory arthritis). Measurement of cutaneous temperature by thermography or infrared thermometer shows difference of $1°C$ between affected and unaffected limb is present in 75% to 98% of patients with reflex sympathetic dystrophy. Autonomic testing of resting skin temperature (RST), resting sweating output test (RSO), and quantitative sudomotor reflex test (QSART) have been reported to have high sensitivities and specificities.

TREATMENT

All treatment should be focused primarily on functional restoration. Blocks, psychotherapy, and drugs are reserved for situations of failure to progress or in significant concomitant problems such as depression. Physical, occupational, recreational therapy, and vocational rehabilitation are geared to minimize edema, normalize sensation (desensitization maneuvers), promote normal positioning, decrease muscle guarding, and increase functional use of each extremity to improve functional use of the extremity to increase independence in work, leisure, and ADLs.

Neuropathic pain is treated with NSAIDs, tricylic antidepressants (amitriptyline and nortriptyline), or anticonvulsants (gabapentin, pregabalin). For severe refractory pain, opioids may be used. Nasal calcitonin (200 IU bid) and bisphosphonates (particularly clodronate IV 300 mg qd for 10 days) can improve motor function and pain control. Palmidronate and alendronate are alternatives. Therapeutic trial with prednisone 1 mg/kg/day for 3 weeks followed by 3-week taper is performed if pain is severe and significant swelling or edema is present.

Postganglionic blocks (intravenous regional blocks), ganglion blocks (lumbar sympathetic and stellate ganglion blocks), and lastly preganglionic blocks (epidural block) may be transiently effective in a selected group. If repeated blocks are required, surgical sympathectomy is an option. Predictors of response to sympathetic blocks include abnormal QSART and RST, cold allodynia, and a positive effect from a single sympathetic block. Dorsal spinal cord stimulator and implantable peripheral nerve stimulator may be used if conventional treatment fails to improve pain control.

REFERENCES

Birklein F: *J Neurol* 252:131–138, 2005.
Harden RN: *Clin J Pain* 16:S26–S32, 2000.

Harden RN, Bruehl SP: *Clin J Pain* 22(5):415–419, 2006.

Harden RN, Swan M: *Clin J Pain* 22(5):420–424, 2006.

COMPUTED TOMOGRAPHY

Computed tomography (CT) combines conventional x-ray with a digitized, computerized reconstruction technique that yields multiple two-dimensional images of the body. Tissues are assigned absorption coefficients by the computer (CT or Hounsfield numbers) and are displayed as shades of gray (Table 28). The range of CT numbers displayed can be manipulated to focus on certain structures (e.g., bony structures or intracranial contents) by "windowing." The *window width* (WW) determines the range of CT numbers displayed, and the *window level* (WL) determines the center of the window width.

Nonenhanced CT (NECT) of the brain is primarily used for the detection of hemorrhage, acute infarcts, or masses. Hemorrhage is initially hyperdense (white) and gradually becomes isodense (gray and equal to brain tissue) and finally hypodense (black) over time. Findings of acute infarction include hyperdensity within vessels (especially the middle cerebral artery), loss of gray-white matter differentiation, effacement of sulci, and hypondensity involving both the gray and white matter (see Table 29). Masses, unless they are hypercellular (i.e., lymphoma, meningioma), can be difficult to detect on NECT. Secondary signs of mass such as midline shift, edema within the white matter, and hydrocephalus are readily seen on NECT. However, a contrast-enhanced CT or MRI is more sensitive in detecting and characterizing masses.

Iodinated IV contrast material enhances (brightens) many normal vascular structures (large vessels, choroid plexus, tentorium, and falx) as well as highly vascular pathologic structures (tumors, metastases, lymphoma). "Ring" enhancement (white rim or dark core) is seen with metastases, abscess, gliomas, late infarcts, contusions, demyelinating disease, or resolving hematomas.

TABLE 28

CT DENSITY

Moiety	Hounsfield Units
Bone	1000
Calcification	100
Acute blood	85
Tumor	30–60
Gray matter	35–40
White matter	25–30
CSF	0
Adipose	−100
Air	−1000

From Woodruff WW: *Fundamentals of neuroimaging*, Philadelphia, WB Saunders, 1993.

TABLE 29

CT FINDINGS IN STROKE

Duration	Infarct		With Contrast
	Infarct Without Contrast		
Hyperacute (<1 day)	Normal or blurring of gray-white junction and/or effacement of gyri		No enhancement
Acute (1–7 days)	Vaguely defined hypodensity, best seen after 3–4 days; maximal edema and mass effect		No enhancement
Subacute enhancement (8–21 days)	Hypodensity less evident; decreased mass effect and edema		Gyral (peaks at week 3)
Chronic (>21 days)	Hypodensity sharply defined and isodense to CSF		Enhancement usually in 6–7 weeks

Intraparenchymal Hemorrhage

Duration	Appearance	Mass Effect
Acute	Homogeneous hyperdensity	Mass effect
Subacute		
Early (3 days to 3 weeks)	Enlarging hypodense periphery with hyperdense center	Mass effect
Late (3–5 weeks)	Hypodense periphery; isodense center	Mass effect
Chronic (>5 weeks)	Hypodense periphery; hypodense center	Mass effect resolves after several months*

In evaluating stroke a negative initial CT should be repeated in 2 to 3 days, when edema (and hypodensity) is maximal, as appropriate.
*Ring enhancement is present from week 1 to week 7.

COMPUTED TOMOGRAPHY

C

CT angiography (CTA) is a relatively new technique that allows visualization of the extracranial vasculature and circle of Willis. It is performed with a rapid bolus of IV contrast agent to enhance the vessels in order to acquire axial images, which can be further reviewed in any plane on a computer workstation. It is useful for the detection of aneurysms, evaluation of vascular dissection, and measuring the degree of stenosis of a given vessel. However, conventional angiography remains the gold standard at this time, particularly for detecting small aneurysms, which can be missed on CTA, revealing vasculitis, and characterizing AVMs.

CT is preferred to MRI for evaluating patients in the *acute* setting (with the exception of cord compression).. However, CT is less sensitive than MRI in the detection of mesial temporal sclerosis, leptomeningeal enhancement, and spinal cord abnormalities. It is the modality of choice for those unable to undergo MRI because they either have metal devices (aneurysm clips, cochlear implants, pacemakers) or are too claustrophobic or agitated to obtain adequate MRI images.

REFERENCES

Schuknecht B: Latest technique in head & neck CTA: *Neuroradiology* 46(Suppl 2): S208–213, 2004.
Woodruff WW: *Fundamentals of neuroimaging*, Philadelphia, WB Saunders, 1993.

CONFUSIONAL STATE

Acute confusional states, also known as delirium, may affect between 20% and 70% of hospitalized patients, depending on the definition. Clinical features are disturbance of attention with (1) disturbance of vigilance, (2) inability to maintain a stream of thought, and (3) inability to carry out goal-directed movements. Mild anomia, dysgraphia, dyscalculia, and constructional deficits may be seen. Perceptual distortions may lead to illusions and hallucinations. Tremor, myoclonus, or asterixis may accompany acute confusional states. Encephalopathy is a nonspecific term for diffuse brain dysfunction and refers to a state similar to delirium, though generally of a more depressed level of consciousness and usually the result of a systemic condition. Initially, there is impaired attention, confusion, and disorientation (i.e., delirium). Later, there may be progression to stupor and coma, or it may present as coma of unknown cause. Associated features may include agitation, hallucination, myoclonus, asterixis, generalized seizures, or EEG slowing or triphasic waves. Complete evaluation of the confusional state includes review of recent medications, metabolic screening (particularly serum glucose), urine toxicology screen, consideration of systemic or CNS infection, and neuroimaging. Metabolic disturbances, toxic exposure, drugs, infection (systemic and CNS), head trauma, and seizures are common causes of confusional states. Because of the potential for nonconvulsive status in this population, an EEG should be obtained, particularly if the initial metabolic testing is unremarkable.

Unilateral or bilateral damage to the fusiform and lingual gyri as well as lesions of the nondominant posterior parietal and inferior prefrontal regions may produce a confusional state.

REFERENCE

Guidotti M, Chiveri L, Mauri M: *Neurol Sci* Suppl 1:S55–56, 2006.

CONGENITAL MALFORMATIONS OF THE BRAIN AND SPINE

I. Dorsal induction
  A. Primary neurulation: 3 to 4 weeks age of gestation (AOG); notochord, chordal mesoderm induce neural plate, neural plate closes forming neural tube, tube closes beginning at medulla, proceeds rostrally and caudally. Defects at this stage may cause *craniorachischisis, myeloschisis* (failure of closure of neural tube or vertebral arch); *anencephaly* (absent calvaria and brain, brainstem and cerebellum present); *encephalocele* (meninges and brain parenchyma protrude through skull defect); *myelomeningocele* (meninges and spinal cord protrude through defect in vertebral arch); *Chiari malformation; hydromyelia* (focal dilation of central spinal cord canal).
  B. Secondary neurulation: 4 to 5 weeks AOG; notochord, mesodermal interactions form dura, pia, vertebrae, skull. Defects at this stage may cause *myelocystocele; diastomyelia* (splitting of spinal cord by mesodermal band); *meningocele/lipomeningocele*; *lipoma*; *dermal sinus with or without cyst; tethered cord/tight filum terminale; anterior dysraphic lesions* (neurenteric cyst); *caudal regression syndrome*.
II. Ventral induction: 5 to 10 weeks AOG; prechordal mesoderm induces face, forebrain; cleavage of prosencephalon; formation of optic vesicles, olfactory bulbs/tracts; telencephalon gives rise to cerebral hemispheres, ventricles, caudate, putamen; diencephalon gives rise to thalami, hypothalamus, and globus pallidus; rhombencephalon gives rise to cerebellar hemispheres, vermis; myelencephalon gives rise to medulla and pons. Defects at this stage may cause *holoprosencephaly* (failure of cleavage of embryonic forebrain into paired cerebral hemisphere with absence of the interhemispheric fissure); *septo-optic dysplasia* (rudimentary septum pellucidum, hypoplasia of optic nerve and chiasm); *arhinencephaly*; olfactory bulb and tract aplasia; facial anomalies; *cerebellar hypoplasias/dysplasias (Joubert syndrome*, rhombencephalosynapsis, tectocerebellar dysplasia); and *Dandy-Walker malformation* (enlarged posterior fossa, hyogenesis or agenesis of the cerebellar vermis, and cystic dilatation of the fourth ventricle).
III. Neuronal proliferation, differentiation, histogenesis: 2 to 4 months AOG; germinal matrix forms at 7 weeks; cellular proliferation forms neuroblasts, fibroblasts, astrocytes, endothelial cells; choroid plexus is formed; CSF production begins. Defects at this stage may cause

microcephaly, megalencephaly, aqueductal stenosis, arachnoid cysts, congenital vascular malformations.

IV. Cellular migration: 2 to 5 months AOG; neuroblasts migrate from germinal matrix along radial glial fibers; cortical layers form from deep to superficial; gyri, sulci form; commissural plates form corpus callosum, hippocampal commissure. Defects at this stage may cause *schizencephaly* (lateral clefts through cerebral hemispheres extending from cortex to ventricles), *lissencephaly* (absence of gyri), *pachygyria* (abnormally wide and thick gyri), *micro/polymicrogyria* (small gyri with increased number and abnormal lamination), *heterotropias* (ectopic collections of gray matter), *Lhermitte-Duclos* syndrome (diffuse enlargement of the cerebelar cortex), *agenesis of the corpus callosum*.

V. Neuronal organization: 6 months postnatal; neuronal alignment, orientation, layering; dendrites proliferate; synapses form.

VI. Normal myelination begins during the fifth fetal month. It proceeds in a highly predictable and orderly manner: caudal to cephalad, dorsal to ventral, and central to peripheral. Sensory tracts myelinate first.

A. Birth (full term): medulla, dorsal midbrain, inferior and superior cerebellar peduncles, posterior limb of internal capsule, ventrolateral thalamus.

B. One month: deep cerebellar white matter, corticospinal tracts, pre/postcentral gyrus, optic nerves, tracts.

C. Three months: brachium pontis, cerebellar folia, ventral brainstem, optic radiations, anterior limb of internal capsule, occipital subcortical U fibers, corpus callosum splenium.

D. Six months: corpus callosum genu, paracentral subcortical U fibers, centrum semiovale (partial).

E. Eight months: centrum semiovale (complete except some frontotemporal areas), subcortical U fibers (complete except for most rostral frontal areas).

F. Eighteen months: essentially like adults.

G. Twenty years: peritrigonal region. Defects at this stage may be due to metabolic, demyelinating, and dysmyelinating disorders.

VII. Acquired degenerative, toxic, or inflammatory lesions may occur at any stage causing injury to otherwise normally formed structures. These may result in defects such as hydranencephaly (remnant cerebral hemisphere is a paper-thin membrane sac composed of glial tissue filled with CSF covered with leptomeninges), hemiatrophy, multicystic encephalomalacia, or periventricular leukomalacia.

REFERENCES

Barkovich AJ: *Pediatric neuroimaging*, ed 3, Philadelphia, Lippincott Williams & Wilkins, 2000.

Bradley WG, Daroff RB et al: *Neurology in clinical practice*, ed 4, Boston, Butterworth-Heinemann, 2004.

CRAMPS

DEFINITION

Cramps (Stiff-Person syndrome, tetanus, Isaac syndrome, and others) are painful muscle contractions, with a characteristic electromyographic signature consisting of crescendo high-frequency, high-amplitude motor unit potentials which cause an interference pattern.

NORMAL CRAMPS

Cramps (Table 30) may be normal/*physiologic*, occurring both at rest and after exercise or stimulant use. Such *common* or *benign* cramps may be attended by fasciculations, but not other neurologic signs, and resolve with passive stretching or fluid and electrolyte repletion. Calcium, magnesium, or quinine may be helpful for frequent, bothersome attacks.

C

CRAMPS

PATHOLOGIC CRAMPS

Pathologic cramps may be accompanied by neurologic signs (weakness or atrophy) and may be classified according to their origin:

I. Central cramps: Cramps originating from CNS dysfunction can be caused by stiff-person syndrome and poisoning by strychnine or tetanospasmin.
   A. Stiff-person syndrome
      1. *Presentation*: Adult onset of rigid, uncontrolled proximal and axial muscle contractions that are present only during wakefulness. Typically, there is fluctuating rigidity, which begins in the axial muscles and propagates over time to the limbs. Focal syndromes with symptoms confined to a limb or two have been reported. The cramps, which may be strong enough to fracture bones, are extremely painful and may be provoked by movement, noise, or other sensory stimuli; they are blocked by curare, general anesthesia, and nerve block. On examination, paraspinal contractions can be palpated and tendon reflexes are generally hyperactive, but spasticity and weakness are absent.
      2. *Laboratory findings*: EMG shows continuous activity in agonist and antagonist muscles with normal motor unit morphology. Antibodies to glutamic acid decarboxylase (GAD) are found in serum and CSF in 80% of cases, though paraneoplastic syndromes associated with thymoma, lymphoma, small cell lung cancer, and breast carcinoma have been noted.
      3. *Treatment*: For cases not caused by malignancy, treatment is with benzodiazepines, often in very high doses, but other agents mediating GABA inhibition such as baclofen, valproic acid, and gabapentin may be helpful. Immunosuppressive therapies with plasma exchange, immunoglobulin, prednisone, azathioprine, and other agents have shown some benefit; and intrathecal baclofen, botulinum toxin injection, and oral dantrolene have been tried for refractory cases.

TABLE 30

COMMON MUSCLE CRAMPS CAUSES

Physiologic benign cramps
    Pregnancy
    Nocturnal leg cramps in the elderly
    Stretch and exercise-related
Lower motor neuron disorders
    Spinal muscular atrophy and amyotrophic lateral sclerosis
    Post poliomyelitis
    Plexopathy and radiculopathy
    Peripheral neuropathy
Metabolic disorders
    Hepatic failure
    Renal failure and uremia
    Hypocalcemia and metabolic alkalosis
    Hypothyroidism
    Hypoadrenalism
Acute extracellular volume depletion
    Perspiration, "heat cramps"
    Hemodialysis
    Diarrhea, vomiting
    Diuretic therapy
Medications
    Hereditary disorders
    Rippling muscle disease
    Neuromyotonia
    Glycogenoses
Autoimmune
    Stiff-person syndrome (anti GAD) and antibodies to voltage-gated potassium channels

   B. *Tetanus* is caused by tetanospasmin, a neurotoxin secreted by *Clostridium tetani*, which interferes with central-mediated GABA and glycine release, producing hyperexcitability of lower motor neurons.
      1. *Presentation*: Rapidly progressive, generalized, continuous tonic contractures with superimposed painful spasms, and autonomic instability. Tonic spasms of the masticatory muscles (trismus or lockjaw) are common. The spasms may be triggered by sensory stimuli or emotional stress.
      2. *Laboratory findings*: EMG is similar to that of stiff-person syndrome.
      3. *Treatment*: Supportive; ventilatory support, tetanus antitoxin, diazepam, or curare may be used, as well as avoidance of stimuli which might provoke symptoms. Intensive care monitoring is necessary to address autonomic dysfunction, manifested by cardiac dysrhythmias and labile blood pressure.
      4. *Prognosis*: Generalized tetanus is fatal in 20% to 50% of cases.
   C. *Strychnine*, a component of rat poison, inhibits glycine release in the CNS causing stiffness and muscle spasms and generalized tonic-clonic seizures.

1. The poison can be detected in urine and gastric fluid.
2. Treatment is supportive; prognosis is good.

II. Peripheral cramps

  A. *Motor axonopathies and motor neuron disease* cause cramps via increased lower motor neuron excitability, in which there is spread of ectopic motor unit potentials to nearby nerve terminals (e.g., radiculopathy, plexopathy and peripheral neuropathy, motor neuron diseases, amyotrophic lateral sclerosis, spinal muscular atrophy, poliomyelitis, and other focal lesions of anterior horn cells).

  B. *Metabolic diseases* include endocrinopathies such as hypothyroidism and adrenal insufficiency, uremia, hepatic insufficiency and fluid or electrolyte imbalance. Significant hypocalcemia, in particular, can cause tetany, as can alkalosis, which results in physiologic hypocalcemia due to depletion of ionized calcium that has left serum to bind proteins vacated by hydrogen ions.

  C. Neuromyotonia (generalized myokymia, continuous muscle fiber activity, and Isaac's syndrome) can occur at any age and is usually sporadic.

    1. *Presentation*: Insidious onset of generalized muscle stiffness. In severe cases stiffness is present at rest and impedes movement. Excessive sweating, dysarthria and dysphagia may occur. Parasthesias may occur, but pain is not usually present. The defect may be an autoimmune channelopathy, and the motor activity is not altered by spinal or proximal nerve block. EMG shows short bursts of motor unit activity at 10 to 100 Hz.

    2. *Treatment*: Phenytoin, carbamazepine, dantrolene, or immunomodulation.

  D. *Cramp-fasciculation syndrome*: Subacute or chronic history of diffuse fasciculations and cramps in unusual places, such as the trunk. Although it is clinically similar to tetany, there is no underlying metabolic disturbance. It may overlap with the hyperexcitable nerve syndrome in which lancinating pain and parasthesias pervade.

III. Myopathic cramps

  A. *Inborn errors of metabolism:* Glycogenoses including myophosphorylase deficiency (McArdle's disease), lipidoses, and carnitine palmityltransferase (CPT) deficiency can cause cramp complaints. Better characterized as contractures (because of electrical silence on EMG), the abnormal muscle activity may be precipitated by exercise (glycogenoses and CPT deficiency) or fasting (CPT deficiency). *Treatment* consists of a high-carbohydrate diet for phosphorylase deficiency and a high-carbohydrate, low-fat diet for CPT deficiency.

  B. *Rippling muscle disease (RMD)* is a rare disease that may be acquired (autoimmune) or congenital (autosomal dominant or recessive).

    1. *Presentation* consists of involuntary muscle stiffness, hypertrophy of large muscles with myoedema, and visible muscle contractions, which spread from one region to another. Cardiac subtype may result in heart failure and dysrhythmias.

C

CRAMPS

2. *Diagnosis*: There is no clinical test; *stretch-induced muscle contractions are sensitive and specific for RMD.*

3. *Treatment* is rarely needed, except in instances of acquired cases; those that lack family history; or those associated with thymoma, which may respond to immunomodulation or thymectomy, respectively.

C. *Cholinesterase intoxication* (e.g., excessive therapy for myasthenia gravis).

REFERENCE

Miller TM, Layzer RB: *Muscle Nerve* 32:431–442, 2005.

CRANIAL NERVES

The cranial nerves and their functions and innervations are listed in Table 31. Table 32 expands on the list to include clinical features of lesions in these nerves.

REFERENCES

Kandel ER et al: *Principles of neural science*, New York, McGraw-Hill, 2000.
White JS: *USMLE road map neuroscience*, New York, Lange/McGraw-Hill, 2004.

CRANIOCERVICAL JUNCTION (See also ARNOLD-CHIARI MALFORMATION)

Dysfunction resulting from lesions at the foramen magnum or craniocervical junction is usually produced by compression or shearing.

Clinical presentation is usually that of a chronic dysfunction, because acute lesions usually become evident with respiratory arrest, and may include various combinations of the following: spastic quadriparesis; cranial nerve palsies such as dysphagia, dysarthria, absent gag, hearing loss, vocal cord paralysis, nystagmus (downbeat and periodic alternating), vertigo, facial weakness or diplopia; hydrocephalus; head and neck pain; extremity weakness or paresthesias; facial pain; drop attacks; syringomyelia; ataxia; papilledema; dorsal column signs; and recurrent apnea or stridor. Some individuals with abnormalities of the craniocervical junction may be asymptomatic.

Evaluation requires MRI of the brain and cervical spine and occasionally a myelogram.

Treatment depends on the underlying cause.

CRANIOSYNOSTOSIS

Craniosynostosis describes the premature closure of suture(s) while the brain is still growing, resulting in an abnormal skull shape. Depending on the suture that closes prematurely, the skull takes on a characteristic shape (Table 33).

TABLE 31

CRANIAL NERVES AND THEIR FUNCTION

Nerve	CNS Nucleus	Function/Innervation
I	Olfactory bulb	Smell
II	Lateral geniculate nucleus	Vision
III	Oculomotor nucleus	Extraocular muscles except superior oblique and lateral rectus
	Edinger-Westphal nucleus	Sphincter pupillae and ciliary muscle
IV	Trochlear nucleus	Superior oblique muscle
V	Spinal and main sensory nucleus	Sensory from face, deep tissues of head and neck, dura mater, and tympanic membrane
	Mesencephalic nucleus	Muscle spindles; mechanoreceptors of face and mouth
	Trigeminal motor nucleus	Muscles of mastication and tensor tympani
VI	Abducens nucleus	Lateral rectus muscle
VII	Facial motor nucleus	Muscles of facial expression and stapedius
	Spinal trigeminal nucleus	Sensory from external ear and tympanic membrane
	Solitary nucleus	Taste from anterior 2/3 of tongue
	Superior salivatory nucleus	Salivary and lacrimal glands
VIII	Cochlear and vestibular nuclei	Balance and hearing
IX	Nucleus ambiguous	Muscles of pharynx
	Spinal trigeminal nucleus	Sensory from external ear, tympanic membrane, and posterior 1/3 tongue
	Solitary nucleus	Taste from posterior 1/3 of tongue
	Solitary and spinal trigeminal	Carotid body and sinus; sensation from nasal nuclei and oral pharynx
	Inferior salivatory nucleus	Parotid gland
X	Nucleus ambiguous	Muscles of larynx and pharynx
	Spinal trigeminal nucleus	Sensory from external ear
	Solitary nucleus	Taste buds of epiglottis
	Solitary and spinal trigeminal	Parasympathetics from thoracic and abdominal viscera; sensory from larynx and pharynx
	Dorsal motor nucleus	Parasympathetics to thoracic and abdominal viscera
XI	Nucleus ambiguous	Muscles of larynx and pharynx
	Accessory nucleus	Sternocleidomastoid and trapezius
XII	Hypoglossal nucleus	Intrinsic tongue muscles

CRANIOSYNOSTOSIS

C

TABLE 32

CRANIAL NERVES: CLINICAL FEATURES OF LESIONS

Nerve	Name	Type	Function	Clinical Features of Lesions
I	Olfactory	Sensory	Smells	Anosmia
II	Optic	Sensory	Sees	Anopsia (visual field defects)
III	Oculomotor	Motor	All eye muscles (except lateral rectis and superior oblique)	Diplopia, external strabismus
			Adduction (medial rectus muscle)	Loss of parallel gaze
			Upper eyelid elevator	Ptosis
			Constricts pupil	Mydriasis; loss of motor limb light reflex with CN II
			Accommodates	Loss of accommodation
IV	Trochlear	Motor	Superior oblique; depresses and abducts eyeball	Weakness looking down when eye adducted
			Intorsion	Head tilts away from lesion side
V	Trigeminal	Mixed		
	V1-ophthalmic		General sensation (touch, pain, temperature) of forehead/scalp, cornea	Sensory loss forehead/scalp
				Loss of sensory limb blink reflex with CN VII
	V2-maxillary		General sensation of palate, nasal cavity, maxillary face, maxillary teeth	Loss of sensation in innervated areas
	V3-mandibular		General sensation of anterior 2/3 tongue, mandibular face, mandibular teeth,	Loss of sensation in innervated areas
			Motor to muscles of mastication (temporalis, masseter, medial & lateral pterygoids) plus anterior belly of digastric, mylohyoid, tensor tympani, tensor palatine	Weakness in chewing; jaw deviates to lesion nerve
VI	Abducens	Motor	Lateral rectus; abducts eye	Diplopia; internal strabismus; loss of parallel gaze, "pseudoptosis"
VII	Facial	Mixed	Muscles of facial expression (orbicularis oculi and oris, platysma, buccinator, stapedius)	Weakness of facial muscles
				Loss of motor limb of blink reflex
				Hyperacusis

VIII	Cochlear	Sensory	Taste anterior 2/3 tongue	Loss or alteration of taste
			Salivates (submandibular and sublingual glands)	Reduction in salivary output
			Tears (lacrimal gland)	Xero-ophthalmia
			Makes mucus (nasal and palatine glands)	Reduction in secretions
			Hears	Sensorineural hearing loss
	Vestibular		Linear acceleration (gravity)	Loss of balance
			Angular acceleration (head turning)	Nystagmus
IX	Glossopharyngeal	Mixed	General sensation of oropharynx, carotid sinus, and carotid body	Loss of sensory limb of gag reflex with CN X
			Taste and general sensation posterior 1/3 tongue	Loss of taste and sensation in innervated areas
			Motor to one muscle: Stylopharyngeus	
			Salivates	Reduction in salivary output
X	Vagus	Mixed	Muscles of palate except tensor palatine (V)	Palate droop, uvula points away from lesion
			Muscles of pharynx except stylopharyngeus (IX)	Dysphagia: loss of motor limb of gag reflex with CN IX
			Muscles of larynx	Hoarseness, dysphonia
			Muscle of tongue (palatoglossus)	
			Senses larynx/laryngopharynx	
			Glands and smooth muscle in thorax, foregut, and midgut	
	Descending hypothalamic nucleus	Motor	Elevates upper eyelid (superior tarsal muscle)	Ptosis
			Mydriasis	Miosis
			Sweat glands face/scalp	Anhidrosis/Horner's syndrome
XI	Accessory	Motor	Turns head to opposite side (sternocleidomastoid)	Weakness turning head to opposite side
			Elevates and rotates scapula	Shoulder droop, difficulty combing hair
XII	Hypoglossal	Motor	All tongue muscles except palatoglossus (X) (hyoglossus, styloglossus, genioglossus, intrinsics)	Tongue deviation on protrusion (toward lesioned nerve)
				Dysarthria

CRANIOSYNOSTOSIS

C

TABLE 33

CRANIOSYNOSTOSIS: SUTURE AFFECTED, HEAD SHAPE, AND DESCRIPTION

Suture Affected	Head Shape	Description
Sagittal	Scaphocephaly	60%; boys > girls; may be familial, neurologically normal
Coronal	Brachycephaly	20%; girls > boys; affected in Apert's and Crouzon's disease (5% of all cases of craniosynostosis)
Single coronal or lambdoidal	Plagiocephaly	Distinguish from deformational plagiocephaly
Metopic	Trigonocephaly	Varies in severity; may results in hypertelorism; may be associated with mental retardation
Multiple	Oxycephaly	Seen in Carpenter's syndrome

Most cases are sporadic and of uncertain etiology. It may be one feature of a larger syndrome of genetic or chromosomal abnormality. Craniosynostosis may be seen in association with metabolic disorders (rickets, mucopolysaccharidoses, hyperthyroidism, hypercalcemia, hypophosphatemia) or hematologic disorders (sickle cell, thalassemia, polycythemia vera). Plagiocephaly must be distinguished from the much more common (1 per 300 births) deformational plagiocephaly. Deformational plagiocephaly has increased as a result of campaigns to prevent sudden infant death syndrome so infants may habitually sleep in a single position.

Clinical presentation depends on the underlying cause, but most cases are associated with hydrocephalus. Evaluation includes palpation of the calvarial bones (palpable ridging) and skull x-rays (band of increased density at site of prematurely closed suture) and CT or MRI.

Treatment depends on the underlying cause; some cases may require surgery or ventriculoperitoneal shunting. Surgery can correct cosmetic appearance and increase cranial vault size. Timing involves a balance of ability to tolerate surgery versus acute and chronic issues to be addressed through surgery (e.g., hydrocephalus, cognitive, cosmetic).

Prognosis depends on the underlying cause. There is no clear data indicating that surgery improves cognitive outcome.

REFERENCES

Aryan HE, Jandial R, Ozgur BM et al: Childs Nerv Syst 21:392–398, 2005.
Kabbani H, Raghuveer TS: Am Fam Physician 69:2863–2870, 2004.
Lekovic GP, Bristol RE, Rekate HL: Semin Pediatr Neurol 11:305–310, 2004.

CREUTZFELDT-JAKOB DISEASE; OTHER HUMAN PRION DISEASES

Prions are protease-resistant proteinaceous infectious agents associated with transmissible spongiform encephalopathy (TSE), which comprises a group of rare, subacute, and fatal neurodegenerative diseases in mammals.

Prions are an aberrant isoform of a protein that is normally expressed and highly conserved in mammals. The normal human cellular prion protein (PrP^c) is encoded by a single gene in the short arm of chromosome 20. All three forms of prion diseases (familial, sporadic, and infectious) are believed to share the same pathogenetic mechanism, which is based on the conversion of the normal PrP^c into the pathogenic prion protein PrP^{Sc}. In human beings PrP^c is a small glycoprotein bound to the cell surface. It is unknown how prion proteins undergo the conformational changes to a self-replicable infectious isoform and cause the typical histopathologic features of spongiform vacuolation, astrocytic proliferation, and neuronal loss. Prions do not evoke an immune response. Human diseases caused by prions include the following:

I. Creutzfeldt-Jakob disease (CJD)
  A. Sporadic CJD (85% of CJD cases) occurs worldwide with an incidence of 0.5 to 1.5 per 1 million people per year. Men and women are equally affected and onset of disease is between 50 and 70 years of age. There is no evidence of geographic or seasonal clustering.
  B. Familial or inherited CJD (15% of CJD cases) affects younger patients and is autosomal dominant (short arm of chromosome 20).
  C. Infectious or iatrogenic CJD has been reported after transplants of cadaver-derived dura mater, injection of cadaver-derived growth hormone and gonadotropic hormone, implantation of stereotactic depth EEG electrodes, inoculation, corneal grafting, and other invasive medical procedures. Initially, CJD presents with fatigue, disordered sleep, cognitive decline, confusion, ataxia, aphasia, visual loss, hemiparesis, or amyotrophy. Signs of cerebellar, pyramidal, and extrapyramidal involvement develop in most patients.
  Diagnosis is suggested by rapid progression of dementia and development of myoclonic jerks, particularly startle myoclonus in response to acoustic or tactile stimulus. EEG findings may be normal in the early stages.
  Workup: Later in the course, periodic biphasic or triphasic (classically 1 Hz activity) synchronous complexes over a slow background rhythm may develop. Periodic complexes carry a sensitivity of 67% and a specificity of 86%, and they are less likely to be present in familial cases. CSF examination is usually normal or may show mildly elevated protein. Immunoassay for 14-3-3 protein in the CSF has a sensitivity and specificity of greater than 90% (false-positive in stroke, SAH, ICH, tumors, meningoencephalitis). Biopsy shows pathologic findings of spongiform changes, neuronal loss, and gliosis.
  There is no therapy.
  Prognosis: The mean survival time is 5 months, with 80% dying within 1 year.
II. Atypical CJD has prominent amyotrophic or ataxic features, with slow progression and longer duration of symptoms and absence of typical

C

CREUTZFELDT-JAKOB DISEASE

EEG changes, and this picture causes diagnostic uncertainty. Differential diagnosis includes amyotrophic lateral sclerosis, multiple sclerosis, and paraneoplastic cerebellar degeneration. Rapid progressive dementia with myoclonus should be differentiated from other neurodegenerative disease such as Alzheimer's disease, infectious diseases such as HIV, tertiary syphilis or subacute sclerosing panencephalitis, and encephalopathies due to heavy metal or other toxins.

III. Variant CJD is a novel form of CJD that is believed to be acquired from cattle affected by bovine spongiform encephalopathy (BSE), also known as "mad-cow disease," which was first reported after an epidemic in the United Kingdom. Patients acquire the disease by eating meat or meat products contaminated with BSE. It affects younger adults (mean age is 29 years) and presents with prominent behavioral manifestations, persistent paresthesias and dysesthesias, with a similar periodic EEG pattern. Ataxia, dementia, and myoclonus appear during the terminal stage of the disease (Table 34 compares variant CJD with sporadic CJD).

IV. Kuru is an endemic form of prion disease associated with cannibalism, as part of the funeral ceremony common to the Fore linguistic group, a tribe of Papua New Guinea. It was first reported by Gadjusek in the 1950s. In Fore language, kuru means "to tremble or shake," which graphically describes a symptom of the disease. Cessation of cannibalism since the 1950s has gradually eliminated the disease.

V. Gerstmann-Sträussler-Scheinker disease (GSS) is familial, with autosomal dominant inheritance (point mutation of *PrP* gene on chromosome 20) and presents with ataxia, dementia, aphasia, and

---

TABLE 34

COMPARISON OF VARIANT AND SPORADIC CREUTZFELDT-JAKOB DISEASE

Clinical Features	Variant CJD	Sporadic CJD
Mean age of onset	29 years	60 years
Mean survival time	14 months	4 months
Early psychiatric symptoms	Common	Unusual
Painful sensory symptoms	Common	Rare
Later cerebellar ataxia	All	Many
Dementia	Commonly delayed	Typically early
Electroencephalogram	Nonspecific slowing	Biphasic and triphasic periodic complexes
MRI (mainly in variant CJD)	Signal in pulvinar region of thalamus	Signal in basal ganglion and putamen
Cerebrospinal fluid 14-3-3 concentration	High in 50% of patients	High in most patients
Histopathology of brain	Many florid plaques	No amyloid plaques
Immunostaining of tonsils	Positive	Negative
Polymorphism at codon 129	All homozygotes (M/M)	Homozygosity and heterozygosity

Adapted from Johnson RT: *Lancet Neurol* 4: 635, 2005.

extrapyramidal symptoms. The course is similar but slower than CJD, and death occurs in 4 to 10 years.

VI. Fatal familial insomnia (FFI) is characterized by disordered sleep, ataxia, and dementia. The disease affects mainly the thalamic nuclei and is associated with an autosomal dominant mutation of codon 178 of the *PrP* gene.

REFERENCES

Gadjusek DC: *Science* 197:943–960, 1977.
Johnson RT: *Lancet Neurol* 4:635–642, 2005.
Prusiner SB: *N Engl J Med* 344:1516–1526, 2001.
Sy M-S et al: *Med Clin North Am* 86:551–571, 2002.

DEGENERATIVE DISEASES OF CHILDHOOD

I. Diseases that predominantly affect white matter (present with long tract signs [spasticity and hyperreflexia], optic atrophy, cortical blindness, or deafness)

A. Metachromatic leukodystrophy: autosomal recessive (AR); arylsulfatase deficiency; metachromatic granules; age of onset 2 to 5 years; with peripheral neuropathy; MRI—arcuate fibers spared.

B. Krabbe's disease: AR; beta-galactosidase deficiency; globoid cells; age of onset 4 to 6 months; optic atrophy, hyperacusis; with peripheral neuropathy; MRI—arcuate fibers spared and parieto-occipital lobes involved early, high-density basal ganglia.

C. Adrenoleukodystrophy: X-linked recessive; acyl-CoA synthetase deficiency and long-chain fatty acids accumulate; single peroxisomal enzyme deficiency; childhood ALD—neurologic symptoms before adrenal insufficiency; adrenoleukomyeloneuropathy—spinal cord and nerves involved, age of onset in 20s to 30s, paraparesis and adrenal dysfunction almost at the same time; MRI—occipital lobes and corpus callosum splenium affected, marked contrast enhancement. Pathologically three zones are identified: innermost zone with necrosis, intermediate zone of active demyelination and inflammatory changes, and peripheral zone of demyelination without inflammation.

D. Pelizaeus-Merzbacher disease: X-linked recessive; deficient proteolipid protein expression; newborn—hypotonia, tongue fasciculations; childhood onset—dementia and choreoathetosis; MRI—perivascular white matter spared producing a "tigroid pattern"; involves arcuate fibers.

E. Alexander disease: sporadic; Rosenthal fibers; macrocephaly; MRI—frontal lobe hyperintensities, (+) contrast enhancement.

F. Canavan disease: AR; *N*-acetylaspartylase deficiency; widespread vacuolation macrocephaly; MRI—near or total lack of myelin, involves arcuate fibers.

G. Cockayne's syndrome: AR; defective DNA repair; large ears, sunken eyes; age of onset 2 years; retinitis pigmentosa progeria; MRI—demyelination, perivascular calcification in basal ganglia and cerebellum.

H. Chédiak-Higashi syndrome: neutrophil dysfunction leading to defective bacterial killing; intracytoplasmic inclusions in neutrophils and neurons, most prominent in pons and cerebellum; albinism, nystagmus, hepatosplenomegaly; mental retardation, cerebellar, and long tract signs, cranial and peripheral neuropathy.

I. Neuroaxonal dystrophy: neuroaxonal spheroids along axons, especially neuromuscular junction; onset at age 2 years, upper and lower motor neuron signs.

J. Phenylketonuria: AR, phenylalanine hydroxylase deficiency. MRI—arcuate fibers spared, optic radiations affected the most. Treatment with low phenylalanine diet; mental retardation results if not treated early.

II. Diseases that predominantly affect gray matter (present with myoclonus, seizures, and cognitive impairment)

A. Lipidoses

1. Tay-Sachs disease (GM2 gangliosidosis): AR; hexosaminidase A deficiency; onset 3 to 6 months, excessive startle, macrocephaly, retinal cherry-red spot; MRI—hyperintense signal in caudate, thalamus, and putamen on T_2-weighted images.

2. Gaucher's disease: AR; glucocerebrosidase deficiency; type III—early to mid-childhood, seizures, dementia, subacute neuronopathy; hepatosplenomegaly.

3. Niemann-Pick disease: AR; sphingomyelinase deficiency. Type A—infantile, hypotonia, pulmonary interstitial disease, organomegaly, retinal cherry-red spot. Type B—neurologically normal. Type C—more than 1 to 2 years of age, presents with spasticity, seizure, vertical gaze paresis, and ataxia.

B. Neuronal lipofuscinosis: "fingerprint" inclusions of lipofuscin within cytosomes on electron microscopy of leukocytes; presents with dementia, vision loss, ataxia, myoclonus, seizures; infantile, late infantile (photoconvulsive response at 3 Hz on EEG), juvenile (Batten disease), adult (Kufs' disease).

C. Mucopolysaccharidoses

1. Hurler syndrome: AR; α-L-iduronidase deficiency; mucopolysaccharides accumulate in neurons (meganeurites) and in histiocytes (gargoyle cells) in perivascular spaces; gargoyle-like facies, dwarfism, kyphosis, hepatosplenomegaly, severe psychomotor deterioration, death within 5 to 10 years of onset;

MRI—macrocrania, thick dura, perivascular "pits"; concave or "hooked" thoracolumbar vertebrae.

2. Hunter syndrome: X-linked recessive; iduronate-2-sulfatase deficiency; thick dura, perivascular "pits."
3. Sanfilippo syndrome: AR; heparan-N-sulfatase deficiency; normal until age 2 to 8 years, then progressive dementia, hyperactive, aggressive, spastic and movement disorder; death in second to third decades of life.

III. Diseases that primarily affect gray and white matter
   A. Leigh's disease (subacute necrotizing encephalopathy): mitochondrial; spongiosis, demyelination, astrogliosis and capillary proliferation in basal ganglia, brainstem, and spinal cord; infantile—onset at age 2 years of hypotonia, vomiting, and seizures; childhood; adult—fifth to sixth decades; MRI—hyperintense foci in globus pallidus, putamen, and caudate.
   B. Myoclonic epilepsy with ragged-red fibers (MERRF): mitochondrial; muscle biopsy—ragged red fibers; myoclonic epilepsy, myopathy, progressive external ophthalmoplegia, multiple infarcts in cortex and white matter.
   C. Mitochondrial encephalomyopathy with lactic acidosis and stroke (MELAS): mitochondrial; myopathy, encephalopathy, lactic acidosis, strokelike episodes, large and multifocal infarcts mainly in occipital lobes.
   D. Kearns-Sayre syndrome: mitochondrial; elevated pyruvate; progressive external ophthalmoplegia, cerebellar ataxia, heart block, and pigmentary retinopathy. Treatment is supportive with pacemaker and coenzyme Q_{10}; prognosis is poor and patients rarely survive past the second decade.
   E. Alper's disease: etiology uncertain: hypoxic injury versus AR inheritance. Onset before age 6 years; myoclonic seizures appear early, then mental retardation and spasticity or opisthotonus.
   F. Menkes' disease: X-linked recessive; defective transmembrane copper transport; seizures, hypotonia develops into spastic quadriparesis; light-colored and brittle hair, hyperextensible joints, skeletal anomalies; susceptible to sepsis, heat-intolerant.
   G. Zellweger syndrome: AR; multiple peroxisomal enzymes; MRI—heterotropia, patchy/polymicrogyria.

IV. Diseases that predominantly affect basal ganglia (present with movement disorders)
   A. Huntington's disease: AD; CAG repeat; chorea and personality changes; atrophy of caudate and enlarged frontal horns of lateral ventricle.
   B. Hallervorden-Spatz disease: iron deposits in globus pallidus (GP) and substantia nigra (SN); mental retardation, stiff gait, equinovarus; low signals in GP and SN on T_2-weighted images MRI, low signal surrounds region of high signal "eye of tiger" sign.

    C. Fahr disease: AR; first 2 years mental retardation and movement disorder; MRI—prominent calcification in dentate nuclei, centrum semiovale, and subcortical white matter.

    D. Wilson disease: chromosome 13, AR; P-type ATPase deficiency, with decrease in ceruloplasmin and serum copper. Copper deposits in liver and basal ganglia; onset 8 to 16 years. Parkinsonism, seizures, ataxia, dementia, hemolytic anemia, liver dysfunction. Treatment is penicillamine and zinc.

    E. Dystonia musculorum deformans (See Dystonia).

    F. Aminoacidurias.

       1. Glutaric aciduria I: AR; glutaryl-CoA dehydrogenase (lysine to tryptophan); dystonia and dyskinesia; MRI—high-signal changes in basal ganglia and caudate; affects mitochondrial activity and preferentially involves basal ganglia leading to "bat wing" dilatation of sylvian fissures.

       2. Methylmalonic acidemia: AR; secondary to blockage of conversion of methylmalonic acid (MMA) to succinyl-CoA leading to MMA accumulation; hyperammonemia and ketoacidosis; MRI—hyperdensities in globus pallidus.

REFERENCES

Bradley WG, Daroff RG, Fenichel GM, Marsden CD: *Neurology in clinical practice*, ed 3, Boston, Butterworth-Heinemann, 2000.

Menkes JH: *Textbook of child neurology*, Philadelphia, Lea & Febiger, 1990.

Osborn AG: *Diagnostic neuroradiology*, St. Louis, Mosby, 1994.

DEMENTIA (See also AAN GUIDELINE SUMMARIES APPENDIX)

Dementia is a clinical syndrome characterized by loss of multiple cognitive functions and emotional abilities in an individual with previously normal intellect and clear consciousness (i.e., in the absence of delirium). *DSM IV-R diagnostic criteria* require memory impairment and abnormalities in at least one of these areas: language, judgment, abstract thinking, praxis, constructional abilities, or visual recognition. This deficit must be sufficient to interfere with activities of daily living, work duties, or other social activities. The term "dementia" does not imply a specific underlying cause, a progressive course, or irreversibility. The definition also excludes patients with isolated deficits, such as aphasia or apraxia, and symptoms that occur during delirium.

    Prevalence is about 1% at age 60 years and doubles every 5 years, to reach 30% to 50% by the age of 85.

    Examination for suspected dementia should include assessment of multiple areas of cognitive performance, including memory, language, perception, praxis, attention, judgment, calculation, and visuospatial functions. The presence of psychiatric features (affective disorder, hallucinations, delusions, and anxiety) must also be sought. Questions about the patient's activities and self-care capabilities should be obtained from collateral sources of information (caregiver). Acquiring family history is essential. Short, standardized mental status tests such as the Mini-Mental Status Examination (MMSE) are widely used. Mild cognitive deficits may require more extensive neuropsychologic testing.

Laboratory evaluation should include electrolyte and screening metabolic panel, complete blood cell count, thyroid function tests, syphilis serologic test, and vitamin B_{12} level. CT or MRI scan of the brain is used to rule out structural lesions. Other tests (EEG, lumbar puncture, HIV titer, serologic testing for vasculitis, heavy metal screening, angiography, brain biopsy, and formal psychiatric assessment) are indicated only if suggested by the history or examination. In younger adults dementia may be caused by late onset childhood metabolic diseases, and special studies may be required.

CONDITIONS CAUSING DEMENTIA
I. Potentially reversible causes of dementia
  A. Neoplasms (gliomas, meningiomas)
  B. Metabolic disorders (hypo/hyperthyroidism, renal failure, hepatic failure, Cushing's disease, Addison's disease, Wilson's disease, hypopituitarism)
  C. Trauma (SDH)
  D. Toxins (alcohol, heavy metals, organic poisons)
  E. Infections (bacterial/fungal/viral/parasitic meningoencephalitis, neurosyphilis, HIV, brain abscess)
  F. Autoimmune disorders (SLE, MS, vasculitis)
  G. Drugs (antidepressants, anxiolytics, sedatives, anticonvulsants, anticholinergics, antiarrhythmics)
  H. Nutritional deficiencies (thiamine, folate, vitamin B_{12} and vitamin B_6)
  I. Psychiatric disorders (depression, schizophrenia, mania)
  J. Other disorders (NPH, Whipple's diseases, sleep apnea and sarcoidosis)
II. Irreversible causes of dementia.
  A. Degenerative diseases (Alzheimer's disease, fronto-temporal dementia, Huntington's disease, progressive supranuclear palsy, Parkinson's disease, diffuse Lewy body disease, olivopontocerebellar atrophy, ALS-parkinsonism-dementia complex, Hallevorden-Spatz disease, Kufs' disease, adrenoleukodystrophy, metachromatic leukodystrophy)
  B. Vascular dementia (multiple small/large infarcts, Binswanger's disease, CADASIL; see later discussion)
  C. Traumatic (dementia pugilistica)
  D. Infectious (CJD, postencephalitic dementia, progressive multifocal leukoencephalopathy).

The most common cause of dementia in adults is Alzheimer's disease (50% to 60%), followed by vascular dementias (20%); in another 15% to 20% of patients, vascular dementias coexist with Alzheimer's disease. Potentially treatable causes account for about 10% of cases.

ALZHEIMER'S DISEASE

Epidemiology

Alzheimer's disease (AD) is the most common cause of dementia. Incidence is 1% per year for individuals over 65 years of age, and prevalence in people 85 years of age and older is about 50%.

Risk Factors

Increased age and family history are the most important risk factors for AD. Less well defined risks include smoking, stroke, female gender, head trauma, endocrine dysfunction, and low educational level. Lower risk has been suggested in those taking nonsteroidal anti-inflammatory drugs (NSAIDs), postmenopausal women on estrogen replacement therapy, individuals with higher education or socioeconomic status, and those with apolipoprotein E epsilon-2 genotype.

Genetic risk: Specific mutations on chromosomes 1, 14, and 21 are associated with autosomal dominant early onset familial AD. Apolipoprotein E4 genotype (Table 35) is associated with both early and late onset familial AD. Apolipoprotein E is a lipid-carrying plasma protein encoded in chromosome 19. It has three allelic forms: epsilon-2, -3, and -4. The epsilon-4 allele is associated with late onset familial AD with the homozygotes developing AD at an earlier age than the heterozygotes. Down syndrome, the clinical manifestation of trisomy 21, is a clearly identified risk factor for AD. Nearly all individuals with Down syndrome develop pathologic evidence of AD if they live to the sixth decade.

Pathologic hallmarks of AD are neurofibrillary tangles, neuritic plaques with amyloid deposition, amyloid angiopathy, and neuronal loss. Secondary association cortex is most heavily involved. The most widespread neurochemical change is a 50% to 90% decline in choline acetyltransferase activity.

Clinical Presentation

Clinical features are variable but include *cognitive decline* due to recent memory loss. The ability to focus attention and recall remote events may initially be subtle and worsen with time and is usually associated with progressive disorientation to time and place. *Language decline* (particularly finding words in spontaneous speech), anomia (especially for parts of objects), and other types of language difficulties appear. *The ability to perform activities*

TABLE 35

GENETIC FACTORS LINKED TO ALZHEIMER'S DISEASE RISK

Genetic Factor	Chromosome Involved	Age at Onset (yr)
Down syndrome	21	>35
Amyloid precursor protein mutation	21	45–66
Presenilin 1 mutation	14	28–62
Presenilin 2 mutation	1	40–85
Apolipoprotein E ε4 allele	19	>60

From Martin JB: *N Engl J Med* 340(25):1970–1980, 1999.

of daily living (ADLs) may be impaired by visuospatial dysfunction, apraxia, or other motor dysfunction such as rigidity or gait disorder. *Behavioral symptoms* are common and include depression, anxiety, and personality changes. Delusions and hallucinations can occur in the later stages of otherwise typical AD. *Other features* such as extrapyramidal signs (rigidity and tremor) may indicate atypical dementia, such as Lewy body dementias, and myoclonus and seizures may indicate Creutzfeldt-Jakob disease.

Diagnosis

Diagnosis of AD is by the typical clinical features and exclusion of other causes of dementia. Definite AD is diagnosed by autopsy. When strict diagnostic criteria (Table 36) are followed, accuracy of antemortem diagnosis of AD reaches 80% to 90%.

D

DEMENTIA

TABLE 36

CRITERIA FOR CLINICAL DIAGNOSIS OF ALZHEIMER'S DISEASE (NINCDS-ADRA)

I. Criteria for *probable* Alzheimer's disease include:
  A. Dementia established by clinical examination and documented by Mini-Mental Test, Blessed Dementia Scale, or some similar examination and confirmed by neuropsychological test.
  B. Deficit in two or more areas of cognition.
  C. Progressive worsening of memory and other cognitive functions.
  D. No disturbance of consciousness.
  E. Onset between ages 40 and 90, most often after age 65.
  F. Absence of systemic disorders or other brain diseases that in and of themselves could account for the progressive deficits in memory and cognition.
II. The diagnosis of *probable* Alzheimer's is supported by:
  A. Progressive deterioration of specific cognitive functions such as language (aphasia), motor skill (apraxia), and perception (agnosia).
  B. Impaired activities of daily living and altered patterns of behavior.
  C. Family history of similar disorders, particularly if confirmed neuropathologically.
  D. Laboratory results of:
    1. Normal lumbar puncture as evaluated by standard techniques.
    2. Normal pattern or nonspecific changes in EEG, such as increased slow wave activity.
    3. Evidence of cerebral atrophy on CT with progression documented by serial observation.
III. Other clinical features consistent with the diagnosis of *probable* Alzheimer's disease, after exclusion of causes of dementia other than Alzheimer's disease, include:
  A. Plateaus in the course of progression of the illness.
  B. Associated symptoms of depression, insomnia, incontinence, delusions, illusions, hallucinations, catastrophic verbal, emotional, or physical outbursts, sexual disorders, and weight loss.
  C. Other neurologic abnormalities in some patients, especially with more advanced disease and including motor signs such as increased muscle tone, myoclonus, or gait disorder.
  D. Seizures in advanced disease.
  E. CT normal for age.

Cont'd

TABLE 36

CRITERIA FOR CLINICAL DIAGNOSIS OF ALZHEIMER'S DISEASE
(NINCDS-ADRA)—Cont'd

IV. Features that make the diagnosis of *probable* Alzheimer's disease uncertain or unlikely include:
  A. Sudden, apoplectic onset.
  B. Focal neurologic findings such as hemiparesis, sensory loss, visual field deficits, and incoordination early in the course of the illness.
  C. Seizures or gait disturbances at the onset or very early in the course of the illness.

V. Clinical diagnosis of *possible* Alzheimer's disease:
  A. May be made on the basis of the dementia syndrome in the absence of other neurologic, psychiatric, or systemic disorders sufficient to cause dementia, and in the presence of variations in the onset, in the presentation, or in the clinical course.
  B. May be made in the presence of a second systemic or brain disorder sufficient to produce dementia, which is not considered to be the cause of the dementia.
  C. Should be used in research studies when a single, gradually progressive severe cognitive deficit is identified in the absence of other identifiable cause.

VI. Criteria for diagnosis of *definite* Alzheimer's disease are:
  A. The clinical criteria for *probable* Alzheimer's disease.
  B. Histopathologic evidence obtained from a biopsy or an autopsy.

VII. Classification of Alzheimer's disease for research purposes should specify features that may differentiate subtypes of the disorder, such as:
  A. Familial occurrence.
  B. Onset before age 65.
  C. Presence of trisomy 21.
  D. Coexistence of other relevant conditions such as Parkinson's disease.

From McKhann G et al: *Neurology* 34:939, 1984.

DIFFERENTIAL DIAGNOSIS

Vascular dementia, the second most common cause of dementia, can be distinguished based on evidence of strokes on neuroimaging, abrupt onset, stepwise deterioration, focal neurologic signs and symptoms, and risk factors for stroke. Pick's disease can be differentiated by early disinhibited behavior and frontal lobe dysfunction and asymmetrical frontal or temporal lobe atrophy on neuroimaging. Creutzfeldt-Jakob disease needs to be excluded in rapidly progressive dementia with myoclonus.

Treatment

Potential pharmacologic approaches to therapy in AD:

  I. Cholinergic enhancements (cholinesterase inhibitors, acetylcholine agonists)
  II. Other neurotransmitter system modifications (NMDA receptor antagonists, SSRIs)
  III. Antioxidants (vitamins C and E, coenzyme Q and selegeline)
  IV. Anti-inflammatory agents (NSAIDs, COX-2 inhibitors)

V. Hormones (estrogen)

To date, only the cholinesterase inhibitors and NMDA receptor antagonists have been demonstrated to have therapeutic efficacy with acceptable side effects in multiple, large, randomized controlled clinical trials.

I. *Donepezil (Aricept)* is a reversible cholinesterase inhibitor with minimal peripheral side effects. It is indicated in mild-moderate dementia. Dosage is 5 mg daily, which may be increased to 10 mg daily after 4 to 6 weeks. The most frequent adverse effects are nausea, diarrhea, vomiting, and insomnia.

II. *Rivastigmine (Exelon)* is a reversible cholinesterase inhibitor indicated in mild-moderate AD. Dosage is 1.5 mg bid and can be increased by 1.5 mg/dose every 2 weeks as tolerated to a maximum of 6 mg bid. Side effects are similar to that of donepezil if titrated slowly.

III. *Galantamine (Razadyne)*, previously called Reminyl, is a reversible cholinesterase inhibitor, and is indicated in mild-moderate dementia. It is started at 4 mg bid and can be increased by 4 mg bid every 4 weeks to 12 mg bid as tolerated. Efficacy and side effects are similar to that of donepezil and rivastigmine.

IV. *Tacrine (Cognex)* is a reversible cholinesterase inhibitor but it is rarely used because of the need for frequent dosing and hepatotoxicity.

V. *Memantine (Namenda)* is a NMDA receptor antagonist and is indicated in moderate-severe dementia, usually in combination with one of the cholinesterase inhibitors, specifically donepezil. Dosage is 5 mg daily and can be increased by 5 mg every week to a maximum total dose of 20 mg daily given bid (i.e., 10 mg bid). It generally has a good side effect profile.

Behavioral symptoms are disruptive and require careful investigation. Treatment for any underlying medical condition (e.g., urinary tract infection) and thorough review of the medication list should be sought before starting any psychoactive drugs. Depression can be treated with tricyclic antidepressants (e.g., imipramine, amitriptyline) or selective serotonin-reuptake inhibitors (e.g., fluoxetine, sertraline). Neuroleptics can be used to treat psychosis and delusions. Oxazepam is useful for episodic anxiety, but benzodiazepines are sometimes associated with paradoxical effect. Chloral hydrate is useful for insomnia. Counseling and social planning in the face of increasing disability is an important facet of long-term management.

VASCULAR DEMENTIA

When dementia is presumed to be caused by vascular disease, the diagnostic term vascular dementia (VaD) is now generally used. Patients diagnosed as having vascular dementia, however, do not constitute a homogeneous group. Types of cerebrovascular brain damage that may cause or contribute to dementia include lacunar infarcts, cortical infarcts, ICH, IVH, SAH, leukoaraiosis, and neuronal loss in the hippocampus, neocortex, and basal ganglia after global cerebral anoxia or ischemia.

Diagnostic criteria for ischemic vascular dementia include the following:

I. Dementia involving memory loss, executive dysfunction, focal cortical signs, personality changes, and affective changes

II. Cerebrovascular disease demonstrated by history, clinical examination, or brain imaging

III. Evidence that the two conditions are causally related by a temporal relationship, abrupt or stepwise deterioration, and specific brain imaging findings, indicating damage to regions important for higher cerebral function

   Supportive *clinical features* include history of cerebrovascular risk factors, early appearance of gait disturbance and urinary incontinence, and frontal lobe, extrapyramidal and pseudobulbar features. Subtypes of vascular dementia worth mentioning include the following:

I. *Multi-infarct dementia* (MID) is caused by multiple infarcts affecting both the cortical or subcortical areas and by multiple lacunar infarcts. The modified *Hachinski scale* (Table 37) may help to differentiate MID from AD.

II. *Binswanger's disease* (subacute arteriosclerotic encephalopathy) consists of periventricular demyelination of the cerebral white matter in demented patients with a history of hypertension. Previously considered rare, it is now diagnosed more often because of brain imaging. Leukoaraiosis is a frequent finding in nondemented elderly patients and therefore the diagnosis should only be considered in patients with leukoaraiosis who are demented with no other obvious cause for the dementia.

III. *CADASIL* (cerebral autosomal dominant arteriopathy with subcortical infarcts and leukoencephalopathy) is a familial nonarteriosclerotic,

TABLE 37

CLINICAL FEATURES OF ISCHEMIC SCORE (MODIFIED HACHINSKI SCALE)

Feature	Point Value[*]
Abrupt onset	2
Stepwise deterioration	1
Fluctuating course	2
Nocturnal confusion	1
Relative preservation of personality	1
Depression	1
Somatic complaints	1
Emotional incontinence	1
History of presence of hypertension	1
History of strokes	2
Evidence of associated atherosclerosis	1
Focal neurologic symptoms	2
Focal neurologic signs	2

[*]Score ≤4 suggests primary degenerative dementia; score >7 suggests vascular dementia.
Adapted from Rosen WG et al: *Ann Neurol* 7:486–488, 1980.

nonamyloid arteriopathy characterized by recurrent subcortical ischemic strokes starting in the third or fourth decade leading to pseudobulbar palsy, subcortical dementia, and early MRI abnormalities and is associated with a high frequency of migraine The inheritance is autosomal dominant and is localized to the notch 3 gene on chromosome 19.

DEMENTIA WITH LEWY BODIES

Pathophysiology

Dementia with Lewy bodies (DLB) is currently the preferred term to describe diffuse Lewy body disease, Lewy body dementia, and cortical Lewy body disease. Lewy bodies are spherical eosinophilic intracytoplasmic neuronal inclusion bodies with a pale halo as seen in the substantia nigra of Parkinson's disease patients. Cortical Lewy bodies contain alpha-synuclein, a presynaptic protein of unknown function, and can be found in association with AD histopathologically, especially in senile plaques.

Clinical Presentation

DLB is the second most commonly encountered type of degenerative dementia after AD. Age of onset is 50 to 70 years. The central feature required for the diagnosis of DLB is progressive cognitive decline of sufficient magnitude to interfere with normal or occupational function. Prominent or persistent memory impairment may not necessarily occur in the early stages but is usually evident with progression. *Core features include fluctuating cognition with pronounced variations in attention and alertness, recurrent visual hallucinations that are typically well formed and detailed, and spontaneous motor features of parkinsonism*.

Diagnosis

Features supportive of the diagnosis include repeated falls, syncope, transient loss of consciousness, neuroleptic sensitivity, systematized delusions, and hallucinations in other modalities. A diagnosis of DLB is less likely in the presence of stroke evident as focal neurologic signs or on brain imaging and evidence on physical examination and investigation of any physical illness or other brain disorder sufficient to account for the clinical picture. Clinical diagnosis is often suspected in patients with *parkinsonism and dementia*, particularly those with visual hallucinations or excess sensitivity to the extrapyramidal effects of neuroleptics. Definitive diagnosis is by autopsy.

FRONTOTEMPORAL DEMENTIA

Frontotemporal dementia (FTD) consists of a clinically and pathologically heterogeneous group of neurodegenerative disorders collectively referred to as "tauopathies," which also includes corticobasal ganglionic degeneration (CBGD) and progressive supranuclear palsy. These have in common degeneration of the frontal and temporal lobes. Behavioral changes, including

D

DEMENTIA

disinhibition, impulsiveness, social inappropriateness, apathy, and withdrawal are early and prominent features. These behavioral changes provide the most important clue allowing the differentiation of this condition from AD. Language disturbances may also appear early, whereas visuospatial function remains intact until later in the disease. Neuroimaging may allow the visualization of focal atrophy, but the disease can often be recognized clinically before changes on routine imaging are apparent. SPECT demonstrates hypoperfusion in the frontal and temporal lobes before atrophy is evident on structural imaging. A panel of experts recently enumerated upon a *Terminology Consensus for Frontotemporal Dementia (Modified)*. The drawback is that frontotemporal dementia refers to the overall name of the group of diseases and the clinical subgroup mainly affecting the frontal lobes. Also, the abbreviation FTD refers to the pathologic name frontotemporal lobe degeneration.

FTD includes the following subtypes:

I. *Frontotemporal dementia* (FTD) also known as Pick's disease (which is also used to refer to the entire entity of FTD), is the third most common degenerative dementia after AD and DLB. Both sexes are affected equally and the age of onset is between 40 and 80 years. It is characterized by motor speech disorders and verbal stereotypy. Language impairments such as abundant unfocused speech (logorrhea), echo-like spontaneous repetition (echolalia), and compulsively uttered repetitive phrases (palilalia) are often seen in conjunction with the behavioral disturbances and represent focal involvement of the frontal lobes. There is marked personality deterioration with antisocial behaviors. Visuospatial skills are remarkably preserved until late in the disease. Pick's cells (chromatolytic ballooned neurons) and Pick's bodies (argyrophilic cytoplasmic inclusions) are classic pathologic findings.

II. *Primary progressive aphasia* (PPA) is characterized by nonfluent speech production with phonologic and grammatical errors in the absence of decline of other aspects of cognition. Difficulties in reading and writing may also occur, but comprehension is relatively preserved. PPA is related to left frontal lobe involvement.

III. *Semantic dementia* (SD) is characterized by progressive loss of word meanings with severe impairment of naming and word comprehension but fluent speech output. SD is primarily related to left temporal lobe involvement, but when the right temporal lobe involvement is out of proportion to other areas, patients present with prosopagnosia, an inability to recognize familiar faces.

IV. *Corticobasal degeneration* (CBD) is frontotemporal dementia with extrapyramidal apractic supranuclear palsy presentation. CBD is a clinical syndrome characterized by asymmetrical rigidity, apraxia, and alien limb phenomenon.

V. *Frontotemporal dementia with parkinsonism* (FTD-P) is a clinical syndrome linked to chromosome 17, with autosomal dominant inheritance. Initially, behavioral abnormalities appear without memory loss, but they are eventually followed by progressive dementia and parkinsonism.

VI. *Frontotemporal dementia with motor neuron disease* (FTD-MND), an increasingly recognized clinical syndrome. In these patients, motor findings may precede, or coincide with, or follow the development of cognitive and behavioral changes.

REFERENCES

Chui et al: *Neurology* 42:473–480, 1992.
Collinge J: *Lancet* 354(9175):317–323, 1999.
Geldmacher DS, Whitehouse PJ: *N Engl J Med* 335(5):330–336, 1996.
Johnson RT, Gibbs CJ Jr: *N Engl J Med* 339(27):1994–2004, 1998.
Kawas CH: *N Engl J Med* 349:1056–1063, 2003.
Lund and Manchester groups: *J Neurol Neurosurg Psychiatry* 57:416–418, 1994.
McKeith IG et al: *Neurology* 47:1113–1124, 1996.
Neary D et al: *Neurology* 51(6):1546–1554, 1998.
Prusiner SB: *Curr Opin Neurobiol* 2:638–664, 1992.
Roman GC et al: *Neurology* 43:250–260, 1993.
Ross GW, Bowen JD: *Med Clin North Am* 86:455–476, 2002.

D

DEMYELINATING DISEASE

DEMYELINATING DISEASE

These CNS disorders—demyelinating disease, neuropathy, and multiple sclerosis (MS, most common)—involve destruction of normally formed myelin and oligodendroglia, in contrast to the dysmyelinating diseases (e.g., leukodystrophies) in which myelin is abnormally formed. MS and the related acute disseminated encephalomyelitis (ADEM) appear to be immune-mediated, although etiopathogenesis remains an enigma.

Demyelinating diseases are classified as follows:

I. Autoimmune
  A. Primary diseases of myelin
    1. Multiple sclerosis (MS) is the most common demyelinating disease and is discussed in greater detail elsewhere in this text.
    2. Devic's disease, possibly a variant of MS, consists of optic neuritis and transverse myelitis.
    3. Schilder's disease, a rapidly progressive sporadic disease, results in bilateral, massive hemispheric demyelination and is seen mainly in children and adolescents.
    4. Balo's sclerosis, also a possible variant of MS, results in acute demyelination in a concentric pattern.
  B. Parainfectious or postvaccination
    1. ADEM, a uniphasic, inflammatory demyelinating disorder, occurs shortly after measles, varicella, rubella, or other viral illnesses, after vaccination, or after immunizations.
    2. Acute hemorrhagic leukoencephalitis, a hyperacute necrotizing form of ADEM, occurs usually after upper respiratory tract infections, and pathologic features are more tissue-destructive.

3. Site-restricted, uniphasic, acute inflammatory demyelinating disorders include transverse myelitis, optic neuritis, cerebellitis, and Bickerstaff's brainstem encephalitis.
   4. Chronic or recurrent parainfectious or postvaccination encephalomyelitis (possibly related to MS).
II. Infectious
   A. Progressive multifocal leukoencephalopathy
   B. Subacute sclerosing panencephalitis
III. Nutritional
   A. Alcohol or tobacco amblyopia
   B. Central pontine myelinolysis
   C. Marchiafava-Bignami syndrome
   D. Vitamin B_{12} deficiency
IV. Toxic or metabolic
   A. Anoxia or hypoxia
   B. Carbon monoxide poisoning
   C. Mercury intoxication (Minamata disease)
   D. Radiation therapy
   E. Methotrexate, especially with radiation therapy
V. Hereditary
   A. Familial spastic paraplegia
   B. Hereditary ataxias
   C. Leber's disease

REFERENCES

Baker D, Davison AN: *Neurochem Res* 16:1067–1072, 1991.
Bradley WG, Daroff RB et al: *Neurology in clinical practice*, ed 4, Boston, Butterworth-Heinemann, 2004.

DERMATOMES

The following summarizes the landmarks for various dermatomes:
I. Cervical
   A. C2—Occiput and tops of ears
   B. C3—The nape of the neck, the throat, and lobe of the ear
   C. C4—The clavicle
   D. C6—The thumb and lateral aspect of the forearm
   E. C8—The "pinky" and medial aspect of the hand
II. Thoracic
   A. T1—The medial aspect of the forearm
   B. T2—Below the clavicle
   C. T5—The nipple
   D. T10—The navel
   E. T12—The iliac crest
III. Lumbar
   A. L1—The groin
   B. L2—The anterior and lateral aspect of the thigh

C. L3—The knee and inner thigh
D. L4—The medial leg and malleolus.
E. L5—The big toe and lateral leg
IV. Sacral
    A. S1—The heel and posterior leg
    B. S2—The posterior thigh
    C. S3—The buttocks
    D. S5—The anus

REFERENCES

Mumenthaler M, Mattle H, Taub E: *Neurology*, ed 4, New York, Thieme, 2004.
O'Brien MD: *Aids to the examination of the peripheral nervous system*, ed 4,
    Philadelphia, WB Saunders, 2000.

D

DIABETES INSIPIDUS

DIABETES INSIPIDUS

Diabetes insipidus (DI) represents a state of vasopressin (AVP, arginine vasopressin) insufficiency due to insufficient release (central) or insufficient renal effect (nephrogenic). AVP is a protein secreted by the magnocellular neurons of hypothalamus. The regulators controlling the AVP release are (1) serum osmolality; (2) intravascular volume; (3) neural factors (stress, pain, emesis); and (4) others (nicotine, morphine, some antidepressants, and chemotherapy, chlorpromazine, phenytoin, reserpine). The two main sites of action of AVP are V2 receptors of the renal collecting ducts, causing water conservation; and V1 vascular receptors, causing vasoconstriction.

    Causes of central DI include primary CNS tumor (15%), postoperative (15%), severe brain injury (18%), idiopathic (25%), others (meningoencephalitis), brain death, ruptured intracranial aneurysm, Sheehan syndrome, cerebral metastases, histiocytosis, and sarcoidosis.

    There are three *clinical stages of central DI*: (1) pituitary injury (decreased AVP release with DI for 4–5 days); (2) pituitary cell death (uncontrolled AVP release with SIADH for 4–5 days); and (3) chronic pituitary depletion of AVP (prolonged DI).

    Clinical features of central DI include polyuria, excessive thirst, polydipsia, seizures, myoclonus (awake patient); dehydration, weakness, fever, prostration, death (in patient with hypothalamic lesion or impaired consciousness).

DIAGNOSIS

  I. Low urine osmolality (50–100 mOsm/L) or specific gravity (<1.005)
  II. Large urinary output (3–4 mL/kg/hour)
  III. Increased serum sodium (>145 mEq/L)

TREATMENT

  I. Hydration, replacing the free water deficit (GI or IV) in an amount
     equivalent with the urinary output
  II. AVP replacement

REFERENCE

Greenberg MS: *Handbook of neurosurgery*, ed 5, Lakeland, FL, Greenberg Graphics, 2001.

DIALYSIS

Two neurologic syndromes are related to dialysis:

I. *Dialysis disequilibrium syndrome* is the acute onset of neurologic manifestations during or after hemo- or peritoneal dialysis. *Clinical features* include seizures (generalized more often than focal), headache, anorexia, nausea, disorientation, cramps, and even coma. The syndrome is probably caused by an accumulation of urea and idiogenic osmoles in the brain during renal failure. With dialysis, plasma osmolality decreases and the subsequent osmotic gradient results in obligatory retention of water by the brain and subsequent brain edema. Slower dialysis offers the brain more time to clear the idiogenic osmoles. EEG changes reflect the degree of uremia before dialysis and consist of bursts of rhythmic delta waves and occasionally spike-and-wave complexes. The syndrome is usually self-limited, and recovery usually occurs in a few days.

II. *Dialysis dementia syndrome* is now rare and occurs almost exclusively in chronic hemodialysis patients. *Clinical features* include subacute development of personality changes, memory difficulties, dysarthria, myoclonus, and seizures. *Dialysis dementia* in part is defined by EEG. There may be 2- to 4-second bursts of high-voltage, irregular, frontally dominated generalized delta waves, accompanied by frontal sharp waves, spikes, and triphasic waves on normal or minimally slow background. The syndrome may be related to elevated aluminum levels in the dialysate fluid. Removal of aluminum from dialysis baths by deionization has markedly reduced the frequency of this syndrome. *Treatment* is with desferrioxamine.

III. *Dialysis encephalopathy* may be part of a multisystem disease that includes vitamin D–resistant osteomalacia, myopathy, and anemia.

IV. *Others:* Subdural hematomas, confusional states from hyperosmolarity, hypercalcemia, hypophosphatemia, drug intoxication, and Wernicke's encephalopathy. Patients with chronic renal failure often have multiple risk factors for cerebrovascular disease.

REFERENCES

Daly DD, Pedley TA: *Current practice of clinical electroencephalography*, ed 2, New York, Raven, 1990, p 376.

Dhondt JL: *N Engl J Med* 318:582–583, 1988.

DISSEMINATED INTRAVASCULAR COAGULATION

DIC is a clotting disorder complicating many diseases and is most commonly associated with obstetric catastrophes, malignancies, massive trauma, and bacterial sepsis. It is less commonly associated with immunologic disturbances, diabetic ketoacidosis, tissue damage (*stroke, brain hemorrhage, meningitis*, etc.), or shock. In each case, potent thrombogenic stimuli, such as tissue factor or endotoxin, trigger the coagulation cascade and activate platelets. Fibrin then deposits in the microcirculation, causing ischemia, RBC damage, hemolysis, and secondary fibrinolysis.

DIC can be either an explosive and life-threatening bleeding disorder or relatively mild and subclinical. Most often, patients have hemorrhagic or thrombotic complications in venipuncture sites or distal extremities. *Neurologic complications* can affect any portion of the brain or spinal cord with hemorrhage or thrombosis, producing a fluctuating encephalopathy, commonly with focal findings. Confusion, delirium, stupor, and coma may occur with hemiparesis, hemianopia, ataxia, aphasia, seizures, and focal brainstem disease.

Laboratory manifestations include an elevated PT and PTT, low platelets, falling fibrinogen (consumptive), and elevated fibrin split products and D-dimer (due to fibrinolysis). Anemia, fragmented RBCs, and schistocytes may be found.

Treatment consists of correcting the underlying cause. Active bleeding requires fresh-frozen plasma and cryoprecipitate to replenish clotting factors and platelet transfusions to correct thrombocytopenia. Thrombotic complications may be treated with heparin. Heparin is sometimes used to treat hemorrhage, when platelets and plasma fail. *Prognosis* is variable, and patients with severe deficits may completely recover.

REFERENCES

Aminoff MJ: *Neurology and general medicine*, Edinburgh, Churchill Livingstone, 1989, pp 204–205.
Bick RL, Arun B et al: *Hemostasis* 29:111–134, 1999.

DIZZINESS

Dizziness is a nonspecific term commonly used to describe a variety of subjective experiences. An accurate description of what the patient means, a detailed medical history, and reproduction of the patient's symptoms by means of provocative maneuvers such as hyperventilation, Barany's maneuver, and stooping over, as well as measuring orthostatic blood pressures, help suggest the following more specific etiologic categories:

I. *Vertigo:* The illusion of self-motion or environmental motion (see Vertigo).
II. *Syncope or presyncope:* The sensation of impending faint or loss of consciousness. Causes include cardiac arrhythmia, carotid sinus hypersensivity, postural hypotension (diabetic autonomic neuropathy or side effect of antihypertensive, diuretic, dopaminergic, or other drugs), anemia, and Addison's disease (see Syncope).
III. *Disequilibrium:* Loss of balance without various subjective movement sensations of head. Causes include cerebellar or proprioceptive disturbances and muscle weakness.

IV. Dizziness that is due to causes other than those previously mentioned may be described as lightheadedness, floating, wooziness, faintness, or some other sense of altered consciousness. Causes include the following:

A. Hyperventilation syndrome. Hyperventilation is one of the most common causes of dizziness or lightheadedness. Circumoral and digital paresthesias are frequently associated. Symptoms may be reproduced during hyperventilation. Occasionally a patient has positional vertigo with hyperventilation (see Hyperventilation, Vertigo).

B. Multiple sensory deficits. Two or more of the following are usually present: visual impairment (often caused by cataracts), neuropathy, vestibular dysfunction (see Vertigo), cervical spondylosis, and orthopedic disorders that interfere with ambulation. Patients may complain of lighheadedness when walking and turning. Holding the examiner's finger lightly may provide enough additional sensory input to relieve the symptoms. Patients are often elderly or diabetic, or both.

C. Psychogenic dizziness (not associated with hyperventilation). Patients complain of vague lightheadedness, mental fuzziness, or difficulty in thinking. They may be depressed or anxious. Dizziness is usually continuous rather than episodic. Patients may state that all or none of the maneuvers performed during physical examination produce dizziness.

D. Severe anemia or polycythemia may cause symptoms of lightheadedness or dizziness.

E. Drugs may produce symptoms of dizziness that are not necessarily related to orthostatic changes in blood pressure or presyncope. These drugs include antiarrhythmics, anticonvulsants, antidepressants, antihistamines, antihypertensives, antiparkinsonian agents, hypnotics, hypoglycemics, phenothiazines, alcohol, and tobacco.

F. Endocrinologic disorders (hypoglycemia, Addison's disease, hypopituitarism, and insulinoma).

Treatment of dizziness depends on the underlying cause. For evaluation and management of vertigo, see Vertigo.

DYSARTHRIA

This disorder of speech is produced by any disturbance of the coordination of the muscles of speech. Six patterns of dysfunction have been distinguished: flaccid, spastic, ataxic, hypokinetic, hyperkinetic, and mixed. Although each has differing sound characteristics to the trained ear, it is often necessary to assess corroborating neurologic deficits such as limb ataxia, involvement of cranial nerves, or brisk jaw jerk or gag reflex to distinguish the speech patterns (ataxic, flaccid, and spastic, respectively). In acute problems producing flaccid ("slurred") speech, it is typically nonlocalizing, as dysfunction at any level from cortex to muscles can produce it.

DYSKINESIA; TARDIVE (See also THERAPEUTIC APPENDIX)

A nonspecific term that refers collectively to the abnormal involuntary movements ascribed to movement disorders. Most commonly the term is utilized to describe the involuntary *nontremorous hyperkinetic* movements associated with L-dopa and dopamine agonist and postneuroleptics (tardive dyskinesia).

DYSPHAGIA

Dysphagia—impaired swallowing—can originate from disturbances in the mouth, pharynx, or esophagus and can involve mechanical, musculoskeletal, or neurogenic mechanisms. Dysphagia can lead to superimposed problems such as inadequate nutrition, dehydration, recurrent upper respiratory infections, and frank aspiration with consequent pneumonia and even asphyxia.

Clinically, dysphagia is divided into two types, oropharyngeal and esophageal, based on characteristics of the symptoms.

I. Oropharyngeal dysphagia is manifested by difficulty in transferring food through the mouth with the following features: occurs immediately, within seconds of swallowing, repetitive swallows, coughing, choking, and nasal regurgitation. There are two important subcategories to consider in oropharyngeal dysphagia: mechanical and neurogenic/neuromuscular (please refer to the following lists).

II. Esophageal dysphagia is characterized by food "sticking in throat" after swallowing and is often localized between the neck and xiphoid process. There is delayed onset of symptoms and there may be pain. The type of esophageal dysphagia is further subdivided into categories based on whether it occurs with solid food only (mechanical) or with both solids and liquids (neurogenic/neuromuscular) (please refer to the following lists).

The four key historical questions are: (1) What types of foods cause symptoms? (2) Is the course progressive or a new onset? (3) Is there a prior history of reflux disease? (4) Is there pain with swallowing? Regurgitation of undigested food and halitosis may be clues to a Zenker's diverticulum.

Therapy for dysphagia is dependent on the specific mechanism responsible for the dysphagia, underlying etiologic disease process, and patient/family desires.

MECHANICAL DYSPHAGIA

I. Oral
   A. Amyloidosis
II. Congenital abnormalities
   A. Intraoral tumors
   B. Lip injuries (burns, trauma)

    C. Macroglossia

    D. Scleroderma

    E. Temporomandibular joint dysfunction

    F. Xerostomia (Sjögren's syndrome)

III. Pharyngeal

    A. Cervical anterior osteophytes

    B. Infection (diphtheria)

    C. Thyromegaly

    D. Retropharyngeal abscess

    E. Retropharyngeal tumor

    F. Zenker's diverticulum

IV. Esophageal

    A. Aberrant origin of the right subclavian artery

    B. Caustic injury

    C. Esophageal carcinoma

    D. Esophageal diverticulum

    E. Esophageal infection (*Candida albicans*, herpes simplex virus, cytomegalovirus, varicella-zoster virus)

    F. Esophageal intramural pseudodiverticula

    G. Esophageal stricture

    H. Esophageal ulceration

    I. Esophageal webs or rings

    J. Gastroesophageal reflux disease

    K. Hiatal hernia

    L. Metastatic carcinoma

    M. Posterior mediastinal mass

    N. Thoracic aortic aneurysm

NEUROGENIC DYSPHAGIA

I. Oropharyngeal

    A. Arnold-Chiari malformation

    B. Basal ganglia disease

        1. Biotin responsive

        2. Corticobasal degeneration

        3. Dementia with Lewy bodies

        4. Huntington's disease

        5. Multiple system atrophy

        6. Neuroacanthocytosis

        7. Parkinson's disease

        8. Progressive supranuclear palsy

        9. Wilson's disease

    C. Central pontine myelinolysis

    D. Cerebral palsy

    E. Drug-related (cyclosporine, tardive dyskinesia, vincristine)

    F. Infectious
       1. Brainstem encephalitis (*Listeria*, Epstein-Barr virus)
       2. Diphtheria
       3. Poliomyelitis
       4. Progressive multifocal leukoencephalopathy
       5. Rabies
    G. Mass lesions (abscess, hemorrhage, metastatic tumor, primary tumor)
    H. Motor neuron disease
       1. Amytrophic lateral sclerosis
    I. Multiple sclerosis
    J. Peripheral neuropathic processes
       1. Charcot-Marie-Tooth disease
       2. Guillain-Barré syndrome (Miller-Fisher variant)
    K. Spinocerebellar ataxias
    L. Stroke
    M. Syringobulbias
II. Esophageal
    A. Achalasia
    B. Autonomic neuropathies
       1. Diabetes mellitus
       2. Familial dysautonomia
       3. Paraneoplastic syndromes
    C. Basal ganglia disorders
       1. Parkinson's disease
    D. Chagas' disease
    E. Esophageal motility disorders
    F. Scleroderma

NEUROMUSCULAR DYSPHAGIA
  I. Oropharyngeal
    A. Inflammatory myopathies
       1. Dermatomyositis
       2. Inclusion body myositis
       3. Polymyositis
    B. Mitochondrial myopathies
       1. Kearns-Sayre syndrome
       2. Mitochondrial neurogastrointestinal encephalomyopathy
    C. Muscular dystrophies
       1. Duchenne's
       2. Fascioscapulohumeral
       3. Limb-girdle
       4. Myotonic
  II. Oculopharyngeal
    A. Neuromuscular junction disorders
       1. Botulism
       2. Lambert-Eaton syndrome

D

DYSPHAGIA

      3. Myasthenia gravis

      4. Tetanus

   B. Scleroderma

   C. Stiff-man syndrome

III. Esophageal

   A. Amyloidosis

   B. Inflammatory myopathies

      1. Dermatomyositis

      2. Polymyositis

   C. Scleroderma

EVALUATION OF DYSPHAGIA

Oropharyngeal Dysfunction

  I. Oral phase dysfunction

   A. Screening tests

      1. Clinical examination

      2. Cervical auscultation

      3. 3-ounce water swallow (i.e., bedside swallow test)

   B. Primary test: modified barium swallow

 II. Pharyngeal phase dysfunction

   A. Screening tests

      1. Clinical examination

      2. 3-ounce water swallow

      3. Timed swallowing

   B. Primary test: modified barium swallow

   C. Complementary tests

      1. Pharyngeal videoendoscopy

      2. Pharyngeal manometry

      3. Electromyography

      4. Videomanofluorometry

ESOPHAGEAL DYSFUNCTION

  I. Primary test

   A. Videofluoroscopy

   B. Endoscopy

 II. Complementary test: esophageal manometry

REFERENCE

Bradley WG, Daroff RB et al: *Neurology in clinical practice*, ed 4, Boston, Butterworth-Heinemann, 2004.

DYSTONIA

Dystonia is an involuntary contraction of muscle groups that manifests as a jerking or twisting movement, or *sustained* abnormal postures. Dystonia is categorized into primary and secondary forms. Primary dystonias refers to those dystonic disorders that are not associated with a presumed or known metabolic, structural, or degenerative abnormality. Primary dystonias in general are worsened with stress or anxiety and are often alleviated with rest, relaxation, or "sensory tricks," such as light touching. Acute onset of dystonia in an adult is often attributable to the initiation of neuroleptics or, less commonly, antidepressants. Hyperglycemia, hypothyroidism, hypoparathyroidism, systemic lupus erythematosus (SLE), and polycythemia rubra vera are a few of the metabolic abnormalities that can be associated with acute onset of dystonia as well as other dyskinesias. Cytologic and chemical evaluation may give a clue to other less common causes for acute onset dystonia and should be obtained in the initial investigations. One should also consider evaluation for Huntington's and Wilson's disease because of the options and implications regarding a positive diagnosis.

D

DYSTONIA

CLASSIFICATION

I. Primary generalized dystonia: idiopathic torsion dystonia (ITD)/dystonia muscularum deformans (DMD).

  Hereditary/sporadic: *DYT1* gene, chromosome 9q32-34, AD/AR, familial forms often found in Ashkenazi Jews. Deep tendon reflexes are preserved and no long tract signs are found. There is also an X-linked form Xq13.1 (*DYT3* gene), which has been described in Filipino males. Patients typically develop symptoms in late childhood involving one limb and progressing to include the other limbs, torso, and neck.

II. Periodic dystonia: AR/AD, hereditary/sporadic, dystonic symptoms precipitated by movement or startle (kinesigenic) or nonkinesigenic.

III. Focal/segmental.

  A. Meige's syndrome (cranial dystonia), orofacial/mandibular manifestations of dystonia; occurs more frequently in women.

    1. Blepharospasm: involuntary spasmodic closure of the eyelids preceded and associated with increased force and frequency of blinking.

    2. Oromandibular dystonia (lingual dystonia): jaw clenching, forced jaw opening, or tongue protrusion, painful grimacing, chewing, lip smacking.

    3. Spasmodic dysphonia (laryngeal dystonia): spasms of the laryngeal muscles that produce strained, harsh, and breathy voice.

  B. Spasmodic torticollis: dystonia limited to the neck muscles, primarily trapezius and sternocleidomastoid. Symptoms manifest as posturing of head in flexion (anterocollis), extension (retrocollis), or to the side (laterocollis) or painful phasic spasmodic alternations. *DYT7* is responsible for autosomal dominant familial torticollis.

  C. Writer's cramp: focal dystonia of the hand precipitated by writing. Symptoms may progress up the arm or include a violent tremor.

Symptoms disappear with cessation of attempt to write. This is one example of task-specific dystonia.

IV. Dystonia-plus syndromes: rapid-onset dystonia-parkinsonism, dopa-responsive dystonia, and myoclonus-dystonia.

V. Secondary dystonias: cerebral palsy, pachygyria, encephalitis, AIDS, Creutzfeldt-Jakob disease, head trauma, anoxia, stroke, multiple sclerosis, hypoparathyroidism, drug-induced (dopamine D_2 antagonists, levodopa, ergotamine, anticonvulsants), toxins (Mn, CO, cyanide, methanol, disulfiram).

VI. Psychogenic: occur in less than 5% of all dystonias.

LABORATORY EVALUATION

Preliminary laboratory evaluation for dystonia may include any of the following:

CBC with differential—wet mount to rule out acanthocytes

Chemistry panel including glucose, BUN/Cr, electrolytes including Ca^{2+}, Mg^{2+}

ESR, LFTs, PTH, thyroid tests, VDRL, ANA profile, lupus anticoagulant, anticardiolipin antibodies

Lactate, pyruvate

Serum Cu/ceruloplasmin

Cholesterol/triglycerides

Acute streptolysin, slit lamp eye examination, ECG, CT/MRI of head

Further investigation may be indicated in the childhood or adolescent onset of dystonic symptoms. Other electrophysiologic tests may be indicated if preliminary tests are inconclusive. EEG may be indicated to exclude epileptic mechanism.

TREATMENT

Treatment for dystonia remains symptomatic. In addition to correcting underlying metabolic abnormalities and deficits, certain pharmacologic therapies have proved effective. Anticholinergic agents, dopaminergic agents (*dopa-responsive dystonia*), benzodiazepines, and muscle relaxants (baclofen) have been moderately efficacious in the symptomatic relief of sustained and painful dystonias. Botulinum toxin injections have been found to be very effective in the treatment of focal dystonias. Botulinum injection needs to be repeated every 3 months, and antibodies against the toxins may develop in 5%. Tests are available commercially to detect these antibodies. Generalized dystonia responds well to stereotactic surgery, such as pallidotomy and thalamotomy.

REFERENCES

Posner JB: *Neurologic complications of cancer*, ed 2, Philadelphia, FA Davis, 1995, p 284.

Thyagarajan D: *J Clin Neurosci* 6:1–8, 1999.

E

ELECTROCARDIOGRAM

Changes in electrocardiographic rhythm and morphology may occur with acute CNS disease in the absence of other etiologies. Although most frequently reported in subarachnoid hemorrhage (SAH), ECG changes can be seen in neuromuscular disorders and muscular dystrophies, migraine, brain tumor, head injury, and stroke.

In epileptic patients, cortical stimulation of the left insula leads to bradycardia and depressor effects, but the opposite effect can be seen with right insular stimulation.

CNS disease is associated with both ventricular and supraventricular dysrhythmias. Morphologic changes include Q waves, ST elevation or depression, and U waves. *In SAH, large upright or deeply inverted T waves and prolonged QT intervals are characteristic*. These changes may be mediated by a sympathetic surge associated with hypothalamic involvement and can cause myocardial ischemia, stunning, and infarction (with CK/tropin elevations and regional wall motion abnormalities).

Abnormal cardiac rhythms, most commonly atrial fibrillation, are associated with embolic strokes. The prevalence of atrial fibrillation below age 55 years in the United States is less than 0.5%, rising to 6% for individuals older than 65 years. Conversely, stroke may lead to atrial fibrillation, brady- or tachyarrhythmias, or myocardial damage.

Patients with muscular dystrophies or mitochondrial myopathies may present with conduction abnormalities with bradycardia and heart block requiring pacemaker. Glycogen storage disease (e.g., Pompe's disease) can cause cardiomyopathy and predispose to fatal arrhythmias.

ELECTROENCEPHALOGRAPHY

The electroencephalogram is a recording of electrical activity originating from extracellular current flow in the superficial layers of cerebral cortex. This activity reflects the major influence of subcortical structures, especially the brainstem reticular formation and intralaminar and reticular nuclei of the thalamus, generating the three normal states of consciousness: waking, non-rapid eye movement (NREM) sleep, and rapid eye movement (REM) sleep. EEG is useful clinically in large part because it provides real-time information regarding brain physiology, rather than structure.

I. The normal adult waking EEG may contain the following.

A. Alpha rhythm (8 to 13 Hz) is present occipitally in nearly all adults. It appears during relaxed wakefulness with eyes closed, and attenuates with eye opening or mental effort; these characteristics distinguish it from *alpha activity*, which merely satisfies the frequency criterion (see alpha coma, below). The alpha rhythm reaches 8 Hz by about age 3 and stays at or above that frequency in the vast majority of normal elderly individuals.

B. Beta activity (>13 Hz) is a normal finding unless its amplitude consistently exceeds 25 mV, which may suggest the presence of benzodiazepines, barbiturates, or chloral hydrate. Beta is enhanced over skull defects (breach rhythm, sometimes quite "spiky" appearing) and depressed in areas of focal brain injury and over subdural, epidural, or subgaleal fluid collections.

C. Theta activity (4 to 7 Hz): Admixed and of low voltage in normal records, theta becomes more sustained and prominent during drowsiness. Normal elderly individuals may have a limited amount of shifting temporal theta. *Activity slower than 4 Hz (delta) should not be present in the waking adult record.*

D. Mu rhythm is a rhythm of alpha frequency that is located centrally, appears with eyes open, and blocks with contralateral extremity movement. It originates from sensorimotor cortex.

E. Lambda waves: These sharp, surface-negative transient waves appear over occipital regions, only with eyes open, especially upon looking at a strong visual pattern.

F. Other benign patterns appearing during waking or drowsiness include rhythmic temporal theta bursts of drowsiness (psychomotor variant), subclinical rhythmic electrographic discharge of adults (SREDA), benign epileptiform transients of sleep (BETS), positive occipital sharp transients of sleep (POSTS), 14- and 6-Hz positive bursts, 6-Hz phantom spike and wave, and wicket spikes.

G. Hyperventilation (HV) response: A physiologic increase in generalized slowing occurs with prolonged HV, particularly in children, and is accentuated with hypoglycemia. Abnormalities during HV include focal slowing or epileptiform discharges.

H. Photic stimulation response: Normal photomyoclonic responses consist of muscular contractions, typically orbicularis oculi, elicited by each flash. Abnormal photoparoxysmal responses, bursts of generalized epileptiform discharges that may outlast the flash stimuli, are indicative of generalized epilepsy or an inherited EEG trait.

II. The normal adult sleep EEG may contain the following.

A. Stage I sleep (drowsiness) is defined by dropout of the waking alpha rhythm, accentuation of frontocentral theta activity, and slow rolling eye movements. *Vertex waves*, large-amplitude, sharp, surface-negative transients maximal at the central vertex, may occur.

B. Stage II sleep is marked by the appearance of sleep spindles, rhythmic 12- to 15-Hz waves with a waxing and waning morphology, and K complexes, large biphasic sharp transients maximal over the vertex, often precipitated by external stimuli.

C. Stages III and IV sleep are defined by the presence of delta waves 2 Hz or slower, greater than 75 μV, occurring between 20% and 50% of a 30-second epoch (stage III) or over 50% (stage IV).

D. REM sleep is defined by relatively low-voltage desynchronized EEG, muscular atonia, and bursts of rapid eye movements.

III. EEG abnormalities (Fig. 15A–F)

A. Epilepsy: Interictal epileptiform activity, consisting of spikes, sharp waves, or spike-wave complexes, is strongly but not absolutely correlated with epilepsy. Thus, their presence does not unequivocally indicate a diagnosis of epilepsy, nor does their absence exclude it. Nevertheless, their presence, in combination with clinical information, frequently allows one to make a diagnosis in terms of recognized electroclinical syndromes (see Epilepsy). Ictal discharges, or electrographic seizures, provide irrefutable evidence of an epileptic seizure disorder. In generalized epilepsies, electrographic seizures may consist of a pronged run of otherwise typical interictal discharges, but in partial epilepsies this is rarely the case, and the ictal patterns have their own morphology. The absence of an ictal EEG pattern during a typical generalized convulsion provides strong evidence of a nonepileptic seizure (see Epilepsy), but this is less true for auras, focal motor or sensory seizures, and complex partial seizures.

B. Focal brain lesions: The presence of continuous, focal, polymorphic delta activity, especially in combination with depression of ipsilateral background rhythms, strongly suggests a focal lesion. However, an area of focal dysfunction, as may be seen following complicated migraine or a focal seizure, should also be considered. Periodic lateralized epileptiform discharges (PLEDs) are frequently associated with irritative lesions such as acute cerebral infarcts or encephalitis.

C. Diffuse encephalopathies: The EEG has a high sensitivity for detecting global cerebral dysfunction but is nonspecific as to etiology. Exceptions include Alzheimer's disease and HIV encephalopathy, in which the EEG may remain normal until late in the course of the disease. Early changes include slowing of the alpha rhythm and the appearance of generalized theta activity; more severe cases show generalized polymorphic delta, frontal intermittent rhythmic delta activity (FIRDA), and lack of normal reactivity. Triphasic waves are seen in hepatic or other metabolic encephalopathies and may be periodic. Other conditions associated with periodic discharges include Creutzfeldt-Jakob disease (most patients have periodic sharp discharges, occurring with a period of about 1 second, within 12 weeks of diagnosis) and subacute

E

ELECTROENCEPHALOGRAPHY

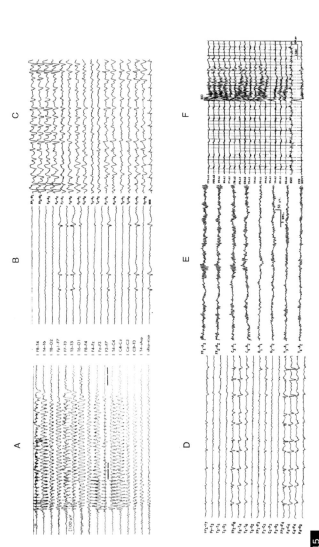

FIGURE 15

Examples of EEG abnormalities. **A,** Typical 3/sec spike and wave seen in absence seizure. **B,** Left mesial temporal epilepsy with interictal focal discharges. **C,** Triphasic waves. **D,** Periodic lateralized epileptiform discharge. **E,** Alpha coma. **F,** Burst suppression.

sclerosing panencephalitis (periodic, generalized slow waves, or sharp and slow complexes, with a period of about 5 to 10 seconds).

D. Coma: Findings include lack of normal background, reactivity, or state changes, in combination with continuous generalized polymorphic delta activity, FIRDA, low-voltage patterns, periodic discharges including PLEDs or triphasic waves, or burst-suppression pattern (bursts of electrical activity separated by periods of diffuse voltage suppression, indicative of severe diffuse cerebral dysfunction). In patients with coma following seizures, electrographic status epilepticus should be ruled out. *Alpha coma*, with generalized invariant unreactive alpha frequency activity, is associated with toxic or metabolic insults and cerebral anoxia, and must be distinguished from normal alpha rhythms present in those with a "locked-in state."

E. Brain death: Confirmatory evidence includes the demonstration of electrocerebral silence (ECS), under proper technical conditions, in the appropriate clinical context. Conditions associated with reversible ECS include overdose of CNS depressants, hypothermia, cardiovascular shock, metabolic and endocrine disorders, and very young age.

REFERENCE

Fisch BY, ed, *Fisch and Spehlmann's EEG primer: Basic principles of digital and analog EEG*, ed 3, St. Louis, Elsevier, 1999.

ELECTROLYTE DISORDERS

Symptoms are usually more severe with acute changes in electrolyte levels. Occasionally, chronic disturbances may produce signs and symptoms opposite from the acute state. In general, CNS dysfunction occurs with abnormalities of sodium, peripheral nervous system dysfunction with abnormal potassium levels, and combinations of both with abnormalities of calcium, magnesium, and phosphate. Management is directed at treatment of the primary disorder and correction of the electrolyte abnormality. Neurologic findings usually disappear with appropriate therapy (Table 38 lists signs and symptoms).

SODIUM

Sodium is the main determinant of serum osmolality (Osm) and extracellular fluid volume. Therefore, neurologic symptoms are dependent on the time lag necessary for the brain to compensate for rapid changes in serum Na^+ concentration, and thus, Osm.

I. *Hyponatremia:* Acute decreases of Na^+ levels to 130 mEq/L may produce symptoms. Chronic changes to 115 mEq/L may be asymptomatic. EEG abnormalities are common but nonspecific, with slowing that correlates with decreased Na^+ levels. Acute hyponatremia (<115 mEq/L) with seizures carries a high mortality rate and

TABLE 38

NEUROLOGIC SIGNS AND SYMPTOMS OF ELECTROLYTE DISTURBANCES

	$\downarrow Na^+$	$\uparrow Na^+$	$\downarrow K^+$	$\uparrow K^+$	$\downarrow Ca^{2+}$	$\uparrow Ca^{2+}$	$\downarrow Mg^{2+}$	$\uparrow Mg^{2+}$	Acute $\downarrow PO^{2-}_4$	Chronic $\uparrow PO_4^{2-}$
Muscle weakness	−	−	+(1)	+/−	−	+/−	+/−	+(2)	+	+(1)
Reflexes	0	0	0	0	0↑	↑	↑	↓	↓	0↑
Cognitive changes	+(3)	+(3)	−	−	+(4)	+(3)	+(4)	+(3)	+(4)	−
Seizures	+	+	−	−	+	+/−	+	−	+/−	−
Tetany	−	−	+(5)	−	+	−	+	−	−	−
Focal signs	+/−	−	−	−	−	+/−	−	−	+(6)	−
Abnormal movements	−	+(7,8,9)	−	−	−	−	+(8,9)	−	−	−
Other	A,B	B(10)		C	D	E				

(1) Proximal > distal.
(2) May be severe.
(3) Lethargy to coma.
(4) Variable or unpredictable.
(5) When associated with alkalosis.
(6) Cranial nerve palsies.
(7) Rigidity.
(8) Tremor.
(9) Myoclonus.
(10) May occur with rehydration.

(A) Cramps.
(B) Cerebral edema.
(C) Cardiac toxicity.
(D) Pseudotumor cerebri.
(E) Headache.
+ Usually present.
− Usually absent.
+/− Occasionally present.
↑ Usually increased.
↓ Usually decreased.
0 Usually normal.

necessitates rapid (over a 6-hour period) correction to 120 to 125 mEq/L (with hypertonic saline or normal saline and furosemide). *Rapid correction to levels greater than 120 to 125 mEq/L may result in central pontine myelinolysis (CPM)*, a disorder described in alcoholics but also occurring in children and adults with liver disease, severe electrolyte imbalances, malnutrition, anorexia, burns, cancer, Addison's disease, and sepsis. There is symmetrical focal myelin destruction predominantly involving the basal central pons. Asymptomatic chronic hyponatremia usually requires no immediate intervention and is managed by correction of the underlying condition.

II. *Hypernatremia:* Neurologic symptoms develop when the serum Na^+ level rises above 160 mEq/L or the serum Osm is greater than 350 mOsm/kg. Level of consciousness correlates well with the degree of hyperosmolality. Sudden increases in serum Osm may produce decreased brain cell volume, with mechanical traction on cerebral vessels causing subcortical, subdural, or subarachnoid hemorrhage. CSF protein levels may be high without pleocytosis, and the EEG is normal or mildly slowed. Hypernatremia resulting from diabetes insipidus may occur with tumors involving the hypothalamus or pineal region, as well as with basilar meningitis, encephalitis, ruptured aneurysms, sarcoidosis, trauma, or surgery.

Treatment: Isotonic solutions should be given to reduce the serum Na^+ level by no more than 1 mEq/L every 2 hours during the first 2 days of treatment. Rapid infusion of hypotonic solutions may cause cerebral edema and seizures.

POTASSIUM

Almost 60% of total body K^+ is located within muscle; therefore, predominantly muscular symptoms occur with altered K^+ levels.

I. *Hypokalemia* most commonly occurs with diuretic use but also occurs with GI losses, mineralocorticoid excess, and rarely, thyrotoxicosis. Muscle weakness usually develops with serum levels of 2.5 to 3.0 mEq/L, with structural muscle damage occurring at levels below 2.0 mEq/L. Hypokalemia and hypocalcemia frequently coexist, with cancellation of neuromuscular manifestations. Treatment of one condition in isolation may produce symptoms of the other. ECG and cardiac abnormalities are common and may require ICU monitoring and treatment.

Treatment: Increasing dietary K^+, supplements of KCl, and the use of K^+-sparing diuretics may be used to correct this imbalance.

II. *Hyperkalemia* is relatively uncommon, but may occur in familial hyperkalemic periodic paralysis (see Periodic Paralysis). Quadriparesis may develop with levels greater than 6.8 mEq/L, and levels greater than 7.0 mEq/L are life-threatening.

Treatment: Levels greater than 6.0 mEq/L require ICU monitoring and immediate therapy with administration of glucose and insulin, cation exchange resins, or calcium gluconate.

CALCIUM

Plasma Ca^{2+} is a stabilizer of excitable membranes in the central and peripheral nervous systems and in muscle. Ca^{2+} concentrations are closely controlled through the combined effects of parathyroid hormone, calciferol, and calcitonin on intestine, kidney, and bone.

I. *Hypocalcemia* is relatively rare, except in neonates, in patients with renal failure, and after thyroid or parathyroid surgery. The "tetany syndrome" originates in the peripheral nerve axon and initially becomes evident with distal and perioral tingling. Distal tonic spasms (carpopedal spasms) may progress to laryngeal stridor and opisthotonus if severe. The EEG is diffusely slow with an exaggerated response to photic stimulation. ECG abnormalities are also common.

Treatment: Oral calcium supplements are given. Tetany or seizures may require 10% IV solutions of calcium gluconate or CaCl. Underlying disorders should be corrected, if possible. Hypocalcemia often coexists with hypomagnesemia. In such cases, total serum calcium levels may be normal, but ionized calcium levels may be low.

II. *Hypercalcemia:* Malignant neoplasms are the most common cause of increased serum Ca^{2+} levels. Mental status alterations occur with total

E

ELECTROLYTE DISORDERS

serum levels greater than 14 mg/dL. Myopathy or carpal tunnel syndrome may occur in association with hyperparathyroidism.
Treatment: Saline hydration and furosemide are recommended. Occasionally, mithramycin (suppresses bone resorption) or calcitonin (suppresses bone resorption and increases urinary Ca^{2+} excretion) is required.

MAGNESIUM

Ninety-eight percent of Mg^{2+} is intracellular. Magnesium is necessary for the activation of various enzymes. Extracellular Mg^{2+} affects central and peripheral synaptic transmission. Changes in serum levels may not reflect total body stores.

I. *Hypomagnesemia* occurs most commonly as a result of excess renal loss (chronic alcoholism, diuretics), but may also be the result of decreased intake or absorption. Neurologic symptoms usually develop at levels below 0.8 mEq/L.
Treatment: The presence of seizures requires treatment with parenteral $MgSO_4$. Oral Mg^{2+} supplements may suffice in less severe cases. Calcium gluconate should be available when giving IV $MgSO_4$, as transient hypermagnesemia may cause respiratory muscle paralysis (see also hypocalcemia, above).

II. *Hypermagnesemia*, an uncommon disorder, usually occurs with increased intake and renal failure. Deep tendon reflexes may be lost at levels of 5 to 6 mEq/L, and CNS depression occurs at levels above 8 to 10 mEq/L. Muscular paralysis is due to neuromuscular blockade.
Treatment: Paralysis treatment may be accomplished by small amounts of parenteral calcium gluconate and hydration. Otherwise, discontinuation of Mg^{2+}-containing preparations is indicated. If renal function is severely impaired, dialysis may be necessary. Magnesium infusions are often given as treatment for seizures associated with eclampsia. Serum magnesium levels need to be closely monitored in this situation.

PHOSPHATE

Hypophosphatemia is often complicated by multiple abnormalities of electrolytes, nutrition, and acid-base balance. The syndrome commonly occurs in malnutrition and chronic alcoholism, especially after the infusion of glucose or hyperalimentation solutions.

Acute hypophosphatemia may not reflect decreased total body stores and may produce neurologic symptoms if severe (<1.5 mEq/L). Chronic hypophosphatemia is usually moderate (1.5 to 2.5 mEq/L) and may not be symptomatic unless acute stresses (alcohol withdrawal, burns, binding of phosphate in the gut) cause sudden decreases below the moderate level.

REFERENCE

Riggs JE: In Aminoff MJ, ed: *Neurology and general medicine*, New York, Churchill Livingstone, 2001.

ELECTROMYOGRAPHY AND NERVE CONDUCTION STUDIES

NCS and EMG examination are used to localize lesions in the peripheral nervous system, to provide insight for underlying pathophysiology of peripheral nervous system disorders, and to assess its severity and temporal course.

I. *Nerve conduction studies* are performed by recording action potentials with a surface electrode over the skin (Table 39).
   A. *Motor nerve conduction studies* involve stimulating a peripheral nerve and recording the action potential from a muscle innervated by that nerve—because this induced action potential conducts in the *same direction* as physiologic motor nerve signals, it is referred to as "orthodromic." Compound muscle action potential (CMAP) is signal recorded as results from depolarization of *all muscle fibers* innervated, hence it is termed compound.
   B. *Sensory nerve conduction studies* are usually done antidromically, by stimulating a peripheral nerve proximally and recording from a distal site innervated by that nerve; for some sensory nerves, orthodromic recording is also possible. The recorded response is called a sensory nerve action potential (SNAP).

The amplitude, duration, shape, and latency of CMAPs or SNAPs are all noted for comparison to expected normalized values or morphology. Conduction velocities are calculated for SNAPs by dividing the distance between stimulator and recording electrode by the latency of (time to) the response; for CMAPs, because the latency recorded includes not only nerve transmission velocity but also neuromuscular junction transmission time, conduction velocity is calculated by dividing (1) the *difference* in distance

TABLE 39

ROUTINE NERVE CONDUCTION STUDIES IN NEUROMUSCULAR DISORDERS

Disorder	Amplitude	Distal Latency	Conduction Velocity	F and H Wave Latencies
Polyneuropathy				
Axonal	↓	NL	>70%	Mild ↑
Demyelinating	NL or ↓	NL or ↑	<50%	↑
Myopathy	NL or ↓motor	NL	NL	NL
Radiculopathy	NL or ↓motor NL sensory	NL	>80%	NL or ↑
Neuromuscular transmission defect				
Presynaptic type	NL or ↓motor NL sensory	NL	NL	NL
Postsynaptic type	NL	NL	NL	NL
Motor neuron disease	↓ motor N1 sensory	NL	>70%	NL or ↑
Upper motor neuron disease	NL	NL	NL	NL

NL, normal.

E

between two stimulation sites (proximal and distal) by (2) the difference in latency between each site's recorded response. Normal values of nerve conduction studies vary with different physiologic factors, most importantly with temperature and age. Normal nerve conduction velocities are approximately 50 m/second in the upper limbs and 40 m/second in the lower.

    C. *Repetitive stimulation and exercise versus rest* may also be studied in special circumstances. Repetitive stimulation focuses on the change in the CMAP amplitude, if any, that results from stimulating the motor nerve multiple times repeatedly, and is useful in diagnosis of disorders of the neuromuscular junction. With slow (3 Hz) repetitive stimulation, which creates progressive decrease in the number of acetylcholine (Ach) vesicles released from the presynaptic terminal, more than a 10% amplitude decrement is often seen in both myasthenia gravis and Lambert-Eaton myasthenic syndrome (LEMS). With fast (50 Hz) stimulation, which causes accumulation of calcium in the presynaptic nerve terminal and results in increased numbers of ACh vesicles being released, over 100% increment can be seen in LEMS (or also, rarely, botulism); this increment is not seen in myasthenia gravis. The order of testing in suspected neuromuscular junction disease is therefore typically first slow then fast repetitive stimulation. These studies are challenging to perform: acetylcholinesterase medications must be withheld, tissue temperature carefully attended to, and for anatomic and technical reasons the study is usually done on facial nerve and musculature or the spinal accessory nerve and trapezius; lastly, 50 Hz stimulation is quite painful.

    D. *The F wave* (or F response) is a "late response" that occurs after a CMAP. This potential results from antidromic conduction of the stimulus up the motor nerve, a resulting discharge ("backfiring") of a small population of alpha motor neuron cell bodies in the spinal cord, and subsequent orthodromic conduction of a motor nerve potential back down the nerve to the muscle. It is recorded as a second CMAP following the first, and is of much lower amplitude. Whereas the initial direct CMAP (the M wave) depends only on the segment between stimulator and recorder, the late response (F wave) depends on the whole length of the nerve—in fact, it is conducted along the length of the nerve *twice*. The latency of the F wave is usually 25 to 32 ms in the upper limbs and 45 to 56 ms in the lower. *In theory, F waves are prolonged by any pathology involving the motor nerve, such radiculopathies, entrapment neuropathies, and hereditary or metabolic polyneuropathies; in practice, F waves have their greatest usefulness in detecting early polyradiculopathies such as in Guillain-Barré syndrome, in which prolonged F waves may be the only detectable abnormalities early on.*

    E. *The H wave* (H response or H reflex) is the other clinically recordable late response. It is the result of a monosynaptic reflex arc:

orthodromic sensory conduction up the nerve, synaptic transmission from the stimulated sensory neurons to a population of alpha motor neurons, firing of those motor neurons as in a muscle stretch reflex, and orthodromic motor conduction to the muscles. For practical and anatomic reasons, the only routinely recordable H reflex is in the S1 segment, recorded after tibial nerve stimulation. Typical latency is 30 ms. As with the clinical analog, the ankle jerk, loss of the H reflex is nonspecific—it can be simply a function of age (it is normally absent over age 60), and it can result from a very large number of disorders.

II. *The EMG needle examination* records electrical activity in muscle, yielding more information on the localization and pathophysiology of peripheral nervous system disorders. Whereas nerve conduction studies record from entire nerves at once and cannot study individual neurons, EMG records from a single muscle, and from only a few muscle fibers within that muscle, at once. An EMG evaluation requires the examiner to carefully select the muscles to be examined on basis of the clinical question remaining after history, physical examination, and nerve conduction studies. The electromyographic needle examination records electrical activity in muscle, yielding more information on the localization and pathophysiology of the peripheral nervous system disorders. For each of the muscles being studied, the first part of the examination is to access insertional and spontaneous activity at rest. Once the insertional and spontaneous activity has been accessed, the examiner will ask the patient to slowly contract the muscle, and the motor unit action potentials (MUAPs) are evaluated. MUAPs are accessed for duration, amplitudes, and numbers of phases. Then, the number of MUAPs and their relationship to the firing frequency (recruitment and activation pattern) are evaluated. The information is obtained in specific order by the electromyographer, as follows:

INSERTIONAL ACTIVITY

Insertional activity occurs when a needle is quickly moved through the muscle and creates depolarization of muscle fiber in a brief burst for several hundred milliseconds; activities lasting longer than 300 ms indicate increased insertional activity. Increased insertional activity may be seen in neuropathic disorders that result in denervation and several myopathic conditions that result in necrosis of the muscle fibers, such as inflammatory myopathies. It is decreased in periodic paralysis during paralytic phases and when normal muscle tissue is replaced by fibrous tissue.

SPONTANEOUS ACTIVITY

Recognition of abnormal spontaneous activity can provide helpful information for the diagnosis:

1. The distribution of abnormal spontaneous activity may suggest the neuroanatomic localization of the lesion (e.g., mononeuropathy, radiculopathy).

2. Certain types of spontaneous activity are associated with specific disorders, for example, myotonic discharges in myotonic dystrophy and hyperkalemic periodic paralysis (see below).
3. The amount of spontaneous activity or the presence of spontaneous activity may provide information regarding the time course and severity of the lesion (e.g., presence of fibrillation potential is seen beginning 2 to 3 weeks after the acute nerve injury).

I. Abnormal spontaneous activity originating from muscle fibers

A. *Fibrillation potentials* (brief, regular-firing, muscle fiber action potentials) and *positive sharp waves* (longer duration with initial positive deflection, regular-firing, muscle fiber action potentials) are due to spontaneous depolarization of the muscle fibers and are electrophysiologic markers of denervation. They typically occur 2 to 3 weeks after denervation in neurogenic disorders (neuropathies, radiculopathies, motor neuron disease, etc.). They may also be seen in muscle disorders, especially in inflammatory myopathy and muscular dystrophies, and can rarely be seen in severe disorders of the neuromuscular junction, as in botulism.

B. *Complex repetitive discharges* (high-frequency, regular-firing, multiserrated repetitive discharges with abrupt onset and termination, creating a characteristic "machine-like" sound) result from the depolarization of a single muscle fiber followed by ephaptic spread to adjacent denervated fibers. This occurs in a wide variety of chronic neurogenic disorders (poliomyelitis, motor neuron disease, radiculopathies, neuropathies) and myopathic disorders (Duchenne and limb-girdle dystrophy, polymyositis, hypothyroidism).

C. *Myotonic discharges* are also spontaneous discharges of a muscle fiber characterized by a waveform with waxing and waning amplitude and frequency, creating a "dive bomber" sound on the recording. They are typically seen in myotonic dystrophy, myotonia congenita, paramyotonia congenita, hyperkalemic periodic paralysis, acid maltase deficiency, diazocholesterol toxicity, clofibrate toxicity, and rarely in polymyositis and colchicine toxicity.

II. Abnormal spontaneous activity originating from the motor unit

A. *Fasciculation potentials* are random single spontaneous discharges from the individual motor unit. On EMG, fasciculations have the morphology of simple MUAP or they can be complex and large if they represent a pathologic motor unit. They are most common in chronic neurogenic disorders (motor neuron disease, peripheral neuropathies, radiculopathies, entrapment neuropathies). Fasciculations may also be seen in normal individuals.

B. *Myokymic discharges* are rhythmic, grouped, spontaneous repetitive discharges of the same motor unit. They may be recorded in facial muscles (facial myokymia) associated with brainstem lesions from multiple sclerosis, brainstem glioma, or vascular disease. Appendicular myokymia is associated with radiation plexopathy.

Rarely, it may be seen in Guillain-Barré syndrome, radiculopathy, chronic entrapment neuropathy, and gold toxicity.

C. *Neuromyotonia* is high-frequency (150 to 250 Hz) decrementing, repetitive discharges of a single motor unit that create a characteristic "pinging" sound on EMG recording. These are rare and are seen only with chronic neuropathic diseases (e.g., poliomyelitis and adult-onset spinal muscular atrophy) and syndromes of continuous motor unit activity, such as in Isaac's syndrome.

D. *Cramp potential* is a painful involuntary muscle contraction that tends to occur with a muscle in shortened position or contracting. Electrically, cramps are high-frequency discharges of motor units. Cramps occur commonly in normal individuals and in many neurogenic and metabolic disorders, including electrolyte imbalances, hypothyroidism, pregnancy, and uremia (see Cramps).

III. Voluntary motor unit potentials: The pattern of MUAP abnormalities will allow determination of whether the disorder is a neuropathic or a myopathic process and often helps to ascertain the time course and severity of the lesion. Assessment of MUAP can be divided into two parts.

A. Morphology

1. *Short-duration, small-amplitude MUAPs* occur in disorders with atrophy or loss of muscle fibers in the motor unit. Thus, they are present in all myopathic disorders and in severe cases of neuromuscular transmission disorders (e.g., botulism). In early reinnervation, after severe denervation in which the newly sprouting axons only begin to reinnervate a few muscle fibers, the MUAP will also be small, short duration, and polyphasic but with reduced recruitment ("nascent" MUAP).

2. *Long-duration, large-amplitude MUAPs* occur with increased number or density of muscle fibers, or a loss of synchrony of fiber firing within a motor unit such as in chronic neuropathic processes (e.g., motor neuron disease, chronic radiculopathies, chronic axonal neuropathies, and chronic entrapment neuropathy).

3. *Polyphasic MUAPs* (≥5 phases). Polyphasia is a measure of synchrony of the firing of muscle fibers within the same motor unit. This is a nonspecific measure and may be abnormal in both myopathic and neurogenic disorders. Increased polyphasia may be seen in up to 5% to 10% of the MUAPs in any muscle and still be normal.

4. *Unstable MUAPs* are fluctuations of amplitude, duration, or shape of a given motor unit potential from moment to moment, and are usually due to blocking of individual muscle fiber action potentials in the motor unit. This may be seen in disorders of neuromuscular transmission, myositis, muscle trauma, reinnervation, and rapidly progressive neurogenic atrophy.

E

ELECTROMYOGRAPHY AND NERVE CONDUCTION STUDIES

B. Recruitment and activation
1. *Recruitment* refers to the relation of firing rate of individual potentials to the total number of motor units firing. *Decreased recruitment* (small number of units firing with a high frequency) occurs when there is a decreased number of available motor units; the remaining motor units will fire at a faster frequency to increase the muscle force as in any *neurogenic disorder or severe myopathy*. *Early recruitment* (an excess of motor units for a given force) occurs in myopathies; when the force generated by each individual motor unit is decreased, more motor units are recruited to generate the same amount of force.
2. *Activation* refers to the ability to increase the firing rate, which is a central process. Poor activation of motor unit action potentials (small number of units firing slowly) is generally due to *upper motor neuron lesions or lack of effort*.

REFERENCES

Katirji B: *Electromyography in clinical practice: A case study approach*, St. Louis, Mosby, 1998.

Preston DC, Shapiro BE: *Electromyography and neuromuscular disorders: Clinical-electrophysiologic correlations*, Boston, Butterworth-Heinemann, 1998.

ENCEPHALITIS

An inflammation of the brain related to infectious, postinfectious, or demyelinating states, encephalitis can occur as an acute febrile illness associated with headache, seizures, lethargy, confusion, coma, ocular motor palsies, ataxia, abnormal movements, and myoclonus. Alternatively it may present as a slowly progressive afebrile disease. With viral infections, the meninges (meningoencephalitis) or the spinal cord (encephalomyelitis) is often involved. Compared to the high frequency of systemic viral infection, encephalitis is an uncommon complication. Prognosis of viral encephalitis depends upon the causative agent and the use of antiviral agents. Variable degrees of residual effects include impaired cognition and memory, behavioral changes, hemiparesis, or seizures. Transmission of viruses can be from humans (e.g., HIV), animals (e.g., rabies), mosquitoes (e.g., St. Louis and Japanese encephalitis), ticks (e.g., Central European encephalitis), or other arthropods. Endemic causes in the United States are herpes simplex, West Nile virus (WNV), and rabies. Japanese B encephalitis is the most common epidemic infection outside North America. Arthropod-born viruses (arboviruses) can be sporadic or epidemic. Viruses enter the CNS by one of two routes—hematogenous (most common) or neuronal. Risk factors are summarized in Table 40.

Diagnosis sometimes is made by history alone (Table 41 discusses the diagnostic workup). The season may help determine the pathogen. CSF usually shows a pleocytosis (mostly mononuclear cells) and mildly elevated protein.

TABLE 40	
RISK FACTORS FOR ENCEPHALITIS	
Risk Factor	**Suspected Pathogen**
Mosquito bites	Alphavirus Western equine, Eastern equine, Venezuelan equine
	Flavivirus: St. Louis, West Nile
	Bunyavirus: La Crosse, California
Tick bite (Apr-June and Oct to Nov)	Colorado tick fever, Powassan virus, Anaplasma (aka *Ehrlichia*), Rocky Mountain spotted fever, tick-borne encephalitis, Lyme disease (borreliosis, spirochete)
Raccoon feces	*Baylisascaris procyonis*
Wild/domestic animals	Leptospirosis
Bats	Rabies
Pigs	Nipah virus
Cats	*Bartonella hensalae*
Rodents	Lymphochoriomeningitis virus
Sheep/goats	Q fever
Travel	
Asia	Japanese encephalitis, Nipah virus
Europe	Tick-borne encephalitis
Africa	Lassa fever
Illness-exposures	
	Chickenpox
	Measles
	Influenza
	Mycoplasma pneumonia
Fresh water	*Naegleria fowleri,* leptospirosis
Soil	*Balamuthia mandrillaris*
Vaccination	Measles-mumps-rubella, vaccinia
Season	
Spring/summer	Mosquito-borne, tick-borne
Drug use, other HIV risk factor	AIDS encephalitis
Other systemic illness	Evaluate as needed for neoplastic and rheumatologic disease

Adapted from Encephalitis. *Pediatr Rev* 26:353–363. 2005.

E

ENCEPHALITIS

Glucose tends to be normal. RBCs can be found in certain types of encephalitis (e.g., herpes simplex). Acute and convalescent antibody levels from serum and CSF typically are only useful retrospectively. PCR testing facilitates the identification of causative agents.

VIRAL ENCEPHALITIS

I. Herpes simplex encephalitis (HSV type 1) is the most common cause of fatal viral encephalitis in the Western world. Most cases represent reactivation of latent trigeminal ganglion infection. HSV-2 causes most cases of encephalitis in newborns. The risk of intrapartum transmission

<table>
<tbody>
</tbody>
</table>

TABLE 41

SUGGESTED LABORATORY TESTING FOR ENCEPHALITIS AND ITS MIMICS

CEREBROSPINAL FLUID

Glucose, protein, cell count, differential count

Routine bacterial culture

Viral culture

Herpes simplex virus polymerase chain reaction (PCR)

Cryptococcal antigen

Enteroviral PCR

Mycoplasma PCR

Tuberculosis culture and PCR

Epstein-Barr virus PCR

West Nile virus IgM

BLOOD

Bartonella henselae IgG

Epstein-Barr virus serology panel

Lyme IgG (in endemic areas if cranial neuropathy present)

Mycoplasma IgM

West Nile virus IgM (during mosquito season)

La Crosse virus IgM (in endemic areas, during mosquito season)

Complete blood count, differential count

Serum to be saved for comparison with convalescent specimen

NEUROIMAGING

Head CT

MRI with seizure protocol

NEUROPHYSIOLOGY

EEG

Evoked potentials

EMG (suspected Lyme disease or demyelinating disease)

OTHER

Viral cultures of nasopharynx and stool

Purified protein derivative skin test

Brain biopsy rarely necessary as a last resort (usually low yield)

Adapted from Encephalitis. *Pediatr Rev* 26:353–363. 2005.

is 30% to 50% in primary maternal infection and less than 3% with recurrent infection.

Clinical presentation consists of subacute onset with fever, headache, behavioral changes, seizures, focal signs, and later stupor and coma.

Diagnosis and evaluation: EEG usually shows periodic lateralizing epileptiform discharges (PLEDs) between the 2nd and 15th days of the illness. Spikes and slow waves are common and are often localized to the temporal lobe. CT scan, although less sensitive than EEG, may show temporal or insular low densities and focal hemorrhages or enhancement. MRI is the neuroimaging procedure of choice and may show increased signal intensity on T_2-weighted image in the medial and inferior temporal lobe extending to the insula. CSF usually shows 5 to 500 cells, elevated protein, normal or mildly decreased glucose, and elevated opening pressure. RBCs may be seen. Antibodies to HSV are detected in the CSF 8 to 12 days after onset of the disease and increase during the first 2 to 4 weeks. Viral cultures are not useful. PCR is greater than 95% sensitive and 100% specific. False-negative results may occur if there are RBCs in the CSF to inhibit PCR or if CSF is collected in the first 24 to 48 hours of symptoms or after 10 days of onset. Brain biopsy should be considered in those who do not respond to therapy or in whom other diagnoses are possible.

Treatment with acyclovir, 10 mg/kg q 8 hr for 2 to 3 weeks, significantly reduces risks of morbidity and death, especially if started early. Acyclovir-resistant HSV infection has been identified in immunodeficient patients.

Prognosis: If untreated, the mortality rate is about 70%, with severe neurologic sequelae in most of the survivors.

II. Rabies: Carriers include skunks, foxes, dogs, bats, and raccoons. The virus is present in saliva and is transmitted by bite. Incubation is from days to months. Not everyone bitten by rabid animals contracts the disease. However, once the infection is established, death almost invariably occurs (usually within 18 days). The prodrome usually consists of headache, malaise, agitation, mental changes, seizures, dysphagia (causing hydrophobia), dysarthria, facial numbness, and spasm. The medulla and pons are most frequently and extensively involved, and paralysis may be secondary to spinal cord involvement.

Treatment consists of mechanically scrubbing wound sites with soap and benzalkonium solution and administering human rabies immunoglobulin or human diploid cell line rabies vaccine. Death is invariable once CNS manifestations occur.

III. Epidemic encephalitis is mostly arthropod transmitted. Peak incidence occurs in late summer and fall. In the United States, St. Louis encephalitis and La Crosse virus (California encephalitis) are the most common. St. Louis encephalitis is found in the Ohio-Mississippi River basin, with 10% to 20% fatality rate. *The La Crosse virus is the most common cause of pediatric arboviral encephalitis.* Venezuelan equine encephalitis is found in the southeastern United States and has a low mortality rate; most infections result in flu-like illnesses. Eastern equine encephalitis occurs along the Gulf of Mexico and Atlantic seaboard, usually affects horses and birds, and is rare among humans. It has 25% to 70% mortality rate, attacking the young and very old with fulminant course. Western equine encephalitis occurs in west, southwest, and central North America. Treatment is aimed at brain edema and seizures. *West Nile virus* is a flavivirus that has birds as a reservoir and is transmitted by mosquitoes. It is endemic in the Middle East, Africa, and southwest Asia. Clinically it is characterized by abrupt onset of flu-like illness. A maculopapular rash occurs in half of the patients.

E

ENCEPHALITIS

Meningitis or encephalitis is most common in older individuals and happens in less than 15% of patients. *Diagnosis* is by PCR or CSF culture, or identification of antibody in the serum and CSF. WNV was first identified in the United States in New York in 1999 and an increase in the death of birds, particularly crows, can be observed during an outbreak. There is no specific treatment, and death may occur in older individuals.

IV. Nonepidemic viral encephalitis: *Enterovirus*, echovirus, coxsackievirus, poliovirus, measles, mumps, Epstein-Barr virus (EBV), rubella, varicella-zoster virus (VZV), and lymphocytic choriomeningitis virus can all cause sporadic encephalitis.

   A. Slow latent viral infections cause slowly progressive disease with insidious onset and lack of fever. These include subacute sclerosing panencephalitis (SSPE), a form of chronic measles virus infection, progressive multifocal leukoencephalopathy (see PML below), and progressive rubella panencephalitis. SSPE has had dramatically decreased prevalence in countries with widespread use of the measles vaccine, but prevalence has increased with the occurrence of AIDS. Usually occurring in children or young adults, onset is insidious, with changes in cognition, vision, and behavior. Malaise and lethargy are common. Myoclonus can occur. Deterioration progresses over weeks to months, with patients becoming markedly demented. CSF shows a mild pleocytosis, increased protein, and occasionally decreased glucose. Neuroimaging shows generalized cortical atrophy. The EEG pattern of periodic discharges is characteristic. Pathologic studies show changes suggestive of viral invasion of gray and white matter, with the hypothalamus and brainstem usually not involved.

   B. AIDS and immune deficiency-related encephalitis. PML caused by a papovavirus designated JC virus (not associated with Creutzfeldt-Jakob disease), usually occurs in patients with lymphoproliferative (leukemia, lymphoma) or granulomatous disease, or during immunosuppression. It is characterized by multifocal white matter signs, such as impaired speech, vision, and cognition, progressing to death in 1 to 18 months. PCR for JC virus in CSF has a sensitivity of 72% to 92% and specificity of 92% to 96%. MRI shows multifocal white matter lesions. Encephalitis in immunosuppressed patients may also be caused by VZV, HSV-1, EBV, human herpesvirus (HHV-6), cytomegalovirus (CMV), measles virus, or enterovirus. In VZV encephalitis, patients may have a history of shingles for days or months previously. Encephalitis CMV is rare in immunocompetent individuals, and a combination of ganciclovir and foscarnet has been used in treatment.

NONVIRAL ENCEPHALITIS OR ENCEPHALOMYELITIS

I. Prion infections: Prion (proteinaceous infectious particle) diseases are sometimes confused with encephalitides, but they are slowly progressive with insidious onset and absence of fever. They include Creutzfeldt-Jakob disease, Gerstmann-Sträussler-Scheinker syndrome, and kuru (see Creutzfeldt-Jakob Disease).

II. *Rickettsia*: epidemic, murine and scrub typhus, Rocky Mountain spotted fever, and Q fever infections.

III. Bacteria: *Listeria* infection, brucellosis, pertussis, legionnaires' disease, tuberculosis, tularemia, typhoid fever, bubonic plague, dysentery, cholera, melioidosis, psittacosis, leprosy, scarlet fever, rheumatic fever.

IV. Spirochetes: relapsing fever, syphilis (meningovascular), rat-bite fever, leptospirosis, Lyme disease.

V. Protozoa/metazoa: *Entamoeba*, *Naegleria*, trypanosomiases, leishmaniasis, malaria, toxoplasmosis.

VI. Helminthic: ancylostomiasis, angiostrongyliasis, ascariasis, cysticercosis, echinococcosis, filariasis, schistosomiasis, toxocariasis, trichinosis.

VII. Miscellaneous: Behçet's disease, CNS Whipple's disease, vasculitis, Rasmussen's syndrome (chronic focal encephalitis).

POSTINFECTIOUS ENCEPHALOMYELITIS

This may follow a CNS or systemic viral infection, nonviral infection, or immunization. In the United States, varicella and upper respiratory infections (especially influenza) are most commonly associated, whereas worldwide it most commonly follows measles. A disturbance of the immune system is the presumed cause, with an irreversible monophasic, demyelinating syndrome. Limited CNS forms may include acute transverse myelitis, acute cerebellitis, and postinfectious optic neuritis. Acute hemorrhagic encephalitis (Hurst's disease) is a severe and usually fatal form. The clinical symptoms and CSF profile are similar to that seen during direct viral infections. *Treatment* is with high doses of intravenous methylprednisolone. Acyclovir and ganciclovir are used if encephalitis by VZV and HHV-6 are in the differential diagnosis.

REFERENCES

Lewis P, Glaser CA: *Pediatr Rev* 26:353–363, 2005.
Marra CM: *Semin Neurol* 20:323–327, 2000.
Roos KL: *Neurol Clin* 17:813–833, 1999.
Steiner I, Budka H, Chaudhuri A et al: *Eur J Neurol* 12:331–343, 2005.

ENCEPHALOPATHY

Encephalopathy is a nonspecific term for diffuse brain dysfunction, usually the result of a systemic condition. Initially, there is impaired attention, confusion, and disorientation. Later, there may be progression to stupor and coma, or it may present as coma of unknown cause. Associated features may include agitation, hallucination, myoclonus, asterixis, generalized seizures, or EEG slowing or triphasic waves. Additional

E

ENCEPHALOPATHY

evaluation should include review of recent medications, metabolic screening, consideration of systemic or CNS infection, and neuroimaging.

ENCEPHALOPATHY, PERINATAL HYPOXIC-ISCHEMIC

Hypoxic-ischemic encephalopathy (HIE) is caused by either diminished oxygen delivery or diminished brain perfusion. Timing of insult may be antepartum (20%; maternal cardiac arrest or hemorrhage), intrapartum (35%; abruptio placentae, uterine rupture, or traumatic delivery), both (35%; maternal diabetes mellitis or infection, intrauterine growth retardation), or postnatal (10%; cardiovascular compromise, persistent fetal circulation, recurrent apnea; more common in premature infants).

CLINICAL FEATURES
The signs of HIE correlate with the severity of the insults. Mild encephalopathy lasts less then 24 hours. It is characterized by hyperalertness or by mild depression of the level of consciousness, which may be accompanied by uninhibited Moro and deep tendon reflexes, signs of sympathetic overdrive, or only slightly abnormal EEG. Infants with moderate to severe encephalopathy show variation in level of alertness in the first 12 to 24 hours. Seizures occur in 70% of these infants during this period. Coma may supervene and progress to brain death by 72 hours. If the infant survives, marked hypotonia and bulbar and autonomic dysfunction persist. Term infants may demonstrate quadriparesis with predominant proximal and arm weakness. This pattern represents involvement of border zones of circulation between the cerebral arteries (ACA-MCA and MCA-PCA). Premature infants manifest spastic diplegia primarily due to injury of motor fibers to the leg that lie dorsal and lateral to the external angles of the lateral ventricles.

NEUROPATHOLOGY
Patterns of injury are influenced by the nature of the insult and the gestational age of the infant at the time of injury. Patterns that occur in term infants include selective neuronal necrosis (CA1 region of hippocampus, deep layers of cerebral cortex, and cerebellar Purkinje fibers), status marmoratus of basal ganglia and thalamus, parasagittal cerebral injury, and focal and multifocal ischemic brain injury. Periventricular leukomalacia (PVL) represents the primary ischemic lesion of the premature infant.

DIAGNOSTIC TESTS
In preterm infants, head ultrasound (HUS) demonstrates periventricular echoes in the first day or two. After 1 to 3 weeks, lateral ventricles enlarge as these areas become cystic and gliosis supervenes. HUS in the term infant is especially accurate when used consecutively in the first weeks of life. Compared to HUS, MRI visualizes HIE injuries of basal ganglia better.

Diffusion-weighted sequence on MRI detects focal cerebral ischemic injury very early in its course.

MANAGEMENT
Supportive care includes ensuring adequate oxygenation and perfusion, and seizure control.

PROGNOSIS
Predictors of poor neurologic outcome include (1) acidosis at birth, (2) persistent moderate or severe HIE, (3) neonatal seizures, (4) interictal background abnormalities such as burst-suppression, persistently low-voltage or electrocerebral inactivity, (5) HUS findings of periventricular intraparenchymal echodensities, and (6) extensive brain edema with effacement of cerebral cortex on MRI.

REFERENCE
Rivkin MJ: *Clin Perinatol* 24:607–625, 1997.

ENDOVASCULAR TREATMENT OF ANEURYSMS

Electrolytically detachable platinum coils (Guglielmi detachable coils, GDCs) have been FDA approved for treatment of intracranial aneurysms since 1995. Embolization requires placement of a microcatheter within the aneurysm itself, the coils are then passed through the catheter, filling the aneurysm lumen, and excluding the aneurysm from the arterial blood flow. The coil is composed of a tight spiral (like a Slinky) of platinum wire, which forms a circle with a predetermined diameter and length when deployed. The coils are available in a variety of sizes, lengths, and shapes. Bioactive coatings on the coils may promote endothelialization across the base of the coil mass, further excluding the aneurysm from the blood flow.

Aneurysm recurrence, either by true enlargement or by coil compaction, depends on the aneurysm size, neck width, and location. Complete embolization of small aneurysms with necks less than 4 mm wide approaches 80% to 90%, with only a tiny neck remnant in most of the remaining aneurysms. In contrast, only 20% to 40% of giant aneurysms are completely embolized during the initial treatment. Incomplete embolization may require repeat treatments. Temporary balloon or permanent stent placement across the aneurysm neck allows treatment of wide-necked aneurysms by preventing coil herniation into the parent artery. These techniques may also allow tighter packing of the aneurysm, reducing their recurrence rate. Higher recurrence rates occur in aneurysms directly in line with the blood stream, such as basilar apex and MCA bifurcation aneurysms. This is from the constant "water hammer" effect on the coil mass. Rerupture of aneurysms in patients presenting with SAH following embolization is about 1% to 3%.

The risk of a major complication during embolization is 6% or less. Intraprocedural rupture occurs in 1% to 2% of embolizations and is treated by further coiling or parent artery sacrifice; 50% of these patients have no significant change in their status, but marked deterioration or death occurs in the other 50%. Intra-arterial thrombus/stroke and parent artery occlusion have an approximate 2% rate each. Intravascular thrombus can be treated with Absciximab (GP IIb/IIIa inhibitor). Significant coil herniation may require balloon remodeling or intra-arterial stent placement to either reposition the coils within the aneurysm, or trap the coils against the vessel wall. Regardless, 6 to 12 weeks of antiplatelet therapy such as Plavix and ASA should be given in this situation.

REFERENCE

International Subarachnoid Aneurysm Trial (ISAT) Collaborative Group: *Lancet* 360: 1267–1274, 2002 and 366:809–817, 2005.

EPILEPSY AND WOMEN (See also CATAMENIAL EPILEPSY, EPILEPSY AND AAN GUIDELINE SUMMARIES APPENDIX)

Epilepsy raises special concerns for women and their clinicians. Hormones alter expression of seizures and can alter a woman's response to antiepileptic drugs (AEDs). For example, pregnant women who have epilepsy have considerations in terms of drug metabolism and teratogenicity. Menopausal women with epilepsy have specific needs such as bone health and changes in weight. Women with epilepsy require tailored care throughout their reproductive cycle.

Women with epilepsy are at increased risk for the following:
 I. Increased frequency of anovulatory menstrual cycles
 II. Abnormal menstrual length
 III. Greater prevalence of polycystic ovarian disease
 IV. Sexual dysfunction
 V. Higher incidence of miscarriages and pregnancy-related complications
 VI. Seizures, which disrupt the cortical regulation of the hypothalamic hormone release, changing the secretory pattern of the pituitary gland, and altering the release of hormones from peripheral sites

CHECKLIST FOR WOMEN WITH EPILEPSY
 I. Be alert to possibility of catamenial epilepsy
 II. Take menstrual history and keep menstrual diary
 III. Ensure adequate daily intake of calcium and vitamin D
 IV. Provide contraceptive counseling and advise barrier method of contraception
 V. Prescribe an oral contraceptive pill (OCP) with 50 μg of estrogen
 VI. Advise prophylactic intake of folic acid 4 to 5 mg/day for women on AEDs of child-bearing age

CONTRACEPTION

I. Women with epilepsy have a high risk for failure of hormonal contraception due to the action of AEDs. Failure rate in women with epilepsy may exceed 6% per year (versus nonepilepsy failure rate of <3%) related to AED enzyme induction reducing efficacy of OCPs.

II. Recommendations for contraception and epilepsy:

A. The 1998 recommendation by AAN advises estradiol dose of 50 µg for 21 days of each cycle.

B. If breakthrough bleeding occurs, then patient should use a barrier method in addition to above.

C. Barrier method is recommended, regardless of bleeding.

D. Norplant and transdermal patch have a higher failure rate.

E. IM medroxyprogesterone needs to be dosed at 8- to 10-week intervals.

PRENATAL CARE

I. Adequate prenatal screening for patients on AEDs

II. Neural tube defect (NTD) screening with serum α-fetoprotein at 15 to 22 weeks

III. Structural ultrasound at 16 to 20 weeks

IV. Offer amniocentesis

V. Ultrasound of fetal heart at 18 to 20 weeks

VI. Folic acid 4 to 5 mg/day for all women of childbearing years

DURING PREGNANCY

I. Measure free AED concentrations and adjust AED dose to maintain stable free AED concentrations (Table 42)

II. Give AED in divided doses when required at high doses to minimize high peak drug concentrations

III. Ensure vitamin K 10 mg/day in final 4 weeks of pregnancy to reduce the risk of neonatal hemorrhage

TABLE 42

CHANGE IN PHARMACOKINETICS OF SELECTED ANTIEPILEPTIC DRUG (AED) DURING PREGNANCY

AED	Reported Inc.Clearance[*]	Reported Dec. in Conc.	Dec.Free Conc.
Lamotrigine	65–230%	—	—
Phenytoin	20–100%	55–61%	18–31%
Carbamazepine	0–20%	0–42%	0–28%
Phenobarbital	—	55%	50%
Primidone	—	55%	—
Valproic acid	35–183%	50%	25–30%[†]

[*]Clearance of almost all AEDs increase during pregnancy. Most AED levels normalize during the first 2 to 3 months post partum

[†]Decreases only during first two trimesters; levels increase or normalize by delivery.

POSTPARTUM CARE
I. Breastfeeding infants are monitored for signs of sedation and poor feeding.
II. Vigilance is needed regarding change in AED levels and sleep deprivation.
III. Precautions to ensure mother and child safety (AEDs and breastfeeding):
   A. The concentrations of AEDs in breast milk are lower than those in maternal serum.
   B. Infant's serum concentration, based on this factor and the AED elimination half-life in neonates, is more prolonged than in adults.
   C. Benefits of AEDs outweigh adverse effects.
   D. Parents should look for lethargy and delayed milestones.

MENOPAUSAL
I. Bone health
II. Measure calcium, vitamin D, PTH
III. Bone density scan first visit and every 2 years thereafter

EPILEPSY (See also AAN GUIDELINE SUMMARIES, NEUROLOGIC EMERGENCY, and THERAPEUTIC APPENDICES)

DEFINITIONS AND CLASSIFICATIONS
The epilepsies are a group of conditions marked by recurrent seizures, which are the clinical manifestations of abnormal brain electrical discharges. Epileptic seizures are classified as focal (partial, local), beginning in a part of one hemisphere; *generalized*, beginning bilaterally; or *unclassified* as to focal or generalized. Focal seizures that subsequently evolve to generalized seizures are said to exhibit secondary generalization.

INTERNATIONAL CLASSIFICATION OF EPILEPTIC SEIZURES
I. Partial
   A. Simple partial seizures
      1. With motor signs
      2. With somatosensory or special sensory symptoms
      3. With autonomic symptoms or signs
      4. With psychic symptoms
   B. Complex partial seizures
      1. Simple partial onset
      2. With impairment of consciousness at onset
   C. Partial seizures evolving to secondarily generalized seizures
      1. Simple partial seizures evolving to generalized seizures
      2. Complex partial seizures evolving to generalized seizures
      3. Simple partial seizures evolving to complex partial seizures evolving to generalized seizures

II. Generalized seizures (convulsive or nonconvulsive)
- A. Absence seizures
  - 1. Typical absence
  - 2. Atypical absence
- B. Myoclonic seizures
- C. Clonic seizures
- D. Tonic seizures
- E. Tonic-clonic seizures
- F. Atonic seizures (astatic seizures)

III. Unclassified seizures

REVISED INTERNATIONAL CLASSIFICATION OF EPILEPSIES, EPILEPTIC SYNDROMES, AND RELATED SEIZURE DISORDERS

I. Localization-related (focal, local, partial)
- A. Idiopathic (primary)
  - 1. Benign childhood epilepsy with centrotemporal spikes ("benign rolandic epilepsy")
  - 2. Childhood epilepsy with occipital paroxysms
  - 3. Primary reading epilepsy
- B. Symptomatic (secondary)
  - 1. Temporal lobe epilepsies
  - 2. Frontal lobe epilepsies
  - 3. Parietal lobe epilepsies
  - 4. Occipital lobe epilepsies
  - 5. Chronic progressive epilepsia partialis continua of childhood (Koshevnikoff's syndrome)
  - 6. Syndromes characterized by seizures with specific modes of precipitation (e.g., reflex epilepsy or startle epilepsies)
- C. Cryptogenic, defined by:
  - 1. Seizure type
  - 2. Clinical features
  - 3. Etiology
  - 4. Anatomic localization

II. Generalized
- A. Primary (idiopathic), in order of age of onset
  - 1. Benign neonatal familial convulsions
  - 2. Benign neonatal convulsions
  - 3. Benign myoclonic epilepsy in infancy
  - 4. Childhood absence epilepsy (pyknoepilepsy)
  - 5. Juvenile absence epilepsy
  - 6. Juvenile myoclonic epilepsy (of Janz)
  - 7. Epilepsy with generalized tonic-clonic convulsions on awakening
  - 8. Other generalized idiopathic epilepsies
  - 9. Epilepsies with seizures precipitated by specific modes of activation

E

EPILEPSY

B. Cryptogenic or symptomatic, in order of age of onset
  1. West's syndrome
  2. Lennox-Gastaut syndrome
  3. Epilepsy with myoclonic-astatic seizures
  4. Epilepsy with myoclonic absences
C. Symptomatic (secondary)
  1. Nonspecific etiology
    a. Early myoclonic encephalopathy
    b. Early infantile epileptic encephalopathy with suppression bursts
    c. Other symptomatic generalized epilepsies
  2. Specific syndromes
    a. Neurologic diseases with seizures as a prominent feature
III. Epilepsies undetermined whether focal or generalized
  A. With both focal and generalized seizures
    1. Neonatal seizures
    2. Severe myoclonic epilepsy of infancy
    3. Epilepsy with continuous spike waves during slow-wave sleep
    4. Acquired epileptic aphasia (Landau-Kleffner syndrome)
    5. Other undetermined epilepsies
IV. Special syndromes
  A. Situation-related seizures
    1. Febrile convulsions
    2. Isolated seizures or isolated status epilepticus
    3. Seizures occurring only with acute metabolic or toxic events due to factors such as alcohol, drugs, eclampsia, and nonketotic hyperglycemia

DIFFERENTIAL DIAGNOSIS OF EPILEPSY

Conditions producing symptoms or signs that may be mistaken for epileptic seizures include the following: (1) syncope, (2) transient ischemic attacks, (3) migraine, (4) metabolic derangements (e.g., hypoglycemia), (5) parasomnias, (6) transient global amnesia, (7) paroxysmal movement disorders (e.g., paroxysmal kinesigenic choreoathetosis), and (8) nonepileptic seizures (pseudo-seizures).

Nonepileptic seizures are common and may coexist in patients with epileptic seizures. They are associated with a variety of psychiatric syndromes, including somatoform disorders, panic disorders, dissociative disorders, psychotic disorders, factitious disorders, and malingering. They may be difficult to distinguish from epileptic seizures, especially of mesial temporal, basal frontal, and supplementary motor area origin. Seizures originating from these areas may not be associated with scalp ictal EEG changes (see Electroencephalography).

SELECTED EPILEPSY SYNDROMES

Idiopathic Syndromes

I. *Benign childhood epilepsy with centrotemporal spikes (benign rolandic epilepsy)* is a common autosomal dominant syndrome producing nocturnal generalized convulsions in otherwise normal children. Focal motor or sensory seizures, often involving the face, may occur. The EEG shows characteristic interictal centrotemporal spikes. Seizures are easily controlled with phenytoin or carbamazepine, and spontaneously disappear before adulthood.

II. *Childhood absence epilepsy* (pyknoepilepsy) occurs in genetically predisposed but otherwise normal children and is marked by typical absence seizures with a corresponding 3-Hz generalized spike-and-wave EEG discharge. Typical absences are not preceded by an aura nor followed by postictal confusion. Generalized tonic-clonic seizures may also occur. Treatment consists of ethosuximide, effective for absence seizures only, and valproic acid, effective for both isolated absence seizures or absence seizures complicated by or with generalized tonic-clonic seizures. Absence seizures rarely persist into adulthood.

III. *Juvenile myoclonic epilepsy (of Janz)* is a genetic epilepsy syndrome whose gene has been mapped to chromosome 6. It presents in normal teenagers with early morning myoclonic jerks and generalized tonic-clonic seizures. Sleep deprivation and photic stimulation are often activating influences. The interictal EEG typically shows 4- to 6-Hz generalized irregular spike-wave or polyspike-wave discharges with normal background. Valproate is highly effective, but relapses are the rule following drug discontinuation.

SYMPTOMATIC OR CRYPTOGENIC SYNDROMES

I. *West's syndrome* consists of the triad of infantile spasms, developmental arrest, and the interictal EEG pattern hypsarrhythmia, consisting of very high voltage multifocal spikes, sharp waves, and slow waves in a chaotic distribution. The syndrome may be cryptogenic or symptomatic of a variety of brain insults and is generally treated with ACTH (typically 40 units IM daily, increasing by 10 units per week as needed to a maximum of 80 units daily) or other corticosteroids. Prognosis is unfavorable and is worse in the cryptogenic than in the symptomatic group.

II. *Lennox-Gastaut syndrome* is characterized by multiple, difficult to control seizure types, especially atonic seizures and atypical absences in addition to generalized convulsions, mental retardation, and an abnormal interictal EEG with generalized 2- to 2.5-Hz slow spike-and-wave discharges. The syndrome often follows West's syndrome in an affected child and is associated with a poor prognosis. Valproate is the drug of choice because of its efficacy against the multiple seizure types, and felbamate is also beneficial. Polytherapy may be necessary.

Surgical section of the corpus callosum is sometimes effective in controlling drop attacks.

SYMPTOMATIC SYNDROMES

Temporal lobe epilepsy (TLE), the most common symptomatic, localization-related epilepsy, causes simple partial, complex partial, and secondarily generalized seizures as a result of ictal discharges typically arising from mesial temporal structures such as the hippocampus or amygdala. The interictal EEG often shows unilateral or bilateral, usually anterior, temporal spikes. The most common associated lesion is hippocampal (mesial temporal) sclerosis; others include hamartomas, neoplasms (especially low-grade gliomas), cortical dysplasia, and vascular malformations. MRI scanning, using thin coronal sections through temporal structures, is the imaging modality of choice and may show unilateral hippocampal atrophy with enlargement of the ipsilateral temporal horn and increased hippocampal signal on T_2-weighted images, suggestive of hippocampal sclerosis. Phenytoin and carbamazepine are equally effective in treating symptomatic partial epilepsies such as TLE. Valproate is as effective in treating secondarily generalized seizures but not as effective for partial seizures. Newer anticonvulsants are also indicated for treating partial complex seizures. Surgical resection, typically anterior temporal lobectomy, eliminates seizures in about 70% of medically refractory patients in whom the epileptogenic lesion can be accurately localized. Vagal nerve stimulation is also effective in treating this syndrome.

Posttraumatic epilepsy typically begins 6 months to 2 years following head trauma. Risk factors include intracranial hemorrhage, depressed skull fracture, early seizures, or duration of posttraumatic amnesia greater than 24 hours. Phenytoin reduces the incidence of seizures within the first week following head trauma but is not effective as prophylaxis against the development of posttraumatic epilepsy.

OTHER SYNDROMES

I. *Febrile seizures* are typically generalized convulsions, occurring in children between 3 months and 5 years of age, associated with fever but without evidence of intracranial infection or defined cause. They are common, occurring in 2% to 5% of children in this country, and tend to run in families. They usually occur during the early, rising temperature phase of an infectious illness. Most febrile seizures are *simple*, lasting less than 15 minutes and without focality; if the seizure is prolonged or focal, it is *complex* and associated with a higher risk of subsequent afebrile epilepsy. Other risk factors for seizure recurrence include more than one seizure in 24 hours, abnormal neurologic examination, and afebrile seizures in a parent or sibling. Overall, 6% to 13% of patients with two or more risk factors will develop afebrile epilepsy, compared to 0.9% without risk factors. There is no evidence that prophylactic treatment with anticonvulsants prevents future epilepsy.

Phenobarbital, diazepam, and valproate (but not phenytoin or carbamazepine) reduce the rate of recurrent febrile seizures, but in most cases they are not recommended, because two thirds of children will never have another febrile seizure and there is no evidence of mental or neurologic impairment due to febrile seizures. Rectal benzodiazepines may be useful for prevention of recurrent complicated febrile seizures.

II. *Neonatal seizures* are nearly always symptomatic, occurring as a result of a large number of brain insults; idiopathic syndromes are rare. The most common causes include hypoxic-ischemic encephalopathy, hypoglycemia, hypocalcemia, hyponatremia and hypernatremia, intraventricular or periventricular hemorrhage, CNS infections, cerebral malformations, inborn errors of metabolism, and drug withdrawal or intoxication. Neonatal seizures are classified clinically as subtle, tonic, clonic, and myoclonic (Volpe, 1989); generalized tonic-clonic convulsions are rare in the neonatal period. Neonatal seizures commonly occur electrographically without clear clinical change and may occur clinically without a clear EEG ictal pattern. Jitteriness is a benign nonepileptic phenomenon consisting of rapid, stimulus-sensitive movements of all four extremities, abolished by passive restraint of the limbs. Treatment of neonatal seizures most commonly involves phenobarbital (loading dose 20 mg/kg followed by maintenance dose of 3 to 4 mg/kg/day to achieve blood level of 16 to 40 mg/mL) or phenytoin (loading dose 15 to 20 mg/kg followed by maintenance dose 3 to 5 mg/kg/day to achieve blood level of 6 to 14 mg/mL). Hypocalcemia is treated with 5% calcium gluconate, 4 mL/kg IV, and hypomagnesemia with 50% magnesium sulfate, 0.2 mL/kg IV. Pyridoxine 50 to 100 mg IV should be given if seizures continue and the cause is uncertain. Duration of treatment once seizures are controlled is controversial.

E

EPILEPSY

STATUS EPILEPTICUS

Generalized tonic-clonic status epilepticus (GTCSE; see Emergency appendix) is a medical emergency diagnosed either when two or more discrete seizures occur without complete recovery of consciousness or when a continuous seizure lasts at least 5 minutes. The likelihood of brain damage or death is directly related to the duration of GTCSE. GTCSE is more easily controlled when no new structural brain insult has occurred, as in withdrawal from anticonvulsants, drugs, or alcohol. More refractory cases may be seen in anoxic encephalopathy, stroke, hemorrhage, neoplasm, trauma, infection, or metabolic derangement. In general, the longer the duration of GTCSE, the more difficult it is to treat. A characteristic progression of EEG patterns in GTCSE has been described: (1) discrete seizures, (2) waxing and waning ictal discharges, (3) continuous ictal discharges, (4) continuous ictal discharges punctuated by flat periods, and (5) bilateral periodic epileptiform discharges on a flat background. In the latter stages, the xspatient may exhibit only subtle or no motor activity. Management of

TABLE 43				

COMPARISON OF MEDICATIONS COMMONLY USED TO TREAT STATUS
EPILEPTICUS

Time	Diazepam	Lorazepam	Phenytoin	Phenobarbital
To reach brain	10 sec	2–3 min	1 min	20 min
To peak brain concentration	<5 min	30 min	15–30 min	30 min
To stop status	1 min	<5 min	15–30 min	20 min
Effective half-life	15 min	6 hr	>22 hr	50–120 hr

GTCSE must be carried out quickly. Treatment protocols are based on the pharmacologic properties of commonly used drugs (see Tables 43 to 48).

Absence status epilepticus (spike-wave stupor) constitutes continuous generalized spike-wave discharges with alteration of consciousness. It occurs more commonly in children with secondarily generalized epilepsy such as Lennox-Gastaut syndrome rather than with pyknoepilepsy. It may also occur sporadically in adults with no prior history of epilepsy. Treatment of the childhood condition consists of IV diazepam (0.3 to 0.5 mg/kg, no faster than 1 to 2 mg/minute) followed by valproic acid. The adult form responds to the protocol listed for GTCSE. Because this condition is not life-threatening and residual brain damage is unproved, use of general anesthesia is not generally recommended.

Simple partial status epilepticus (epilepsia partialis continua) most commonly involves continuous clonic focal motor seizures, but other manifestations such as aphasia, head and eye deviation, somatosensory changes, visual disturbances, and autonomic symptoms may occur. Ictal EEG may be normal. Focal motor status is often seen in the setting of metabolic derangements, particularly nonketotic hyperglycemia. Treatment in this case consists of correcting metabolic abnormalities. Slow loading with IV diazepam or lorazepam to avoid respiratory depression, followed by phenytoin, may also be used.

Complex partial status epilepticus may consist of repeated discrete complex partial seizures without full clearing of consciousness or as a more continuous clouding of consciousness, mimicking a confusional state. EEG is diagnostic. Treatment initially is identical to the protocol listed for GTCSE, although the use of general anesthesia (e.g., thiopental, midazolam, propofol) if initial maneuvers fail may be indicated.

Generalized convulsive status epilepticus in children is treated as in adults with the following modifications: use diazepam 0.25 mg/kg IV, no faster than 1 to 2 mg/minute. If there is a delay in obtaining an IV line in a small child, this dose may be administered rectally via a feeding tube flushed with saline. Phenytoin 18 to 20 mg/kg is given IV over 20 minutes. If seizures persist, be prepared to intubate, and give phenobarbital 15 to 20 mg/kg IV no faster than 60 mg/minute, with additional doses of

Text continued on p. 191

TABLE 44

AN APPROACH TO THE TREATMENT OF GENERALIZED TONIC-CLONIC STATUS EPILEPTICUS (GTCSE)

Action	Cumulative Time Frame
1. *Stabilization and diagnosis:* Secure an airway, administer oxygen, and be prepared to intubate quickly; assess vital signs, including rectal temperature, and treat hyperpyrexia appropriately; Insert 2 large-bore IVs; obtain ECG, blood glucose, anticonvulsant levels, CBC, BUN, electrolytes, calcium, magnesium, phosphorus, serum and urine toxicology screens, and arterial blood gases; administer 100 mg thiamine IV and 50 mL of 50% glucose IV if necessary; obtain history and perform neurologic examination; consider possibility of nonconvulsive seizures.	0–15 min
2. *Stop seizures:* Through one IV, administer phenytoin 20 mg/kg no faster than 50 mg/min. Contraindications to phenytoin include documented allergy, significant heart block, or severe bradycardia. (If phenytoin is contraindicated, administer phenobarbital as described below or valproic acid at 20–25 mg/kg IV). ECG should be monitored continuously, and blood pressure taken frequently. If significant rhythm disturbances or hypotension occur during phenytoin infusion, reduce the rate to 25 mg/min. Fosphenytoin, a prodrug, can be used IM or IV, infusing at 20 mg/kg phenytoin equivalents, with a maximum rate of 150 mg/min. If additional seizures occur while phenytoin is being infused, administer either diazepam (no faster than 2 mg/min, to maximum 20 mg) or lorazepam (the preferred agent due to its longer half-life) no faster than 2 mg/min, to maximum 0.1 mg/kg, no more than 8 mg through the second IV, to avoid interrupting the phenytoin infusion. Benzodiazepines may cause respiratory depression.	15–60 min
3. *If seizures persist:* Following infusion of phenytoin, administer an additional 10 mg/kg phenytoin/fosphenytoin IV, no faster than 50 mg/min or try valproic acid at 20–25 mg/kg IV, at a maximum rate of 50–100 mg/min.	
4. *If seizures persist:* Intubate the patient, if not already done. Obtain emergency EEG monitoring; administer phenobarbital IV 20 mg/kg at a rate of 50–75 mg/min, until seizures stop. Carefully monitor blood pressure and ECG.	60–120 min
5. *If seizures persist:* Induce general anesthesia with short (thiopental) or intermediate (pentobarbital) half-life barbiturates. Pentobarbital is given IV as a 5- to 10-mg/kg loading dose (no faster than 25 mg/min), followed by initial maintenance dose of 1–3 mg/kg/hr. Midazolam (loading dose 0.2–0.3 mg/kg or propofol (loading dose 1–2 mg/kg with a maintenance of 2–10 mg/kg/hr) anesthesia can also be employed in refractory cases. Adjust doses to achieve burst-suppression pattern on EEG with minimal blood pressure reduction. Pressor support may be required. Infusions should be utilized for at least 12 hours and used in conjunction with other antiepileptic agents.	120 min
6. *Other maneuvers:* Concurrently with above, treat metabolic or toxic conditions; ensure adequate hydration, keep blood glucose between 100 and 150 mg/dL and core body temperature <37.5°C. If there is clinical suspicion for new brain insult, obtain neuroimaging once GTCSE is aborted. Perform LP following neuroimaging and treat appropriately in cases suggestive of CNS infection.	

E

EPILEPSY

TABLE 45

COMMON ANTIEPILEPTIC DRUGS: PRESCRIBING INFORMATION

Drug	Preparations	Average Target Plasma Concentrations (mg/L)*	Monotherapy Dose	Approximate Half-Life	Protein Binding
Phenytoin (Dilantin)	30 mg, 100 mg caps, 50 mg tabs, 30 or 125 mg/5 mL elixirs	10–20 (6–14 in neonates to 12 weeks)	Neonates: 15–20 mg/kg, then 3–5 mg/kg/day in divided doses Infants: 15 mg/kg, then 3–5 mg/kg/day in 3–4 doses Children: 15 mg/kg, then 5–15 mg/kg/day in 2 doses Adults: 15 mg/kg, then 5 mg/kg/day, once daily	Variable	90%
Phenobarbital (Luminal)	15, 30, 60, 130 mg tabs 20 mg/5 mL elixir	15–40	Infants, children: 6–16 mg/kg, then 3–8 mg/kg/day Adults: 4–8 mg/kg, then 2–4 mg/kg/day, single dose	40–70 hr 50–120 hr	50%
Primidone (Mysoline)	50, 250 mg tabs 250 mg/5 mL elixir	5–12 (metabolized also to phenobarbital)	Children: 50 mg/day, increasing 50 mg q 3 days to 15–25 mg/kg in 2–4 doses Adults: 250 mg/day in 2 doses; start with 100 mg at bedtime and increase by 100 mg q 3 days to 10–20 mg/kg/day in 2–4 doses	10–12 hr	<5%
Carbamazepine (Tegretol)	100, 200 mg tabs 100 mg/5 mL suspension	4–12	Children: 100 mg bid, increasing 100 mg qod to 15–20 mg/kg/day in 3–4 doses Adults: 200 mg bid, increasing 100 mg qod to 7–15 mg/kg/day in 3–4 doses	5–27 hr	75%

Drug	Preparation	Therapeutic level	Dosage	Half-life	Protein binding
Ethosuximide (Zarontin)	250 mg caps 250 mg/5 mL elixir	40–100	Children: 250 mg/day, increasing 250 mg q 4–7 days to 15–40 mg/kg/day in 3–4 doses Adults: 250 mg bid, increasing 250 mg q 4–7 days to 15–30 mg/kg/day in 3–4 doses	30 hr 50–60 hr	0%
Valproic acid (Depakene)	250 mg tabs 250 mg/5 mL elixir	50–100	Children: 10–15 mg/kg/day, increasing 5–10 mg/kg/day q 1 week to 15–100 mg/kg/day in 3–4 doses Adults: 10–15 mg/kg/day, increasing 5–10 mg/kg/day q 1 week to 15–45 mg/kg/day in 3–4 doses	4–14 hr 6–16 hr	75–90% (inverse to concentration)
Divalproex Sodium (Depakote)	125, 250, 500 mg tabs	50–100	Same as valproic acid except given in 2–3 doses	Same	75–90% (inverse to concentration)
Clonazepam (Klonopin)	0.5, 1, 2 mg tabs	Not usually monitored	Children: 0.01–0.03 mg/kg/day, increasing 0.25–0.5 mg q 3 days to 0.1–0.2 mg/kg/day in 3 doses Adults: 0.5 mg/day, increasing 0.5–1.0 mg/day q 3 days	18–50 hr 18–50 hr	85%
Felbamate (Felbatol)	400, 600 mg tabs 600 mg/5 mL elixir	Not usually monitored	Children (adjunctive): 15 mg/kg/day 3 or 4 times daily Adult: 1200 mg/day, increasing 600 mg q 2 weeks up to 3600 mg/day	14–20	25%
Lamotrigine (Lamictal)	25, 50, 100, 200 mg tabs	0.5–3.0 mg/mL	50 mg hs increasing 50 mg q 2 weeks, as tolerated, divided into 2 doses	12–50 hr	55%

cont'd

TABLE 45

COMMON ANTIEPILEPTIC DRUGS: PRESCRIBING INFORMATION—Cont'd

Drug	Preparations	Average Target Plasma Concentrations (mg/L)*	Monotherapy Dose	Approximate Half-Life	Protein Binding
Levetiracetam (Keppra)	250, 500, 750 mg tabs	Not usually monitored	Children: 20–40 mg/kg Adults: 500 mg bid increasing up to 1500 mg bid	6–8 hr	<10%
Tiagabine (Gabitril)	2, 4, 12, 16, 20 mg tabs	Not usually monitored	4 mg q days, increasing at weekly intervals by 4–8 mg up to 56 mg/day	4–9 hr (shorter if on hepatic inducing AEDs)	95%
Topiramate (Topamax)	25, 100, 200 mg tabs 15, 25 mg sprinkle capsules	Not usually monitored	Initial 25–50 mg/day increasing by 25–50 mg increments to 20 mg bid as tolerated	20 hr	
Oxcarbazine (Trileptal)	150, 300, 600 mg tabs	4–12 (10-monohydroxy metabolite)	Children: 8–10 mg/kg/day increasing up to 20–40 mg/kg/day Adults: 150–300 mg bid up to 1200 mg bid	2 hr	40%
Zonisamide (Zonegran)	100 mg capsules	Not usually monitored	Children: 2–4 mg/kg/day Adults: 100–200 mg/day increasing up to 400–600 mg/day	60 hr	<10%
Gabapentin (Neurontin)	100, 300, 400 mg tabs 600, 800 mg tabs	Not usually monitored	300 mg/day, increasing up to 900–1800 mg/day over 2–3 days divided into 3–4 doses	5–7 hr	0%

* Many patients will respond at different plasma concentrations, below or above the average plasma concentrations.

TABLE 46

DOSE-RELATED ADVERSE EFFECTS OF ANTIEPILEPTIC DRUGS

Drug	Side Effects
Phenytoin	*Acute*: Drowsiness, ataxia, diplopia, GI complaints, choreoathetosis, nausea, hypotension (after parenteral use), heart block
	Chronic: Gingival hyperplasia, hirsutism, folate deficiency, megaloblastic anemia, osteomalacia with vitamin D deficiency, peripheral neuropathy, encephalopathy, cerebellar dysfunction, pseudolymphoma, hemorrhage in the newborn
Phenobarbital	*Acute*: Sedation, behavior disturbance, ataxia
	Chronic: Attentional difficulty, hemorrhage in the newborn rheumatic syndrome
Primidone	*Acute*: Sedation, nausea, vertigo, ataxia
	Chronic: Behavior disturbances (in children), loss of libido, attentional difficulties, hemorrhage in the newborn
Carbamazepine	*Acute*: Diplopia, vertigo, blurred vision, sedation, dry mouth stomatitis, hyponatremia (SIADH), headache, diarrhea, constipation, paresthesias
	Chronic: Liver enzyme induction, leukopenia, nervousness, hemorrhage in the newborn
Ethosuximide	*Acute*: Nausea, vertigo, vomiting, hiccups, headache
	Chronic: Insomnia, nervousness
Valproate	*Acute*: Sedation, GI disturbances
	Chronic: Weight gain, hepatic enzyme elevation, hyperammonemia, granulopenia, thrombocytopenia, alopecia, tremor
Clonazepam	*Acute*: Sedation, ataxia, irritability, hypersalivation
	Chronic: Behavior disturbances, tolerance, and withdrawal syndrome
Felbamate	*Acute*: GI disturbances, insomnia, headache, fatigue, nausea, vomiting
	Chronic: Weight loss
Lamotrigine	Rash, diplopia, sedation, dizziness, ataxia, headache, nausea, vomiting
Topiramate	Somnolence with confusion, psychomotor slowing, weight loss, speech disorders, ataxia, paresthesias, renal calculi
Oxcarbazine	Hyponatremia, headache, somnolence, nausea, vomiting, diplopia
Tiagabine	Somnolence, dizziness, attentional difficulties
Levetiracetam	Dizziness, somnolence, fatigue
Zonisamide	Renal calculi, kidney dysfunction, somnolence, fatigue, confusion, anorexia, ataxia, dizziness
Gabapentin	Sedation, fatigue, dizziness, nausea, weight gain, ataxia, headache and diplopia

E

EPILEPSY

TABLE 47

FACTORS AFFECTING SERUM CONCENTRATIONS OF ANTICONVULSANTS AND OTHER DRUG INTERACTIONS

Drug	Increased by AEDs	Increased by Other Drugs	Increased in Clinical State	Decreased by AEDs	Decreased by Other Drugs	Decreased by Clinical State	Interacts with Other Drugs
Phenytoin	Diazepam	Alcohol (acute)	Hepatic disease	Phenobarbital	Alcohol (chronic)	Acute hepatitis	Corticosteroids
	Ethosuximide	Amiodarone		Carbamazepine	Antineoplastics	Mononucleosis	Cyclosporine
	Felbamate	Amphetamines		Clonazepam	Loxepine	Pregnancy	Ketoconazole
	Oxcarbazine	Aspirin			Nicotine	Renal disease	Methadone
	Phenobarbital	Chloramphenicol			Nitrofurantoin		Oral contraceptives
	Primidone	Chlordiazepoxide			Sucralfate		Protease inhibitors
	Topiramate	Chlorpheniramine			Theophylline		Rifampin
	Valproic acid	Cimetidine			Tube feedings		Tacrolimus
		Diazepam					Trazodone
		Disulfiram					Warfarin
		Dicumarol					
		Estrogens					
		H² antagonists					
		Isoniazid					
		Methylphenidate					
		Omeprazole					
		Phenylbutazone					
		Phenothiazines					
		Propoxyphene					
		Sulfonamides					
		Tolbutamide					
		Trazodone					
Phenobarbital	Valproid acid	Alcohol	Acidic urine	Clonazepam	Chloramphenicol	Alkaline urine	Chloramphenicol
	Phenytoin	MAO inhibitors	Hepatic disease		Dicumarol		Cimetidine

Drug					
Felbamate		Renal disease		Phenylbutazone	
Primidone	Valproic acid, Clonazepam	—		—	Folic acid, Haloperidol, Oral contraceptives, Phenylbutazone
Carbamazepine	Felbamate (↑10, 11 Epoxide); Cimetidine, Diltiazem, Erythromycin, Fluoxetine, Fluvoxamine, Grapefruit juice, Isoniazid, Propoxyphene, Sertraline, Verapamil	Hepatic disease	Carbamazepine, Phenytoin, Ethosuximide, Felbamate, Phenobarbital, Phenytoin, Primidone, Valproic acid	Pregnancy	Same list as Phenytoin, Corticosteroids, Doxycycline, Ketoconazole, Lithium, Oral contraceptives, Protase inhibitors, Quinidine, Rifampin, Tacrolimus, Thyroid hormone, Warfarin
Valproic acid	Felbamate; Salicylates	Hepatic disease	Carbamazepine, Phenytoin, Phenobarbital, Primidone, Valproic acid	Rifampin	Amitryptyline, Nortriptyline, Tolbutamide, Warfarin, Zidovudine
Ethosuximide	—	—	Carbamazepine, Phenytoin, Phenobarbital, Primidone	—	—
Clonazepam	—	—	Carbamazepine, Phenobarbital	Antifungal agents, Phenytoin (possibly)	—

cont'd

TABLE 47

FACTORS AFFECTING SERUM CONCENTRATIONS OF ANTICONVULSANTS AND OTHER DRUG INTERACTIONS—Cont'd

Drug	Increased by AEDs	Increased by Other Drugs	Increased in Clinical State	Decreased by AEDs	Decreased by Other Drugs	Decreased by Clinical State	Interacts with Other Drugs
Felbamate	—	—	—	Phenytoin Carbamazepine All hepatic inducing AEDs	—	—	—
Lamotrigine	Valproic acid	—	Hepatic disease Renal failure	Phenytoin Carbamazepine	—	—	Methotrexate
Topiramate	—	—	Renal disease Hepatic disease (possibly)	Phenytoin Carbamazepine	—	—	Carbonic anhydrase inhibitors
Tiagabine	—	—	Hepatic disease	Phenytoin Phenobarbital Carbamazepine	—	—	—
Zonisamide	—	—	—	Phenytoin Carbamazepine Lamotrigine	—	—	—
Levetiracetam	—	—	Renal failure	—	—	—	—
Oxcarbazine	—	—	Renal failure	Phenytoin Carbamazepine Lamotrigine Phenobarbital Valproic acid	—	—	Oral contraceptives See list for Carbamazepine
Gabapentin	—	—	Renal failure	—	Antacids	—	—

TABLE 48

IDIOSYNCRATIC ADVERSE EFFECTS OF ANTIEPILEPTIC DRUGS

Effect	Drug Type
Skin rash	All antiepileptic drugs
Erythema multiforme	All; more likely with ethosuximide
Stevens-Johnson syndrome	All
Exfoliative dermatitis	All
Systemic lupus erythematosus	Phenytoin, ethosuximide
Bone marrow depression	Most, including phenytoin, primidone, carbamazepine, ethosuximide, valproic acid, felbamate
Thrombocytopenia	Valproic acid; rare with phenytoin, phenobarbital, clonazepam
Lymphadenopathy	Phenytoin, ethosuximide
Hepatic toxicity	Valproic acid (usually in first 6 months of therapy), phenytoin, carbamazepine
Pancreatic toxicity	Valproic acid

Adapted from Dreifuss FE: In Ward AA, Penry JK, Purpura D, eds: *Epilepsy*, ed 1, New York, Raven, 1983.

E

EPILEPSY

10 mg/kg as needed to control seizures. Recent studies have shown the benefit of valproic acid at 20 to 25 mg/kg IV in patients allergic to phenytoin or phenobarbital, or as an adjunct to these agents in convulsive status epilepticus.

Neonatal status epilepticus must be diagnosed using EEG monitoring because of the frequent dissociation between electrographic and clinical seizure activity. Treatment is as previously outlined for neonatal seizures. Diazepam 0.3 to 0.5 mg/kg IV or lorazepam 0.1 mg/kg IV may be given in refractory cases but these drugs are contraindicated in jaundiced neonates.

ANTIEPILEPTIC DRUGS (See Also AAN GUIDELINE SUMMARIES APPENDIX)

Selection of an AED is based on clinical and electrographic identification of seizure type. The dose is increased until seizures are controlled or clinical toxicity develops. If the drug is ineffective when taken in toxic doses, it is generally recommended to switch to another monotherapy with another agent before using drug combinations. Drug levels may be useful to answer specific questions regarding compliance, toxicity, or individual pharmacokinetics. Free levels of highly protein-bound drugs such as phenytoin, carbamazepine, and valproic acid may be helpful during hypoalbuminemic states, renal or hepatic disease, pregnancy, malignancy, sepsis, burns, or in the presence of other drugs that displace protein binding. The use of serial laboratory monitoring to prevent serious idiosyncratic reaction is of little value. It may be implemented in high-risk patients (children under age 2, especially those treated with polytherapy, patients with urea cycle defects, organic acidurias, mitochondrial disorders,

GMI gangliosidosis, and neurodegenerative diseases) and in those with a history of adverse drug reactions. Abnormalities such as mild leukopenia or elevated hepatic enzymes are not predictive of severe complications. Current recommendations include the following: (1) obtain initial baseline blood work prior to initiation of therapy, including CBC with differential count, liver and kidney function tests, lipid profile, PT, PTT; (2) refrain from subsequent routine monitoring in asymptomatic patients; (3) counsel patients and family to notify you immediately should any of the following develop: bruising, bleeding, rash, abdominal pain, vomiting, jaundice, lethargy, coma, or marked increase in seizure frequency; (4) for multiply handicapped, institutionalized patients who may not be able to communicate the preceding information, annual routine blood monitoring may be of value.

REFERENCES

Browns TR: *Neurology* 40:S28–S32, 1990.

Dodson WE: *Neurology* 39:1009–1010, 1989.

Engel J Jr: *Seizures and epilepsy*, Philadelphia, FA Davis, 1989.

Gates JR, Roman AJ, eds: *Non-epileptic seizures*, Boston, Butterworth-Heinemann, 2000.

Mattson RH et al: *N Engl J Med* 327:765–771, 1992.

Temkin NR: *N Engl J Med* 323:497–502, 1990.

Treiman DM: *Adv Neurol* 34:377–384, 1983.

Treiman DM et al: *Epilepsy Res* 5(1):49–60, 1990.

Volpe JL: *Pediatrics* 84:422–428, 1989.

Wyllie E, ed: *The treatment of epilepsy, principles and practice*, ed 3, Philadelphia, Lippincott Williams & Wilkins, 2001.

Zaidat OO, Suarez JI: In *Geriatric neurosurgery*, Park Ridge, AANS, 1999.

ERECTILE DYSFUNCTION; IMPOTENCE

PATHOPHYSIOLOGY

Penile erection is mediated by the cavernous nerves from *S2–4 roots* and is dependent on the integrity of both the paired deep arteries, which supply the corpora cavernosa, and the plexus of veins that drain it. Nitric oxide release from cavernous nerves and vascular endothelium promotes formation of cGMP, which stimulates smooth muscle relaxation, allowing increased arterial flow into the corpora cavernosa and resultant compression of outflow veins, facilitating rigidity. Sympathetic input from T11–L2 constricts arterioles, reducing inflow and permitting venous drainage; this promotes detumescence and explains how sympathetic overactivity produces psychogenic impotence.

EPIDEMIOLOGY

Erectile dysfunction may affect up to 30 million men in the United States. The prevalence and severity increase with age, tripling in incidence from the 20s to the 50s.

ETIOLOGY

An organic cause may be found in more than 80% of cases lasting more than a year. Organic causes fall into several categories:

1. *Neurologic:* multiple sclerosis (MS), spinal cord injury, pelvic nerve trauma (prostatectomy, pelvic injury, radiation)
2. *Arterial:* atherosclerosis, aortoiliac disease (Leriche syndrome) trauma
3. *Venous:* diabetes, Peyronie's disease, normal aging
4. *Endocrine:* low testosterone (primary or secondary), high prolactin
5. *Pharmacologic: Drugs* affecting any of these systems can exacerbate the problem, and the same vascular risk factors implicated in coronary and cerebrovascular disease (diabetes, hypertension, hyperlipidemia, smoking) increase the risk of erectile dysfunction.

DIAGNOSIS

Diagnosis is greatly eased if the patient reports achieving even very occasional firm, persistent erections (nocturnal, morning, with masturbation)—*this removes concern for a vascular basis and suggests a psychogenic etiology.* Sphincter or sensory dysfunction suggests a neurologic basis; *difficulty maintaining erection suggests venous insufficiency; delay in achieving erection suggests arterial insufficiency;* and painful erection suggests Peyronie's disease or priapism. Examiners should look for evidence of feminization (hormonal basis) or peripheral vascular disease, abnormalities of the external genitalia, and adequacy of anal sphincter tone and the bulbocavernosus reflex.

EVALUATION

In addition to a history and physical examination, serum prolactin, testosterone, fasting glucose, and lipid panel should be evaluated. Additional workup may include penile-brachial index, penile ultrasonography, cavernosometry, and pelvic arteriogram.

TREATMENT

Medications such as *sildenafil, tadalafil, and vardenafil* have an overall efficacy of around 50%. These drugs inhibit the phosphodiesterase specific to the corpora cavernosa, thereby increasing cGMP. They are particularly effective in psychogenic cases and less severe organic dysfunction (including diabetes) and are also effective to a lesser extent in cases of severe organic dysfunction including spinal cord injury. *They are absolutely contraindicated in patients taking nitrates*, as the associated hypotension has been associated with myocardial infarction and stroke. *Many case reports exist of onset of nonarteritic anterior ischemic optic neuropathy (NAION) within 36 hours of taking sildenafil*. Other therapies include *alprostadil penile injection* (estimated efficacy for organic disorders is 80%), *alprostadil intraurethral pellet* (much less efficacious), and *penile prosthesis* (requiring surgery but effective and reliable). *Testosterone supplements* may help, particularly in cases of decreased libido. *Yohimbine* is a mixed α_1- and α_2-adrenergic receptor antagonist that works by a dual mechanism; it facilitates sexual arousal by acting on α_2-adrenergic receptors in the CNS and blocks adrenergic influences at the peripheral level.

REFERENCE
Morgentaler A: *Lancet* 354:1713–1718, 1999.

EVOKED POTENTIALS

Evoked potentials (EPs) are recordable changes in the electrical activity of the nervous system in response to an external stimulus. They are an adjunct to the history and physical examination and may provide corroborative evidence of disease of the nervous system. EPs utilize the functional integrity of the nervous system to provide information about the anatomic location of lesions. They may detect the presence of lesions that are not clinically apparent, but are of little value in providing clues to the origin or cause of the lesions.

The clinically useful EPs are derived from stimulation of one of the modalities of the sensory system—visual (VEP), brainstem auditory (BAEP), and somatosensory (SEP)—and are recorded from electrodes on the scalp. Because of the low voltage of EPs (100 times smaller than the scalp EEG), multiple stimulations with averaging and filtering are necessary to separate the signal from background noise. The actual signal recorded may be either "near-field" (the electrode is placed *near* the generator of the signal in the cortex, for example, the P100 wave of the VEP generated by the occipital cortex) or "far-field" (the electrode is placed *far* from the generator of the signal, which is volume conducted through the tissues of the body to the recording electrodes on the scalp, for example, P11 wave of the SEP generated by the dorsal root entry zone). In general, the latency from stimulus to recorded potential is more important than signal amplitude. The potentials are usually designated by the letter "P" or "N" followed by a number. "P100" is a wave of *positive* deflection occurring at a latency of 100 ms. "N20" is a wave of *negative* deflection occurring at a latency of 20 ms. By convention, "positive" is a downward and "negative" an upward needle deflection. It should be remembered that *absolute latencies and standard deviations are quite laboratory specific* (Fig. 16).

Electroretinograms (ERGs) are derived from stimulation of the retina with light while recording electrical activity directly from the cornea. When combined with VEPs, ERGs can be useful in prognosis for recovery of visual function and differentiation of retinal from optic nerve disease.

Motor evoked potentials (MEP) are derived from stimulating the CNS motor system with magnetically induced or directly applied electrical current. Recordings are made from electrodes placed over muscles. MEPs have yet to gain significant clinical use and will not be discussed further.

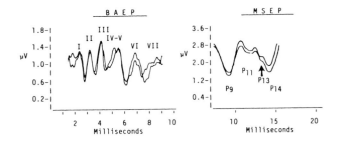

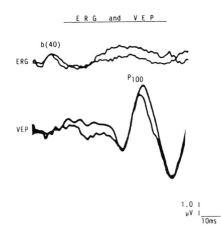

EVOKED POTENTIALS

FIGURE 16

Normal evoked potentials.

VISUAL EVOKED POTENTIALS

Visual evoked potentials (VEPs) are primarily used to detect
anterochiasmatic lesions of the visual system. Their usefulness in
retrochiasmatic lesions is minimal. The most useful VEPs are generated by
checkerboard pattern-reversal stimuli that evoke large, reproducible
potentials. Check sizes subtending greater than 40 degrees of arc
preferentially stimulate retinal luminance channels. Those less than
30 degrees stimulate contrast and spatial frequency detectors, and those
less than 15 degrees mainly stimulate the fovea. *P100* is the most useful
and reproducible wave. It is generated by the striate cortex as a near-field
potential and recorded from electrodes placed over the occipital cortex.
A significant prolongation of latency between eyes with alternate *full-field
monocular* stimulation is evidence for anterochiasmatic disease on the side

with prolonged latency. P100 may be bilaterally absent or prolonged with chiasmatic lesions. Refractive errors and macular disease can affect both the latency and amplitude of VEPs (see also Electroretinograms, following).

BRAINSTEM AUDITORY EVOKED POTENTIALS

Brainstem auditory evoked potentials (BAEPs) detect lesions of the auditory system and mid-upper brainstem. Click stimuli of 50 to 100 μs square-wave pulses to headphones or ear-insert transducers are used to elicit seven recordable potentials at the scalp. Waves I through VII occur within 10 ms after stimulation and are generated by propagating action potentials within the eighth cranial nerve (CN VIII) and central auditory pathways. They are volume conducted to the scalp and recorded there as far-field potentials. The specific generators of the waves are controversial, but most authorities agree with the following schema: I—distal CN VIII; II—proximal CN VIII; III—bilateral superior olivary complex; IV—ascending auditory fibers in the rostral pons; V—inferior colliculus; VI—medial geniculate nucleus; VII—distal auditory radiations. Waves VI and VII are often unobtainable or inconsistent and are clinically useless. Waves II and IV may be buried in or fused to other waves and are not as important as waves I, III, and V. Absolute latencies are not as important as the I-III-V interpeak latencies (IPLs).

Commonly recognized abnormal BAEP patterns include the following:

 I. *Absence of all waves:* Peripheral hearing loss, excessive background noise, technical error (rarely in Friedreich's ataxia, distal CN VIII lesions, or system atrophies).
 II. *Wave I only (or increased I-III IPL)*: Lesions of the proximal acoustic nerve or pontomedullary junction near the root entry zone (peripheral demyelination or inflammation, cerebellopontine [CP] angle tumors, pontine glioma, MS, leukodystrophies, neonatal anoxia, or brainstem infarct).
III. *Waves I-III only (or increased III-V IPL):* Lesions sparing the pontomedullary junction but affecting the pons to low midbrain (most commonly seen with MS, any disorder of pontine tegmentum, or large extrinsic masses compressing the brainstem—especially CP angle tumors opposite the stimulated ear).
IV. *Increased I-III, III-V, and I-V IPL:* Diffuse or multifocal disease such as demyelination, brainstem glioma, and especially hypothermia. (*Note*: BAEPs are extremely stable over wide ranges of metabolic derangement. Diffuse prolongation of IPLs should not be explained by metabolic abnormality.)

SOMATOSENSORY EVOKED POTENTIALS

Somatosensory evoked potentials (SEPs) are obtained from electrical stimulation of the median nerve at the wrist (MSEP) or the posterior tibial nerve at the ankle (PTSEP). Analysis of SEPs can give information about the integrity of the sensory component of peripheral nerves, spinal cord, brainstem, and to a lesser extent, the cortex. Recordings of far-field potentials are made over the scalp, and both near- and far-field potentials may be obtained at other points along the proximally propagating action potential.

I. *MSEP*: Four clinically useful "early" components of MSEPs and their presumed generators have been identified and are consistent and reproducible regardless of position of scalp electrodes. *P9* originates from the distal brachial plexus, *P11* from the dorsal root entry zone, *P13* from the dorsal columns of the cervical cord, and *P14* from the medial lemniscus of the brainstem. It can be seen that absence of a component or increased IPL provides evidence of a lesion along the course of propagation. Other "late" components (approximately N19, P23, N32, P40, and N60) have been identified and probably correspond to thalamic or suprathalamic generators. They are prolonged with decreasing levels of arousal and are not reproducible from person to person, or from the same person at different times or with changes of state. They also vary with different recording montages. Their usefulness is seen only when simultaneous bilateral stimulation produces asymmetries.

II. *PTSEP*: This is the most "laboratory specific" EP, with widely differing waveform designations and terminology. *PV* (propagated volley) is the designation given to the near-field potential recorded over the lower spine, which roughly corresponds to the cauda equina and lower gracile tract. It increases in latency with more proximal recording sites. *N22* is probably generated by axon collaterals in the dorsal columns near the thoracolumbar junction. Later components can be recorded from the scalp and represent more rostral brainstem, thalamic, and cortical generators. Their usefulness is proportional to the technique and reliability of the given laboratory. As with MSEPs, PTSEPs can give localizing information pertaining to lesions along the course of propagation.

ELECTRORETINOGRAMS

Two types of ERGs are in common use. Flash ERGs are useful for detecting retinal lesions and will not be discussed. Pattern ERGs (P-ERGs) utilize a checkerboard pattern-reversal stimulus. When a small enough check size is used (less than 2.4 degrees of arc), the major positive wave recorded from the cornea (b-wave) represents retinal ganglion cell function. The latency of "b" is about 40 ms and is prolonged or abolished by disease processes in or distal to the ganglia. When "b" is subtracted from the simultaneously recorded P100 of the VEP, retinocortical time (RCT) can be determined (RCT = P100 − b). RCT is a more accurate reflection of optic nerve integrity proximal to the retinal ganglia and is independent of macular disease.

Three abnormal patterns of P-ERG/VEP have been identified:

I. *Normal P-ERG, delayed VEP, and RCT:* Demyelination of the optic nerve.

E

EVOKED POTENTIALS

II. *Normal P-ERG, absent VEP:* Acute total block of optic nerve fibers.
III. *Absent P-ERG, absent VEP:* Severe macular disease or long-standing severe optic nerve disease with retrograde degeneration of retinal ganglion cells.

There is also evidence that decreased amplitude of P-ERGs in recent optic neuritis has a poor prognosis for visual recovery, and progressive loss of P-ERG amplitude correlates with the development of optic nerve atrophy.

EVOKED POTENTIALS AND MULTIPLE SCLEROSIS

EPs are most useful in the evaluation of MS (1) to demonstrate sensory abnormalities when the history or physical examination is equivocal and (2) to demonstrate clinically unapparent lesions when demyelination is suspected in other areas of the nervous system. Less important uses are (3) to define the distribution of the disease process and (4) to monitor changes in a patient's status. *When the diagnosis of MS is clinically definite, EPs will add little additional information.*

Abnormal VEPs are present in about 95% of cases of optic neuritis, regardless of how remote and regardless of whether vision has returned. About 50% of MS patients have abnormal VEPs even without clinical evidence of optic nerve involvement. Whereas about 35% of patients with progressive myelopathy have abnormal VEPs, only about 10% show abnormality after a single episode of transverse myelitis.

Forty-six percent of patients with MS have abnormal BAEPs, regardless of clinical classification. Thirty-eight percent of patients without clinical findings of brainstem involvement show abnormalities. The most common abnormalities are decreased or absent wave V or increased III-V IPL.

Of 1000 MS patients with varying classifications, 58% had abnormal MSEPs and 76% had abnormal PTSEPs.

The differential sensitivity of EPs in detecting white matter lesions in MS is related to the length of fiber tract being tested (i.e., the order of sensitivity is SEP greater than VEP and BAEP). As the degree of clinical certainty of the diagnosis increases from possible to probable to definite, the detection rate of lesions will be greater but the usefulness of the information obtained will be less.

EVOKED POTENTIALS AND OTHER NEUROLOGIC DISEASES

Many attempts have been made to use EPs as prognostic indicators of disease and trauma. In general, results comparing the quality, size, or shape of the potentials are conflicting and no better than following clinical examination. A more recent study has demonstrated that the complete absence of SEPs bilaterally more than 3 days after brain injury is very highly predictive of poor outcome or death. However, there is currently no definite role for EPs in the evaluation of brain death or recovery from coma. *Intraoperatively*, SEPs (during spinal cord surgery or endovascular embolization; brain or spine) and BAEPs (during posterior fossa surgery or endovascular embolization) may provide an early indication of compromise of neural tissue. In cervical spondylosis, PTSEPs may eventually help predict which patients are more likely to develop a significant cord deficit so that early surgical intervention can be considered. Flash VEPs have been used by some centers to monitor changes in intracranial pressure, but this is controversial.

REFERENCE

Gilmore R, ed: *Neurologic clinics*, Philadelphia, WB Saunders, 1988.

EXTRACRANIAL ULTRASONOGRAPHY

The carotid and vertebral arteries and their branches can be evaluated with ultrasound, that is, sound with frequency higher than 20,000 Hertz. *B-mode* (brightness modulation) is based on the transmission of ultrasound through tissues and reflection from tissue interfaces. This imaging technique produces a real-time two-dimensional picture of examined extracranial vessels in longitudinal or transverse view. It allows measurement of vessel diameter and reveals the presence of stenosis or occlusion. High-resolution scans can also determine plaque morphology, such as ulceration, calcification, or hemorrhage. In *Doppler ultrasonography*, the ultrasound is reflected off moving targets (erythrocytes). Increased blood flow velocity in a narrowed segment of arterial lumen (stenosis) is associated with higher frequency shift, which correlates with flow velocities. The best result in vascular ultrasonography can be obtained by combination of these two techniques, *duplex ultrasonography*. It combines the advantages of B-mode with exact sampling of the site, and systolic, diastolic, and mean velocities are measured in Doppler mode. Carotid duplex ultrasonography has an excellent accuracy for detection of stenotic process compared with angiography. For arteries with more than 50% stenosis, sensitivity is approximately 94% to 100%; for occlusions, sensitivity is 80% to 96% and specificity is 95%. However, these results vary considerably with the experience of the ultrasonographer. Examination of vertebral arteries allows determination of flow direction (for example, subclavian steal syndrome), but morphologic evaluation is not always possible.

REFERENCES

Babikian VL et al: *J Neuroimaging* 10:101–115, 2000.
Beletsky VY, Kelley RE: *J La State Med Soc* 148:467–473, 1996.

EYE MUSCLES

Because of their insertional properties, the six extraocular muscles affect eye movements in the three planes relative to primary position (Table 49). In testing muscle strength, the optical axis is aligned with a muscle's main vector. The superior and inferior rectus muscles insert on

TABLE 49

ACTIONS OF EYE MUSCLES IN PRIMARY POSITION

Muscle	Primary Action	Secondary Action	Tertiary Action
Lateral rectus	Abduction		
Medial rectus	Adduction		
Superior rectus	Elevation	Intorsion	Adduction
Inferior rectus	Depression	Extorsion	Adduction
Superior oblique	Intorsion	Depression	Abduction
Inferior oblique	Extorsion	Elevation	Abduction

the anterior globe at 23 degrees temporal to the primary position. Therefore, these muscles function solely in the vertical plane only when the eye is abducted 23 degrees. The oblique muscles insert on the posterior globe at 51 degrees nasal to the primary position. Thus, adduction maximizes the depressor effect of the superior oblique, whereas abduction maximizes intorsion (Fig. 17).

Diplopia testing in paralytic strabismus begins with measurement of visual acuity, confrontation visual fields, and observation of any abnormal head posture. *Head tilt occurs in the direction of action of the weak muscle.* Range of motion in each eye is tested in the nine cardinal positions of gaze with the opposite eye covered (ductions) and with both

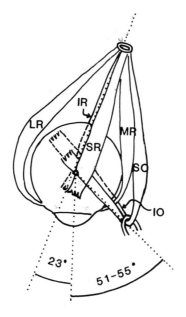

FIGURE 17

Insertion of ocular muscles of the globe. LR, lateral rectus; MR, medial rectus; SR, superior rectus; IR, inferior rectus; SO, superior oblique; IO, inferior oblique.

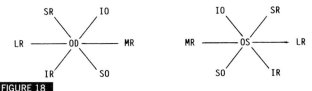

FIGURE 18

Main field of action of individual eye muscles.

eyes viewing (versions). *Misalignment can be seen in the corneal reflection of a penlight* and can be tested in all directions of gaze (Hirschberg's test).

Subjective diplopia testing relies on the principles that the disparate images are maximally separated in the main field of action of the paretic muscle and that *the more peripheral image belongs to the paretic eye* (Fig. 18). The Maddox rod tests primarily for phoria because it disrupts fusion; therefore, only the noncomitant deviations (unequal in different fields of gaze) should be considered abnormal. The paretic eye and the position of gaze producing the maximum separation of the images can be determined; the paretic muscle can be identified.

Objective tests include the cover-uncover test for tropia and the alternate cover test for phoria, which are performed in the primary position and in each cardinal position. Deviation of the nonparetic eye when covered (secondary deviation) is always greater than the deviation of the paretic eye when covered (primary deviation).

REFERENCE

Leigh RJ, Zee DS: *The neurology of eye movements*, ed 3, New York, Oxford University Press, 1999.

FACIAL NERVE, HEMIFACIAL SPASM

NEUROANATOMY

The *course of the facial nerve* (CN VII) is depicted in Figure 19. The numbers in the figure refer to the following *locations of the lesions*:

1. Peripheral to chorda tympani in facial canal or outside stylomastoid foramen. Peripheral upper and lower facial weakness (motor aspects of CN VII) only. Usually related to trauma.
2. Facial canal (mastoid), involving chorda tympani. In addition to upper and lower facial weakness, patients have loss of taste over the anterior two thirds of tongue and decreased salivation.

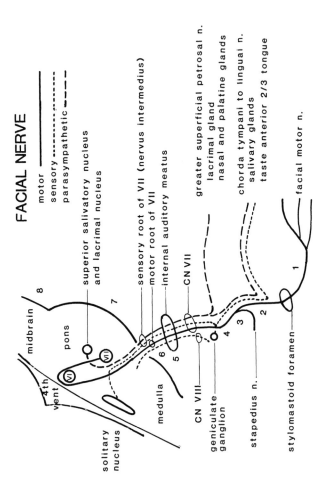

FIGURE 19
Facial nerve.

3. Facial canal, involving the stapedius nerve. Upper and lower facial weakness as in 1 and 2, plus hyperacusis.
4. Geniculate ganglion. Usually associated with pain in the ear. May have decreased lacrimation.
5. Internal auditory meatus. Complete CN VII (facial weakness; decreased taste, salivation, and lacrimation) plus CN VIII dysfunction (deafness or vestibular symptoms).
6. Extrapontine, subarachnoid. May have other cranial nerve involvement. Hemifacial spasm is more commonly associated with more proximal lesions of CN VII.
7. Pontine (nuclear or infranuclear). Millard-Gubler, Foville's, and Brissaud's syndromes (see Ischemia).
8. Supranuclear. Lesions may occur anywhere from mid-pons to motor cortex and are usually associated with other findings such as hemiparesis, hemisensory deficit, language disturbance, or homonymous hemianopia, depending on location. Taste, salivation, and lacrimation are not involved. Lower facial weakness is much more prominent than upper because of bilateral input to the portions of the facial nucleus controlling the upper face; input for the lower face is from contralateral cortex. Mild weakness may appear only as slight drooping of the angle of the mouth, slight widening of the palpebral fissure, or flattening of the nasolabial fold. (Table 50 compares clinical findings in the upper and lower motor neuron facial nerve weakness.)

DIFFERENTIAL DIAGNOSIS OF PERIPHERAL FACIAL PARALYSIS

Idiopathic Facial Paralysis or Bell's Palsy

Idiopathic facial paralysis or Bell's palsy is the most common form (60% of cases) and is probably a result of HSV-1 infection. Typified by a sudden, unilateral onset often preceded by a viral prodrome, the paralysis often regresses spontaneously in 8 to 10 weeks with complete recovery in 85% to 90% of patients. Acyclovir and prednisone are often prescribed to treat the condition but their use is controversial. Exposure keratitis may be ameliorated by lubricating ointment but rarely requires tarsorraphy. Melkersson's syndrome represents episodes of recurrent facial palsy with a deeply furrowed tongue (lingua plicata) and recurrent facial edema. Overall prognosis for this condition is good, but permanent paralysis may result after many recurrences.

Aberrant regeneration of the facial nerve with resolution of the paralysis has several variations. The most common of these is involuntary tearing of the eye on the involved side when eating ("crocodile tears") or synkinesis of the facial musculature when chewing. This often takes the form of a jaw-winking phenomenon, wherein the lid closes on the involved side when the jaw opens (Marin-Amat syndrome).

F

FACIAL NERVE, HEMIFACIAL SPASM

TABLE 50

CLINICAL FEATURES OF UPPER MOTOR NEURON VERSUS LOWER MOTOR NEURON FACIAL WEAKNESS

Upper Motor Neuron Lesions	Lower Motor Neuron Lesions
Unilateral paresis of voluntary movements of lower face with sparing of frontalis muscle	Unilateral paresis of all mimetic muscles, including the frontalis muscle
Facial muscle weakness *less* apparent with emotional than with voluntary action	Degree of facial weakness *similar* with emotional and voluntary movements
Preservation or accentuation of facial reflexes	Suppression of facial reflexes
Preserved taste, anterior two thirds of tongue	Possible impairment of taste
Normal lacrimation	Possible abnormality of lacrimation

Posttraumatic Facial Paralysis

Trauma is the second most common cause of peripheral facial paralysis in adults. Most often injury occurs in the intrapetrous portion. Nevertheless, traumatic lesions along the brainstem, the cerebellopontine angle, or in the parotid gland also occur.

Infectious Disorders

I. Ramsay-Hunt syndrome is the third most frequent cause of peripheral facial paralysis. It is caused by herpes zoster oticus and the symptoms are more severe than in idiopathic facial paralysis, often including dizziness, perception deafness (due to involvement of the vestibulocochlear nerve), and intense otalgia. A vesicular eruption in the external auditory canal, pinna, tragus, or soft palate confirms the diagnosis.

II. Inflammatory lesions of the middle ear include otitis media. Acute otitis media can cause a peripheral facial paralysis that resolves after antibiotic treatment or myringotomy. In chronic otitis media facial paralysis indicates compression of the nerve by a cholesteatoma or osteitis and necessitates surgery.

III. Necrotic otitis externa (malignant otitis externa) is due to *Pseudomonas aeruginosa* infection in diabetics. The nerve is invaded through the stylomastoid foramen.

IV. Other infectious causes: Lyme disease is complicated by facial paralysis in 10% of cases; paralysis is bilateral in 25% of cases and may be the initial symptom of the disease. Involvement of CN VII during the course of AIDS is also nonspecific.

Tumors

Tumors may cause sudden or relapsing facial paralysis, but progressive facial paralysis with a slow onset of more than 3 weeks strongly indicates the presence of a tumor.

I. Brainstem primary or secondary tumors produce impairment in a number of cranial nerve pairs.

II. Cerebellopontine angle (CPA) and the internal acoustic meatus (IAM) can be sites of tumors. Most frequently, lesions are neurinomas of CN VIII and mengiomas (consider neurofibromatosis-2). Epidermoid tumors have CSF signal on T_1 and T_2 sequences of MRI (Table 51). Arachnoid cysts are isointense to the CSF, have sharp contours, and remain confined to the subtentorial space. FLAIR can help detect epidermoid tumors; diffusion sequences show reduced diffusion within an epidermoid cyst compared with an arachnoid cyst.

III. IAM and the region of the ganglion geniculi may be sites for hemangiomas, which are small lesions associated with notable clinical manifestations: perception deafness, rigidity, or facial paresis.

IV. Tympanic cavity and mastoid: otoscopic examination can suggest tumor in the tympanic cavity and the mastoid by showing a whitish (primary cholesteatoma), grayish, or bluish (glomus) retrotympanic mass.

F

FACIAL NERVE, HEMIFACIAL SPASM

TABLE 51

TOPOGRAPHIC DIAGNOSIS OF LESIONS TO THE FACIAL NERVE: CHOICE OF IMAGING PROCEDURE

Segment	Clinical Aspect/Test	Imaging Procedure	Lesions
Nuclear: Pons	CN VII + CN VIII	MRI	Infarction, hematoma, multiple sclerosis, tumor, arteriovenous malformation, cavernous angioma, abscess
Cerebellopontine angle + internal acoustic meatus	CN VII + CN VIII; audiometry: perception deafness, vestibular examination	MRI	Neurinoma of CN VIII, meningioma, epidermoid cyst, vascular compression, neurinoma of the CN VII, hemangioma, glomus tumor, inflammation, fracture
Ganglion geniculi	Schirmer test	CT or MRI	Neurinoma and hemangioma of CN VII, primary or secondary cholesteatoma, cholesterol granuloma, metastasis, infection, fracture
Tympanic membrane or mastoid	Audiometry: transmission deafness, otoscopic examination, stapes reflex, gustometry	CT	Acute otitis, mastoiditis, cholesteatoma, fracture, neurinoma of CN VII, necrotic otitis externa, metastasis, glomus tumor
Parotid and endings	Often partial involvement	MRI	Often malignant parotid tumor, infection, sarcoidosis, trauma (forceps, penetrating lesion, surgery)

Primary or secondary bone tumors can be seen in the petrosal bone. Metastatic tumors are the most common type.

V. Parotid gland: Every parotid mass associated with facial paralysis should suggest a malignancy.

BILATERAL PERIPHERAL FACIAL PARALYSIS

I. Sarcoidosis: facial diplegia and uveitis
II. Guillian-Barré syndrome: facial diplegia, velopharyngeal involvement, and impairment in the sensory and motor nerves of the extremities
III. Lyme disease: facial diplegia in the presence of aseptic meningitis or with a slightly erythematous indurated face resembling painless cellulitis (also referred to as *Bannwarth's syndrome*)
IV. Leukosis/lymphomas: search for associated parenchymal or meningeal lesions
V. Melkersson-Rosenthal syndrome: see earlier mention under Idiopathic Facial Paralysis
VI. Ethylene glycol (antifreeze) toxicity: facial diplegia (temporary or permanent)

Neonatal Facial Paralysis

I. Obstetric facial paralysis is most often related to the use of forceps, but injury can be seen after spontaneous delivery or as a result of a pathologic intrauterine position. The facial paralysis usually resolves in a couple of weeks. CT scanning is indicated when there is no regression after 2 months to exclude a dishpan fracture that requires early surgical decompression (before age 3 months) to be efficacious.
II. Facial paralysis due to malformations
   A. Isolated hypoplasia of CN VII
   B. Möbius syndrome is typically associated with facial diplegia and paralysis of the abducens nerves, but there are unilateral forms associated with impairment in other ipsilateral cranial nerves. It is probably caused by antenatal ischemia of the nuclei of the nerves in the brainstem.
   C. Hypoplasia of the ear often has coexistent malposition of CN VII.

HEMIFACIAL SPASM

This entity is characterized by sudden, painless, involuntary contraction of the muscles innervated by CN VII. It is most often due to a conflict between vascular structures and the nerve at the root exit zone (REZ), which is an approximately 3-mm area beginning at the emergence of CN VII from the brainstem, at the junction of the central-type and peripheral-type myelin fibers. The vascular structures involved are, by decreasing order of frequency, the posteroinferior cerebellar artery, the vertebral artery, the anteroinferior cerebellar artery, and a vein (respectively 70%, 40%, 28%, and 21% in Magnan's series of 183 patients). Treatment usually consists of surgical decompression.

REFERENCES

Bradley WG, Daroff RB, et al: *Neurology in clinical practice*, ed 4, Boston, Butterworth-Heinemann, 2004.

Caces F et al: *Rev Laryngol Otol Rhinol (Bord)* 117:347–351, 1996.

Doyon D et al: *The cranial nerves* (English), Paris, Masson, Icon Learning Systems, 2004.

FEMORAL NERVE

The femoral nerve is formed by the combination of the posterior divisions of the ventral rami of L2, L3, and L4 spinal roots. The obturator nerve is formed by the ventral divisions of the same roots. The course of the femoral nerve runs through the psoas muscle. The femoral nerve innervates the psoas muscle, which additionally receives other branches directly from the L3 and L4 nerve roots. The nerve emerges from the psoas muscle and passes between it and the iliacus muscle. The femoral nerve is tightly covered by the iliacus fascia and is within the iliacus compartment. The femoral nerve innervates the iliacus approximately 4 to 5 cm proximal to the inguinal ligament, passes beneath the inguinal ligament just lateral to the femoral artery, and then emerges from the iliacus compartment. Just distal to the inguinal ligament, the femoral nerve ends by dividing into terminal motor and sensory branches. Motor branches supply the four heads of the quadriceps (rectus femoris, vastus lateralis, vastus medialis, vastus intermedius) and the sartorius muscles. The sensory branches are the medial and intermediate cutaneous nerves of the thigh and the saphenous nerve. The medial and intermediate cutaneous nerves of the thigh almost immediately enter the subcutaneous space and supply sensation to the anterior and medial thigh. The saphenous nerve travels through the thigh in the adductor canal deep to the sartorius muscle, gives off the infrapatellar branch to supply cutaneous sensation to the anterior patella, emerges from the canal approximately 10 cm proximal and medial to the patella, and then runs subcutaneously along the medial leg until reaching the medial arch of the foot.

NERVE INJURY

Because the femoral nerve is actually quite short, injuries usually occur either in the retroperitoneal pelvic space or at the inguinal ligament. Most femoral neuropathies are iatrogenic. Pelvic surgical procedures are the most common cause. Injury to the nerve within the pelvis may occur when a retractor is held tightly against the pelvic wall for a prolonged period of time. Injury to the nerve at the inguinal ligament may occur with prolonged use of the lithotomy position. Femoral artery catheterization with subsequent hematoma formation may compress the femoral nerve at the inguinal ligament. Spontaneous hematomas in the iliacus compartment or the psoas muscle may compress the femoral nerve or the lumbar plexus and usually occur with excessive anticoagulation. Non-iatrogenic femoral nerve neuropathies may occur in diabetes mellitus, usually as part of a more widespread polyradiculoplexopathy (i.e., diabetic amyotrophy).

F

FEMORAL NERVE

NEUROPATHY

Femoral neuropathy must be distinguished from L2–L4 polyradiculopathy and lumbar plexopathy. A lesion in any of these areas may cause weakness of knee extension, loss of quadriceps reflex, and sensory loss in the anterior and medial thigh and medial calf. In both L2–L4 polyradiculopathy and lumbar plexopathy, weakness of hip adduction, weakness of ankle dorsiflexion, and sensory loss in the very proximal medial thigh (obturator nerve) and lateral thigh (lateral femoral cutaneous nerve) may be present, but these findings will not occur in an isolated femoral neuropathy. If the site of femoral nerve injury is intrapelvic, weakness of hip flexion is expected, while if the site is at the inguinal ligament, hip flexion will be spared. Electromyography is useful both to confirm the lesion localization and to give information about prognosis for recovery. If more than 5 or 6 days have passed since the injury (allowing wallerian degeneration to occur) and the quadriceps CMAP amplitude is preserved, this suggests a predominantly demyelinating process with potential for recovery within several weeks. A low CMAP amplitude suggests an axonal process and a slower recovery.

REFERENCES

Katirji B et al: *Neuromuscular disorders in clinical practice*, Boston, Butterworth-Heinemann, 2002.

Preston DC, Shapiro BE: *Electomyography and neuromuscular disease*, ed 2, St. Louis, Elsevier, 2005.

FONTANEL

The anterior fontanel is an interosseous space located at the juncture of the sagittal and coronal sutures; the posterior fontanel is located at the juncture of the sagittal and lambdoidal sutures. At birth both fontanels are open. *The posterior fontanel becomes fused between 4 and 6 months of age. The anterior fontanel closes between 7 and 19 months of age* with an average closing time around 17 months. The anterior fontanel may be quite large at birth; this has little significance unless associated with palpably split sutures. If the infant has been delivered vaginally, the cranial bones may override each other and the fontanel may be difficult to palpate. When the infant cries, the fontanel may be tense and bulging. At other times it should be soft and flat and may pulsate. *A "full" or "tense" fontanel when the infant is quiet is a sign of increased intracranial pressure*. Causes of delayed closure of the anterior fontanel (persistently large) include prematurity, malnutrition, increased intracranial pressure, chromosomal abnormalities (trisomies 13, 18, and 21), metabolic disorders (hypothyroidism, rickets, and hypophosphatasia), and primary bone disorders (achondroplasia, cleidocranial dysostosis, and osteogenesis imperfecta).

FRONTAL LOBE

The frontal lobe consists of the precentral gyrus and superior, middle, and inferior frontal gyri and contains several different functional areas: the motor, premotor, supplementary motor, and prefrontal areas. The motor cortex (Brodmann's area 4) with somatotopic representation of the contralateral body (so-called homunculus) controls the voluntary movement. The giant pyramidal cells (Betz cells) in the motor cortex contribute 30% of the corticospinal tract and corticobulbar tract. The premotor and supplementary areas (Brodmann's area 6) participate in programming, preparation of movement, and control of posture. The premotor cortex also includes the frontal eye field (Brodmann's area 8) and Broca's area (Brodmann's areas 44 and 45). The prefrontal areas lie anterior to the premotor area with extensive connections to parietal, temporal, and occipital cortices. These areas help coordinate intellect, judgment, and planning of behavior.

FRONTAL LOBE LESIONS

Partial seizures, contralateral hemiplegia, and neurobehavioral syndromes may arise from different lesions of the frontal lobe. Expressive aphasia is associated with dominant frontal lobe lesion. Three behavioral syndromes have been described with prefrontal lesions. These syndromes may exist in pure or mixed forms:

   I. *Orbitofrontal syndrome:* disinhibition, impulsiveness, emotional lability, euphoria, poor judgment, and distractibility
   II. *Frontal convexity syndrome:* apathy, psychomotor retardation, poor word-list generation, motor perseveration and impersistence, and inability to execute multistep behaviors
   III. *Medial frontal syndrome*: paucity of spontaneous movement, sparse verbal output, lower extremity weakness, and incontinence

FUNCTIONAL MAGNETIC RESONANCE IMAGING

PET and SPECT imaging, under the rubric of nuclear medicine, had been the only types of functional imaging available until the relatively recent advent of functional magnetic resonance imaging (fMRI). Unlike traditional MRI, which provides exquisite anatomic imaging, fMRI provides an avenue into imaging actual brain physiology. Compared to PET and SPECT, fMRI has better spatial resolution with less total scan time. In addition, fMRI does not require the injection of any material, let alone a radioactive isotope.

A detailed explanation of the technical parameters of fMRI is beyond the scope of this work. In brief, among the various factors affecting signal intensity on MRI is local magnetic inhomogeneity with greater inhomogeneity leading to more rapid loss of signal. Deoxyhemogolobin, unlike oxyhemoglobin, is paramagnetic. Paramagnetic substances increase inhomogeneity and, as expected, result in accelerated loss of signal. Autoregulation of cerebral blood flow causes increased blood flow to active regions of the brain. The increase in blood flow far exceeds the increase in oxygen extraction, resulting in a net decrease in deoxyhemoglobin in the capillary bed and venules. With the net decrease in deoxyhemoglobin comes an improvement in the local magnetic homogeneity and thus a net increase, approximately 2%, in signal intensity from the active region of the brain. That 2% can be used to map brain function.

The effective genesis of fMRI occurred in 1990, when Ogawa noted the blood oxygen level dependent (BOLD) effect on signal intensity just described. By 1992, Ogawa and associates and Kwong and associates had published the first functional images using the BOLD technique.

A cursory search of the literature reveals that fMRI has a potential role to play in seizure localization, pain management, understanding the physiologic basis of cognition and perception, identifying psychiatric disorders, and differentiating the various forms of dementia, as well as assessing myriad other functional abnormalities of the brain.

fMRI has already improved our understanding of the organization of the brain in addition to providing a powerful tool in evaluating neurologic status. fMRI continues to make inroads into assessing neurosurgical risk; neurosurgery, in particular, depends on defining both brain structure and function.

fMRI may well become the optimal method for studying brain function in the normal, diseased, and injured states in addition to being the least intrusive and most accurate way for assessing the potential risks of neurosurgery or radiation therapy.

REFERENCES

Buxton RB: *Introduction to functional magnetic resonance imaging: Principles and techniques*, Cambridge, Cambridge University Press, 2002.

Huettel SA, Song AW, McCarthy G: *Functional magnetic resonance imaging*, Sunderland, Sinauer Associates, 2004.

G

GAIT DISORDERS

Gait depends on both maintenance of equilibrium and mechanisms of locomotion. Abnormal gait, especially in the elderly, is due to a combination of factors. A useful approach to assessing contributors to gait disorder is by localizing the level of the sensorimotor deficit and differentiating them into three groups: low, middle, and high sensorimotor level gait disorders.

Low sensorimotor level gait disorders can be divided into peripheral sensory and peripheral motor dysfunction. In peripheral sensory impairment, unsteady and tentative gait is commonly caused by vestibular disorders, peripheral neuropathy, proprioceptive deficits, or visual ataxia. Peripheral motor impairment results from arthritic, myopathic, and neuropathic conditions causing deformity of the extremities, painful weight bearing (e.g., antalgic gait), and focal weakness (e.g., Trendelenburg gait in hip adductor weakness and "steppage" gait in footdrop). The resulting gait disorders are primarily compensatory, allowing patients to adapt well to the deficit.

Middle sensorimotor level gait disorders encompass hemiplegic, paraparetic, cerebellar ataxic, parkinsonian, choreic, hemiballistic, and dystonic gaits. Pyramidal, cerebellar, and basal ganglia motor systems dysfunction results in faulty execution of centrally selected postural and locomotor responses, resulting in the disruption of the sensory and motor modulation of gait. Despite the abnormal stepping pattern, gait initiation and postural reflexes are usually intact.

High sensorimotor level gait disorders have more nonspecific gait characteristics. They are due to difficulties in frontal planning and execution and include cautious gait, frontal and subcortical disequilibrium, gait ignition failure (gait apraxia), frontal gait disorders, primary progressive freezing gait (PFG) disorder, and psychogenic gait disorder. Cognitive dysfunction and behavioral aspects such as fear of falling play a role, particularly in cautious gait. The severity of frontal-related disorders runs a spectrum from gait ignition failure to frontal gait disorder to frontal disequilibrium, in which gait initiation difficulty and small shuffling steps progress to the point at which unsupported stance is not possible. They are difficult to differentiate clinically and are usually the result of a lesion that affects the corticobasal ganglionic-thalamocortical loop caused by bilateral infarction, hemorrhage, neoplasm, hydrocephalus, or a degenerative process.

The anatomic or neurochemical abnormality in primary progressive freezing gait disorder remains unknown. This disorder is restricted to the legs and is characterized by start hesitation, motor blocks or freezing spells, and recurrent falls. The patient walks as if the feet were glued to the floor, while the upper part of the body is normally mobile. Progression of this disorder may lead to total inability to walk and to severe functional disability. Imaging studies are usually normal and response is poor to dopaminergic drugs.

Gait disorder in the elderly frequently results from an overlap of deficits in the three sensorimotor levels. Two mechanisms appear to precipitate gait disorder particularly in the elderly. First, "benign disequilibrium of the elderly" is a multiple sensory deficit syndrome (combination of impairments in position and tactile sense, vision, hearing, and vestibular or baroreceptor function) causing vague dizziness or disequilibrium ("dizziness of feet") while standing, walking, or turning but not while sitting or lying, and equilibrium improves with holding or leaning onto a wall. These patients benefit from gait training and use of an assistive device (cane or walker) and should not be medicated (meclizine, benzodiazepines) for presumed vestibular disease. A second common problem is acute deterioration in gait, balance, and postural adjustments in acutely ill elderly patients. The ensuing "toxic-metabolic encephalopathy" (caused by medications, organ failure, dehydration, electrolyte imbalance, or systemic infection) may result in varying gait difficulty and altered postural reflexes, gegenhalten (paratonia involving an involuntary resistance to passive movement) of limb and neck, diffuse myoclonus, and bilateral asterixis. Acute gait disorder may in turn be the presenting feature of acute systemic decompensation in the elderly and warrants further evaluation (i.e., stroke, myocardial infarction, or infection).

Diagnosis of gait disorders is based on history and associated neurologic findings. Isolated gait disorders in the elderly are frequently due to treatable disorders such as Parkinson's disease, cervical myelopathy, or normal-pressure hydrocephalus. Gait evaluation and training by physical therapy should be initiated early. Discontinuing unnecessary medication use and home safety evaluations are pertinent in preventing future falls.

REFERENCES

Alexander NB, Goldberg A: *Cleveland Clin J Med* 72:586–600, 2005.
Nutt JG, Marsden CD, Thompson PD: *Neurology* 43:268–279, 1993.
Rubino FA: *Neurologist* 8(4):254–262, 2002.

GAZE PALSY

Horizontal gaze palsies: A unilateral gaze (for both saccadic and pursuit movements) palsy may indicate a contralateral cerebral hemispheric (frontoparietal), contralateral midbrain, or ipsilateral pontine lesion. Except when the pontine lesion is at the level of the abducens nucleus, either involving the nucleus itself or the paramedian pontine reticular formation, the eyes can be driven toward the side of the palsy with cold caloric stimulation of the ipsilateral ear or oculocephalic maneuvers. Hemispheric lesions characteristically produce transient defects; brainstem lesions may be associated with enduring defects. An acute cerebellar hemispheric lesion can result in an ipsilateral gaze palsy that can be overcome with calorics. Unilateral saccadic palsy with intact pursuit is unusual and indicates an acute frontal lesion. Unilateral impaired pursuit with normal saccades is usually due to an ipsilateral deep posterior hemispheric lesion with a contralateral hemianopia.

Vertical gaze palsies: The rostral interstitial nucleus of the medial longitudinal fasciculus (riMLF) in the upper midbrain contains the cells that generate vertical eye movements. A medially placed lesion will result in both an up-gaze and down-gaze palsy. An isolated down-gaze palsy is due to a bilateral or lateral midbrain lesion. Isolated up-gaze palsies occur with lesions of the posterior commissure, bilateral pretectal regions, and large unilateral midbrain tegmental lesions. In the dorsal midbrain (Parinaud's) syndrome the paralysis of upward gaze is usually associated with convergence-retraction nystagmus, lid retraction, and light-near dissociation of the pupils. An acute bilateral pontine lesion at the level of the abducens nucleus may result in a transient up-gaze paralysis in addition to bilateral horizontal gaze palsy.

Conjugate eye deviations: Horizontal deviations are associated with acute gaze palsies as described above and with irritative cerebral foci (seizure or intracerebral hemorrhage), which usually drive the eyes to the side opposite the lesion. Ipsiversive eye and head movements, however, are reported with focal seizures. Tonic upward deviations occur in the oculogyric crisis of postencephalitic parkinsonism and, more commonly, as an idiosyncratic reaction to phenothiazines. They may also occur in coma, usually as a result of anoxic encephalopathy. Downward deviations may occur transiently in normal neonates but also in infantile hydrocephalus and in adults with metabolic encephalopathy, bilateral thalamic infarction, or hemorrhage.

GERSTMANN'S SYNDROME

I. *Definition*. The clinical tetrad of agraphia, acalculia, agnosia to fingers, and agnosia to right-left (disorientation) defines Gerstmann's syndrome. Finger agnosia may manifest as bilateral difficulties in finger naming, moving fingers to command, matching of fingers to demonstration, or recognizing stimuli ("wiggle the finger that I touch"). When all features are present, a *dominant inferior parietal or posterior perisylvian lesion* is highly likely. Aphasia, alexia, and constructional apraxia almost always accompany this syndrome.

II. *Etiology*. Developmental Gerstmann's syndrome occurs in children with or without dyslexia. Verbal IQ among such children is often significantly higher than performance IQ. This syndrome can also manifest in the context of global disease such as SLE, AIDS, or multiple sclerosis.

REFERENCES

Devinsky O: *Behavioral neurology: 100 maxims*, St. Louis, Mosby, 1992.
Mesulam MM: *Principal of behavioral and cognitive neurology*, New York, Oxford University Press, 2000.

GLOSSOPHARYNGEAL NEURALGIA

Glossopharyngeal neuralgia is similar to trigeminal neuralgia in etiology and pathogenesis.

CLINICAL FEATURES

Clinical features also are similar, although distribution is different and the pain may be more variable with longer duration and is associated with autonomic dysfunction (salivation, lacrimation, bradycardia, and syncope). Pain distribution is to the throat, posterior one third of the tongue, tonsillar pillars, eustachian tube, and ear. Trigger points are variable, most commonly associated with swallowing, chewing, speaking, laughing, coughing, or touching particular areas in the distribution of the glossopharyngeal nerve and upper sensory fibers of the vagus nerve. Onset is after age 40, with males and females affected equally.

DIFFERENTIAL DIAGNOSIS
The differential diagnosis includes underlying causes such as oropharyngeal carcinoma, peritonsillar abscess, enlarged styloid process (Eagle's syndrome), or enlarged tortuous vertebral or posterior inferior cerebellar arteries, and SUNCT syndrome (short-lasting, unilateral, neuralgiform headache attacks with conjunctival injection and tearing). Evaluation for glossopharyngeal neuralgia should include a thorough ear, nose, and throat examination.

TREATMENT
Treatment is aimed at underlying causes of "symptomatic" neuralgias. Otherwise, carbamazepine or phenytoin or both may be used, although the response rate to these drugs is less than 50%. Surgical therapy has included microsurgical decompression of the glossopharyngeal and vagal root entry zones, and sectioning of the glossopharyngeal nerve almost always produces complete relief.

REFERENCE
Bradley WG, et al: *Neurology in clinical practice*, ed 4, Philadelphia, Butterworth Heinemann, 2004.

GLUCOSE IMBALANCE

In contrast to other tissues, the brain normally derives its energy from carbohydrates only. A significant drop in blood sugar will diminish oxygen utilization and intracellular energy production. Typical constellation of signs and symptoms resulting from hypo- or hyperglycemia are described here.

I. *Hypoglycemia*: Symptoms arise from neuroglycopenia and endogenous release of catecholamines. Mild hypoglycemia produces hunger, weakness, dizziness, blurred vision, anxiety, tremor, tachycardia, pallor, diaphoresis, headache, and mild confusion. With more severe hypoglycemia, the preceding symptoms are followed by seizures (glucose <30 mg/100 dL) with progression to coma, pupillary dilation, hypotonia, and extensor posturing (glucose <10 mg/100 mL). The presence of hyperventilation may lead to paresthesias. *Focal findings may mimic cerebrovascular disease*. Symptoms, signs, and residual neurologic deficit depend on the rate of onset, duration, and severity of hypoglycemia. Patients with chronic hypoglycemia may have no sympathetic symptoms but present with cognitive or behavioral disturbances. Repeated severe attacks of hypoglycemia may result in dementia because of damage to hippocampal neurons. The degree of slowing on EEG correlates well with the severity of hypoglycemia, but *enhanced response to hyperventilation appears first*. Epileptiform discharges are rare even if hypoglycemic convulsions occur.

II. Hyperglycemia

    A. Diabetic ketoacidosis is the most common cerebral complication of diabetes and is frequently accompanied by stupor or coma. Muscle cramps, dysesthesias, and diffuse abdominal pain may occur. The neurologic changes correlate best with serum osmolarity, although dehydration, acidosis, and associated electrolyte disorders contribute. *The treatment of diabetic ketoacidosis may lead to fatal cerebral edema if blood osmolarity is rapidly lowered relative to brain osmolarity*. Treatment may also cause hypophosphatemia, hypokalemia, and hypoglycemia. In diabetic ketoacidosis, generalized slowing on EEG parallels declining consciousness.

    B. Hyperglycemic nonketotic states result in CNS complications due to extracellular hyperosmolarity. Neurologic manifestations are variable and include hallucinations, depression, apathy, irritability, seizures (typically transient focal or epilepsia partialis continua), flaccidity, diminished deep tendon reflexes, tonic spasms, myoclonus, meningeal signs, nystagmus, tonic eye deviations, and reversible loss of vestibular caloric responses. As the blood glucose rises above 600 mg/dL, coma may develop. Studies indicate that hyperglycemia can lead to poor outcome in stroke patients during the acute phase, and tight control of blood sugar is recommended. Seizures generally improve within 24 hours of rehydration and correction of hyperglycemia. EEG may show corresponding focal abnormalities, including periodic lateralized epileptiform discharges.

    In both ketotic and nonketotic hyperglycemia, care should be placed in recognizing and treating the underlying stressor, which may include stroke, myocardial infarction, infection, or other acute medical illnesses.

III. *Hypoglycorrhachia*, low CSF glucose, is usually associated with infection, either bacterial or chronic meningitis. It may also be seen in meningeal carcinomatosis. Persistent low CSF glucose with normal serum glucose levels in a patient with seizures and developmental delay may be a result of a genetic defect in glucose transport across the blood-brain barrier. These long-term neurologic sequelae may be prevented by a ketogenic diet.

REFERENCES

De Vivo et al: *N Engl J Med* 325:703–709, 1991.
Jorgenson HS et al: *Stroke* 25:1977–1984, 1994.

GRAVES' OPHTHALMOPATHY

Graves' ophthalmopathy refers to any thyroid-associated ophthalmopathy. Approximately 50% of patients with Graves' disease will manifest ophthalmopathy. The mean presenting age of thyroid ophthalmopathy is 43 years, ranging between 8 and 88 years. Cigarette smoking is a well-established risk factor for more severe ophthalmopathy; the risk is proportional to the amount of cigarette consumption. Alterations in cellular immunity (CD4/CD8 T lymphocyte ratio) are thought to initiate the orbital changes associated with thyroid ophthalmopathy. Activated CD4 T-helper lymphocytes may bind to orbital fibroblasts that express thyroid-type receptors and antigens, subsequently producing edema and fibrosis. Also, loss of CD8 T-suppressor cells may contribute to the inflammatory process, plasma cell proliferation, and production of autoantibodies specific for extraocular tissues.

CLINICAL FEATURES AND DIAGNOSIS

Clinical features include dryness, "gritty" sensation, lacrimation, photophobia, blurring of vision, deep orbital pressure, or diplopia. Diplopia is due to fibrosis of ocular muscles that do not extend fully when their antagonist contracts. Fibrosis of the inferior rectus, the most frequently affected muscle, causes diplopia on upgaze. Other findings on examination are periorbital and lid edema, lid retraction, lid lag, conjunctival chemosis and injection, and corneal exposure ranging from minor lagophthalmos to complete decompensation and corneal perforation. Some patients have compressive optic neuropathy with decreased visual acuity, optic disk changes, visual loss, dulling of color perception, and visual field defects.

Diagnostic evaluation of thyroid eye disease includes thyroid function tests, serum thyrotropin receptor antibody, and serum antimicrosomal and antithyroglobulin antibodies. Enlarged extraocular muscles can be demonstrated by ultrasonography, CT, or MRI.

TREATMENT

Most cases of thyroid ophthalmoplegia resolve spontaneously. The therapeutic intervention is separated into acute and chronic phases. Acute intervention is prompted by the development of the vision-threatening conditions of optic neuropathy and corneal exposure. Compressive optic neuropathy is usually treated with high-dose corticosteroids and, less commonly, emergent surgical decompression. Orbital radiation therapy is proved to be safe and effective in acute ophthalmopathy; high-dose IVIG is equal in efficacy to systemic corticosteroids. In preexisting ophthalmopathy, 67% of people who received radioiodine followed by a 3-month course of oral prednisone showed improvement. In minor corneal exposure, conservative measures such as lubrication and taping of the lids or use of a moisture chamber while sleeping are often sufficient. In more severe cases, tarsorrhaphy may be necessary and the use of botulinum toxin has been suggested.

REFERENCE

Zobian J, Mans M: *Curr Opin Ophthalm* 9:105–110, 1998.

GUILLAIN-BARRÉ SYNDROME (See also NEUROPATHY)

GBS is an acute autoimmune polyneuropathy encompassing a heterogeneous group of pathologic and clinical entities. The annual incidence is around 1 to 3 in 100,000 population. Although it can affect both sexes and any age group, there is a bimodal distribution with peaks in young adults and the elderly and a predilection for males.

CLINICAL FEATURES

Clinical features (Table 52) includes limb weakness, areflexia, and albuminocytologic dissociation. Antecedent infections such as *Campylobacter jejuni*, cytomegalovirus, Epstein-Barr virus, *Mycoplasma* pneumonia, *Haemophilus influenzae*, influenza A and B viruses, parinfluenza virus, adenovirus, varicella-zoster, and parvovirus B19 have been associated with GBS. HIV infection, herpes simplex 1 and 2 infections, and Lyme disease can cause GBS with pleocytosis in CSF. Vaccines are possible additional factors associated with GBS. Although 10% of GBS cases present as atypical forms (pure sensory, pure Guillain-Barré syndrome dysautonomic, pharyngeal-brachial-cervical, and paraparetic), there are four major clinical variants (Table 53).

G

GUILLAIN-BARRÉ SYNDROME

TABLE 52

CLINICAL FEATURES OF GUILLAIN-BARRÉ SYNDROME

Motor Dysfunction
Symmetrical limb weakness (proximal, distal, global)
Neck muscle weakness
Respiratory muscle weakness
Cranial nerve paralysis: III-VII, IX-XII
Areflexia
Wasting of limb muscles

Sensory Dysfunction
Pain, numbness, paresthesiae
Loss of position sense, vibration, touch and pain
Ataxia

Autonomic Dysfunction
Sinus tachycardia and bradycardia
Other cardiac arrhythmias
Hypertension and orthostatic hypotension
Wide fluctuation of pulse and blood pressure
Tonic pupils, hypersalivation, anhidrosis or excessive sweating, urinary sphincter disturbances, constipation, gastric dysmotility, abnormal vasomotor tone with venous pooling and facial flushing

TABLE 53

CLINICOPATHOLOGIC FORMS OF GULLAIN-BARRÉ SYNDROME

Forms of GBS	Pathology	Electrophysiologic features	Comments
AIDP (acute inflammatory demyelinating polyneuropathy)	Lymphocytic infiltration of the peripheral nerves, segmental demyelination macrophages mediated	Segmental slowing, absent or prolonged F reflexes, increased distal latency, conduction block or abnormal temporal dispersion	Good strength recovery, permanent areflexia
AMAN (acute motor axonal neuropathy)	Lengthening of the Ranvier nodes, distortion of paranodal myelin, axonal dissection	Distal latencies, motor conduction velocities, F waves and sensory nerve action potentials are normal, but CMAP are reduced.	Anti-GM1, GD1a and GD1B antibodies can be present Normo- or hyperreflexia are possible, common association with *Campylobacter* infection; usually good recovery
AMSAN (acute motor sensory axonal neuropathy)	Wallerian-like degeneration of sensory and motor fibers, little demyelination or lymphocytic infiltration	Very low M responses amplitude, inexcitable motor nerves, sensory and motor axonal dysfunction	Fulminant course, associated with *Campylobacter* infection; poor prognosis—slow and incomplete recovery
Miller-Fisher syndrome	Positive immunostain for antibodies in the paranodal region of CN III, IV, and VI, inflammation and demyelination	Reduced or absent sensory and motor nerve action potentials, absent H reflex; motor and sensory conduction velocities are normal or minimally reduced	Although the ophthalmoplegia, areflexia, and ataxia constitute the typical picture, weakness can be occasionally seen; anti-GQ1b antibodies are usually present

TREATMENT

Immunotherapy with plasma exchange (PE) or intravenous immunoglobulin (IVIG) hastens recovery from GBS. PE is recommended for nonambulant patient with GBS within 4 weeks of the onset, or for ambulant patients within 2 weeks of onset. IVIG is recommended for nonambulant patients with GBS within 2 to 4 weeks of the onset. The effects of PE and IVIG are equivalent, and combination of the two or sequential treatment is not recommended. Corticosteroids have no role in GBS treatment. Pain control, hemodynamic monitoring, deep-vein thrombosis prophylaxis, and physical therapy are warranted.

REFERENCES

Hughes RAC, Wijdicks EFM, Barohn R, et al: *Neurology* 61:736–740, 2003.
Senevirante U: *Postgrad Med J* 76:774–782. 2000.

H

HALLUCINATIONS

The DSM IV-R defines hallucinations as a "sensory precept without external stimulation of the relevant sensory organ." Some distinguish true hallucinations (experiences perceived as real and outside the body) from pseudohallucinations (perceived as occurring within the body or known to be unreal). Phenomena include lilliputian (small animals or people), brobdingnagian (giants), and autoscopic (seeing oneself from outside) characteristics, as well as palinopsia, voices, palinacusis, crawling sensations, shooting pains, smells, and other features.

I. Differential diagnosis of visual hallucinations
  A. Ocular disorders: Hallucinations may be associated with reduced vision. These are usually formed, bright, colored images. *Charles Bonnet syndrome* is isolated visual hallucinations, usually of ocular cause. These ocular disorders include enucleation; cataracts; macular, choroidal, and retinal disease; vitreous traction.
  B. CNS disorders: Hallucinations may be due to lesions anywhere along the optic pathways and visual association cortices. They are also seen with midbrain disease ("peduncular hallucinosis"; complex forms, usually with other brainstem signs), dementias, epilepsy, migraine, and narcolepsy. Hypnagogic hallucinations occur just before falling asleep, and hypnopompic hallucinations occur on awakening.
  C. Medical disorders: Hallucination may be seen in 40% to 75% of delirious patients; usually they are brief, nocturnal, and emotionally charged. Causes include alcohol and drug withdrawal, hallucinogens, sympathomimetics, and metabolic encephalopathies.

    D. Psychiatric disorders: Schizophrenia, mania or depression, and hysteria can produce hallucinations.

    E. Normal individuals may experience hallucinations during dreams, falling asleep (hypnagogic hallucinations), hypnosis, childhood (imaginary companion), sensory deprivation, sleep deprivation, intense emotional experiences.

II. Differential diagnosis of auditory hallucinations

    A. Diseases of the ears or peripheral auditory nerves

    B. CNS diseases: epilepsy, neoplasms, and occasionally, vascular lesions

    C. Toxic or metabolic: alcoholic hallucinosis, encephalopathies

    D. Psychiatric: schizophrenia (60% to 90% of patients), affective disorders, conversion reactions, multiple personality disorder

III. Tactile, somatic, and phantom limb hallucinations

    A. Phantom limb is the sensation of persistent presence of an amputated extremity and is found in almost all amputees; patients usually describe the phantom limb as being numb or tingling, of normal size, correctly aligned, with peripheral areas more prominent; the sensation recedes gradually.

    B. Tactile hallucinations occur commonly in patients with schizophrenia (15% to 50%) and affective disorder (25%).

    C. Formication (the sensation of insects crawling) is found in alcohol and drug withdrawal (especially sympathomimetics) and dementias.

IV. Olfactory and gustatory hallucinations

    A. Medial temporal lobe lesions and complex partial seizures ("uncinate fits") may produce olfactory hallucinations. They may also occur in migraine, dementias, toxic and metabolic conditions, depression, and Briquet's syndrome (20% to 25% of patients).

    B. Gustatory hallucinations may be seen in manic-depressive illness, schizophrenia, Briquet's syndrome, and partial seizures.

REFERENCE

Trimble MR, Cummings JL, eds: *Contemporary behavioral neurology*, Boston, Butterworth-Heinemann, 1997.

HEAD TRAUMA

EPIDEMIOLOGY

Traumatic brain injury (TBI) is a leading cause of disability and death affecting over 5 million people in the United States alone. Severe TBI is defined by a Glasgow Coma Score under 9. TBI involves an initial injury and is followed by further neurologic damage that occurs over days following the initial trauma. All geographic areas should have an organized trauma system and follow published guidelines for managing TBI.

TREATMENT

Initial management of the trauma patient includes ABCI: airway, breathing, circulation, and spine immobilization. Patients with severe TBI (GCS < 9) should be intubated for airway patency/protection and ventilatory support. The goals of TBI management are to prevent secondary insults (hypoxia, hypotension) that lead to secondary neuronal injury. To date, we have no therapies that can reverse the primary neurologic injury. Maintenance of normal hemodynamic and respiratory parameters prevents secondary injury from hypotension and hypoxemia. Even a single episode of hypotension (SBP < 90 mm Hg) worsens outcomes in TBI, as does hypoxia ($PaO_2 < 60$ mm Hg). Cerebral perfusion pressure (CPP = MAP − ICP) should be kept greater than 60 mm Hg.

Intracranial pressure should be monitored in comatose patients with TBI (Glasgow coma score <9). The incidence of elevated ICP increases with the depth of coma and greater neuroimaging abnormalities. There is no predictable relationship between BP and ICP. Treat ICP greater than 20 mm Hg. *Hyperventilation* can be used to acutely decrease elevated ICP but has no role in chronic management. *Osmotic therapy* with mannitol or hypertonic saline can be used to control ICP along with ventricular CSF drainage. *Hemicraniectomy* should be considered in patients with life-threatening unilateral cerebral edema. *Prophylactic antiepileptic drugs* should be used for the first 7 days following injury. There is no role for steroid use in TBI.

Fever should be aggressively treated over the first few days with the goal being normothermia. There is currently no proven benefit to hypothermia. *Glycemic control* is also a priority in acute TBI. Brain tissue oxygenation ($PbtO_2$) and jugular venous oxygen saturation ($SjvO_2$) can be monitored to ensure adequate brain oxygenation.

Following the initial injury, physical and cognitive rehabilitative services will likely be needed on an ongoing basis. The incidence of chronic cognitive-behavioral impairment is high.

REFERENCE

Dutton RP, McGunn M: *Curr Opin Crit Care* 9:503–509, 2003.

HEADACHE: MIGRAINE AND OTHER TYPES (See also AAN GUIDELINE SUMMARIES APPENDIX)

Headache is one of the most common reasons for neurologic consultation. Given the range of disorders that present with headache, a systematic approach to headache classification and diagnosis is essential. Since 1988, the classification of International Headache Society (IHS) has been the accepted standard for headache diagnosis. *The International Classification of Headache Disorders*, 2nd edition (ICHD-2, Table 54), groups headache disorders into primary and secondary headaches. The four categories of primary headache include migraine, tension-type

---

TABLE 54

THE INTERNATIONAL CLASSIFICATION OF HEADACHE DISORDERS, 2ND
EDITION (ICHD-2)

I. The primary headaches
   A. Migraine
   B. Tension-type headache (TTH)
   C. Cluster headache and other trigeminal autonomic cephalalgias
   D. Other primary headaches
II. The secondary headaches
   A. Headache attributed to head or neck trauma
   B. Headache attributed to cranial or cervical vascular disorder
   C. Headache attributed to nonvascular intracranial disorder
   D. Headache attributed to a substance or its withdrawal
   E. Headache attributed to infection
   F. Headache attributed to disorder of homoeostasis
   G. Headache or facial pain attributed to disorder of cranium, neck, eyes, ears,
      nose, sinuses, teeth, mouth, or other facial or cranial structures
   H. Headache attributed to psychiatric disorder
III. Cranial neuralgias, central and primary facial pain, and other headaches
   A. Cranial neuralgias and central causes of facial pain
   B. Other headache, cranial neuralgia, central or primary facial pain

From Lipton; *Neurology* 63:427, 2004.

---

headache (TTH), cluster headache (CH) and other trigeminal autonomic
cephalalgias (TACs), and other primary headaches. There are also eight
categories of secondary headache, and a third group that includes central
and primary causes of facial pain and other headaches.

PRIMARY HEADACHE TYPES
Migraine
An estimated 27.9 million Americans suffer from migraine, with a 1-year
prevalence of 18.2% among females and 6.5% among males aged 12 and
older. The prevalence of migraine peaks between the ages of 25 and 55,
during patients' most productive years. Migraine costs the United States
about $13 billion per year in lost productivity. Migraine also adversely
affects quality of life and ability to function.

Migraine is classified into five major categories:
 I. *Migraine without aura*
   A. At least five attacks fulfilling criteria B through D
   B. Headache attacks lasting 4 to 72 hours (untreated or unsuccessfully
      treated)
   C. Headache has at least two of the following characteristics:
      1. Unilateral location
      2. Pulsating quality
      3. Moderate or severe pain intensity
      4. Aggravation by or causing avoidance of routine physical activity
         (e.g., walking or climbing stairs)

D. During headache at least one of the following:
   1. Nausea or vomiting
   2. Photophobia and phonophobia
E. Not attributed to another disorder
F. In addition, when attacks occur on at least 15 days per month, the diagnoses are chronic migraine plus migraine without aura.

II. *Migraine with aura:* The typical aura of migraine is characterized by focal neurologic features that usually precede migrainous headache but may accompany it or occur in the absence of the headache.
   A. At least two attacks fulfilling criteria B through D under type I
   B. Aura consisting of at least one of the following, but no motor weakness:
      1. Fully reversible visual symptoms including positive features (e.g., flickering lights, spots, or lines) or negative features (i.e., loss of vision)
      2. Fully reversible sensory symptoms including positive features (i.e., pins and needles) or negative features (i.e., numbness)
      3. Fully reversible dysphasic speech disturbance
   C. At least two of the following:
      1. Homonymous visual symptoms or unilateral sensory symptoms
      2. At least one aura symptom develops gradually over at least 5 minutes or different aura symptoms occur in succession over at least 5 minutes
      3. Each symptom lasts between 5 and 60 minutes
   D. Headache fulfilling criteria B through D for type I. Migraine without aura begins during the aura or follows aura within 60 minutes.
   E. Not attributed to another disorder
   F. Typical aura symptoms develop over at least 5 minutes and last no more than 60 minutes, and visual aura is overwhelmingly the most common. Typical visual aura is homonymous, often having a hemianopic distribution and expanding in the shape of a crescent with a bright, ragged edge, which scintillates. Scotoma, photopsia, or phosphenes and other visual manifestations may occur. Visual distortions such as metamorphopsia, micropsia, and macropsia are more common in children. Sensory symptoms occur in about one third of patients who have migraine with aura. Typical sensory aura consists of numbness (negative symptom) and tingling or paresthesia (positive symptoms). The distribution is often cheiro-oral (face and hand). Dysphasia may be part of typical aura but motor weakness, symptoms of brainstem dysfunction, and changes in level of consciousness, all of which may occur, signal particular subtypes of migraine with aura (hemiplegic and basilar-type). Typical aura occurring in the absence of any headache is a disorder most often reported by middle-aged men. Differentiating this benign disorder from TIA, a medical emergency, may require investigation, especially when it first occurs after age 40, when negative features (i.e., hemianopia) are predominant, or when the aura is of atypical duration.

H

HEADACHE: MIGRAINE AND OTHER TYPES

Familial hemiplegic migraine is the first migraine syndrome to be linked to a specific set of genetic polymorphisms. In this disorder aura includes some degree of motor weakness (hemiparesis) and may be more prolonged than 60 minutes (up to 24 hours); additionally, at least one first-degree relative has had similar attacks (also meeting these criteria). The two known loci for FHM are on chromosomes 1 and 19. Migraine meeting these criteria but without a family history is classified as sporadic hemiplegic migraine.

In *basilar-type migraine* (basilar migraine) symptom profile suggests posterior fossa involvement and requires at least two of the following fully reversible symptoms: dysarthria, vertigo, tinnitus, decreased hearing, double vision, visual symptoms simultaneously in both temporal and nasal fields of both eyes, ataxia, decreased level of consciousness, and simultaneously bilateral paresthesias. About 60% of patients with FHM have basilar-type symptoms.

III. *Childhood periodic syndromes* that are commonly precursors of migraine: Cyclical vomiting occurs in up to 2.5% of school-age children with episodes of intense but otherwise unexplained nausea and vomiting lasting 1 hour to 5 days in children free of symptoms interictally. Abdominal migraine afflicts up to 12% of school-age children with recurrent attacks of abdominal pain associated with anorexia, nausea, and sometimes vomiting. Physical examination and investigations exclude other causes of these symptoms. Benign paroxysmal vertigo is a disorder characterized by recurrent (at least five) attacks resolving spontaneously after minutes to hours with normal neurologic examination, normal audiometric and vestibular functions, and normal EEG between attacks.

IV. *Retinal migraine:* This disorder is rare. Recurrent attacks (at least two) of fully reversible scintillations, scotomata, or blindness, affecting one eye only, are accompanied or followed within 1 hour by migrainous headache. Other causes of monocular visual loss, including TIA, optic neuropathy, and retinal detachment, must be ruled out.

V. *Probable migraine:* Between 10% and 45% of patients with features of migraine fail to meet all criteria for migraine (or any of its subtypes). Probable migraine is when a single criterion is missing (and the full set of criteria for another disorder are not met).

Complications of migraine. Chronic migraine (CM) is considered when headache is both present and meets criteria for migraine on at least 15 days per month for at least 3 months, in the absence of medication overuse. Most cases evolve from episodic migraine. When medication overuse is present (acute antimigraine drugs or opioids or combination analgesics taken on 10 days per month, or simple analgesics on at least 15 days per month), it is a likely cause of chronic headache. Medication-overuse headache (analgesic rebound headache) cannot be diagnosed with confidence until the overused medication has been withdrawn and improvement within 2 months occurs. *Status migrainosus* refers to an attack of migraine with a headache phase lasting over 72 hours. Persistent aura without infarction is diagnosed when aura symptoms, otherwise typical of past attacks, persist for over 1 week. Investigation shows no evidence of infarction. *Migrainous infarction* is an uncommon occurrence. One or more otherwise typical aura, which exactly mimics the previous attacks, persists beyond 1 hour and neuroimaging confirms ischemic infarction. Other causes of stroke must be excluded.

Headaches are common in the postictal period, but epilepsy can be triggered by migraine (*migralepsy*). The criteria for migraine-triggered seizure require that a seizure fulfilling diagnostic criteria for one type of epileptic attack occur during or within 1 hour after a migraine aura.

Tension-type Headache

TTH is the most common type of primary headache, with 1-year period prevalence ranging from 31% to 74%. The ICHD-2 distinguishes three subtypes: infrequent episodic TTH (ETTH) with headache episodes on less than 1 day per month, frequent ETTH with headache episodes on 1 to 14 days per month, and chronic TTH (CTTH) with headache on 15 days per month, perhaps without recognizable episodes.

The ICHD-2 diagnostic criteria for TTH are as follows:

I. *Infrequent episodic TTH*
   A. At least 10 episodes occurring on less than 1 day per month on average (<12 days per year) and fulfilling criteria B through D
   B. Headache lasting from 30 minutes to 7 days
   C. Headache has at least two of the following characteristics:
      1. Bilateral location
      2. Pressing/tightening (nonpulsating) quality
      3. Mild or moderate intensity
      4. Not aggravated by routine physical activity such as walking or climbing stairs
   D. Both of the following:
      1. No nausea or vomiting (anorexia may occur)
      2. No more than one of photophobia or phonophobia
   E. Not attributed to another disorder
II. *Frequent episodic TTH:* At least 10 episodes occurring on at least 1 but less than 15 days per month for at least 3 months (between 12 and 180 days per year) and fulfilling foregoing criteria B through E.
III. Chronic TTH
   A. Headaches happening on at least 15 days per month on average more than 3 months (180 days per year and fulfilling criteria B through D).
   B. Headache lasts hours or may be continuous
   C. Headache has at least two of the following characteristics:
      1. Bilateral location
      2. Pressing/tightening (nonpulsating) quality
      3. Mild or moderate intensity

      4. Not aggravated by routine physical activity such as walking or climbing stairs
- D. Both of the following:
   1. No more than one of photophobia, phonophobia, or mild nausea
   2. Neither moderate nor severe nausea or vomiting
- E. Not attributed to another disorder
- F. Like chronic migraine, CTTH cannot be diagnosed in patients overusing acute medication.

IV. Probable tension-type headache. When headache fulfills all but one of the criteria for TTH and does not fulfill criteria for migraine without aura.

Cluster Headache and Other Trigeminal Autonomic Cephalalgias

This group of primary headache disorders is characterized by trigeminal activation coupled with parasympathetic activation.

  I. *Cluster headache (CH):* Men are affected more commonly than women, with a peak age of onset between 25 and 50 years. This disorder manifests as intermittent, short-lasting, excruciating unilateral head pain accompanied by autonomic dysfunction. The pain is described variously as sharp, boring, drilling, knife-like, piercing, or stabbing, in contrast to the pulsating pain of migraine. It usually peaks in 10 to 15 minutes but remains excruciatingly intense within a duration range of 15 to 180 minutes. During this pain, patients find it difficult to lie still, exhibiting often marked agitation and restlessness, and autonomic signs are usually obvious. After an attack, the patient remains exhausted for some time. Attacks of episodic CH occur in cluster periods lasting from 7 days to 1 year separated by attack-free intervals of 1 month or more. Approximately 85% of CH patients have the episodic subtype. In chronic CH, attacks recur for longer than 1 year without remission, or with remissions lasting less than 1 month.

  II. *Paroxysmal hemicrania:* As a group, the paroxysmal hemicranias have three main features: (1) at least 20 frequent (more than five per day) attacks that are short-lasting (2 to 30 minutes); (2) severe and strictly unilateral orbital, supraorbital, or temporal pain and symptoms of parasympathetic activation ipsilateral to the pain (as in CH); (3) absolute response to therapeutic doses of indomethacin. ICHD-2 subclassifies PH to episodic paroxysmal hemicrania and chronic paroxysmal hemicrania (CPH), which are distinguished by the presence or absence of attack-free intervals lasting 1 month or more.

  III. *Short-lasting unilateral neuralgiform headache attacks with conjunctival injection and tearing (SUNCT):* SUNCT syndrome is a very rare primary headache. The diagnostic criteria require at least 20 high-frequency attacks (3 to 200 per day) of unilateral orbital, supraorbital, or temporal stabbing or pulsating pain, lasting 5 to 240 seconds and accompanied by ipsilateral conjunctival injection and lacrimation.

  IV. *Probable trigeminal autonomic cephalalgia:* This headache fulfills all but one of the diagnostic criteria for TACs.

Other Primary Headaches

This group of miscellaneous primary headache disorders includes some mimics of potentially serious secondary headaches, which need to be carefully evaluated by imaging or other appropriate tests.

I. *Primary stabbing headache*. Episodic localized stabs of head pain (jabs and jolts) occurring spontaneously in the absence of any structural cause. Pain is predominantly in the distribution of the first division of the trigeminal nerve (orbit, temple, and parietal area). It lasts for up to a few seconds and recurs one to many times per day.

II. *Primary cough headache*. Brought on suddenly by coughing, straining, or Valsalva maneuver, and not otherwise, in the absence of any underlying disorder such as cerebral aneurysm or, especially, Arnold-Chiari malformation. Neuroimaging, with special attention to the posterior fossa and base of the skull, is mandatory to rule out secondary forms of cough headache.

III. *Primary exertional headache*. Triggered by physical exercise, pain is pulsating and lasts from 5 minutes to 48 hours. After the first occurrence of any exertional headache of sudden onset, appropriate investigations must exclude subarachnoid hemorrhage and arterial dissection. Must be distinguished from primary cough headache and headache associated with sexual activity

IV. *Primary headache associated with sexual activity*. Precipitated by sexual activity, it usually begins as a dull bilateral ache as sexual excitement increases, and suddenly becomes intense at orgasm. Two subtypes are preorgasmic headache and orgasmic (explosive) headache. Diagnosis of the latter requires exclusion of subarachnoid hemorrhage and arterial dissection.

V. *Hypnic headache*. Characterized by short-lived attacks (typically 30 minutes) of nocturnal head pain that awaken the patient at a constant time each night. It's a disorder of the elderly and does not occur outside sleep. It is usually bilateral and mild to moderate without autonomic features.

VI. *Primary thunderclap headache*. Severe headache of abrupt onset, which mimics the pain of a ruptured cerebral aneurysm. Intensity peaks in less than 1 minute. Pain lasts from 1 hour to 10 days and may recur within the first week after onset but not regularly over subsequent weeks or months. This diagnosis can be established only after excluding subarachnoid hemorrhage.

VII. *Hemicrania continua*. This daily and continuous strictly unilateral headache is defined by its absolute response to therapeutic doses of indomethacin. Pain is moderate, with exacerbations of severe pain, and autonomic symptoms accompany these exacerbations, although less prominently than in CH and CPH.

VIII. *New daily persistent headache (NDPH)*. The essence of this headache, which otherwise resembles CTTH, is that it is daily and unremitting from or very soon (<3 days) after onset. There is no history of evolution from episodic headache. Diagnosis is not confirmed until it has been present for over 3 months and cannot be made if this manner of onset is not clearly recalled by the patient. Nor can it be made in the presence of medication overuse.

Note: Chronic daily headache (CDH) of long duration is a clinical syndrome not included in the ICHD-2, defined by headaches that occur for at least 4 hours a day on at least 15 days a month over more than 3 months. CDH is one of the more common headache presentations to headache specialty care centers and afflicts 4% to 5% of the general population. CDH includes CM, CTTH, NDPH, and CH, and subtypes with or without medication overuse.

HEADACHE THERAPY

Three components of a systematic approach to treating headache are psychological, physical, and pharmacologic. Psychological therapy involves reassurance and counseling, as well as stress management, relaxation therapy, and biofeedback as appropriate. Physical therapy involves identifying headache triggers, such as diet, hormone variations, and stress, and whether alteration may be helpful in treating selected cases. The patient should record a headache calendar documenting the occurrence, severity, and duration of headaches; the type and efficacy of medication taken; and any triggering factors.

Pharmacotherapy can be divided into two approaches, abortive and prophylactic.

Abortive Therapy of Migraine

Migraine specific agents (e.g., triptans, DHE, ergotamine) are used in patients with more severe migraine and in those whose headaches respond poorly to NSAIDs or combination of analgesics. Select a nonoral route of administration for patients whose migraines present early with significant nausea or vomiting.

I. Routine analgesics (aspirin, acetaminophen, and NSAIDs, including ibuprofen, naproxen, indomethacin, ketorolac, and others) are given for less severe headaches.

II. Triptans: Begin specific migraine therapy with a triptan for clinic patients with severe migraine or those who do not respond to analgesics. A number of randomized, controlled trials and systematic reviews have found all of the triptans to be effective for the treatment of acute migraine.

III. Narcotic analgesics should be avoided (especially as the first-line treatment) but are useful for occasional, severe headaches.

IV. Ergotamine preparations are available for oral, sublingual, and rectal administration and by inhalation.

A. Ergotamine 1 mg PO q 30 minutes up to 5 mg per attack

B. Ergotamine 1 mg and caffeine 100 mg (Cafergot), 1 or 2 tabs PO q 30 minutes up to 5 tabs per attack.

C. Ergotamine 2 mg sublingually q 30 minutes up to three doses per day.

D. Ergotamine 2 mg and caffeine suppository 1000 mg, 1 PR, may repeat in 1 hour.

E. Dihydroergotamine intranasal (Migranal) 1 spray (0.5 mg) into each nostril; if needed, repeat after 15 minutes, up to a total of 4 sprays.

F. Dihydroergotamine (DHE 45) IV (Table 55).

V. Metoclopramide 10 mg IM, IV, or PO 15 minutes before other analgesic agents have proved useful.

VI. Prochlorperazine 10 mg IM, IV or chlorpromazine 25 to 50 mg IM, IV.

VII. Prednisone 40 to 60 mg PO qd over a short course may break "status migrainosus."

Prophylactic Treatment of Migraine

I. Avoid inciting dietary factors such as red wine, aged cheese, chicken liver, pickled herring, tuna, sour cream and yogurt, ripe avocado and banana, smoked meats, and foods with monosodium glutamate or nitrates.

II. Conduct trial when patient is not using oral contraceptives and nitrates, if possible.

III. Prophylactic medication for those with frequent or disabling attacks includes the following. Start with low dose and gradually increase. Should inform patients of potential side effects.

A. Beta blockers

1. Propranolol, starting at 20 mg PO bid and gradually increasing prn to 80 mg tid

H

HEADACHE: MIGRAINE AND OTHER TYPES

TABLE 55

PROTOCOL FOR SEVERE, PERSISTENT HEADACHES

I. Dihydroergotamine (DHE 45) and metoclopramide protocol is tried initially. It is contraindicated in pregnancy and in Prinzmetal's angina. For patients over 60 years of age, monitor cardiac status during first two doses of DHE 45. Side effects include diarrhea, leg pains, vasospasm, chest pain, and supraventricula arrhythmia.

A. Metoclopromide 10 mg IV plus DHE 45, 0.5 mg IV over 2 to 3 min.

B. If nausea and headache are absent, continue DHE 45, 0.5 mg IV q 8 hr for 3 days with metoclopramide 10 mg IV. Stop metoclopromide after sixth dose.

C. If no nausea is present and headache is persistent, repeat DHE 45, 0.5 mg IV in 1 hour without metoclopramide; if nausea does not recur, give DHE.45 1 mg q 8 hr for 3 days with six doses of metoclopramide. If nausea recurs with the second dose of DHE 45, reduce DHE 45 dose to 0.75 mg.

D. If nausea and headache persist, hold DHE 45 for 8 hours, then give DHE 45, 0.3 to 0.4 mg q 8 hr for 3 days, with metoclopramide for six doses.

II. Protocol for those unable to tolerate DHE 45.

A. Prednisone 80 mg/day (short, rapidly tapering dosage).

B. Neuroleptics: Haloperidol 5 mg PO or IM, thiothixene 5 mg PO or IM, or chlorpromazine 10 to 50 mg PO or 25-mg suppository.

C. Opiate analgesics: Meperidine 75 to 100 mg, hydromorphone 4 mg, or morphine 10 mg.

From Raskin NH: *Neurol Clin* 8:857–865, 1990.

    2. Others: nadolol (80 to 240 mg/day); atenolol (50 to 100 mg/day); timolol (20 to 100 mg/day), metoprolol (50 to 300 mg/day)

B. Antidepressants
  1. Tricyclic antidepressant: amitriptyline starting at 10 mg PO qhs and increasing to 150 mg qhs; nortriptyline 10 to 125 mg/day; desipramine 10 to 200 mg/day; doxepin 10 to 250 mg/day
  2. SSRIs: fluoxetine 10 to 80 mg/day; paroxetine 10 to 40 mg/day; sertraline 25 to 200 mg/day
  3. Other: bupropion 75 to 300 mg/day.

C. Antiepileptics
  1. Depakote, 250 tid to 1500 mg/day
  2. Gabapentine, start with 100 mg tid or 300 mg qhs and increase to 3600 mg/day
  3. Topiramate start with 25 mg bid and increase to 200 mg/day
  4. Phenytoin 200 to 400 mg/day; especially useful in children

D. Calcium channel blockers
  1. Verapamil 120 mg to maximum 720 mg/day
  2. Others: nifedipine 30 to 180 mg/day; diltiazem 60 to 360 mg/day; nimodipine 20 to 60 mg/day

E. Serotonin antagonist
  1. Methysergide 2 mg PO tid or qid (need drug holiday every 6 months for 1 month to prevent fibrotic retroperitoneal or mediastinal changes; now off the market in United States)
  2. Cyproheptadine 4 to 8 mg PO tid

F. MAO inhibitors: phenelzine sulfate 15 mg PO qd, qod, or bid

G. Ergot derivatives: ergonovine 0.2 mg PO tid up to 2 mg qd

Treatment of Tension-Type Headache

  I. Simple analgesics such as acetaminophen, aspirin, and other NSAIDs are the drugs of choice for abortive therapy.
  II. Prophylactic therapy is indicated for patients with chronic headaches requiring daily analgesics.

Treatment of Cluster Headache

  I. Treat as for migraine (triptan, intranasal DHE, ergotamine).
  II. 100% O_2 by mask at 6 L/minute up to 15 minutes per attack.
  III. Octrotide 100 mg SC especially for patients with cardiovascular risk factor.
  IV. Lidocaine 4% intranasal; 15 drops ipsilateral to headache with head extended and rotated away from side of headache.
  V. Prednisone 40 to 60 mg PO qd over short course (slow taper in 3–4 weeks); rebound headaches can occur after discontinuation.
  VI. Lithium carbonate 300 mg PO bid-qid titrated to lithium levels (0.6 to 1.2 mEq/L) is especially useful for prophylaxis in chronic cluster headaches.

VII. Verapamil 120 mg tid for prophylaxis in chronic cluster headaches.

Treatment for Indomethacin-Responsive Headaches
Indomethacin 75 to 250 mg daily in divided doses for primary exertional, cough, and stabbing headaches and also episodic and chronic paroxysmal hemicrania.

Treatment of Chronic Daily and Medication Overuse Headache
I. Discontinue the offending medications, especially analgesics used to excess.
II. Use of pharmacotherapeutic agents in attempt to break the cycle of continuous headache.
III. Initiation of prophylactic pharmacotherapy (often valproic acid, tricyclic antidepressants, or beta blocker).
IV. Concomitant behavioral intervention, including biofeedback therapy, individual behavioral counseling, family therapy, physical exercise, and dietary instruction.
V. Adequate instruction on ill effects of medications with special focus on analgesics.

REFERENCES
Aukerman G: *Am Fam Phys* 66, 2002.
Landy S: *Neurology* 62:S2–S8, 2004.
Lipton RB: *Neurology* 63:427–435, 2004.
Silberstein SD: *Neurology* 55:754–762, 2000.

H

HEARING

HEARING

I. *Bedside testing of hearing* should include examination of the external ear and the tympanic membranes. Auditory acuity can be grossly assessed by whispering into each ear while closing the other and by comparing the distance from the ear at which the patient and the examiner can hear a ticking watch or fingers rubbing together. *Tuning fork tests* are commonly used. In *Weber's test* a 256-Hz tuning fork is placed at the midline vertex of the skull; sound referred to an ear with decreased acuity indicates conductive hearing loss. In *Rinne's test* a tuning fork placed on the mastoid and one held in front of the ear are compared; if bone conduction is greater, conductive loss is implied.
II. *Audiologic tests* are used to quantitate and localize (conductive, sensorineural, cochlear, and retrocochlear) hearing loss. *Pure-tone threshold* determines auditory threshold for tones over various frequencies and intensities for both air and bone conduction. Impairment of both air and bone conduction, especially at high frequencies, indicates sensorineural hearing loss. When bone conduction is greater than air conduction, conductive hearing loss is present. Other tests of loudness function are the alternate binaural

loudness balance and the short-increment sensitivity index. Bekesy audiometry, tone decay tests, speech discrimination tests, the stapedius reflex (pathway from cochlea to eighth cranial nerve to facial nerve to stapedius muscle), and brainstem auditory evoked potentials (BAEPs) help distinguish retrocochlear from cochlear lesions. Rarely, cortical deafness or auditory agnosia occurs with bitemporal lesions and BAEPs are normal.

III. *Causes of nonretrocochlear hearing loss*
   A. Infections: bacterial, viral, or fungal of the external, middle, or inner ear
   B. Presbycusis; otosclerosis
   C. Tumor: glomus tumor, cholesteatoma
   D. Ototoxic drugs, such as aminoglycosides, aspirin, and diuretics
   E. Meniere's disease
   F. Trauma

IV. *Causes of retrocochlear (eighth cranial nerve and CNS) hearing loss*
   A. Tumors: acoustic neuroma, cholesteatoma, meningioma, pontine glioma
   B. Vascular: vertebrobasilar ischemia and inferior lateral pontine infarction or basilar occlusion
   C. Demyelinating diseases
   D. Congenital malformations: Arnold-Chiari, Klippel-Feil syndromes
   E. Degenerative diseases: hereditary ataxias, hereditary neuropathies; Refsum's disease, xeroderma pigmentosum, Cockayne's syndrome, Usher's syndrome (retinitis pigmentosa and deafness), and other rare hereditary degenerative disorders
   F. Infectious: meningitis, encephalitis, syphilis
   G. Inflammatory: Vogt-Koyanagi-Harada syndrome, Behçet's syndrome; sarcoidosis
   H. Mitochondrial diseases: Kearns-Sayre syndrome

REFERENCE

Rudge P: *Clinical neuro-otology*, New York, Churchill-Livingstone, 1983.

HEMIFACIAL SPASM

Hemifacial spasm is a syndrome of involuntary contraction of the muscles innervated by the facial nerve. The estimated incidence is 0.78/100,000, and it is more common in women than men. Onset is usually between 40 and 50 years of age.

I. *Clinical presentation*. Patients usually present with a complaint of one eye closing involuntarily. In 90% of patients, the orbicularis oculis is the first muscle affected, but eventually, other muscles innervated by the ipsilateral facial nerve become affected as well. The resulting spasms occur in all ipsilateral affected muscles synchronously. In about 5% of cases, bilateral facial nerves will be affected; in these cases, the spasms of the right facial muscles are not synchronous with those of the left.

II. *Etiology.* It is presumed to be related to vascular compression of the ipsilateral facial nerve as it emerges from the pons. It is thought that this compression results in demyelination, and that adjacent demyelinated fibers of the facial nerve trigger each other to fire through ephaptic coupling.

III. *Evaluation.* If the diagnosis is not clear from the history and physical examination, MRI and MRA may be helpful, but these results are neither sensitive nor specific. Vascular abnormalities are seen in 88% in hemifacial spasm patients versus 25% of control subjects. The differential diagnosis includes tic disorders, blepharospasm, tardive dyskinesia, and facial myokymia.

IV. *Treatment.* Neurosurgical treatment involves microvascular decompression of the offending artery. This procedure is still done, and has a high success rate. However, some patients do suffer recurrence of symptoms, and ipsilateral hearing loss is a known complication of the surgery.

Recently, the use of botulinum toxin injections has emerged as a nonsurgical treatment. It is widely used, and has a high rate of patient satisfaction. It is not a permanent solution, and injections must be repeated every few months. Less than 10% of cases resolve without treatment.

REFERENCE

Tan NC, Chan LL, Tan EK: *Q J Med* 95:493–500, 2002.

HERNIATION

Herniation is defined as displacement of the cerebral or cerebellar structures from their normal compartments owing to pressure differences. Most commonly, increased pressure is due to a focal lesion (e.g., tumor with cerebral edema, extra/intra-axial hemorrhage, infarct, abscess). Some diffuse elevations of ICP, such as pseudotumor cerebri, rarely produce herniation. Other conditions produce diffuse cerebral edema, elevated ICP, and frequent herniation (e.g., hepatic coma, meningoencephalitis, hypoxic brain injury, diffuse traumatic brain injury).

HERNIATION SYNDROMES

I. *Central (transtentorial) herniation*—diencephalon is forced down through the tentorial incisura; most often seen in the setting of diffuse cerebral edema.

II. *Uncal (lateral) herniation*—usually rapid (acute), often from a temporal lobe mass, pushing uncus and hippocampal gyrus over the edge of tentorium, entrapping the oculomotor nerve, and later directly compressing midbrain. The posterior cerebral arteries may be pinched on the tentorium and cause occipital infarction (as with central herniation).

H

HERNIATION

III. *Cingulate (subfalcine) herniation*—the cingulate gyrus herniates under the falx cerebri; often asymptomatic and preceding central/transtentorial herniation; can lead to bifrontal infarctions when anterior cerebral arteries become compromised.

IV. *Upward cerebellar herniation*—the cerebellar vermis herniates upward through the transtentorial notch compressing the midbrain; with sylvian aqueduct compression it can cause hydrocephalus and occlusion of superior cerebellar arteries leading to cerebellar infarctions; can occasionally be seen with posterior fossa masses and may be exacerbated by ventriculostomy.

V. *Tonsillar herniation*—cerebellar tonsils herniate downward through the foramen magnum, compressing medullary respirator centers, which may be fatal; rarely may be precipitated by lumbar puncture in the presence of intracranial mass lesions.

These syndromes are accompanied by characteristic clinical signs that correspond to the anatomic structures involved (Table 56). Decreased level of consciousness or coma is usually the first clinical finding. There is a rostral-caudal progression of clinical signs seen with both central and lateral transtentorial herniation, indicating worsening herniation (Table 57). This begins with diencephalic involvement, followed by mesencephalic, pontine, and finally medullary involvement. Two infrequent exceptions to this orderly progression, in which signs skip from the hemispheres or

---

TABLE 56

HERNIATION SYNDROMES

Syndromes	Anatomy	Signs
Central transtentorial herniation: Caudal displacement of diencephalon through tentorial notch	Reticular formation or diencephalon initially, then rostral-caudal progression	Altered consciousness
Lateral transtentorial herniation (uncal)	Ipsilateral CN III	Ipsilateral pupil dilation, then external ophthalmoplegia
	Ipsilateral posterior cerebral artery	Contralateral homonymous hemianopia
	Contralateral cerebral peduncle (false localizing); then follows rostral-caudal progression but may skip diencephalic stage	Ipsilateral hemiparesis
Cerebellar tonsillar herniation	Medullary respiratory center	Respiratory arrest
Cingulate herniation under falx cerebri	Anterior cerebral artery	Leg weakness

TABLE 57

ROSTRAL-CAUDAL PROGRESSION OF TRANSTENTORIAL HERNIATION

	Diencephalon	Midbrain-Upper Pons	Low Pons-Upper Medulla	Medulla
Consciousness, systemic	Agitated or drowsy to coma, diabetes insipidus	Hypothermia or hyperthermia, comatose	Comatose	Fluctuating pulse, blood pressure falls Coma
Breathing	Yawns, pauses, Cheyne-Stokes respirations	Central hyperventilation	Tachypnea (20–40 breaths per min) shallow	Slow and irregular or hyperapnea alternating with apnea, then breathing stops
Pupils	Small (1–3 mm) reaction, small but brisk	Irregular, midposition, (3–5 mm), fixed	Small midposition fixed	Dilated, fixed
Eye movements	Roving, VOR weak or brisk, fast-phase caloric response lost, loss of vertical movement	Intact VOR, may be dysconjugate response	No VOR, no caloric response	No VOR, no caloric response
Motor	Preexisting hemiplegia worsens, decorticate posturing to noxious stimuli, plantars extensor	Bilateral decerebrate posturing to noxious stimuli	Flaccid flexor response in LEs to noxious stimuli	Flaccid, no deep tendon reflexes

VOR, vestibulo-ocular reflex; LE, lower extremity.

H

HERNIATION

diencephalon to the medulla, bypassing the rostral brainstem, are as follows: (1) acute cerebral hemorrhage, with extravasation into the ventricles, compresses the medullary respiratory center in the floor of the fourth ventricle, and (2) when lumbar puncture is performed on patients with incipient transtentorial herniation, it may induce enough of a pressure gradient change to produce tonsillar herniation.

For treatment of herniation, see Intracranial Pressure.

HICCUPS (SINGULTUS, HICCOUGHS)

I. *Definition:* A reflex myoclonic contraction of the diaphragm with a forceful inspiration, associated with laryngeal spasm and closure of the glottis, producing a characteristic sound. It is mediated by the phrenic (afferent), vagus, and thoracic nerves (efferent). Gastrointestinal, pulmonary, and cardiovascular signs and symptoms may be present.

II. *Causes:* Carcinoma, achalasia, and hiatal hernia are common pathologic causes. Other pathologic causes include intrathoracic distention, pulmonary or pleural irritation, pericarditis, mediastinitis and mediastinal mass, intrathoracic abscess or tumor, and aortic aneurysms. There are several *CNS causes* as well, including metabolic (acetonemia, uremia), drugs (sulfonamides), infection (encephalitis), hypothalamic disease (also associated with yawning), tumors of the fourth ventricle, and cerebrovascular disease (vertebrobasilar insufficiency). Chronic idiopathic and psychogenic hiccups are also common.

III. *Treatment:* Usually treatment is not required, because hiccups tend to be self-limited. If intractable, there is likely to be an underlying cause. Drug therapies include phenothiazines (prochlorperazine, chlorpromazine), valproic acid, phenytoin, carbamazepine, benzodiazepines (clonazepam, diazepam), and baclofen. Surgical sectioning of the phrenic nerve or selective vagotomy is occasionally required; more recently acupuncture and sertraline have been used.

REFERENCES

Macdonald J: *BMJ* 319:976, 1999.
Moretti R et al: *Eur J Neurol* 6:617, 1999.

HORNER'S SYNDROME, COCAINE TEST

I. *Pathophysiology:* Horner's syndrome (oculosympathetic paresis) is due to disruption at any point along the course of the sympathetic pathway from the hypothalamus to the orbit (Fig. 20). Signs are ipsilateral pupillary miosis (resulting from iris dilator weakness) most evident in dim illumination, blepharoptosis (weakness of Müller's muscle), and facial anhidrosis. Heterochromia of the iris occurs in congenital Horner's syndrome.

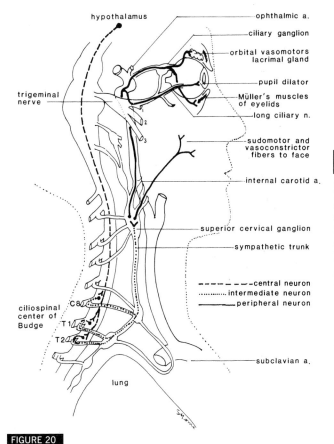

hypothalamus

ophthalmic a.

ciliary ganglion

orbital vasomotors lacrimal gland

pupil dilator

Müller's muscles of eyelids

long ciliary n.

trigeminal nerve

sudomotor and vasoconstrictor fibers to face

internal carotid a.

superior cervical ganglion

sympathetic trunk

– – – – – central neuron
.... intermediate neuron
——— peripheral neuron

ciliospinal center of Budge

C8
T1
T2

subclavian a.

lung

H

HORNER'S SYNDROME, COCAINE TEST

FIGURE 20

Oculosympathetic pathways.

II. *Etiology:* The cause of Horner's syndrome can be determined in about 60% of cases. Lesions of the first-order neuron (central) are myriad and may be due to *stroke, tumor, hemorrhage, and demyelinating disease*. Second-order neuron (preganglionic) causes include *apical lung tumor, tuberculosis, radical neck dissection, trauma, and neck masses*. Third-order neuron (postganglionic) lesions include *internal carotid aneurysms, carotid dissection, cluster headaches, and migraine, and do not have anhidrosis*.

III. *Evaluation:* Cocaine eye drops (10%) are used to differentiate Horner's syndrome from simple anisocoria on a pharmacologic basis. By preventing norepinephrine reuptake at sympathetic nerve endings, the eyedrops cause normal pupils to dilate. Lesions of any part of the sympathetic pathway cause failure of pupillary dilation because of lack of norepinephrine at the nerve terminal. The day after confirming with topical cocaine, hydroxyamphetamine (no longer commercially available) or pholedrine can be used to distinguish central and preganglionic from postganglionic sympathetic lesions. This causes mydriasis by releasing norepinephrine from the synaptic terminal, but only if the third-order neuron is intact.

Evaluation for central and preganglionic lesions should include careful neck palpation, apical lordotic chest x-ray views, and possibly CT of the neck and chest. New-onset postganglionic Horner's syndrome suggests carotid artery disease. Isolated postganglionic Horner's syndrome is generally benign. Because localization through pharmacologic testing can be incorrect and misleading, imaging of the entire sympathetic pathway is warranted if the accuracy of localization cannot be ensured. Imaging studies to consider include MRI brain, CT chest, and for carotids, an ultrasound, CTA, or MRA.

IV. *Treatment:* Treatment should be directed at underlying disease. Blepharoptosis may be corrected surgically or with topical phenylephrine drops.

REFERENCES

Loewenfield IE: *The pupil anatomy, physiology and clinical applications*, vol. 1, Ames, IA, Iowa State University Press, 1993.
Walton KA: *Curr Opin Ophthalmol* 14:357–363, 2003.

HUNTINGTON'S DISEASE

Huntington's disease (HD) is an autosomal dominant neurodegenerative disease that belongs to the family of polyglutamine diseases (such as Kennedy's disease, dentatorubropallidoluysian atrophy, and some of the autosomal dominant inherited spinocerebellar ataxias that result from an increased number of CAG nucleotide repeats that encode polyglutamine tracts within the corresponding gene products).

Clinical presentation includes progressive choreoathetosis, psychological or behavioral changes, and dementia. Although chorea is generally thought to be the first sign of HD, behavioral changes may occur a decade or more before the movement disorder, with depression the most common symptom. Patients may become erratic, irritable, impulsive, and emotionally labile.

The reported mean age of onset ranges from 35 to 42 years, with an average duration from onset to death of 17 years. Three percent of patients develop signs and symptoms before the age of 15, with rigidity, myoclonus, dystonia, and seizures more evident than chorea; in these cases, the course is rapid and there is often paternal transmission. Longer expansions correlate with earlier onset and more severe disease.

Neuropathologic changes consist of neuronal loss with a glial response that is more severe in the caudate and putamen. Several neurotransmitters are altered, with abnormally increased or decreased levels of neurotransmitters, biosynthetic enzymes, and receptor-binding sites.

Genetic testing has been based on linkage analysis of affected families. The gene has now been identified and the disease state correlated with excess copies of a trinucleotide CAG repeat. CT and MRI reveal atrophy of the caudate nucleus and cortex. PET studies have revealed relative hypometabolism in the striatum of some patients at risk for the disease.

Treatment is symptomatic for the movement disorder when it is disabling or embarrassing. Haloperidol is quite effective at doses of 1 to 40 mg/day but may cause dyskinetic and chorea movements if usage is prolonged. Fluphenazine is another alternative and recently olanzepine has been given. Possibly useful drugs are L-dopa and pramipexole for rigidity; amitryptiline and mirtazapine for depression; risperidone for psychosis; and olanzapine, haloperidol, and buspirone for behavioral symptoms in HD. Amantadine, riluzole, and tetrabenazine may be considered for unresponsive chorea, although more studies are needed. Agents under study for potential neuroprotection are coenzyme Q_{10}, minocycline, and unsaturated fatty acids.

REFERENCES

Berman SB, Greenamyre JT: *Curr Neurol Neurosci Rep* 6(4):281–286, 2006.
Bonelli RM, Wenning GK: *Curr Pharm Des* 12(21):2701–2720, 2006.

HYDROCEPHALUS

Hydrocephalus (HCP) is the increase in volume of CSF associated with dilatation of the ventricles. Three mechanisms can cause HCP: (1) obstruction of CSF pathways, (2) defective absorption of CSF, and (3) oversecretion of CSF (rare, but seen with choroid plexus papilloma).

I. Noncommunicating hydrocephalus is due to intraventricular obstruction of the foramen of Monro, the third ventricle, the aqueduct, or the foramina of Luschka or Magendie. Aqueductal stenosis, cysts, intra- and extraventricular tumors, inflammation, and congenital malformations are some of the causes.

II. Communicating hydrocephalus is most often due to obstruction of CSF pathways in the subarachnoid space, arachnoid villi, or draining veins. *Causes* include inflammation of the leptomeninges from prior infection or hemorrhage, tumors, posttraumatic obstruction, and congenital malformations (most commonly Arnold-Chiari malformation).

III. Normal pressure hydrocephalus (NPH) is a syndrome of communicating hydrocephalus without evidence of intracranial hypertension by definition. However, pressure is believed to fluctuate from normal to high throughout the course of the disease.

    A. Clinical presentation: triad of (1) apractic gait characterized by slow velocity short steps with low height, (2) subcortical dementia, and (3) urinary incontinence.

    B. Diagnosis depends on the history and physical examination, LP with normal opening CSF pressure and improvement, and imaging with cisternogram.

    C. Treatment requires surgical shunting. *The most favorable responses occur in nondemented patients.*

IV. Hydrocephalus ex vacuo describes the phenomenon of an increase in volume of CSF under normal pressure in compensation for loss of brain mass (cerebral atrophy).

Overall clinical presentation will vary depending on age and whether the HCP is acute or chronic. *In an infant*, the most common symptoms are irritability, poor feeding, and lethargy. On examination, there may be bulging, tense fontanel, separation of sutures, increased head circumference, frontal bossing, globular but symmetrical head shape, "setting sun" sign due to paralysis of upward gaze, and loss of developmental milestones. In older children (>6 years of age) and adults, the most common symptoms are headache and emesis that are worse in the morning, diplopia, loss of gross and fine motor coordination usually manifested as a gait abnormality, CN VI palsy, absent retinal pulsation, and papilledema.

Diagnosis requires CT or MRI (Fig. 21). A small or normal fourth ventricle usually implies obstruction proximal to it. A dilated fourth ventricle implies obstruction distally, either at the outflow of the foramina of the fourth ventricle or in the subarachnoid space. In the infant with an open anterior fontanel, ultrasonography is useful for assessing ventricular size and presence of blood. CSF examination may be helpful in diagnosing the etiology of HCP, but LP is contraindicated when imaging studies show evidence of mass effect, midline shift, effacement of cortical sulci, or effacement of the suprachiasmatic, basilar, quadrigeminal, or cerebellar cisterns.

Surgical treatment of hydrocephalus is mainly extraventricular shunting (see discussion under Shunts). Improvement with LPs in NPH may be diagnostic in some cases and has some predictive value in assessing shunt responsiveness. The most common symptom to improve is incontinence and then gait disturbance. However, this has shown to be less effective through the course of the disease and has a high complication rate. Dementia is less likely to respond. Medical treatment of CSF overproduction includes carbonic anhydrase inhibitors, such as acetazolamide and furosemide.

REFERENCES

Fishman RA: *Cerebrospinal fluid in diseases of the nervous system*, Philadelphia, WB Saunders, 1992.

Greenberg MS: *Handbook of neurosurgery*, ed 5, Lakeland, FL, Greenberg Graphics, 2001.

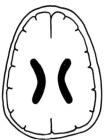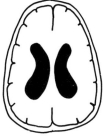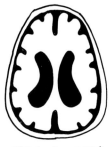

normal   **hydrocephalus**   **atrophy (ex vacuo)**

FIGURE 21

MR or CT appearance of normal and enlarged ventricles.

H

HYPOTONIC INFANT

HYPERVENTILATION

Inspiratory patterns reflect many factors and may provide localizing information.

I. *Involuntary hyperventilation* resulting from autonomic hyperactivity of brainstem respiratory centers is rare; hypoxemia, acid-base disorders, CSF acidosis, increased intracranial pressure, pulmonary disease, drug effects, and voluntary hyperventilation are more common causes.

II. *Voluntary hyperventilation* is usually related to anxiety. Symptoms include chest pain, palpitations, dyspnea, lightheadedness, perioral and fingertip numbness or paresthesias, cramps, GI distress, insomnia, a feeling of fright, and occasionally syncope. Arterial blood gas levels should show a respiratory alkalosis during an attack. Reproduction of symptoms by hyperventilation is diagnostic.

III. *Posthyperventilation changes: Apnea* is characterized by an exaggerated apneic response to lowered $Paco_2$ seen with bilateral hemispheric dysfunction. The diagnosis is made when more than 12 seconds of apnea follows 20 to 30 seconds of voluntary hyperventilation (normal response, less than 10 seconds of apnea). *Induction of absence seizures* may occur (see Epilepsy for further discussion).

Cheyne-Stokes breathing, central neurogenic hyperventilation, and apneustic and ataxic respirations may occur during coma (see Coma for a discussion of these entities).

REFERENCE

Colice GL: *Clin Chest Med* 10(4):521–543, 1989.

HYPOTONIC INFANT

Hypotonia in infancy can be caused by lesions at any level of the nervous system. The history and examination help determine the site of dysfunction and identify the cause of the hypotonia (Fig. 22).

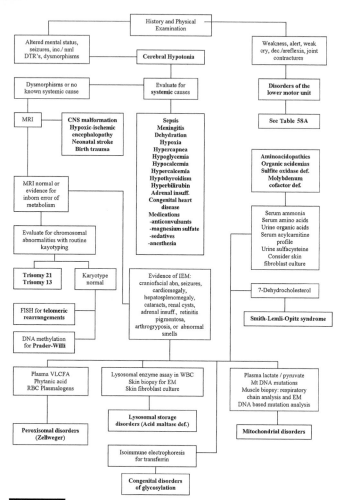

FIGURE 22

Evaluation of the hypotonic infant. abn, abnormal; DTRs, deep tendon reflexes; IEM, inborn errors of mechanism; VLCFA, very long fatty acid chains.

TABLE 58A

DIFFERENTIAL DIAGNOSIS OF THE HYPONOTIC INFANT

I. CNS disease.
   A. Perinatal hypoxia-ischemia.
   B. Congenital infection.
   C. Encephalitis, meningitis.
   D. Trauma.
   E. Hydrocephalus.
   F. Tumors.
   G. Trisomies 21 and 13.
   H. Aminoacidopathy.
   I. Storage diseases.
   J. Werdnig-Hoffmann syndrome.
   K. Poliomyelitis.
   L. Leigh disease.
   M. Prader-Willi syndrome.
II. Neuropathy.
   A. Guillain-Barré syndrome.
   B. Infantile neuropathy.
III. Neuromuscular junction.
   A. Myasthenia gravis.
   B. Infantile botulism.
IV. Muscle disease.
   A. Congenital myopathies.
   B. Myotonic dystrophy.
   C. Carnitine deficiency.
V. Nonneurologic.
   A. Ehlers-Danlos syndrome.
   B. Sepsis.
   C. Dehydration.
   D. Hypothyroidism.
   E. Hypothermia.
   F. Rickets.

H

HYPOTONIC INFANT

HISTORY AND PHYSICAL EXAMINATION

History: Specific emphasis should be placed on the following: prenatal toxin/teratogen exposure, maternal diabetes, parental age, decreased fetal movement, and family history of neuromuscular disease. Perinatal history of trauma, breech presentation (possibly indicative of poor fetal mobility), and low Apgar scores are very important in terms in determining onset of hypotonia.

Physical examination: In a classic case, the hypotonic ("floppy") infant assumes a frog-leg posture (hips abducted and externally rotated and the entire length of the limbs in contact with the flat surface). There is decreased resistance to passive movement and marked head lag with traction from the supine position. In horizontal suspension, neck extension is absent, and elbow and knee flexion is minimal. In vertical suspension at the shoulders, hypotonic infants will often slide through your hands.

DETERMINING THE CAUSE

Cerebral hypotonia: Decreased alertness, poor response to external stimuli, seizures, apnea, dysmorphic features, poor suck or grasp reflex, suppressed brainstem reflexes, and increased or normal deep tendon reflexes in the hypotonic infant suggest CNS disease.

Anterior horn cell and peripheral hypotonia: Concomitant weakness, hypo/areflexia, and appropriate level of consciousness are more indicative of lesions of the lower motor unit. Muscle fasciculations occur with neuropathy and anterior horn cell disease.

Beyond the neonatal period hypotonic infants frequently come to medical attention with delay in achieving motor milestones. Assessment of nonmotor-dependent activity such as social response, smiling, and vocalization is important in determining associated intellectual delay. Mental retardation in association with hypotonia suggests a CNS origin.

Benign congenital hypotonia is a diagnosis of exclusion, with a generally good prognosis, although some affected children remain clumsy throughout development.

REFERENCES

Prasad AN, Prasad CP: *Brain Devel* 25(7):457–476, 2003.
Swaimann KF, Ashwal S: *Pediatric neurology: Principles and practice*, ed 3, St. Louis, Mosby, 1999.

IDIOPATHIC INTRACRANIAL HYPERTENSION

Idiopathic intracranial hypertension (IIH) was originally named "meningitis serosa" in 1893 in patients with increased intracranial hypertension without a brain tumor. Other names have included benign intracranial hypertension and pseudotumor cerebri. The syndrome of IIH is characterized by clinical signs and symptoms of increased intracranial pressure (ICP) but no evidence of intracranial mass, infection, hydrocephalus, or other apparent structural CNS pathology on neuroimaging studies and CSF examination.

EPIDEMIOLOGY
The incidence of IIH is 0.9/100,000. The typical patient with IIH is an obese (94%) but otherwise healthy woman (94%) of childbearing age (mean age 31 years).

CLINICAL PRESENTATION
Symptoms include headache (92%), transient visual obscurations (72%), intracranial noises (60%), visual loss (26%), nausea/vomiting, photophobia, diplopia, dizziness, neck or shoulder pain, and pulsatile intracranial sounds.

Signs most commonly noted are papilledema, CN VI palsy, and visual disturbances: contrast sensitivity deficits (50%), color vision loss, constricted visual fields, abnormal automated perimetry (92%), contrast sensitivity defects (50%), and abnormal visual acuity (22%). Blind spot enlargement is characteristic.

ETIOLOGY
Idiopathic by definition. Conditions associated with IIH are obesity, pregnancy, and hypertension. Other causes of generalized intracranial hypertension that are *not idiopathic* include venous sinus thrombosis, endocrinopathies, hyper/hypovitaminosis A, anemia, recent use of certain medications (tetracycline, indomethacin, nalidixic acid, nitrofurantoin, oral contraceptives, lithium), and prolonged use of corticosteroids. Other systemic conditions include COPD, right-sided heart failure, renal failure, SLE, and hyperthyroidism.

DIAGNOSIS
I. If symptoms (of increased intracranial pressure) present, they may only reflect those of *generalized* intracranial hypertension or papilledema.
II. If signs (of increased intracranial pressure) present, they may only reflect those of *generalized* intracranial hypertension or papilledema.
III. Documented elevated intracranial pressure (greater than 250 mm H_2O) measured in the lateral decubitus position.
IV. Normal CSF composition (no pleocytosis, cellular atypia, or hypoglycorrhachia, normal protein).
V. No evidence of hydrocephalus, mass, structural, or vascular lesion on MRI or contrast-enhanced CT for typical patients, and MRI and MRV for all others.
VI. No other cause of intracranial hypertension identified. Other radiologic findings, not part of formal criteria, include flattening of the posterior globe (80%), empty sella turcica (70%), and distention of the perioptic nerve sheath (45%).

MANAGEMENT
I. Baseline and follow-up neuro-ophthalmologic evaluation includes visual field perimetry, optic disk stereophotographs, visual acuity, and contrast sensitivity testing.

IDIOPATHIC INTRACRANIAL HYPERTENSION

II. Initial medical treatment is with acetazolamide (250 to 1000 mg PO daily to tid). Although usually well tolerated, side effects include metabolic alkalosis, paresthesias of the extremities, liver dysfunction, and allergic reactions. Furosemide may be used.

III. Weight loss is essential.

IV. Repeated high volume lumbar punctures may provide relief, and in some cases remission.

V. Optic nerve sheath fenestration or ventriculoperitoneal shunting in cases with rapidly progressing visual loss or intractable headaches.

VI. Steroids provide symptomatic relief but the myriad side effects make these drugs undesirable for chronic treatment.

REFERENCES

Friedman D, Jacobson D: *Neurology* 59:1492-1495, 2002.
Wall M, George D: *Brain* 114:155-180, 1991.

IMMUNIZATION, VACCINATION

Many neurologic symptoms are blamed on antecedent immunizations, but it is difficult to evaluate true causality. A common concern is when patients hear about small studies suggesting causal relationships between a vaccination and a particular disease. Studies and vaccine modification (such as the acellular pertussis vaccine) are ongoing to minimize risk to patients.

Vaccines against the following diseases and infections are currently available:

I. Anthrax: Recent studies among immunized military personnel have shown no increase in disability among those receiving the vaccine.

II. Japanese encephalitis: There is increased risk of acute disseminated encephalomyelitis (ADEM).

III. *Haemophilus influenzae* type B: no complications have been reported.

IV. Hepatitis B: There has been public concern about increased risk of MS, but this was disproved in a large study.

V. Influenza: There may an increased frequency of Guillain-Barré syndrome following influenza vaccination. Incidence of giant cell arteritis may also be increased.

VI. Measles: This vaccine is ordinarily combined with mumps and rubella (measles, mumps, and rubella [MMR]) vaccine. Except for febrile seizures in children who are genetically predisposed, neurologic complications are uncommon but controversial. There are case reports of ADEM after measles vaccine, but that risk is very minor compared to the high risk of encephalopathy (subacute sclerosing panencephalitis) from natural measles. In a very large study, MMR vaccine was shown to have no increase in risk of neurologic complications, refuting a prior, small study suggesting increased rates of autism.

VII. Pertussis: The new, acellular pertussis vaccine (DTaP) has replaced the DTP (diphtheria, tetanus toxoid, pertussis) vaccine after many concerns about increased neurologic complications. These complications appear to be much less frequent with the new vaccine. Simple febrile seizures, with no long-term effects, can occur within 24 hours of administration. Autism, epilepsy, and hypotonic/hyporesponsive episodes, all previously related to the DTP vaccine, are much less common now.

VIII. *Pneumococcus* conjugate: There is a small increase in the frequency of seizures, usually febrile, in children.

IX. Poliomyelitis: Paralytic poliomyelitis is the only known complication of oral polio vaccine (OPV). It is especially a concern for immunodeficient contacts. The inactivated vaccine (IPV) is now replacing it in most countries to reduce this risk.

X. Rabies: Whole-virus vaccines that contain myelin basic protein are associated with ADEM and polyneuritis within 2 weeks after immunization.

XI. Rubella: Transient arthralgias may develop in up to 40% of patients. No causal evidence exists for association with polyneuritis or other neuropathies.

XII. Toxoids: These vaccines contain antigens from toxins, not from the microbes themselves. Tetanus and diphtheria are the most common and are often given together. Allergic hypersensitivity is the most common (though rare) complication. Demyelinating neuropathy with complete recovery has also been reported.

XIII. Smallpox: Severe, usually transient headaches are common after vaccination.

XIV. Varicella: A new vaccine. There have not been any serious neurologic complications. The theoretic concern of a shift to more serious adult zoster infections as childhood immunization wanes will be tested in the years to come.

XV. Other agents: Chemical vehicles, preservatives, and contamination have caused complications. Aluminum, commonly in diphtheria, tetanus, and hepatitis A and B vaccines, rarely causes a myofascitis. Mercury was used until 1999 in several preparations. Bovine products carry the risk of prion diseases but have been well monitored in the United States.

REFERENCES

Aminoff MJ: *Neurology and general medicine*, ed 3, New York, Churchill Livingstone, 2001.

Haber P et al: *JAMA* 24:292(20):2478–2481, 2004.

Piyasirisilp S, Hemachudha T: Curr Opin Neurol 15:333, 2002.

INTRACRANIAL PRESSURE

BASIC CONCEPTS

Normal values of intracranial pressure range from 5 to 15 mm Hg (torr), which equals 65 to 200 mm CSF or H_2O (conversion: 1 torr = 13.6 mm

INTRACRANIAL PRESSURE

H_2O). Factors that determine the level of ICP are the volume of intracranial contents, and arterial and venous pressures. After the cranial sutures fuse, the skull becomes an inelastic, closed container with fixed total intracranial volume consisting of three components: brain, CSF, and blood. The *Monroe-Kellie doctrine* states that the sum of intracranial brain tissue, CSF, and blood volumes is constant; therefore, an increase in the volume of one must be compensated by an equal decrease in another compartment. Slow increases in the volume of one compartment can be compensated by decreases in the others, but a rapid rise in ICP is not well tolerated and increases the risk of herniation or the occurrence of global ischemia and is a neurologic emergency. Cerebral perfusion pressure (CPP) is critical to maintain adequate cerebral blood flow (CBF) and is calculated as a difference between mean arterial pressure (MAP) and ICP (CPP = MAP − ICP). CPP less than 50 mm Hg is detrimental to brain function and survival. Following any major cerebral injury, ICP should be maintained as close to normal as possible, to provide a margin of safety. Continuous ICP monitoring provides useful information about "pressure waves" and may be used to guide treatment. Plateau waves, consisting of episodic surges in ICP sometimes exceeding 450 mm H_2O, can occur several times an hour, especially with pain and iatrogenic maneuvers such as suctioning, and are associated with increased risk of herniation.

Clinical presentation of increased ICP depends on the underlying process, compartmentalized or diffuse, and whether it is acute or chronic. Manifestations of headache, papilledema, diplopia, or focal signs may occur. *Cushing's triad of bradycardia, hypertension, and slowing of respiration* may occur, as may cardiac arrhythmias such as atrial fibrillation, nodal and ventricular bradycardia, large T waves, prolonged QT intervals, and changes in ST segments.

CAUSES OF INCREASED ICP

Space-occupying lesions, cerebral edema, trauma, intra/extra-axial hemorrhages, infections, venous sinus thrombosis, and pseudotumor cerebri may increase ICP. An acute rise in blood pressure beyond the autoregulatory curve causes an elevated ICP, as seen in hypertensive encephalopathy; chronic hypertension does not cause a change in ICP. Processes that increase venous pressures cause increases in ICP and include jugular compression (as reflected by *Queckenstedt's test* during LP), superior vena cava obstruction, congestive heart failure (CHF), or Valsalva maneuvers. Postural effects alter the pressures in the intracranial venous sinuses, which in turn alter the CSF pressure.

TREATMENT

I. *General measures:* Elevate the head to 30 to 45 degrees above horizontal, with the neck in straight position to optimize the jugular venous drainage; equalize fluid balance, control fever (hyperthermia markedly increases CBF as a reflection of increased cerebral energy metabolism), and avoid hypotonic IV solutions. Avoid hypotension (SBP <90 mm Hg); aim for a CPP above 60 mm Hg. If blood pressure control is necessary, use beta blockers and calcium channel blockers, avoiding antihypertensives with known effect of increasing ICP: nitroprusside or nitropaste. Avoid hypoxia ($Po_2 < 60$ mm Hg) and ventilate to normocarbia (Pco_2 35–40 mm Hg).

II. Active measures:

  A. Hyperventilation results in cerebral vasoconstriction and rapidly decreases ICP. The Pco_2 should be maintained between 30 and 35 mm Hg.

  B. Mannitol is given as a 20% IV solution, 0.5 to 1 g/kg over 15 minutes, and repeated at 3- to 6-hour intervals. Mannitol is best used when ICP can be directly monitored; otherwise, it should be titrated to produce a serum osmolality of 315 to 320 osmol/L. Urine output should be monitored. Side effects include renal failure, CHF, and pseudohyponatremia.

  C. When mannitol cannot be used owing to a high serum osmolality, rescue doses of hypertonic saline (NaCl 23.4%) in boluses of 30 mL for persistently increased ICP can be used, titrating for a maximum serum Na concentration of 160 mg/dL; furosemide (10 to 20 mg IV q 6 hr) and dexamethasone 0.25 to 0.5 mg/kg IV q 6 hr) are also useful.

  D. Glucocorticoids are used in controlling brain edema associated with brain tumors and meningitis, but are of uncertain value in treating other forms of cerebral edema.

  E. Hypothermia (27° to 36°C) decreases ICP by 50%, but peak effect takes several hours, and it may also decrease cerebral perfusion.

  F. Neuromuscular blockade may be necessary, using short-acting agents such as cisatracurium.

  G. Barbiturate coma with burst suppression can decrease ICP and is a last resort medical therapy; complications include further sedation of comatose patients, hypotension often requiring vasopressors to maintain blood pressure, and sepsis.

III. Surgical evacuation when possible offers rapid and definitive relief of intracranial hypertension. Although intraparenchymal, epidural, subdural, and subarachnoid ICP monitors can be used, the intraventricular catheter is the most accurate and allows therapeutic CSF extraventricuar drainage (EVD), resulting in immediate ICP reduction, especially in cases with hydrocephalus. Indications for EVD include severe brain insult with Glasgow Coma Scale (GCS) score less than 8 and an abnormal head CT. EVD is indicated, even with a normal CT, when additional factors are present, such as age over 40 years, SBP below 90 mm Hg, and decerebrate or decorticate posturing. Hemicraniectomy has been used after massive middle cerebral stroke and appears to be promising.

INTRACRANIAL HYPOTENSION

Decreased ICP may occur in the setting of CSF leakage, either spontaneously through openings in the dura to sinuses or mastoid, after lumbar puncture or neurosurgery, or through overshunting. Postural headache, similar to that observed after lumbar puncture, is a frequent symptom. Diagnosis is confirmed by demonstration of CSF leak on cisternogram or other evidence of CSF leak (positive glucose test in pharyngeal secretions). MRI may show meningeal enhancement. Spontaneous remission may occur, and treatment depends on the cause; occasionally dural graft may be necessary.

REFERENCES

Brain Trauma Foundation: Guidelines for the management of severe traumatic brain injury, 2003, accessed at http//www2.braintrauma.org.

Greenberg MS: *Handbook of neurosurgery*, ed 5, Lakeland, FL, Greenberg Graphics, 2001.

Qureshi AI, Suarez JI et al: *Crit Care Med* 26:440–446, 1998.

INTRACRANIAL STENOSIS

I. *Epidemiology.* Intracranial artery stenosis (ICS) secondary to atherosclerosis is a significant cause of ischemic stroke, accounting for 5% to 10% of all ischemic strokes. The annual risk of stroke in patients with ICS was estimated at 3% to 15%, although the warfarin versus aspirin for intercranial disease (WASID) trial showed a risk of recurrent vascular events at 15% to 17%. Patients with severe stenosis of the vertebral artery, the basilar artery, or both, are at particularly high risk of recurrent stroke despite antithrombotic therapy.

II. *Clinical presentation.* Stroke type can vary and depends on the artery involved and if it is related to hypoperfusion and the extent of collateral, perforator involvement, or progression to complete occlusion. The majority presents with deep infarct and watershed infarcts.

III. *Diagnosis.* In order of sensitivity and specificity, the gold standard conventional angiogram, CTA, MRA, and transcranial Doppler ultrasound are used for diagnosis.

IV. *Treatment.* A recent study (Chimowitz et al) showed no difference between ASA (325–1300 mg daily) and warfarin, although subsequent subgroup analysis showed minor benefit of warfarin over aspirin in basilar artery and intracranial vertebral artery stenosis. Intracranial balloon angioplasty and stenting can be an option in refractory cases that continue to have symptoms despite medical therapy.

REFERENCE

Chimowitz MI, Lynn MJ, Howlett-Smith H, Stern BJ: *N Engl J Med* 352(13): 1305–1316. 2005.

ISCHEMIA (STROKE)

A thorough medical evaluation is required for the diagnosis and management of cerebrovascular injury. The history should include age, race, family history, handedness, comorbidities, medications, time of onset, and prior pattern of neurologic deficits. History, physical examination, and imaging studies determine risk factors, localize lesions, delineate underlying pathophysiologic conditions, and guide treatment. In the United States, stroke of all types ranks third as a cause of death, after heart disease and cancer.

STROKE CLASSIFICATION

Cerebral ischemic events are classified by anatomic location, size of blood vessels (small and large vessel disease), duration of deficit, and mechanism (cardioembolic, atherosclerotic, lacunar).

Transient ischemic attacks (TIAs) and reversible neurologic deficits (term not used as often any more) have duration lasting up to 24 hours and 3 weeks, respectively. Typically TIAs last less than 30 minutes and commonly resolve within an hour. *Attacks lasting only a few seconds are rarely TIAs, with the exception of amaurosis fugax, which can resolve in 30 to 60 seconds.* When TIA deficits do not resolve completely after 1 to 2 hours, they are frequently associated with strokes on pathologic examination or imaging.

Completed stroke indicates that the patient has a stable neurologic deficit without evidence of progression or resolution. Completed stroke refers to the acute onset and persistence of neurologic dysfunction resulting from cerebrovascular disease (hemorrhagic or ischemic infarction).

Progressing stroke is defined as waxing and waning neurologic deficit with ultimate worsening.

Classification by duration is of limited value, as it does not provide detailed insight into the pathophysiologic characteristics of the injury.

Central nervous system ischemia or infarction may be described in terms of vascular anatomy (Table 58B). The cerebral vasculature is divided into *anterior* (carotids) and *posterior* (vertebrobasilar) distributions. There are many variants in cerebrovascular anatomy. In about 5% of patients, the circle of Willis is congenitally absent. Brainstem cross-sectional anatomy that correlates with many of the syndromes described in Table 59 is shown in Figures 23 to 25.

STROKE MECHANISM AND DIFFERENTIAL DIAGNOSIS

Identification of the ischemic mechanism is necessary for therapy selection. The characteristic clinical profile of *embolic* infarction is sudden onset of maximal neurologic deficit. Other cerebral injuries with sudden onset include intraparenchymal and subarachnoid hemorrhages, which often involve sudden headache and changes in mental status. Cerebral injury due to *small vessel disease* is often characterized by a "stuttering" course from time of onset.

TABLE 58B	
SIGNS AND SYMPTOMS OF ISCHEMIC VASCULAR OCCLUSION	
Artery	Signs and Symptoms
Common carotid artery (CCA) or internal carotid artery (ICA)	Ipsilateral eye; distal vessels; may be asymptomatic
Middle cerebral artery (MCA)	Contralateral hemiparesis (face and arm greater than leg); horizontal gaze palsy; hemisensory deficits; homonymous hemianopia; language and cognitive deficits (aphasia, apraxia, agnosia, neglect)
Anterior cerebral artery (ACA)	Contralateral hemiparesis (leg greater than arm and face); contralateral grasp reflex and gegenhalten; abulia; gait disorders; perseveration; urinary incontinence; may produce bilateral signs caused by involvement of a single vessel of common origin
Posterior cerebral artery (PCA)	Contralateral homonymous hemianopia (or quadrantanopia); may produce memory loss, dyslexia without dysgraphia, color anomia, hemisensory deficits, and mild hemiparesis; may be supplied by the anterior circulation
Cerebellar infarction	Dizziness, nausea, vomiting, nystagmus, ataxia; recognition is important to detect brainstem compression caused by swelling; neurosurgical decompression may be lifesaving

TIAs may result from emboli of ulcerated carotid plaques, but imaging and pathologic studies reveal many patients with asymptomatic ulcerations. Serial arteriography in embolic infarction reveals vascular occlusion that may vanish despite persistence of neurologic deficit. In addition, recurrent TIAs correlate more with the presence of carotid stenosis and frequently manifest as border zone ("watershed") ischemic injury distal to areas of critical stenosis. *Watershed infarcts* are also seen secondary to clinically significant decrease in blood pressure.

Differential diagnosis of transient neurologic deficits includes syncope, hyper/hypoventilation syndromes, Ménière's disease, transient global amnesia (TGA), migraine, metabolic disease (hypercalcemia, hypoglycemia), psychogenic disorders, and seizures. Patients with a history of migraine may have transient neurologic deficits with or without headache. Late-life migraine may cause fleeting visual or sensory loss in the elderly. However, in this age group, careful workup is necessary to exclude vascular causes. For instance, isolated transient vertigo or the feeling of lightheadedness in the absence of brainstem signs may indicate labyrinthine disease or orthostatic hypotension. However, particularly in patients older than 55 years, cerebrovascular disease of the posterior circulation must be seriously considered. Transient deficits may be a manifestation of seizure; when there is involuntary motor activity or a jacksonian-like march of symptoms, TIA is a less likely diagnosis, although stroke may be heralded by a seizure.

TABLE 59

BRAINSTEM SYNDROMES

Syndrome	Localization	Clinical Features		
		Ipsilateral	Contralateral	
Benedikt's	Midbrain tegmentum, red nucleus, cranial nerve CN III, cerebral peduncle	CN III palsy	Hemiataxia, tremor, hemiparesis, hyperkinesia	
Claude's	Paramedian midbrain tegmentum, red nucleus, ND III, superior cerebellar peduncle	CN III palsy	Hemiataxia, tremor, hemiparesis	
Weber's	Ventral midbrain, CN III, cerebral peduncle	CN III palsy	Hemiparesis	
Parinaud's	Dorso rostral midbrain, posterior commissure and its interstitial nucleus	Paralysis of upward gaze and accommodation, light-near dissociation of pupil lid retraction, convergence-retraction nystagmus		
Nothnagel's	Dorsal midbrain, brachium conjunctivum, CN III nucleus, medial longitudinal fasciculus	Ataxia, CN III palsy, vertical gaze palsy		
Raymond-Cestan	Medial mid-pons (paramedian branch, mid-basilar artery), middle cerebellar peduncle, corticobulbar tract, corticospinal tract, variable medial lemniscus	Ataxia	Hemiparesis (face, arm, and leg), variable sensory, variable oculomotor	
	Lateral mid-pons (short circumferential artery, middle cerebellar peduncle, CN V	Ataxia, paralysis of muscles of mastication, facial hemihypesthesia		
One and a half	Paramedian pontine reticular formation or CN VI nucleus, medial longitudinal fasciculus	Horizontal gaze palsy	Internuclear ophthalmoplegia	
Foville's	Paramedian pontine reticular formation, CN VI, and VII, corticospinal tract	Horizontal gaze palsy, CN VII palsy	Hemiparesis, hemisensory loss, internuclear ophthalmoplegia	
Millard-Gubler	Ventral paramedian pons, CN VI and VII fascicles, corticospinal tract	CN VI palsy, facial palsy	Hemiparesis	
Raymond's	Ventral pons, CN VI fascicles and corticospinal tract	CN VI palsy	Hemiparesis	
Babinski-Nageotte	Dorsolateral pontomedullary junction	Ataxia, hemihypesthesia in face, Horner's syndrome	Hemiparesis, hemihypesthesia in body, vertigo, vomiting, nystagmus	

cont'd

ISCHEMIA (STROKE)

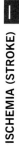

TABLE 59
BRAINSTEM SYNDROMES—cont'd

Syndrome	Localization	Clinical Features		
		Ipsilateral	Contralateral	
Wallenberg's	Dorsolateral medulla, vestibular nucleus, restiform body, CN V nucleus and spinal tract, CN IX and X, lateral spinothalamics, descending sympathetics	Lateropulsion; ataxia; loss of pain and temperature in face; paralysis of soft palate, posterior pharynx, and vocal cord; Horner's syndrome.	Loss of pain and temperature in body	
Cestan-Chenais	Lateral medulla	Ataxia; paralysis of soft palate, posterior pharynx, and vocal cord; Horner's syndrome, hemihypesthesia in face	Hemiparesis, hemihypesthesia in body	
Avellis'	Lateral medulla, CN IX and X, lateral spinothalamics	Paralysis of soft palate, posterior pharynx, and vocal cord	Hemiparesis, hemihypesthesia	
Vernet's	Lateral medulla, CN IX, X, and XI	Paralysis of soft palate; paralysis of vocal cord, posterior pharynx, and sternocleidomastoid; decreased taste over posterior third of tongue; hemihypesthesia of pharynx	Hemiparesis	
Jackson's	Lateral medulla, CN IX, X, XI, and XII	Paralysis of soft palate, posterior pharynx, vocal cords, sternocleidomastoid, upper trapezius, and tongue	Hemiparesis, hemihypesthesia	
Tapia's	Lateral medulla, CN IX, X, XII (more commonly, there is extracranial involvement)	As in Jackson's syndrome, except that sternocleidomastoid and trapezius are not involved		
Preolivary	Anterior medulla, CN XII, pyramid	Tongue atrophy or weakness	Hemiparesis	

Vertebrobasilar artery (VBA) brainstem syndromes are best described in terms of neuroanatomic localization. Eponymic descriptions in the literature vary.

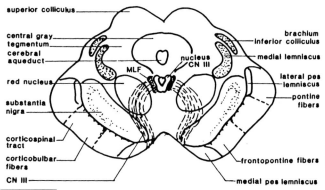

FIGURE 23

Midbrain cross-section. MLF, Medial longitudinal fasciculus.

NATURAL HISTORY AND RISK FACTORS

The recognition and reduction of risk factors is the most effective way to prevent stroke. Risk factors may be modiflable or nonmodifiable and vary with age and race. In young adults, trauma, drugs, oral contraceptives, migraine, and spontaneous arterial dissection are the most common causes of stroke. In patients 55 and older, hypertension, prior stroke or TIAs, coronary artery

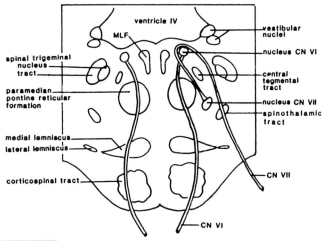

FIGURE 24

Pons cross-section. MLF, Medial longitudinal fasciculus.

ISCHEMIA (STROKE)

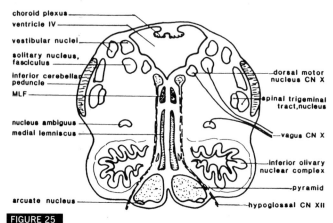

choroid plexus
ventricle IV
vestibular nuclei
solitary nucleus, fasciculus
inferior cerebellar peduncle
MLF
nucleus ambiguus
medial lemniscus
arcuate nucleus

dorsal motor nucleus CN X
spinal trigeminal tract, nucleus
vagus CN X
inferior olivary nuclear complex
pyramid
hypoglossal CN XII

FIGURE 25

Medulla cross-section (MCS).

disease, congestive heart failure, and diabetes mellitus are important independent risk factors. Smoking, obesity, increased fibrinogen level, family history of premature death from stroke, and excessive alcohol use are also recognized as risk factors. Studies show that *atrial fibrillation (AF) is associated with a sixfold increased risk for stroke.* Of all these risk factors, AF and TIAs are most commonly associated with large vessel ischemia.

The prognosis in individuals with TIAs varies considerably. Up to one third of patients who have had a TIA will develop a disabling stroke within 5 years. Overall incidence of stroke after a TIA is 10% to 20% in the first year and thereafter 5% each year (five times the normal age-adjusted risk).

CLINICAL AND LABORATORY EVALUATION

The clinical evaluation and management during the first 72 hours of stroke onset usually determine outcome from ischemic brain injury. The National Institutes of Health Stroke Scale (NIHSS) is an effective means of measuring the total neurologic deficit. Careful attention should be given to supine blood pressure in both upper extremities, orthostatic blood pressure, cardiac examination, presence of carotid or cranial bruits and facial pulses, funduscopic examination, and evidence of peripheral emboli. Patients with carotid bruits have a higher incidence of TIA, stroke (2% per year on either side and 0.1% to 0.4% per year on the ipsilateral side of the bruit), myocardial infarction, and vascular death as compared to those without a bruit.

Radiographic evaluation: A CT scan should be performed on all patients to exclude the presence of hemorrhage. Unless a subarachnoid hemorrhage is suspected (10% have negative CT results), MRI is more sensitive for the detection of small strokes, particularly in the brainstem and posterior fossa. Additional techniques include MRI with diffusion-weighted images (DWI) and perfusion-weighted images (PWI), as well as MRA. Cerebral angiography is still considered to be the "gold standard" for studying the intracranial and extracranial vasculature when there is either an unclear or a potentially treatable condition. As a general guideline, patients with TIA in the carotid distribution should have angiography if they are considered candidates for surgery.

Transcranial Doppler is useful for noninvasive evaluation of the large cerebral arteries. It can demonstrate large vessel occlusion and help assess collateral flow in ischemic territories. Duplex carotid ultrasonography is also useful as an initial screening examination, especially for patients with carotid-distribution ischemic events. Operator dependency is ultrasonography's main disadvantage.

Laboratory evaluation: Complete evaluation includes complete blood counts, erythrocyte sedimentation rate, blood chemistries, prothrombin time (PT), and partial thromboplastin time (PTT). One may also include syphilis screening (test CSF for neurosyphilis if syphilis is highly suspected), lipid profile, urinalysis, chest x-ray, and hemoglobin electrophoresis in patients at risk for sickle cell disease (SCD). Because anticoagulation (AC) is contraindicated in established endocarditis, serial blood cultures should be obtained if there is suspicion of endocarditis (especially in patients with artificial valves or a history of intravenous drug abuse and those with congenital heart disease).

Cardiac evaluation of stroke patients: History and examination consistent with an embolic event or history of heart disease necessitates an evaluation of possible source for artery-to-artery embolus as well as cardioembolic sources. Cerebral and cardiac atherosclerosis share many pathogenic mechanisms and risk factors. Atherosclerotic stroke survivors are more likely to die from coronary artery disease than recurrent stroke. Evaluations identify possible cardiogenic sources of embolism and detect occult coronary artery disease. Besides intracardiac sources, proximal aortic atheroma, especially mobile aortic plaques larger than 4 mm, is a strong risk factor for stroke. Transesophageal echocardiogram (TEE) is most useful in identifying the cardioembolic source. Holter monitoring is used when arrhythmia is implicated in stroke pathogenesis.

Stroke in the Young

Additional evaluation for patients under the age of 55 and those with no clear risk factors includes cardiac evaluation as just discussed. Cardiac sources in young adults may include patent foramen ovale and atrial septal aneurysm. Mitral valve prolapse is not clearly correlated with increased stroke in the young. A search for causes of increased coagulability should be initiated before starting anticoagulation (antiphospholipids antibodies, anticardiolipin antibodies, heparin cofactor II deficiency, antithrombin III, protein C and S, activated protein C, factor V Leiden), antinuclear antibodies, serum viscosity, protein electrophoresis, ANA/rheumatologic profile, and serum homocystine and amino acid levels. Mitochondrial studies may be indicated in selected cases such as MELAS (mitochondrial encephalopathy with lactic acidosis and stroke). Peripheral blood sample may be diagnostic, searching for mutation, but muscle biopsy may be needed. Skin biopsy or genetic testing for notch-3 mutation in cases of suspected CADASIL (cerebral autosomal dominant arteriopathy with subcortical infarct and leukoencephalopathy) may prove to be helpful.

TREATMENT
General Measures
Prevention of secondary complications: Secondary complications in stroke patients, primarily deep vein thrombosis (DVT), urinary tract infection (UTI), and pneumonia, may be minimized by prophylactic measures. Venous stasis may be prevented by the use of Jobst stockings, sequential compression devices, and subcutaneous heparin (when not medically contraindicated). Both decubiti and stasis may be prevented by patient mobilization. Depressed gag reflexes or dysphagia should be carefully evaluated to avoid the risk of aspiration pneumonia. Alterations in bladder function are common after stroke and are treated as needed. Intermittent catheterization reduces the risk of infection compared to an indwelling urinary catheter.

General measures to minimize ischemia: Once prolonged ischemia occurs, little can be done to reverse neuronal death. However, the area surrounding an ischemic injury, the so-called "ischemic penumbra," is at continued risk secondary to impaired autoregulation and perfusion. Damage to this area may be reversed and is critically influenced by management choices in the first 72 hours of stroke onset. In hypertensive patients, rapid lowering of blood pressure should be avoided. Although considerable controversy exists regarding optimal blood pressure control in the period immediately after stroke, there is greater risk in lowering blood pressure than in allowing it to remain at high levels (within 20 to 40 mm Hg of baseline). Blood pressure reduction is indicated by symptoms of hypertensive crisis (e.g., acute renal failure, convulsions, or myocardial infarction). Bed rest is recommended during and immediately after a stroke to prevent postural changes in blood pressure, which coupled with impaired autoregulation may exacerbate ischemia. Although blood pressure management remains under debate, there are now clear indications for tight control of body temperature and glucose level. Avoiding lactic acidosis may prevent secondary worsening of noninfarcted tissue in the ischemic penumbra.

Anticoagulation Therapy
I. *Acute stroke and TIAs.* There are a number of relative indications for AC therapy in the presence of acute ischemia, including the following: aortic arch mobile plaque greater than 4 mm, ventricular

aneurysm/thrombus, atrial fibrillation, atrial septal aneurysm, valvular disease/replacement, and spontaneous echocardiographic contrast that suggests low blood flow velocity. Other potential indications for AC include stenosis of a major vessel in an inoperable location, distal stump thrombus, or ulceration of an atheromatous plaque. Only one prospective trial in acute stroke used IV heparin regardless of cardiac status, and no clear benefit was demonstrated. Thus, heparin use remains controversial. Heparin has been traditionally used in critical large cerebral vessel stenosis, in crescendo TIAs, and in progressing and fluctuating stroke. Because recurrent stroke is relatively uncommon, particularly in the first 7 days, physicians still have no clinical basis for early initiation and use of heparin beyond anecdotal success. Complications of heparin AC include symptomatic intracranial hemorrhage, asymptomatic hemorrhagic transformation of infarction, major and minor extracranial bleeding, thrombocytopenia, and thrombophlebitis. Contraindications for heparin use include recent surgery, trauma, seizure, recent gastrointestinal bleed, and the presence of a large, acute infarct or hemorrhage. Strokes affecting greater than two thirds of the MCA territory on the CT scan have an increased risk for hemorrhagic transformation during heparin therapy. The advent of DWI and PWI may improve the prediction of the risk of hemorrhage with heparin therapy.

II. *Cardioembolic stroke*. There is good evidence that AC therapy reduces the risk of future embolization. Because the risk of stroke in patients with AF and sinus node disease is six times greater than in those without AF, patients with AF should receive AC therapy. Long-term AC therapy with warfarin requires monitoring (PT) and international normalized ratio (INR) to ensure values of 1.2 to 1.5 times the control value of PT, which translates to INR between 2 and 3. Even without a history of TIA or stroke, candidates for AC include patients with asymptomatic/symptomatic atrial fibrillation, atrial fibrillation with coexisting cardiomyopathy, mechanical prosthetic cardiac valves, symptomatic mitral valve prolapse, and intracardiac mural thrombus. When not medically contraindicated cardioversion should be considered. Short-term AC therapy is recommended in the setting of cardioversion for AF.

Many large embolic strokes (i.e., greater than two thirds of an arterial territory) occur in association with a known cardiac source (e.g., mural thrombus). A completely satisfactory course of action is difficult to select because AC therapy may worsen the neurologic deficit and morbidity/mortality outcome through hemorrhagic transformation. Unfortunately, withholding AC therapy may lead to repeated embolization. Management of such cases must be highly individualized. AC therapy provides no benefit in patients with embolism resulting from marantic endocarditis, calcific valves, or atrial myxoma. When embolic stroke is associated with prosthetic valve, AC therapy should be withheld while arteriography and contrasted CT scans are performed to exclude ruptured mycotic aneurysm.

III. *Use of anticoagulants.* Anticoagulation therapy is usually achieved with IV heparin administration and then maintained with oral administration of warfarin, due to transient protein C and S deficiency with initiation of warfarin.

Unlike the use of heparin in thromboembolic diseases, bolus administration is avoided with cerebral embolism because of the risk of hemorrhagic complications. The heparin infusion rate is adjusted every 4 to 6 hours until obtaining a maintenance level with activated PTT of 1.5 times the control value. Patients should be monitored for evidence of excessive anticoagulation (petechiae, microscopic hematuria, occult blood in stool, signs and symptoms of retroperitoneal bleeding). Heparin can be reversed with protamine sulfate (use 10 to 15 mg IV protamine sulfate; 1 mg neutralizes 100 USP units of heparin).

The necessity of warfarin loading is controversial. Loading may result in supratherapeutic levels. Warfarin dose is typically 2 to 10 mg/day. PT is determined daily, and the dosage is adjusted to maintain an INR of 2 to 3. Valve replacement patients require an INR of 3 to 4. Higher levels of anticoagulation are associated with a greater incidence of hemorrhagic complications. Numerous factors, including many drugs and liver disease, influence the response to warfarin. After satisfactory anticoagulation is attained with warfarin, the PT should be determined at least every 2 weeks. Excessive prolongation of PT can be corrected with vitamin K; however, vitamin K reversal significantly prolongs the time required to re-attain therapeutic AC levels with warfarin. Immediate reversal is accomplished by the use of fresh-frozen plasma.

Antiplatelet Agents

Platelets play a central role in the development of thrombi and subsequent ischemic events. In one study, the rate of infarction and death with TIAs and stroke was reduced by treatment with 1200 mg/day of aspirin. Other trials show no clear evidence that aspirin doses higher than 80 mg/day show improved benefit. In addition, lower doses are associated with decreased risk of bleeding complications. Antiplatelet agents are frequently used in small vessel, noncardioembolic infarcts; however, there is no prospective data to prove efficacy of this management. Ticlopidine (Ticlid) is an antiplatelet agent that is slightly more efficacious (at 150 mg bid) than aspirin. The use of ticlopidine necessitates initial monitoring of complete blood cell counts every other week for the first 3 months of therapy because of the risk of neutropenia. Clopidogrel (Plavix), another antiplatelet agent, is reportedly slightly more efficacious (at 75 mg qd) than aspirin and has relatively little gastrointestinal side effects. Clopidogrel-associated thrombotic thrombocytopenic purpura has been reported. Dipyridamole is another antiplatelet agent. The slow release form in combination with 25 mg aspirin bid (Aggrenox) is more efficacious than either aspirin or dipyridamole monotherapy alone.

Ancrod is an intravenous antiplatelet agent that has been shown to be slightly more effective than placebo in treating acute stroke patients.

Thrombolytic Therapy in Acute Stroke

Since 1996, IV tissue plasminogen activator (tPA) has been approved in the United States for use in ischemic stroke patients within 3 hours of onset in a dose of 0.9 mg/kg (10% as a bolus and the remainder over 1 hour). The main risk with tPA administration is brain hemorrhage. Although reports reveal a ten-fold increased risk of symptomatic brain hemorrhage within the first 36 hours after tPA, patients receiving tPA were at least 30% more likely to have only minimal or no disability at 3 months.

Current recommendations include the following: (1) emergency medical support (EMS) recognition of stroke as an emergency to be able to identify more patients within the critical 3-hour window; and (2) minimal standards for stroke care facilities should include access to physician evaluation within 10 minutes, stroke expertise within 15 minutes, cranial CT scan within 25 minutes, interpretation of CT scan within 45 minutes, and intravenous tPA administration within 60 minutes of presentation. Unfortunately, only 5% of stroke victims receive tPA. Increased effort is needed to offer and administer thrombolytic therapy to qualified patients.

Direct *intra-arterial thrombolysis* (*IAT*) demonstrates a recanalization rate two to three times higher than IV thrombolysis. However, IAT requires angiographic documentation of vessel occlusion and administration within 6 hours after onset. In PROACT I and II (intra-arterial thrombolysis with Pro-Urokinase in Acute Cerebral Thromboembolism Trials) 40% of patients had slight or no neurologic disability compared to 25% of control subjects. Recanalization rate was 67% versus 18% for control subjects.

Contraindication to thrombolysis includes early signs of infarction on head CT, minor/improving symptoms, seizure at onset, stroke/head trauma within 3 months, major surgery within 14 days, known intracranial hemorrhage, sustained systolic blood pressure >185 mmHg, sustained diastolic blood pressure higher than 110 mm Hg, gastrointestinal or genitourinary hemorrhage within 21 days, arterial puncture at noncompressible site within 7 days, heparin within 48 hours and elevated PTT and PT more than 15 seconds or INR >1.7, platelet count <100,000 mL, and serum glucose under 50 mg/dL or over 400 mg/dL. Also, there is a 1% to 2% incidence of anaphylactoid reactions and angioedema to tPA. Patients on angiotensin-converting enzyme may be at increased risk for angioedema with concomitant tPA therapy.

Surgical Treatment of Stroke

Carotid endarterectomy (CEA): Carotid endarterectomy is indicated in patients with retinal or hemispheric stroke coupled with ipsilateral high-grade stenosis (70% to 90%). The rate of fatal and nonfatal stroke was reduced significantly when compared to medical therapy according to the North American Symptomatic Carotid Endarterectomy Trial (NASCET). Timing for surgery following acute stroke is most commonly 4 to 6 weeks; occasionally this may be shorter in unstable patients.

The Asymptomatic Carotid Atherosclerosis Study (ACAS) found that patients with asymptomatic carotid artery stenosis of 60% or greater reduction in diameter and whose general health makes them good candidates for elective surgery will have a reduced 5-year risk of ipsilateral stroke if carotid endarterectomy performed with less than 3% risk of perioperative morbidity and death is added to aggressive management of modifiable risk factors.

Hemicraniectomy: Decompressive craniectomy may involve removal of a portion of the calvaria with durotomy or a more aggressive approach with removal of the infarcted tissue as a lifesaving procedure. This procedure can reduce the compartmentalization in the intracranial pressure and prevent brainstem herniation and death. This procedure is currently experimental. Prior to such an intervention, close monitoring is required. Placement of either intracranial pressure monitors or an intraventricular catheter is used in planning for possible surgical intervention.

Bypass surgery: Previous trials of bypass surgery have been discouraging. Recent interest in bypass surgery has emerged in selected cases; those may include moyamoya disease and hemodynamic-dependent occlusion and/or stenosis in the carotid arteries with pressure-dependent neurologic deficits in patients without an alternative procedure to augment cerebral blood flow.

Endovascular therapy: stenting and angioplasty: The role of these interventions is still unclear, but they may be used in patients who are at high risk to undergo CEA or if the site of the stenosis is not amenable for surgical intervention.

Neuronal tissue transplantation: There has been an increasing interest in transplanting cultured neuronal cells at the site of the injured brain cells using stereotactic surgical guidance, aiming at restoring neurologic function. This novel technique is still in its infancy, and it is premature to predict the real potential and outcome for this kind of intervention.

REHABILITATION

Rehabilitation decreases the long-term economic cost of stroke. Rehabilitation should be initiated 24 to 48 hours after the onset of stroke. The goals of stroke rehabilitation include restoration of lost abilities (motor and psychological), prevention of stroke-related complications, quality of life improvement, and education regarding secondary stroke prevention. New techniques in rehabilitation are on the horizon, including functional electrical stimulation and constraint-induced therapy.

RECOVERY AND PROGNOSIS

Approximately 10% of stroke survivors are without disability. Another 10% of patients are institutionalized because of markedly severe disability and inability to achieve functional independence. Factors that favor a poor prognosis include hemorrhagic stroke, impaired consciousness, heavy alcohol use, older age, male sex, hypertension, heart disease, and leg weakness. Negative predictors for functional outcome include incontinence, severe inattention, severe cognitive deficits, previous stroke, global aphasia, and complex comorbidities. The mortality rates at 1 month are 17% for patients with carotid distribution and 18% for patients with vertebrobasilar territory infarction.

Most rapid neurologic and functional recovery occurs by 3 months after a stroke. Recovery is categorized in stages, and a particular stage may be prolonged or recovery may stop at any stage. Stages include the following: (1) flaccidity, (2) spasticity, (3) synergistic movements (flexor and extensor), (4) isolated movements, (5) increased muscle strength, endurance, and coordination, and (6) return of muscle tone to prestroke state. Recovery from stroke may be prolonged and late functional improvements are possible.

DIFFERENTIAL DIAGNOSIS OF CEREBRAL INFARCTION

I. Cerebrovascular thrombosis associated with vascular disease
  A. Atherosclerosis
  B. Lipohyalinosis
  C. Dissection
  D. Chronic progressive subcortical encephalopathy (Binswanger's disease)
II. Cerebral embolism
  A. Cardiac source
    1. Valvular (mitral stenosis, prosthetic valve, infective endocarditis, marantic endocarditis, Libman-Sacks endocarditis, mitral annulus calcification, mitral valve prolapse, calcific aortic stenosis)
    2. Atrial fibrillation, sick sinus syndrome
    3. Acute myocardial infarction, left ventricular aneurysm, or both
    4. Left atrial myxoma
    5. Cardiomyopathy
    6. Acute and subacute bacterial endocarditis
    7. Prosthetic valve dysfunction
    8. Chagas' disease, trichinosis
  B. Paradoxical embolism and pulmonary source
    1. Pulmonary arteriovenous malformations (including Osler-Weber-Rendu syndrome)
    2. Atrial and ventricular septal defects with right-to-left shunts
    3. Patent foramen ovale with right-to-left shunt
    4. Pulmonary vein thrombosis
    5. Pulmonary and mediastinal tumors
  C. Artery-to-artery embolism
    1. Cholesterol emboli
    2. Atheroma thrombus
    3. Complications of vascular and neck surgery
    4. Idiopathic carotid mural thrombus, emboligenic aortitis

        5. Emboli distal to unruptured aneurysm
        6. Arterial dissection
    D. Other
        1. Fat embolism syndrome
        2. Air embolism
        3. Foreign body embolism (e.g., bullets, catheter tips, etc.)
III. Arteriopathies, *inflammatory*
    A. Takayasu's disease
    B. Allergic granulomatosis (Churg-Strauss syndrome)
    C. Granulomatosis, polyarteritis nodosa, rheumatoid arthritis, Sjögren's syndrome, scleroderma, Behçet's syndromes, acute rheumatic fever, inflammatory bowel disease

LACUNAR SYNDROMES

Lacunar infarcts are described as small, deep lesions on CT or MRI usually 10 mm or less in diameter with density or signal consistent with infarct. Between 10% and 24% of all strokes are lacunar. There is a greater incidence of lacunes in Asians, blacks, and Hispanics than in whites. Lacunar infarcts are characteristically located in the subcortical cerebrum or brainstem. Pathophysiology of lacunes can be categorized by four different mechanisms: (1) small vessel lipohyalinosis and fibrinoid degeneration, (2) decreased perfusion of penetrating arteries from proximal narrowing of larger vessels, (3) branch artery atheromatous occlusion, and (4) embolism.

    Patients with lacunes frequently have a history of hypertension, diabetes, hypercholesterolemia, smoking, and atherosclerosis of large and mid-sized intracranial arteries, but there is no increased incidence of these risk factors in patients with lacunar infarcts versus other ischemic strokes. Lacunes are infrequently associated with embolism and extracranial carotid occlusive disease. Lacunes occur in the lenticular nuclei (37%), caudate nucleus (10%), thalamus (14%), internal capsule (10%), and pons (16%). Lacunes are also seen in the corona radiata, external capsule, pyramids, and other brainstem structures.

    Clinical presentations of lacunar infarction (Table 60) are related to size and site of the lesion and range from asymptomatic to classic lacunar syndromes. Onset is often gradual or stepwise. Approximately 30% are preceded by transient ischemic attacks. Defined lacunar syndromes include pure motor hemiparesis, pure sensory syndrome, sensorimotor syndrome, ataxic hemiparesis, dysarthria-clumsy hand, and hemichorea/ballism.

    Head CT demonstrates up to 70% of lesions within 7 days. Multiple lacunes are present in 30% of patients. MRI is more sensitive than CT. Thirty percent of lesions on imaging studies are asymptomatic. Treatment consists of antiplatelet agents, control of hypertension, and management of other vascular risk factors. Cerebral angiography is not recommended in pure lacunar syndromes. However, the absence of history or signs of hypertension (such as retinopathy and left ventricular hypertrophy) requires an aggressive workup for sources of embolus, large vessel disease, or unusual causes of stroke. Prognosis is usually favorable, but the probability of recurrence is high.

TABLE 60

MOST COMMON LACUNAR SYNDROMES

Syndrome	Localization	Clinical Features
Pure sensory stroke	Venticular posterior thalamus	Sensory loss face, arm, leg—same side; no weakness; no visual field deficits; no "cortical" signs
Pure motor hemiparesis	Posterior limb interior capsule, basis pontis, cerebral peduncle	Weakness face, arm, leg—same side; no sensory loss; no visual field deficits; no "cortical" signs
Ataxic hemiparesis	Basis pontis, ventricular anterior thalamus and adjacent interior capsule	Cerebellar ataxia and weakness—same side; often leg >face
Dysarthria—clumsy hand syndrome	Basis pontis, genu interior capsule	Facial weakness, dysarthria, dysphagia, slight weakness and clumsiness of hand—same side

THALAMIC SYNDROMES

Cerebrovascular disease is the most common cause of discrete thalamic lesions. The thalamic arteries arise from the posterior communicating arteries and from the perimesencephalic segment of the posterior cerebral arteries. The following thalamic syndromes result from infarctions and each corresponds to a different arterial territory:

Inferolateral artery (thalamogeniculate artery) infarcts with posterolateral thalamic lesions involve mainly the ventral posterior, ventral lateral, and subthalamic nuclear groups. These most commonly include hemisensory loss and pain, hemiataxia, disequilibrium, athetoid posture, and paroxysmal pain.

Tuberothalamic artery supplies the anterior regions. Neuropsychologic dysfunction occurs most commonly. Other symptoms include facial paresis for emotional movement, occasional hemiparesis, dysphasia with left-sided lesions, and hemineglect and visuospatial dysfunction with right-sided lesions. Bilateral lesions lead to lethargy, apathy, abulia, and impaired memory.

Posterior choroidal arteries supply the lateral geniculate body. With infarction, visual field deficits occur, most commonly quadrantanopia.

Paramedian arteries supply the paramedian midbrain and thalamus, including the intralaminar group and most of the dorsomedial nucleus. The triad of common changes is somnolent apathy, memory loss, and abnormalities in vertical gaze. Also, this triad is occasionally associated with akinetic mutism.

The syndrome of *Dejerine and Roussy (inferolateral thalamic syndrome)* is due to a vascular lesion in the territory of the thalamogeniculate artery. It is characterized by a mild hemiparesis, persistent hemianesthesia for touch, slight hemiataxia and astereognosis, choreoathetotic movements, and pain. *Thalamic pain syndrome* occurs contralateral to the lesion and is described as burning, aching, or boring. It is constant, but often there are paroxysmal increases, spontaneous or observed in patients with lesions in brainstem, internal capsule, basal ganglia, and subcortical parietal lobe. Treatment with tricyclic antidepressants (amitriptyline 10 to 100 mg qhs) or anticonvulsants (carbamazepine or dilantin) is sometimes effective. Conventional analgesics are ineffective.

REFERENCES

Glucose in Ischemia
Auer R: *Neurology* 51(Suppl 3):S39–S43, 1998.

Anticoagulation
Harrison L et al: *Ann Intern Med* 126:133–136, 1997.
Korczyn AD: *Neurol Clin* 10:209–217, 1992.
Swanson RA: *Neurology* 52:1746–1750, 1999.

Cardioembolic Stroke
Fatkin D et al: *Am J Cardiol* 73:672–676, 1994.
Hart RG, Halperin JL: *Ann Intern Med* 131:688–695, 1999.

Antiplatelet Therapy
Bennett CL et al: *Ann Intern Med* 128:541–544, 1998.
CAPRIE Steering Committee: *Lancet* 348:1329–1339, 1996.
Diener HC et al: *J Neurol Sci* 143:1–13, 1996.

Thrombolytic Therapy
Adams H et al: *Stroke* 27:1711–1718, 1996.
Hacke W et al: *Lancet* 352:1245–1251, 1988.
Hakim AM: *Neurology* 51(Suppl 3):S44–S46, 1998.
Hill MD et al: *Can Med Assoc J* 162:1281–1284, 2000.

Surgical Therapy
Chaturvedi S, Halliday A: *Curr Atheroscler Rep* 2(2):115–119, 2000.
Executive Committee for the Asymptomatic Carotid Atherosclerosis Study: *JAMA* 273(18):1421–1428, 1995.
Gomez CR: *Semin Neurol* 18(4):501–511, 1998.
Kondziolka D, Wechsler L et al: *Neurology* 55(4):565–569, 2000.
North American Symptomatic Carotid Endarterectomy Trial Collaborators: *N Engl J Med* 325(7):445–453, 1991.

Stroke Risk Factors
Gilon D et al: *N Engl J Med* 341:8–13, 1999.
Hart RG, Halperin JL: *Ann Intern Med* 131:688–695, 1991.
Sacco R: *Neurology* 51(Suppl 3):S27–S30, 1998.
Wilterdink JL et al: *Neurology* 51(Suppl 3):S23–S26, 1998.

Lacunar Syndromes
Gan R et al: *Neurology* 48:1204–1211, 1997.
Horowitz D et al: *Neurology* 48:325–327, 1997.

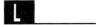

LAMBERT-EATON MYASTHENIC SYNDROME

Lambert-Eaton myasthenic syndrome (LEMS) is an autoimmune disorder of neuromuscular transmission. Antibodies directed at the voltage-gated calcium channels (VGCCs) on presynaptic cholinergic nerve terminals are responsible for the disease. Calcium entry via VGCCs is required to facilitate docking and release of presynaptic acetylcholine vesicles. Antibodies to VGCCs lead to a decrement in the release of presynaptic acetylcholine (ACh) vesicles. Presynaptic ACh stores and the postsynaptic response to individual quanta are normal.

LEMS is a rare disease and usually occurs in older adults with mean age of onset of 50 and ratio of men to women of 1.8:1. LEMS is associated with small cell lung carcinoma (SCLC) in approximately two thirds of cases. The remaining third of cases are mainly idiopathic. Other neoplasms associated with LEMS include carcinomas of the rectum, kidney, stomach, and breast and leukemia. Autoimmune diseases such as systemic lupus erythematosus, rheumatoid arthritis, and Sjögren's syndrome may be related to LEMS. LEMS may precede the diagnosis of cancer by an average of 10 months.

CLINICAL FEATURES

Clinical features include proximal leg or arm weakness; muscle aching and stiffness worsened by prolonged exercise; and difficulty with certain movements, such as combing hair or rising from a chair. Unlike myasthenia gravis, initial symptoms due to cranial nerve dysfunction are rare. However, transient diplopia, ptosis, dysphagia, dysarthria, and neck flexion weakness can develop in later stages. Eighty percent of patients will experience autonomic involvement, usually dry mouth and impotence, and occasionally constipation, blurred vision, and impaired sweating. Sensory complaints are rare.

On examination, proximal weakness of the lower limbs greater than the upper limbs is the most consistent finding. A progressive increase in strength after a few seconds of sustained contraction is usual, with fatigue after continued contraction. Muscle wasting is rare. Limb reflexes are decreased or absent in over 90% of cases. However, a potentiation of reflexes after maximal contraction of the involved muscle for 10 to 15 seconds is usually present.

LABORATORY FINDINGS

On nerve conduction studies, the amplitude of the compound muscle action potentials (CMAP) is reduced. The sensory responses are normal. Nerve conduction velocities and latencies are normal. Slow repetitive stimulation (2 Hz) produces a decremental response of the CMAP amplitude similar to myasthenia gravis. In contrast, the repetitive stimulation performed at high frequencies (>10 Hz) creates a profound incremental response (100% to 200% increase in amplitude of CMAP) due to calcium accumulation in the presynaptic terminal with subsequent enhancement of the release of ACh vesicles. A similar phenomenon is present after a brief (10-second) sustained voluntary exercise (postexercise facilitation). Antibodies to VGCCs can be tested in blood. LEMS patients sometimes respond to edrophonium but not consistently, and it usually is not useful for the diagnosis.

TREATMENT

Treatment is directed at the responsible tumor or underlying autoimmune disorder. Response to cholinesterase inhibitors is variable. Plasmapheresis, immunosuppressive agents (azathioprine), and prednisone (100 mg/day for 1 week followed by a gradual taper to 60 mg every other day) may help, particularly if the LEMS is due to autoimmunity. A drug that facilitates synaptic transmission, *3,4-diaminopyridine (DAP)*, which prolongs the duration of presynaptic action potentials by blocking delayed rectifier potassium channels and leads to increased calcium entry to the presynaptic terminal, may improve strength in LEMS patients in doses of 15 mg qid (1 mg/kg/day). Anticholinesterases may facilitate the effect of DAP. Guanidine 10 mg/kg/day may improve strength but is not well tolerated owing to severe side effects including bone marrow suppression and renal failure.

The survival rate for those with tumor-associated LEMS is low owing to progression of the underlying malignancy, although patients with both SCLC and LEMS generally have longer survival time in comparison to patients with SCLC alone. In LEMS without underlying disease the prognosis is good and clinical remission can be achieved in 40% of patients with immunosuppressive agents.

REFERENCES
Lennon VA et al: *N Engl J Med* 332:1467–1474, 1995.
Saunders DB: *Ann Neurol* 37:S63–S73, 1995.

LEARNING DISABILITIES

A learning disability (LD) is an unexpected difficulty in the acquisition and use of language, reading, mathematical abilities, or social skills in a patient with otherwise normal intelligence. The most common learning disorder (80%), dyslexia, occurs in 5% to 17% of school-age children. Dyslexia is a chronic condition in which there is impaired ability to break down words into their basic phonologic parts, resulting in difficulties in decoding and identifying the words. This will often present as a child (unexpectedly) having difficulty learning to read. Approximately 50% of children with LD have associated attention deficit hyperactivity disorder (ADHD), conduct disorder, anxiety disorders, and to a lesser extent, mood disorders.

In preschoolers, LD usually becomes evident as language delay. A child who has no meaningful words by age 18 months, no meaningful phrases by age 24 months, or speech unintelligible to strangers by age 3 years should be evaluated for hearing loss and referred for speech therapy. In school-age children, LD usually becomes evident as unexpected school failure. There is often a family history of learning problems. Psychometric evaluation should be administered to every child who is having difficulties in school to verify normal intelligence and failure to achieve the expected level of performance.

In the United States; the clinician should assure parents that, under the Individuals with Disabilities Education Act, public schools are mandated to meet the educational needs of all developmentally disabled children. This act further mandates the proper assessment of educational needs (including psychometric testing) and enactment of an individual education plan (IEP). All of this assessment should be performed in a timely fashion.

Counseling for associated social, behavioral, and psychiatric symptoms should be tailored to take into account the child's specific language and cognitive deficit. Parent support and consultation may be needed to help the family develop a supportive home environment and a consistent home-school behavioral reinforcement program.

REFERENCE
Wolraich ML: *Development and learning, ed 3,* London, BC Decker, 2003.

LIMBIC SYSTEM

The limbic system is a brain network subsystem that integrates endocrine function and autonomic activity with social behaviors. It consists of paralimbic cortex (the cingulate, parahippocampal and paraterminal gyri, and the caudal orbitofrontal, insular, and temporal pole cortices), limbic cortex (hippocampal formation and primary olfactory cortex), and the corticoid areas (amygdala, septal area, and substantia innominata). These limbic regions have two different sets of connections: (1) intracortical networks for emotion, attention, and memory; and (2) subcortical pathways through the hypothalamus and brainstem for homeostasis and social behaviors. Lesions and disease in the limbic system lead to abnormalities of memory, emotion, motivation, behavior, and autonomic and endocrine control.

REFERENCE
Gilman S, Newman SW: *Manter and Gatz's essentials of clinical neuroanatomy and neurophysiology*, ed 10, Philadelphia, FA Davis, 2003, pp 193–203.

LUMBOSACRAL PLEXOPATHY

The lumbosacral plexus comprises the anastomoses derived from the ventral primary rami of T12–S4 (Fig. 26).

L

LUMBOSACRAL PLEXOPATHY

ETIOLOGY

Lumbosacral dysfunction may be caused by neoplasms (cervix, prostate, bladder, colorectal, kidney, breast, ovary, and lymphoma), retroperitoneal hemorrhage, psoas abscess (from osteomyelitis), diabetes, inadvertent injections into the gluteal artery or umbilical artery, intravenous heroin, idiopathic retroperitoneal fibrosis, herpes zoster infections, pyelonephritis, appendicitis, retroperitoneal masses, aortic aneurysms, and trauma.

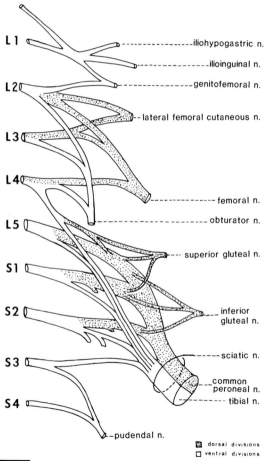

FIGURE 26

Lumbosacral plexus.

CLINICAL PRESENTATION

Pain, weakness, loss of deep tendon reflexes, and sensory changes may occur in the appropriate distribution (see also Dermatomes, Myotomes). Some variants of lumbar plexus disease are described here:

  I. *Peripartum lumbosacral plexus neuropathy* (less common than idiopathic brachial plexopathy) occurs during labor and delivery, when the descending fetal head may compress the lumbosacral trunk and S1 root at the point where they join and pass over the pelvic rim. It is characterized by a *sudden onset of severe pain in the thigh or buttock* followed 5 to 10 days later by weakness in the distribution of the involved plexus and elevated erythrocyte sedimentation rate.

 II. *Radiation plexopathy* usually occurs 1 to many years after radiation. Findings include unilateral or bilateral distal leg weakness, mild pain, and EMG showing myokymic discharges (50%). In contrast, plexopathy due to *tumor is associated with severe pain at onset and weakness involving proximal and unilateral leg muscles.*

III. *HIV/AIDS-related lumbosacral polyradiculopathy*, sometimes associated with CMV infections, is becoming a more common phenomenon. These radiculopathies occur in the late stages of the disease and include weakness, pain, paresthesias, and urinary retention.

IV. Idiopathic lumbar plexopathy

 V. Paraneoplastic disease

DIAGNOSIS

EMG may be performed, and MRI is the imaging procedure of choice for visualizing the lumbosacral plexus.

TREATMENT

Treatment consists of identifying and treating the underlying cause. Steroids and intravenous immunoglobulin have been used in treatment of idiopathic lumbosacral plexopathy.

REFERENCES

Triggs WJ et al: *Muscle Nerve* 20:244–246, 1997.
Ismael SS et al: *J Neurol Neurosurg Psychiatry* 68:771–773, 2000.

LYME DISEASE, NEUROBORRELIOSIS (See also AAN GUIDELINE SUMMARIES APPENDIX)

Lyme disease, also called Lyme borreliosis, is a multisystem disease (dermatologic, neurologic, rheumatologic, and cardiac manifestations) caused by a tick-transmitted spirochete, *Borrelia burgdorferi.*

CLINICAL PRESENTATION

Lyme disease may be divided into three stages:

Stage I: Localized infection (3 days to 1 month) usually begins shortly after a tick bite with a flulike syndrome. Skin lesion manifests as a red macule or papule and expands centrifugally to form an annular red lesion with central clearing (*erythema chronicum migrans*) (Fig. 27). Regional adenopathy and mild systemic symptoms of headache, neck stiffness, lethargy, or mild encephalopathy may occur. The CSF is usually normal.

Stage II: Disseminated infection (up to 9 months) occurs within days or weeks. The spirochete may spread hematogenously. This stage manifests clinically as meningoradiculitis, migratory musculoskeletal pain, acute arteritis, generalized adenopathy, splenomegaly, carditis, severe malaise, and fatigue. Weeks to months after illness the most common neurologic abnormality is lymphocytic meningitis with or without accompanying CNS parenchymal involvement. Radiculoneuritis, when present, may be asymmetrical, painful, and with dermatomal sensory and myotomal motor abnormalities. Variations include mononeuritis, mononeuritis multiplex, brachial or lumbosacral plexopathy, and Guillain-Barré-like syndrome. Electrophysiologic testing usually points to axonal degeneration in distal nerves and roots. Cranial neuropathies develop in about 60% of patients. Facial palsy is most common and is seen in 70% to 80% instage II and 10% of all patients. Cranial nerves III, IV, VI (13%), V (6%), VIII (5%), and II (3%) may also be involved. CSF findings in stage II include increased WBC count (100 to 200 WBC/mm^3 with >90% lymphocytes), decreased glucose (<66% of normal serum glucose value), and increased protein (35% of patients, usually 100 to 300 mg/dL).

Stage III: Late or persistent infection occurs months to years after initial infection. It manifests as attacks of arthritis in large joints, persistent skin

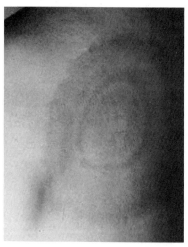

FIGURE 27
Erythema migrans.

infection, and persistent, often progressive, neurologic abnormalities sometimes with a long latency. Neurologic manifestations include chronic progressive encephalomyelitis (meningitis, encephalitis, myelitis, cranial neuritis, radiculoneuritis), focal encephalitis, mild encephalopathy, dementia, seizures, distal axonopathy, and asymmetrical polyneuropathy. CSF findings are similar to those in stage II.

DIAGNOSIS

There may be a history of erythema migrans, tick bite, or exposure to travel in an endemic area, and examination may show extraneural involvement or suggestive neurologic syndromes (i.e., unilateral or bilateral Bell's palsy, aseptic meningitis, atypical Guillain-Barré syndrome, and mild polyneuropathy). Not all patients recall the tick bite or the rash. Serologic evidence of IgM and IgG antibodies are measured by ELISA as an initial screen and confirmed by Western blot. CSF Lyme antibody index confirms neurologic Lyme disease but is not invariably elevated. *B. burgdorferi* is virtually impossible to culture, and routine biopsy is not helpful. Polymerase chain reaction may be used in the future.

TREATMENT

Stage I and II with facial palsy: Doxycycline 100 mg PO bid for 21 to 30 days or amoxicillin (with probenecid) 500 mg PO qid 21 to 30 days or cefuroxime 500 mg PO bid for 21 to 30 days. *Stage II with neurologic involvement other than facial palsy*: Penicillin G 24 MU/day IV for 14 to 21 days or ceftriaxone 2 g/day IV for 30 days or cefotaxime 2 g IV q 8 hr for 30 days or doxycycline 100 to 200 mg PO bid for 21 to 28 days. *Stage III:* Same as for stage II, except doxycycline is given for 30 days. Parenteral antibiotics are preferred for CNS Lyme syndromes. Nonspecific problems (fatigue, joint pain, muscle ache) may persist for months after treatment.

REFERENCES

Halperin JJ et al: *Neurology* 46:619–627, 1996.
Halperin JJ: *Curr Neurol Neurosci Rep* 5:446–452, 2005.

Macrocephaly is defined as head circumference greater than 2 standard deviations above the normal distribution for age.

ETIOLOGY

Hydrocephalus (communicating or noncommunicating), megalencephaly, thickening of the skull, and hemorrhage into the subdural or epidural spaces may cause macrocephaly. *Anatomic megalencephaly* includes conditions in which the brain is enlarged because the number or size of cells increases. These children are macrocephalic at birth but have normal intracranial pressure. Children with *metabolic megalencephaly* are normocephalic at birth and develop megalencephaly during the neonatal period because of storage of abnormal substances or by producing cerebral edema.

The causes of anatomic megalencephaly include genetic megalencephaly or megalencephaly (with gigantism, typical facial changes, and learning difficulties, as seen in Sotos' syndrome or associated with mutations or deletions in the nuclear receptor-binding SET domain containing protein), neurocutaneous disorders (e.g., macrocephaly cutis marmorata telangiectatica congenital), or other neurologic disorders.

Examples of metabolic megalencephalies include leukodystrophies. Glutaric aciduria type I (glutaryl-CoA dehydrogenase deficiency) may present with macrocephaly before the individual goes on to develop severe leukoencephalopathy, at a potentially treatable stage. Megalencephalic leukoencephalopathy with subcortical cysts is a rare leukodystrophy characterized by macrocephaly and a slowly progressive clinical course marked by spasticity and cognitive decline. Macrocephaly is also frequently seen in autism, but its relationship to the pathogenesis is unclear.

EVALUATION

Evaluation involves review of prior head circumference measurements to assess rate of head growth (a rapidly growing head that is crossing percentile lines suggests hydrocephalus), assessment of head shape (frontal bossing is associated with hydrocephalus, lateral bulging with infantile subdural hematoma), measurement of head circumference of parents and siblings (*benign familial megalencephaly*), and CT, MRI, or ultrasound. If the infant is neurologically and developmentally normal, close observation may be all that is necessary.

A useful rule of thumb for normal rate of head growth follows:
Premature infants: 1 cm/week
1 to 3 months: 2 cm/month
3 to 6 months: 1 cm/month
6 to 12 months: 0.5 cm/month

REFERENCES

Kulkens S, Harting I, Sauer S et al: *Neurology* 64:2142–2144, 2005.
Lapunzina P, Gairi A, Delicado A et al: *Am J Med Genet A* 130:45–51, 2004.

MAGNETIC RESONANCE IMAGING

MRI creates images based on behavior of various tissues exposed to strong magnetic fields, controlled magnetic field gradients, and radiofrequency (RF) pulses. Image intensity and contrast depends upon the concentration of unpaired protons, typically from hydrogen nuclei, the motion of these nuclei, nuclear magnetic relaxation parameters, and the type of sequence or acquisition being performed.

When tissue protons are placed in a magnetic field, they tend to align themselves either parallel in a low-energy state or antiparallel in a high-energy state to the vector of the imposed magnetic field, although they flip periodically between the two states. Because low-energy states are preferred, more protons align parallel than antiparallel at any given moment, creating a net magnetization vector. An RF pulse can then be applied, exciting the protons, changing them from longitudinal to transverse alignment. As these protons return to equilibrium within the magnetic field (i.e., longitudinal alignment), they emit energy (as an RF signal), which can be detected and converted into meaningful data—the image—by means of certain manipulations.

TECHNICAL PARAMETERS

Repetition time (TR) defines the duration of a cycle as the time between successive RF pulses.

Echo time (TE) defines a sampling interval during the cycle and is the time between giving the RF pulse and measuring the amount of RF signal being emitted by the tissue, the "echo." There may be single or multiple echoes sampled during a given cycle.

Relaxation time is the time it takes the protons to return to equilibrium within the magnetic field after an RF pulse has been given.

COMMON MRI SEQUENCES

I. T_1 relaxation is based upon how fast protons return to equilibrium (longitudinal alignment) after being excited by an RF pulse. At any given time after the RF pulse is given (TE), those substances whose protons re-equilibrate fastest (lipids, for example, with the highest percentage of protons in the longitudinal position) appear brightest on T_1-weighted images (T1WI) where the T_1 characteristics are emphasized. Those substances whose protons re-equilibrate slower (water, for example) will appear darker (Table 61). The shorter the TE, the greater the difference between various substances and tissues. At short TE, a large percentage of the lipid protons have regained their longitudinal position, whereas few water protons have done so. At longer TE, a greater percentage of both lipid and water protons have regained their longitudinal position. The greater the difference between the two substances (the shorter the TE), the greater the contrast on T1WI. Therefore, T_1-weighted images have both short TR and short TE.

II. T_2 relaxation is determined by how fast transverse magnetization decays. The longer transverse alignment is maintained, the stronger the signal that is emitted on T_2-weighted images (T2WI) (Table 62). At shorter TE, a higher percentage of both lipid and water protons are in transverse alignment. At a longer TE, most of the lipid protons have lost their transverse magnetization (fast decay), whereas most of the

TABLE 61

T$_1$-WEIGHTED IMAGE

DARK (LOW SIGNAL, LONG T$_1$)

CSF

Liquids

Cortical bone

Air

Edema

Most pathologic lesions

BRIGHT (HIGH SIGNAL, SHORT T$_1$)

Lipid

Gadolinium, other paramagnetic substances such as copper and manganese

Proteinaceous substances

Melanin

water protons remain in transverse alignment (slow decay). Therefore, for greatest contrast on T2WI images, a longer TE should be chosen. Consequently, T2WI have long TE and long TR.

The degree of brightness or darkness on T1WI and T2WI can thus be determined by tissue content (Tables 61 to 63). In general, pathologic conditions are dark on T1WI, bright on T2WI, and bright on proton density images. The acquisition of data may be performed in a variety of patterns or sequences, which emphasize differences in tissue properties.

III. A typical example is the spin echo (SE) sequence in which an initial 90-degree pulse is given, and the echo is assessed at a predetermined point with an additional 180-degree pulse. The 180-degree pulse is necessary because of "dephasing" or spreading of the magnetic vectors of individual protons as they decay. If dephasing is not corrected, the vectors would eventually cancel each other out until the net vector becomes so weak that the signal emitted would be undetectable. The 180-degree pulse "rephases" or brings back together the individual proton vectors so the echo emitted can be detected. T1WI images,

TABLE 62

T$_2$-WEIGHTED IMAGE

DARK (LOW SIGNAL, LONG T$_2$)

Cortical bone

Air

Melanin

Dense fibrous tissue

BRIGHT (HIGH SIGNAL, SHORT T$_2$)

CSF

Liquids

Edema

Most pathologic lesions

TABLE 63

INTRAPARENCHYMAL HEMATOMA

	T1WI	T2WI	Time Course	Type
Hyperacute	Isointense	Isointense or bright	Minutes to hours	Intracellular oxyhemoglobin
Acute	Isointense	Dark	Hours to days	Intracellular deoxyhemoglobin
Early subacute	Bright	Dark	Days to weeks	Intracellular methemoglobin
Late subacute	Bright	Bright	Few to several weeks	Extracellular methemoglobin
Chronic	Dark	Dark	Months	Hemosiderin

T2WI images, and proton density images (PDIs) may be obtained with this sequence. PDIs emphasize tissue characteristics between T1WI and T2WI (long TR, short TE). Fluid attenuated inversion recovery (FLAIR) is another sequence that takes advantage of T1WI and T2WI.

IV. Another frequently used acquisition sequence is the gradient echo (GRE), a relatively fast scanning technique. The sequence takes less scanning time and is useful for imaging flowing blood (flow-related enhancement), for detecting calcification or hemorrhage, and for moderate myelogram effect (white CSF) in the spinal canal. GRE images, like SE, may be either T_1-weighted or T_2-weighted, but usually only T2WI or PDIs are obtained.

V. Perfusion-weighted images (PWIs) are useful in evaluating cerebral blood flow using a bolus-tracking method whereby repeated images are acquired at the same location during the passage of a high volume of intravenous gadolinium. These are T_2-weighted sequences and because gadolinium produces decreased signal intensity on T_2-weighted scans, areas of diminished blood flow are bright on PWI.

VI. Diffusion-weighted images (DWIs) are reflective of water motion in brain tissue. Areas with low diffusion appear bright. For example, DWI reveals cerebral infarcts as bright areas within 30 minutes of onset, with the increased signal intensity lasting 7 to 21 days.

VII. Quantitative measurement using apparent diffusion coefficient (ADC) maps can be performed. ADC maps may be helpful in cases of suspected T_2 shine-through artifact on DWI, where bright signal on T_2 appears bright on DWI and ADC versus acute infarct (bright on DWI and dark in ADC).

DWI and PWI images are vital in taking care of acute stroke patients. Combining both imaging sequences enables the clinician to identify the penumbra area, which represents potentially salvageable tissue.

CLINICAL USES OF MRI

I. Vascular: Strokes appear earlier and in better detail on MRI (particularly DWI) than on CT. For vascular malformations, MRI and MRA are fine diagnostic tools. For aneurysms, MRA is excellent for screening, but conventional angiography can exclude smaller aneurysms. In addition, the sensitivity of CT angiography is greater than MRA. MR venography is superb for diagnosing dural venous sinus thrombosis. Although MRI can detect all types of hemorrhage, unenhanced CT is the appropriate screening examination, in particular for subarachnoid hemorrhage. In cases of suspected diffuse axomal injury, MRI may prove of diagnostic value, especially with the addition of a GRE pulse sequence.

II. Tumors: MRI is the procedure of choice to rule out small tumors or for tumor delineation. The ability to map the extent of a tumor (especially with the use of gadolinium) and the multiplanar capability of MRI make it very useful in surgical planning.

III. Infections: Cerebritis is well visualized with MRI. Abscess is well delineated with MRI.

IV. Meningeal processes: MRI is more sensitive than CT for visualizing both infected and neoplasm-infiltrated meninges.

V. Trauma: Acutely, MRI is not the examination of choice because of the lack of bony detail and the length of time needed to obtain images. CT should be used.

VI. Demyelinating disease: MRI is the procedure of choice because of the excellent delineation of white matter disease. Active lesions of multiple sclerosis will enhance with gadolinium.

VII. Congenital/structural abnormalities: Multiplanar MRI is excellent for showing heterotopias and other anatomic abnormalities.

VIII. Spine imaging: Because the spinal cord is a thin, inherently low contrast structure, MRI is the noninvasive examination of choice for the spine. Vertebral bone is well imaged on spinal MRI because it contains fatty marrow. However, small spinal column fractures are better seen on CT. MRI also allows good visualization of the soft tissue and ligaments.

IX. Pregnancy: The safety of MRI in pregnancy has yet to be determined; therefore, risk versus benefit must be considered. Gadolinium should not be administered during pregnancy.

ADVANTAGES OF MRI

I. Multiplanar capability: The magnetic field can be adjusted to image in any plane without moving the patient.

II. No ionizing radiation.

III. Superior soft tissue contrast: Subtle differences in soft tissue proton relaxation characteristics enable visual distinction between soft tissues. This is considered "inherent" contrast of the soft tissue that can be significantly better appreciated with MRI than with any other modality.

IV. Vascular anatomy: Flowing blood has different characteristics than stationary soft tissue. Vessels can be imaged in detail with MRI. Magnetic resonance angiograms and magnetic resonance venograms can be reconstructed by subtracting out the background tissue signal.

V. MRI can easily image areas that are poorly visualized by CT (e.g., areas encased in thick bones, such as the posterior fossa and anterior temporal lobes).

VI. Gadolinium is a paramagnetic IV contrast agent, which enhances tissues that are highly vascular or have a damaged blood-brain barrier. Unlike traditional contrast agents, gadolinium has very few contraindications. Adverse reactions are extremely rare. Contrast-enhanced MRI is generally obtained with T1WI, where gadolinium enhancement appears bright.

DISADVANTAGES AND LIMITATIONS OF MRI

I. MRI has a longer imaging time than CT. This has improved markedly with newer generation machines.

II. Sensitivity to motion is very high, resulting in degraded image quality with patient movement. Chloral hydrate, benzodiazepines, barbiturates, or other medications can be used as a sedative, but timing and dosage and possible respiratory depression are important parameters to monitor.

III. Claustrophobia is often due to tighter confinement and longer imaging times than CT. Sedation may be necessary. Consider using an open MRI.

IV. Metal and electronic devices, such as pacemakers, cochlear implants, and foreign bodies, often contraindicate MRI. A list may be obtained from the manufacturer, but it is becoming less problematic since the newest metal devices are being made MRI compatible.

V. Calcium is not well visualized. Dense cortical bone appears as a signal void. Therefore, bone signal is restricted to that given off by marrow fat. Areas of parenchymal calcification identified on CT may not be seen on MRI and, if seen, are often of variable signal intensity.

VI. Artifacts are common on MRI because of the complex interactions of several types of information, any of which can distort the final image.

INTRAOPERATIVE MRI

The use of open MRI units in the operating room has contributed to an increased extent of tumor removal and a parallel improvement in survival times. In addition, preoperative MRI with the patient's head in a stereotactic frame or with fiducial markers can be used for surgical planning.

REFERENCES

Burgener FA, et al: *Differential diagnosis in magnetic resonance imaging*, New York, Thieme, 2002.

Vlaardingerbroek MT, den Boer JA: *Magnetic resonance imaging: Theory and practice*, New York, Springer-Verlag, 2003.

MAGNETOENCEPHALOGRAPHY

Magnetoencephalography (MEG) records the extracranial magnetic fields produced by electrical current which is the basis of EEG and measures vectors tangential to the cortical surface. *MEG signal is very small, but it*

M

MAGNETOENCEPHALOGRAPHY

is not subject to the distortion from dura, skull, and scalp. MEG and EEG are complementary in obtaining cerebral electrical activity. MEG is used in localizing epileptiform spiking activity in patients and in localizing eloquent cortex for surgical planning in patients with brain tumors intractable epilepsy. Currently, MEG has limited availability because of its cost.

MEMORY

Memory comprises the mental processes of registration, encoding, and storage of experiences and information. It is divided into short-term or working memory (active holding and manipulation of information) and long-term memory (information stored for periods of minutes to decades). Other classifications include declarative (explicit) and nondeclarative (implicit) memory. The anatomy of memory involves many widely distributed neural structures. The medial temporal lobe memory system (hippocampus, amygdala, and adjacent related entorhinal, perirhinal, and parahippocampal cortices and their connections to neocortex) is involved in the processing and storage of long-term memory. Papez circuit plays a critical role in the transfer of information into long-term memory and its emotional components. Damage to basal forebrain structures (septum, nucleus basalis of Meynert, and orbitofrontal regions), as occurs in Alzheimer's disease, is associated with memory disorder, often accompanied by other frontal lobe abnormalities.

Damage to diencephalic structures, particularly dorsomedial and other thalamic nuclei, as in Korsakoff's syndrome, leads to amnesia, possibly by disconnection of cortical areas involved in memory processing. Bilateral damage of the limbic system causes severe memory disturbance. Bilateral damage to the amygdaloid region and anterior temporal lobes may produce the *Klüver-Bucy syndrome*, which is characterized by behavioral and cognitive deficits, placidity, apathy, hypersexuality, hyperorality, and visual and auditory agnosia.

Amnestic syndromes include retrograde or antegrade amnesia. Retrograde amnesia commonly follows head injury and involves loss of memory for a variable time before the event. Antegrade amnesia, the inability to incorporate ongoing experience into memory stores, is seen in head trauma, Wernicke-Korsakoff's psychosis, or bilateral limbic lesions to the hippocampal-amygdala complex. The latter is usually due to occlusive vascular disease, hypoxic encephalopathy, or encephalitis. Total global retrograde amnesia, in which an individual loses all prior memory, is never due to organic dysfunction.

REFERENCE

Mesulam MM: *Principles of behavioral and cognitive neurology*, New York, Oxford University Press, 2000.

MENINGITIS (See also NEUROLOGIC EMERGENCY APPENDIX)

DEFINITION
Meningitis is an infectious or inflammatory process involving the subarachnoid space. Bacterial meningitis (invariably associated with a cortical encephalitis and often with a ventriculitis) is a medical emergency.

CLINICAL PRESENTATION
Meningitis should be suspected in any patient with an acute onset of nuchal rigidity, headache, altered mental status, fever, emesis, and photophobia. *Meningeal signs are often absent in infants younger than 6 months of age and in elderly individuals.*

DIAGNOSIS AND EVALUATION
If the diagnosis of acute bacterial meningitis is suspected, blood cultures and head CT are obtained immediately. Antibiotic therapy should begin before the patient leaves the emergency room for the CT. Antibiotics are chosen based on patient age, severity of clinical situation, and possible organisms (Table 64). If the CT result is normal, a CSF examination must be performed and sent for blood cell and differential cell counts, glucose and protein levels, and cultures (bacterial, viral, fungal, and mycobacterial, as appropriate). Organism-specific studies, including cryptococcal antigen studies and counterimmunoelectrophoresis specific for some strains of *Haemophilus influenzae, Neisseria meningitidis, Streptococcus pneumoniae*, fl-hemolytic streptococci, and *Escherichia coli* are often useful, especially if results of initial CSF cultures are negative (Table 65). Laboratory evaluation of CSF includes a Gram stain and India ink examination of centrifuged CSF sediment. Cell counts greater than 1000/mm^3, protein levels greater than 50 mg/dL, and glucose levels less than 30 mg/dL suggest bacterial infection. There is overlap with ranges

TABLE 64

WIDE-COVERAGE ANTIBIOTICS USED IN INITIAL TREATMENT OF ACUTE MENINGITIS BEFORE RETURN OF CULTURES

Patients	Antibiotic Therapy
Neonates	Ampicillin or penicillin G IV IM; aminoglycoside or ampicillin and cefotaxime; appropriate dosages depend on age and weight
Children 1–3 mo	Ampicillin 200 mg/kg/day IV divided q 6 hr and cefotaxime 200 mg/kg/day IV divided q 6 hr
Children >3 mo	Cefotaxime 200 mg/kg/day IV divided q 6 hr or ceftriaxone 100 mg/kg/day IV divided q 12 hr
Adults	Cefotaxime 1 g IV q 8 hr to 2 g IV q 4 hr or ceftriaxone 1 to 2 g IV q 12 hr

Note: For severe penicillin allergy consider giving chloramphenicol and trimethoprim-sulfamethoxazole. If methicillin-resistant *Staphylococcus* organisms are a consideration, vancomycin 1 g IV q 12 hr is recommended.

TABLE 65

CAUSATIVE ORGANISMS IN MENINGITIS ACCORDING TO PATIENT
AGE AND CLINICAL SETTING

Infants < 6 wk old: group B streptococci, *E. coli, S. pneumoniae, L. monocytogenes,*
 Salmonella organisms, *P. aeruginosa, S. aureus, H. influenzae, Citrobacter*
 organisms, herpes simplex 2

Children 6 wk to 15 yr old: *H. influenzae, S. pneumoniae, N. meningitidis, S. aureus,*
 viruses

Older children and young adults: *N. meningitidis, S. pneumoniae, H. influenzae, S.*
 aureus, viruses

Adults > 40 yr old: *S. pneumoniae, N. meningitidis, S. aureus, L. monocytogenes,*
 gram-negative bacilli

Diabetes mellitus: *S. pneumoniae,* gram-negative bacilli, staphylococci, *Cryptococcus*
 organisms, *Mucor*

Alcoholism: *S. pneumoniae*

Sickle cell anemia: *S. pneumoniae*

Pneumonia or upper respiratory infection: *S. pneumoniae, N. meningitidis,* viruses,
 H. influenzae

AIDS or other abnormal cellular immunity: *Toxoplasma, Cryptococcus, Coccidioides,*
 and *Candida* organisms; *L. monocytogenes, M. tuberculosis* and
 M. avium-intracellulare, T. pallidum, Histoplasma organisms, *Nocardia,*
 S. pneumoniae, gram-negative bacilli

Abnormal neutrophils: *P. aeruginosa, S. aureus, Candida* and *Aspergillus* organisms,
 Mucor

Immunoglobulin deficiency: *S. pneumoniae, N. meningitidis, H. influenzae*

Ventricular shunt infections: *S. epidermidis, S. aureus,* gram-negative bacilli

Penetrating head trauma, skin lesions, bacterial endocarditis or other heart disease,
 severe burns, IV drug abuse: *S. aureus,* streptococci, gram-negative bacilli

Closed head trauma, CSF leak, pericranial infections: *S. pneumoniae,* gram-negative
 bacilli

Following neurosurgical procedures: *S. aureus, S. epidermidis,* gram-negative bacilli

Tick bites: *B. burgdorferi*

Swimming in fresh water ponds: *Naegleria* organisms

Contact with water frequented by rodents or domestic animals: *Leptospira* organisms

Contact with hamsters or mice: Lymphocytic choriomeningitis virus

Exposure to pigeons: *Cryptococcus* organisms

Travel in southwestern United States: *Coccidioides* organisms

Adapted from Mandell GL et al: *Principles and practice of infectious diseases,* ed 2, New York,
John Wiley & Sons, 1985.

---

more typical of fungal, tuberculous, and viral meningitis (see Cerebrospinal
Fluid). A polymorphonuclear (PMN) predominance is more common with
bacterial meningitis, and a lymphocytosis with aseptic meningitis.
Approximately 10% of bacterial meningitides show a lymphocytosis. Early viral
meningitis, especially as a result of mumps, may show a PMN predominance.
Hypoglycorrachia (low CSF glucose level) occurs in bacterial, tuberculous,
fungal, carcinomatous, or chemical meningitis. In the subacute presentation
(more than 24 hours of symptoms), unless mental status is impaired, a more
detailed workup may be done before starting antibiotic therapy.

Chronic meningitis is meningoencephalitis lasting for > 4 weeks with persistently abnormal CSF study.

Recurrent meningitis describes repetitive episodes of meningitis with an abnormal CSF followed by symptom-free periods and normal CSF (Table 66).

Mollaret's meningitis is a benign recurrent aseptic meningitis associated with herpes simplex virus, type 2, and may improve on administration of prophylactic acyclovir.

TABLE 66

CAUSES OF ASEPTIC, CHRONIC (C), AND RECURRENT (R) MENINGITIS

INFECTIOUS

Actinomyces sp. (C)*
Amebas
Blastomyces sp. (C)*
Brucella sp. (C)
Borrelia sp. (C, R)
Candida sp. (C)
Coccidioides sp. (C)
Cryptococcus sp. (C)
Cysticercosis (C)*
Fungi (C, R)
Herpes simplex 1 and 2
Histoplasma sp. (C)
Human immunodeficiency virus (C)
Leptospira sp. (C, R)
Listeria sp.
Mycobacterium tuberculosis (C, R)
Mycoplasma sp.
Nocardia sp.*
Parameningeal suppurative foci (R)
Partially treated meningitis (R)
Rickettsia sp.
Treponema pallidum (C)
Toxoplasma sp. (C)*

NONINFECTIOUS

Behçet's syndrome (C, R)
Chemical
Drugs (ibuprofen, isoniazide, sulindac, sulfamethoxazole)
Granulomatous angitis (C)
Lupus erythematosus (R)
Meningitis-migraine syndrome (R)
Mollaret's meningitis (R)
Neoplasm (C, R)
Rupture of cyst (R)
Sarcoidosis (C, R)
Uremia
Uveomeningoencephalitis (C, R)
Viruses (R)

* More commonly cause brain abscess or focal lesion.

M

MENINGITIS

TREATMENT

Tailored to the underlying cause, initial broad-spectrum wide coverage may include ceftriaxone 2 g q 24 hr, ampicillin 2 g IV q 4–6 hr, vancomycin 1 g q 12 hr, and metronidazole 500 mg IV q 6 hr. Glucocorticoid administration suppresses the inflammatory response, with resultant decreased brain edema and lowered intracranial pressure. Children with meningitis who receive treatment with dexamethasone 0.6 mg/kg/day in four divided doses for the initial 4 days of antibiotic therapy have lower rates of sensorineural hearing loss and neurologic sequelae. The advantages of corticosteroids in the treatment of adults with meningitis are unclear, although such treatment may benefit those with increased intracranial pressure.

PROGNOSIS

The major complications from meningitis acutely are seizure, stroke, abscess, hydrocephalus, and herniation with death (Fig. 28). Mortality rates for the different forms of meningitis are variable. The three most common bacterial meningitides (pneumococcal, meningococcal, and *H. influenzae*) have an average mortality rate of 10%; neurologic deficits occur in about 20% of survivors. The less common bacterial meningitides

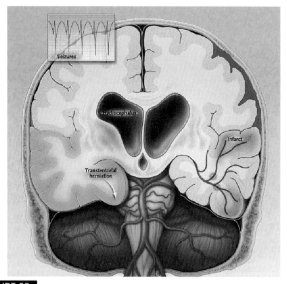

FIGURE 28

Cranial complications in bacterial meningitis. (Adapted from van de Beek D et al: *N Engl J Med* 354:44–53, 2006.

can have much higher mortality rates. The frequency of complications correlates with increased duration of symptoms before treatment. Mental status changes, in particular agitation and confusion, are poor prognostic signs, as is an underlying malignancy, alcoholism, diabetes, or pneumonia. Common sequelae include hearing loss, vestibular dysfunction, cognitive and behavioral changes, and seizures.

REFERENCES

Durand ML et al: *N Engl J Med* 328:21–28, 1993.
Quagliarello V, Scheld WM: *N Engl J Med* 327:864–872, 1992.
van de Beek D, de Gans J, Tunkel AR, Wijdicks EF: *N Engl J Med* 354:44–53, 2006.

MENTAL STATUS TESTING

Routine clinical mental status examination should allow for quick screening of focal and global abnormalities. Elements of the mental status examination include state of awareness, attention, mood and affect, speech and language, memory, visual spatial function, praxis, and other aspects of cognition such as calculations, thought content, and judgment. Patients who appear to have difficulties on screening examinations should have a more detailed survey of their cognitive abilities, ranging from short, standardized tests such as the Mini-Mental Status Examination or the short Blessed Test to more detailed neuropsychological evaluation (Fig. 29).

Interpretation of mental status testing cannot be performed in isolation. An inattentive patient may not perform well on memory tasks or language comprehension, but this is not indicative of primary language or memory disturbance. Visual impairment may complicate constructional testing and naming. General information and proverb testing, although useful as a screening test, is highly dependent on educational level, socioeconomic status, and cultural background.

REFERENCES

Crum R et al: *JAMA* 269(18):2386–2391, 1993.
Katzman R et al: *Am J Psychiatry* 140:734–739, 2000.
Strub RL, Black FW: *The mental status examination in neurology*, ed 4, Philadelphia, FA Davis, 2000.

METABOLIC DISEASES OF CHILDHOOD

A metabolic disorder should be suspected under the following conditions: (1) neurologic disorder is replicated in sibling or close relative, (2) recurrent episodes of altered consciousness or unexplained vomiting in an infant, (3) recurrent unexplained ataxia or spasticity, (4) progressive CNS degeneration, (5) mental deterioration in sibling or close relative, and (6) mental retardation in the absence of major congenital anomalies.

Actual	Possible	Orientation
_____	5	What is the date, year, month, day, season?
_____	5	Where are we: state, county, town, hospital, floor?

		Registration
_____	3	Name three objects: 1 second to say each. Then ask the patient to name all three after you have said them. Give one point for each correct answer. Then repeat them until patient learns all three. Count trials and record. Trials _____

		Attention and calculation
_____	5	Serial 7's. One point for each correct. Stop after five answers. As an alternative, spell "world" backwards.

		Recall
_____	3	Ask for the names of the three objects repeated above. Give 1 point for each correct name.

		Language
_____	2	Name a pencil and a watch.
_____	1	Repeat the phrase "No ifs, ands, or buts."
_____	3	Follow a three-stage command: "Take the paper in your right hand, fold it in half, and put it on the floor."
_____	1	Read and obey the following: "Close your eyes."
_____	1	Write a sentence.
_____	1	Copy the design shown here.

_____ **Total** (maximum score, 30)

Assess level of consciousness along the following continuum:

Alert Drowsy Stupor Coma

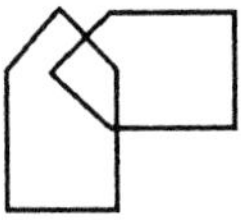

FIGURE 29

Mini mental state examination (From Folstein MF, Folstein SE, McHugh PR: *Psychiatr Res*: 189–198, 1975.)

The following procedures may be performed: (1) urine screen, (2) serum ammonia, fasting blood glucose, pH, Pco_2, and lactic and pyruvic acid, (3) serum amino and organic acids, (4) x-ray, (5) serum lysosomal enzyme screen, (6) tissue biopsy for structural and biochemical alterations, and (7) CT or MRI.

CLASSIFICATION BY CLINICAL PRESENTATION

I. *Acute encephalopathy* presents shortly after birth or during early infancy with recurrent vomiting, lethargy, poor feeding, and dehydration. It initially affects the gray matter, and, hence, presents with cognitive impairment, seizures, or vision impairment. Course is rapidly progressive. This presentation is usually caused by "small-molecule diseases" (amino acids, organic acids, and simple sugars) and represents an "intoxication" or toxic encephalopathy. Intoxications result from accumulation of toxic compounds proximal to the metabolic block. Serum lactate and ammonia, blood gas, and urine ketones permit classification of the metabolic disorders into those with (1) ketosis (maple syrup urine disease [MSUD]), (2) ketoacidosis and acidosis (organic acidurias), (3) lactic acidosis, (4) hyperammonemia with ketoacidosis (urea cycle disorders), and (5) no ketoacidosis or hyperammonemia (nonketotic hyperglycinemia [NKH], sulfite oxidase deficiency, and peroxisomal/lysosomal disorder) (Table 67).

II. *Chronic or progressive encephalopathy* manifests during late infancy, childhood, or adolescence. It initially affects white matter and presents with gradual onset of long-tract signs such as spasticity, ataxia, or hyperreflexia. Dementia may develop later. Liver, heart, muscle, or kidneys are frequently involved. This clinical presentation is caused by large-molecule (glycogen, glycoprotein, lipids, and mucopolysaccharides) or storage diseases and represents intoxication, energy deficiency, or both. Glycogen storage diseases, congenital lactic acidosis, fatty acid oxidation defects, mitochondrial respiratory disorders, and peroxisomal disorders belong to this group. Routine metabolic screening tests are seldom helpful. Neuroimaging and EEG, evoked potentials, electromyography and nerve conduction studies, and specialized genetic/metabolic testing are often necessary to elucidate the diagnosis.

The following metabolic disorders require early recognition and prompt treatment:

I. Phenylketonuria (PKU): autosomal recessive (AR); defect of phenylalanine hydroxylase; 2 months, vomiting and irritable; 4 to 9 months, mental retardation; later seizures, eczema, reduced hair pigmentation; early treatment with phenylalanine-restricted diet can preserve normal IQ.

II. MSUD: AR; defect in branched-chain amino acids (valine, leucine, isoleucine); first week, opisthotonos, intermittent hypertonia, and irregular breathing; 50% with hypoglycemia; sweet-smelling urine; if a diet restricted in branched-chain amino acids is started within first 2 weeks of life, normal or near-normal IQ may be achieved.

III. Homocystinuria: AR; cystathionine synthase defect; presents between 5 and 9 months; strokes or seizures; ectopia lentis; sparse, blond, and brittle hair; treatment is methionine-restricted diet with or without pyridoxine 250 to 1200 mg/day.

IV. Bassen-Kornzweig disease (abetalipoproteinemia): AR; first year, steatorrhea; second year, ataxia, retardation, retinitis pigmentosa; hypocholesterolemia, acanthocytosis; treat with vitamins E, A, and K.

V. Galactosemia: AR; defect in galactose-1-uridyl transferase; normal at birth; first week, listless, jaundice, vomiting, diarrhea, and no weight gain; second week, cataracts, hepatosplenomegaly; may be hypotonic and have pseudotumor cerebri; treat with lactose-free diet;

TABLE 67

DETECTION OF NEUROMETABOLIC DISORDERS: A PRACTICAL CLINICAL APPROACH

History (early infancy)	Routine Laboratory Studies				Special Laboratory Studies			Enzyme Studies			Disorder
	Blood Gases	Ketone	Lactic Acid	Ammonia	Organic Acids	Amino Acids	Sulfites	WBC	Fibroblasts	Tissue	
Acute encephalopathy	−	+	−	−	+	+	−	+	+	+	Maple syrup urine disease
	+	+	−	−	+	−	−	+	+	−	Organic aciduria
	+	+	+	−	+	−	−	+	+	+	Lactic acidosis
	−	−	−	+	−	+	−	−	−	+	Urea cycle disorder
	−	−	−	−	−	+	−	+	+	−	Nonketotic hyperglycinemia
	−	−	−	−	−	−	+	+	+	−	Sulfite oxidase deficiency

History (older child)	Urine MPS	Urine Oligosaccharides	Lysosomal Enzymes	VLCFA	Inclusion Bodies	WBC	Fibroblasts	Tissue	Disorder
Chronic encephalopathy	−	−	+	−	−	+	+	+	Sphingolipidosis
	+	−	+	−	−	+	+	+	Mucopolysaccharidoses
	−	+	+	−	−	+	+	+	Glycoprotein degradation disorder
	−	−	−	+	−	+	+	+	Peroxisomal disorder
	−	−	−	−	−	+	+	+	Fatty acid oxidation disorder
	−	−	−	−	+	−	−	−	Neuronal ceroid lipofuscinosis

visual-perceptual deficits persist despite early treatment; susceptible to *Escherichia coli* sepsis.

VI. Hypothyroidism: post-term, macrosomia, jaundice, large posterior fontanel, mottled skin, big belly; second month, hypotonia, grunting cry, macrocephaly, coarse hair; later, developmental delay, deaf-mutism, and spasticity; if thyroid replacement not started within first 3 months of life, cerebellar and speech defects may persist.

VII. Pyridoxine deficiency: neonatal seizures and EEG abnormalities respond only to pyridoxine; requires lifelong treatment.

REFERENCE

Menkes JH: *Textbook of child neurology*, Baltimore, Lippincott Williams & Wilkins, 2000.

MICROCEPHALY

Microcephaly refers to head circumference smaller than 2 standard deviations (SD) below the normal distribution for age, sex, and race. It is important to note familial trends (measure the heads of both parents), as it can be a normal variant and normal intelligence and development are not uncommon. Head circumference smaller than 3 SD of age norms usually indicates later mental retardation. About 34 cm is the mean for head circumference at birth.

Microcephaly usually results from a small brain except in the case of craniosynostosis, in which premature closure of sutures occurs despite a normal brain. Primary microcephaly refers to diminished brain size due to abnormal development early in the pregnancy.

Causes include inherited disorders (usually autosomal recessive), abnormal structural development (schizencephaly, lissencephaly, pachygyria, micropolygyria, agenesis of corpus collosum), and chromosomal abnormalities. Damage caused by irradiation or TORCH infections early in the pregnancy are also common causes. Secondary microcephaly implies that the brain was forming normally but a disease process impaired further growth. It usually occurs late in the pregnancy. Causes include intrauterine disorders (infection, toxins, vascular), perinatal brain injuries (hypoxic-ischemic encephalopathy [HIE], intracranial hemorrhage, encephalitis, stroke) and postnatal systemic diseases (chronic cardiopulmonary or renal disease, malnutrition).

Evaluation involves determining primary versus secondary causes, with special attention to identifying infectious causes (i.e., TORCH infections). MRI is useful to distinguish the two forms, as secondary microcephaly often has identifiable abnormalities.

REFERENCES

Fenichel GM: *Clinical pediatric neurology*, Philadelphia, WB Saunders, 2001.
Menkes JH: *Textbook of child neurology*, Philadelphia, Lippincott Williams & Wilkins, 2000.

MITOCHONDRIAL DISORDERS

Mitochondrial diseases (MDs) are a clinically heterogeneous group of disorders that arise as a result of dysfunction of the mitochondrial respiratory chain as a result of nuclear or mitochondrial DNA (MDNA) mutation. Mitochondrial disease may affect a single organ, but many involve multiple organ systems and often present with prominent neurologic and myopathic features. Nuclear MD presents commonly in childhood and MDNA presents in late childhood or adult life.

CLINICAL FEATURES

Many mitochondrial diseases display a cluster of clinical features that fall into a known clinical syndrome, such as the Kearns-Sayre syndrome (KSS), chronic progressive external ophthalmoplegia (CPEO), mitochondrial encephalomyopathy with lactic acidosis and stroke-like episodes (MELAS), myoclonic epilepsy with ragged-red fibers (MERRF), neurogenic weakness with ataxia and retinitis pigmentosa (NARP), or Leigh syndrome (LS) (Table 68). Clinical variability exists and many individuals do not fit neatly into one particular category. Common clinical features of mitochondrial disease include ptosis, external ophthalmoplegia, proximal myopathy and exercise intolerance, cardiomyopathy, sensorineural deafness, optic atrophy, pigmentary retinopathy, and diabetes mellitus. The CNS findings are often fluctuating encephalopathy, seizures, dementia, migraine, stroke-like episodes, ataxia, and spasticity. A high incidence of mid- and late pregnancy loss is a common occurrence that often goes unrecognized.

EVALUATION AND MANAGEMENT

The clinical picture is characteristic and confirmed by molecular genetic blood testing. If it is not one of the well known mitochondrial diseases, then family history, blood or CSF lactate concentration, neuroimaging, cardiac evaluation, and muscle biopsy for histologic or histochemical evidence of mitochondrial disease and genetic testing may be warranted.

The management of mitochondrial disease largely consists of genetic counseling and supportive care. Management issues may include early diagnosis and treatment of diabetes mellitus, cardiac pacing, ptosis correction, and intraocular lens replacement for cataracts. Individuals with complex I or complex II deficiency may benefit from oral administration of riboflavin.

REFERENCE

Schapira AH: Mitochondrial disease. *Lancet* 368(9529):70–82, 2006.

MOTOR NEURON DISEASE, AMYOTROPHIC LATERAL SCLEROSIS (See also AAN GUIDELINE SUMMARIES APPENDIX)

AMYOTROPHIC LATERAL SCLEROSIS

ALS is a progressive neurodegenerative disease primarily affecting the motor neurons. Annual incidence varies from 0.2 to 2.4 per 100,000.

TABLE 68

COMMON MITOCHONDRIAL CLINICAL SYNDROMES

Disorder	Main Clinical Characteristics	Other Clinical Features
Mitochondrial encephalomyopathy with lactic acidosis and stroke-like episodes (MELAS)	Stroke-like episodes before age 40 years Seizures and/or dementia Ragged red fibers and/or lactic acidosis	Diabetes mellitus Cardiomyopathy (initially hypertrophic; later dilated) Bilateral deafness Pigmentary retinopathy Cerebellar ataxia
Myoclonic epilepsy with ragged-red fibers (MERRF)	Myoclonus Seizures Cerebellar ataxia Myopathy	Dementia Optic atrophy Bilateral deafness Peripheral neuropathy Spasticity Multiple lipomata
Leber hereditary optic neuropathy (LHON)	Subacute painless bilateral visual failure Males:females ~4:1 Median age of onset 24 years	Dystonia Cardiac pre-excitation syndromes
Chronic progressive external ophthalmoplegia (CPEO)	External ophthalmoplegia Bilateral ptosis	Mild proximal myopathy
Kearns-Sayre syndrome (KSS)	PEO onset before age 20 years Pigmentary retinopathy One of the following: CSF protein greater than 1 g/L, cerebellar ataxia, heart block	Bilateral deafness Myopathy Dysphagia Diabetes mellitus Hypoparathyroidism Dementia
Leigh syndrome (LS)	Subacute relapsing encephalopathy Cerebellar and brainstem signs Infantile onset	Basal ganglia lucencies Maternal history of neurologic disease or Leigh syndrome
Pearson syndrome	Sideroblastic anemia of childhood Pancytopenia Exocrine pancreatic failure	Renal tubular defects
Infantile myopathy and lactic acidosis (fatal and non-fatal forms)	Hypotonia in the first year of life Feeding and respiratory difficulties	Fatal form may be associated with a cardiomyopathy and/or the Toni-Fanconi-Debre syndrome
Neurogenic weakness with ataxia and retinitis pigmentosa (NARP)	Late childhood or adult-onset peripheral neuropathy Ataxia Pigmentary retinopathy	Basal ganglia lucencies Abnormal electroretinogram Sensorimotor neuropathy

M

MOTOR NEURON DISEASE

The majority of cases are sporadic. Five percent to 10% of cases are familial, with 20% of familial cases related to the mutation in the Cu/Zn superoxide dismutase (*SOD1*) gene located on *chromosome 21*. A combination of ALS, parkinsonism, and dementia occurs in several western Pacific islands, and may not have the same underlying pathogenesis as sporadic ALS. Onset of ALS is typically from age 55 to 75 years, with onset at a younger age in the familial cases. Male-female ratio is in the range of 1.4:1 to 2.5:1.

Clinical Presentation

Both upper motor neuron (UMN) and lower motor neuron (LMN) signs are present. Classic ALS accounts for the vast majority of cases, although onset is frequently initially limited to either the lower or upper motor neurons, or to the bulbar muscles. Painless weakness and atrophy of distal muscles in the limbs are common symptoms. The distribution of weakness may be asymmetrical and over time progresses to adjacent myotomes in the same limb and the opposite limb. Upper motor neuron complaints such as loss of fine movement and stiffness are also present. An initial bulbar onset occurs in 19% to 28% of all cases, resulting in dysarthria, dysphagia, and sialorrhea. In general, bulbar onset portends a worse prognosis. On clinical examination, patients with classic ALS have upper motor neuron signs (spasticity, increased tone, hyperreflexia) and lower motor neuron signs (muscle atrophy, weakness, and fasciculation) in bulbar or spinal innervated muscles or both (Table 69). Death is usually caused by respiratory insufficiency or aspiration pneumonia. Mean survival time from symptom onset to death is approximately 3 years, although roughly 10% of patients have a prolonged survival.

ALS subtypes include the very rare *progressive bulbar palsy* (PBP), in which involvement does not progress beyond the bulbar region at all. From 2% to 3.7% of all ALS cases present as *primary lateral sclerosis* (PLS), a condition involving only the UMN and progressing slowly over many years. *Progressive muscular atrophy* (PMA) involves only the LMN. It occurs in approximately 2.4% of ALS patients and has a better prognosis than classic ALS.

Diagnosis

El Escorial revised criteria are the standard for *diagnosis*. These criteria divide the neuraxis into bulbar, cervical, thoracic, and lumbar regions.

TABLE 69

CLASSIFICATION OF MOTOR NEURON DISEASE BY INITIAL PRESENTATION

Disease	Spinal Cord	Brainstem
Lower motor neuron (atrophic)	Spinal muscular atrophy	Progressive bulbar palsy
Upper motor neuron (spastic)	Primary lateral sclerosis	Progressive pseudobulbar palsy

Definite ALS requires UMN and LMN involvement in three regions. *Probable ALS* requires UMN and LMN signs in two regions with at least some UMN signs rostral to the LMN signs. *Probable laboratory-supported ALS* can be diagnosed if EMG confirms LMN involvement in two regions in cases that would otherwise only meet criteria for possible ALS. *Possible ALS* is diagnosed if (1) UMN and LMN involvement are present in only one region, (2) UMN signs alone are present in two regions, and (3) UMN and LMN signs are present in two regions, but some LMN signs are rostral to the UMN signs. *Suspected ALS* is the diagnosis if only LMN findings are present.

Differential Diagnosis
1. Diseases affecting the brain, including stroke, Parkinson's disease, multiple system atrophy (MSA), and HIV infection;
2. Disorders affecting the brainstem and spinal cord, including cervical spondylosis, syringomyelia, multiple sclerosis, adrenomyeloneuropathy, vitamin B_{12} and copper deficiencies, familial spastic paraparesis, HTLV-1 infection, HIV infection;
3. Disorders affecting anterior horn cells, including adult-onset spinal muscular atrophy, Kennedy's disease, hexosaminidase A deficiency, and infection with the polio and West Nile viruses;
4. Polyradiculopathies such as those caused by syphilis, CMV and HIV, and neuropathies such as multifocal motor neuropathy (MMN), CIDP, and POEMS syndrome;
5. Muscle diseases such as inclusion body myositis (IBM), myotonic dystrophy, and oculopharyngeal muscular atrophy; and
6. Rarely, systemic disorders such as hyperparathyroidism.

Laboratory Evaluation
Laboratory tests include CBC, ionized Ca, PO_4, Mg, CK, VDRL, ESR, TSH, vitamin B_{12}, and SPEP/UPEP. Testing for HIV may be indicated, as an ALS-like presentation has been reported to be treatable with antiretroviral therapy in at least one case. Anti-GM1 antibodies may be useful if a pure LMN presentation for possible MMN. Extensive electrodiagnostic evaluation is indicated in all cases. MRI of the neck and brain may be necessary to evaluate for cervical spondylosis and other structural lesions.

Management of ALS
I. *Supportive management.* Daytime sialorrhea can be treated with anticholinergic medications such as trihexyphenidyl, atropine, or glycopyrrolate. Botulinum toxin injection of the parotid gland may also be helpful. Depression and pain should be treated. Pseudobulbar affect is difficult to treat, but may respond to amitriptyline or dextromethorphan. Nutritional support is vital, particularly in patients with dysphagia. PEG tube placement may prolong survival by few months, and should be done before the forced vital capacity (FVC) falls below 50% of normal. Serial pulmonary function tests (PFTs) can help in planning ahead.

M

MOTOR NEURON DISEASE

BIPAP should be offered when FVC falls to below 50% of normal. Dyspnea and progressive FVC decline predict poor prognosis, and the issue of resuscitation and whether the patient wishes to be on a mechanical ventilator should be discussed.

II. *Antiexcitotoxicity*. Riluzole 50 mg bid, when used early, slows ALS progression, and in bulbar onset group, prolongs survival by a few months. However, riluzole provides little benefit with more advanced disease and does not show any positive impact on patient's quality of life or muscle strength. Monthly follow-up of LFTs and CBC is necessary every 3 months. Other antiexcitotoxicity agents are under investigation.

ATYPICAL MOTOR NEURON DISEASES

ALS mimickers are disorders that primarily affect the motor system. These disorders are often referred to as atypical motor neuron diseases (Table 70). Most are distinguished from ALS clinically, while others have different

---

TABLE 70

ATYPICAL MOTOR NEURON DISEASES

Immune-mediated motor neuropathies
    Multifocal motor neuropathy with conduction block (MMN)
Nonimmune-mediated lower motor neuron syndromes
    Spinal muscular atrophy (SMA)
    Distal spinal muscular atrophy
    X-linked bulbospinal muscular atrophy (Kennedy's disease)
    Monomelic amyotrophy (benign focal amyotrophy)
    Fazio-Londe disease
Multiple system disorders with motor signs
    Adult hexosaminidase A deficiency
    Spinocerebellar degenerations
        Machado-Joseph disease (SCA III)
        Autosomal dominant cerebellar ataxia
Other multiple system disorders
    Shy-Drager syndrome
    Guamanian Parkinson-Amyotrophic lateral sclerosis-dementia complex
    Hallervorden-Spatz disease
    Creutzfeldt-Jakob disease
    Huntington's disease
    Pick's disease
Hyperparathyroidism
Electrical injury associated with motor neuron disease
Infectious/postinfectious
Retroviral-associated syndrome
Post-radiation motor neuron disease
Paraneoplastic disorders with motor neuron dysfunction (anti-Hu)
Toxins/drugs
Postpolio syndrome

laboratory, electrophysiologic, and pathologic characteristics. *Clinical clues* that may help differentiate these conditions from ALS include long duration of illness, lack of bulbar involvement after 1 year, onset before age 35 years, presence of family history (although familial ALS does occur), and absence of concurrent upper and lower motor neuron signs in the same spinal segment. Absence of muscle wasting in chronically weak limbs may suggest that the weakness is a consequence of focal conduction block with preservation of motor axon, as seen in MMN. The presence of sensory involvement, bowel or bladder dysfunction, cerebellar or extrapyramidal dysfunction, extraocular muscle weakness, and involvement of other organ systems such as endocrine disorders should suggest ALS is not the diagnosis. A correct diagnosis is important to avoid missing a treatable disorder such as MMN or a familial disorder for which others are at risk.

REFERENCES

Katirji B et al: *Neuromuscular disorders in clinical practice*, Boston, Butterworth-Heinemann, 2002.
Motor neuron disease: ALS I, ALS II, and familial ALS. *Continuum* 3:48–74, 1997.
Quality Standards Subcommittee of the AAN: *Neurology* 49:657–659, 1997.

MOYAMOYA DISEASE

Moyamoya disease was first described in 1957 by Takeuchi and Shimizu as "hypogenesis of bilateral internal carotid arteries." In 1969, Suzuki and Takaku gave the Japanese name "moyamoya," meaning "puff of smoke," to the disease based on the angiographic appearance of fine, collateral blood vessels arising from the large vessels at the base of the brain.

EPIDEMIOLOGY

Moyamoya disease mainly affects people of Asian descent, but it is seen worldwide. About 3000 cases have been reported in Japan from 1969 to 1998, whereas about 239 cases had been reported in the United States up to 1996. Mean age of diagnosis is bimodal (largest peak 10–14 years of age and smaller peak in the 40s), and there is female preponderance (1.8:1 female-male ratio).

PATHOGENESIS

A *chronic cerebral vasculopathy* results in the gradual occlusion of *large intracranial arteries* arising from the circle of Willis. Over time, a sprouting of myriad, thin, fragile collateral vessels distal to the stenotic arteries occurs (Fig. 30). These collaterals are highly susceptible to rupture, resulting in intracranial hemorrhage. The genetic and environmental factors involved in the moyamoya disease process are unknown. Moyamoya may be a heterogeneous disease, as similar findings may be seen in patients with sickle cell disease, Down syndrome, neurocutaneous syndromes, Fanconi's anemia, cyanotic congenital heart disease, cranial irradiation, and other vasculitides.

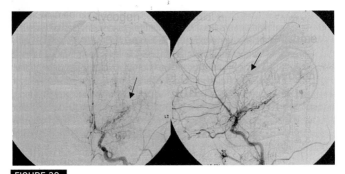

FIGURE 30
Moyamoya disease.

CLINICAL PRESENTATION

Based on a study of 35 U.S. patients with angiographically proven moyamoya disease, the following initial clinical presentations were observed: ischemic stroke—18 (51%), TIA—8 (23%), hemorrhagic stroke—6 (17%), headache—1 (3%), growth factor deficiency—1 (3%), metastatic carcinoma—1 (3%). The mean age of presentation in this group was 32 years (range 6–59 years). The initial clinical diagnosis in patients with Asian ethnicity is likely different than in this population. Based on a study of moyamoya patients in Hawaii, in which most patients had Asian ancestry, 29% had intracranial hemorrhage as their initial clinical presentation. Furthermore, in general it is thought that moyamoya in children presents more often with ischemic stroke and hemorrhagic stroke in adults.

DIAGNOSIS

Radiographic diagnosis of moyamoya disease requires cerebral angiography; however, MRA or CTA may be used as noninvasive alternatives. The angiography must demonstrate stenosis or occlusion at the terminal portions of the intracranial ICA, and at the proximal portions of the anterior and middle cerebral arteries. There should also be a characteristic abnormal network of fine collateral vessels stemming from the circle of Willis. Occasionally, there may be only unilateral carotid involvement. There is a high association of aneurysms and arteriovenous malformations with moyamoya disease.

MANAGEMENT

Surgical treatment is generally preferred and in some cases has improved cerebral blood flow and allowed resolution of the affected collateral vessels. One of the more widely used surgical procedures is encephaloduroarteriosynangiosis (EDAS). EDAS involves rerouting a branch of the external carotid (EC) artery intradurally through nonanastomotic means. This allows for the development of more stable intracranial collateral circulation. Other surgical procedures including EC-IC bypass have been used, but EDAS is the most common for treating moyamoya. The complication rate of EDAS has been cited at 4%.

Medical management of moyamoya has included antiplatelets, pentoxifylline, and calcium channel blockers, but no definitive data are available for their use. Dehydration and hypotension should probably be avoided because of the precarious blood supply. Anticoagulants are not generally used because of the association of moyamoya with ICH. There are no studies comparing medical to surgical management.

PROGNOSIS

The stroke recurrence rate based on the previously mentioned study of 35 U.S. patients diagnosed with moyamoya was 18% in the first year, then 5% per year to the fifth year for a cumulative risk of 40% at 5 years. Of the 31 patients who had follow-up data available, 58% had no disability (modified Rankin's scale [mRS] 0-1), 29% had mild to moderate disability but were able to walk (mRS 2-3), and 18% had died.

REFERENCES

Chiu D, Shedden P et al: *Stroke* 29:1347–1351, 1998.
Mohr JP et al, eds: *Stroke: Pathophysiology, diagnosis and management*, ed 4. New York, Churchill Livingston, 2004.

MULTIPLE SCLEROSIS (See also AAN GUIDELINE SUMMARIES AND THERAPEUTIC APPENDICES)

EPIDEMIOLOGY

Multiple sclerosis (MS) is the most common demyelinating disease, affecting 250,000 to 350,000 people in the United States and over 1 million people worldwide. Onset of the disease is usually between the ages of 10 and 60 years, with peak age between 20 and 30. The cause remains unknown but is suspected to be autoimmune. The incidence of MS increases with latitude in temperate climates. Risk for development of the disease correlates with the latitude at which one lived before the age of 15 years. There is a familial predisposition for its development; women are more affected than men and whites more than blacks or Asians. Approximately 80% of patients will have relapsing-remitting MS, while 20% follow a primary progressive course. Of the patients with relapsing-remitting disease, 50% will develop secondary progressive MS (Fig. 31).

CLINICAL PRESENTATION

Fatigue, limb weakness, spasticity, hyperreflexia, paresthesias, Lhermitte's sign (sensation of "electricity" down the back associated with neck flexion), ataxia, tremor, nystagmus, optic neuritis, internuclear ophthalmoplegia, diplopia, vertigo, bowel or bladder dysfunction, impotence, depression,

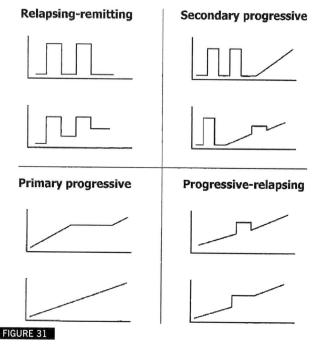

FIGURE 31

Clinical classification of multiple sclerosis.

emotional lability, and cognitive abnormalities. The *Uhthoff phenomenon* is the worsening of a sign or symptom with exercise or increased temperature.

DIAGNOSIS

MS is a clinical diagnosis that aims at proving dissemination in space and in time. For diagnostic purposes, symptomatic attacks should have objective dysfunction lasting at least 24 hours and occurring in different CNS locations involving primarily white matter and should be separated by a period of at least 1 month (separated by space and time). Diagnostic criteria have been used since 1982 and rely on clinical characteristics and laboratory studies such as CSF evaluation and evoked potentials. New diagnostic criteria for MS were formulated by the international panel on MS diagnosis in 2001.They are called the McDonald criteria and are intended to replace the older Poser criteria and Schumacher criteria, and incorporate MRI with clinical evaluation and laboratory studies (Table 71). These criteria help in the early diagnosis of MS even after the first clinical event. The true onset of MS is now believed to be long before the onset of clinical

M

MULTIPLE SCLEROSIS

TABLE 71

REVISED MCDONALD DIAGNOSTIC CRITERIA FOR MULTIPLE SCLEROSIS (MS)

Clinical Presentation	Additional Data Needed for MS Diagnosis
Two or more attacks[a]; objective clinical evidence of two or more lesions	None[b]:
Two or more attacks[a]; objective clinical evidence of one lesion	Dissemination in space, demonstrated by: • MRI[c] or • Two or more MRI-detected lesions consistent with MS plus positive CSF[d] or • Await further clinical attack[a] implicating a different site
One attack[a]; objective clinical evidence of two or more lesions	Dissemination in time, demonstrated by: • MRI[e] or • Second clinical attack[a]
One attack[a]; objective clinical evidence of one lesion (monosymptomatic presentation; clinically isolated syndrome)	Dissemination in space, demonstrated by: • MRI[e] or • Two or more MRI-detected lesions consistent with MS plus positive CSF[d] and Dissemination in time, demonstrated by: • MRI[c] or • Second clinical attack[a]
Insidious neurologic progression suggestive of MS	One year of disease progression (retrospectively or prospectively determined) and two of the following: • Positive brain MRI (nine T_2 lesions or four or more T_2 lesions with positive visual evoked potential)[f] • Positive spinal cord MRI (two focal T_2 lesions) • Positive CSF[d]

MRI demonstrations of dissemination in SPACE and TIME

MRI DISSEMINATION IN SPACE IN 3 OF THE FOLLOWING:	MRI DISSEMINATION IN TIME IN 2 WAYS TO SHOW USING IMAGING:
1. At least one gadolinium-enhancing lesion or nine T_2 hyperintense lesions if there is no gadolinium-enhancing lesion	1. Detection of gadolinium enhancement ≥3 mo after the onset of the initial clinical event, if not at the site corresponding to the initial event
2. At least one infratentorial lesion	2. Detection of a *new* T_2 lesion if it appears at any time compared with a reference scan done ≥30 days after the onset of the initial clinical event

3. At least one juxtacortical lesion

4. At least three periventricular lesions

A spinal cord lesion can be considered equivalent to a brain infratentorial lesion: an enhancing spinal cord lesion is considered to be equivalent to an enhancing brain lesion, and individual spinal cord lesions can contribute together with individual brain lesions to reach the required number of T_2 lesions

cont'd

TABLE 71

REVISED MCDONALD DIAGNOSTIC CRITERIA FOR MULTIPLE
SCLEROSIS (MS)—*cont'd*

CRITERIA

1. If criteria indicated are fulfilled and there is no better explanation for the clinical presentation, the Dx is MS.
2. If suspicious, but the criteria are not completely met, the Dx is "possible MS."
3. If another Dx arises during the evaluation that better explains the entire clinical presentation, the Dx is not MS.

[a] An attack is defined as an episode of neurological disturbance for which causative lesions are likely to be inflammatory and demyelinating in nature with subjective report (backed up by objective findings) or objective observation that the event lasts ≥ 24 hr.

[b] No additional tests are required; however, if tests (MRI, CSF) are undertaken and are *negative*, extreme caution needs to be taken before making a diagnosis of MS. Alternative diagnoses must be considered. There must be no better explanation for the clinical picture and some objective evidence to support a diagnosis of MS.

[c] MRI demonstration of space dissemination must fulfill the criteria at the bottom of the table.

[d] Positive CSF determined by oligoclonal bands different from any such bands in serum, or by an increased IgG index.

[e] MRI demonstration of time dissemination must fulfill the criteria at the bottom of the table.

[f] Abnormal visual evoked potential of the type seen in MS.

Adapted from *Ann Neurol* 58:840–846, 2005.

---

symptoms, and axonal damage usually occurs early in MS. Earlier diagnosis allows earlier treatment with disease-modifying drugs.

Radiologic and laboratory studies support the clinical diagnosis. CT results are usually normal but can show areas of decreased attenuation in the white matter, areas of contrast enhancement, or both. MRI is far more sensitive than CT for detecting MS plaques and is the imaging procedure of choice. Enhancement with gadolinium is considered evidence of an "active" plaque. T_2 imaging frequently demonstrates finger-like extensions along the small or medium-sized blood vessels ("Dawson's fingers"), and T_1 imaging reveals areas of decreased signal "black holes." CSF shows normal to mildly elevated protein, normal glucose, moderate lymphocytic pleocytosis (5 to 20 cells/mm³), *elevated IgG index, and oligoclonal IgG bands in 90% of cases*. Free kappa light chains or myelin basic protein are elevated during flares. Visual, auditory, and somatosensory evoked potentials may reveal abnormalities in their respective pathways. Cystometry may show an uninhibited, spastic, or flaccid bladder or detrusor-sphincter dyssynergia.

TREATMENT

General management includes avoidance of heat and excessive fatigue. *A small, spastic bladder* can be treated with oxybutynin, propantheline, imipramine, or tolterodine (long acting). Sphincter dyssynergia and a spastic bladder often coexist and are treated with phenoxybenzamine, or diazepam, or both. A large, flaccid bladder is treated with Valsalva or Credé maneuvers, catheterization (intermittent or permanent), or pharmacologic agents such as bethanechol and phenoxybenzamine. *Spasticity* is treated most commonly with baclofen at doses of 40 to 80 mg/day or tizanidine in doses up to 24 mg/day with diazepam or dantrolene as needed to control spasms. *Chronic pain or neuralgia* is treated with carbamazepine, gabapentin, phenytoin, or amitriptyline. *Depression* is treated with selective serotonin reuptake inhibitors (SSRIs) and *fatigue* with amantadine.

Disease-modifying agents (see AAN Guideline Summaries) for treatment of relapsing-remitting MS include interferon beta-1b (Betaseron) 8 million units SC every other day, interferon beta-1a (Avonex) 30 μg IM weekly, Rebif 22 or 44 μg every other day, or glatiramer acetate (Copaxone) 20 μg SC daily. These agents reduce relapses and the formation of new lesions on MRI. New trials on early treatment with interferon beta-1a after the first clinical event or clinically isolated syndrome (CIS), with disseminated lesions on brain MRI, showed increase in time to a second clinical attack and decreased relative risk of relapses, with decreased MRI activity. This implies that treatment should be started after the first clinical attack in high-risk patients. There are no evidence-based recommendations regarding the duration of treatment. Interferon beta-1b is also being used in the treatment of secondary progressive MS, but it is controversial whether treatment has any proven benefit. *Side effects* of interferon beta include flu-like symptoms, erythema or tenderness of injection site, elevated liver function tests, depressed lymphocyte counts, and depression. Glatiramer acetate injections also may cause irritation at the injection site or brief episodes of chest tightness, palpitations, or shortness of breath. The timing for initiation of therapy is still a source of debate. Neutralizing antibodies may also reduce effectiveness.

Mitoxantrone (Novantrone), an antineoplastic agent with immune-modulating effect, has been approved for treating patients with secondary progressive MS. The cumulative maximum dose is 120 mg/m$_2$ over a 3-year period to limit its cardiac toxicity. Many variables must be weighed, including individual lifestyle, cost, side effects, and disease course, before initiating therapy.

Methylprednisolone (Solu-Medrol) is used for acute relapses. The usual dose of 1000 mg daily for 3 to 5 days with oral prednisone taper (1 mg/kg/day) shortens the time to recovery. Plasma exchange has been used in patients not responding to steroids based on one small study. The recommended approach for a patient who fails to improve enough from IV Solu-Medrol after 2 weeks is to give a second course, and if this fails also, then plasmapheresis should be considered. In patients with severe symptoms not responding to steroids, plasmapheresis should be considered earlier. A variety of other immunosuppressive therapies including azathioprine, methotrexate, cyclophosphamide, and cyclosporine have been tested, but none have been shown to alter the course of the disease.

Natalizumab (Tysabri) is a new therapeutic agent that was approved by the FDA for treatment of immune-mediated disorders such as MS in June 2004. It is a humanized monoclonal antibody against α_4 integrins.

M

MUSCULAR DYSTROPHY

It inhibits the binding and migration of lymphocytes and immune cells into the CNS. Unfortunately, the drug was subsequently withdrawn from the market after finding an association between treatment and the occurrence of PML. This was seen in three patients, two with MS and one with Crohn's disease.

REFERENCES

Drazen MJ: *N Engl J Med* 1:2, 2005.
McDonald WI et al: *Ann Neurol* 50(1):121–127, 2001.
Noseworthy JH et al: *N Engl J Med* 343:938–952, 2000.
Rieckmann P et al: *J Neurol* 251:1329–1339, 2004.
Rudick RA et al: *N Engl J Med* 337:1604–1611, 1997.

MUSCLE DISEASES AND TESTING

Bedside examination of the muscles involves assessment of *bulk*, *tone*, and *strength*. In certain neurologic diseases, *fatigue* of muscular response may be important. Subtle weakness may not be demonstrated by action against resistance but may be revealed with provocative postures or movement, such as pronator drift or arm-rolling. Quantitative measures of force generation by specific muscle groups may be helpful in the context of rehabilitation and physical/occupational therapy (Table 72). In addition to clinical muscle testing, histopathologic classification to different types of muscle fibers (Table 73) is vital for sorting out the various muscle diseases (Table 74). Location of muscle weakness may provide invaluable information about the underlying disease and pathophysiology (Table 75).

REFERENCES

Wolf JK: *Segmental neurology*, Baltimore, University Park Press, 1981.
The guarantors of brain: Aids to the examination of the peripheral nervous system, ed 4, Philadelphia, WB Saunders, 2000.

MUSCULAR DYSTROPHY

DEFINITION

Muscular dystrophy (MD) refers to a group of hereditary diseases that cause progressive muscle weakness, generally with evidence of muscle fiber degeneration and regeneration on muscle biopsy. In general, evaluation of the weakness includes the time course, distribution, and a family history.

LABORATORY TESTING

Laboratory evaluation includes CK level and may include genetic testing without a muscle biopsy. An EMG and muscle biopsy may be necessary. Immunostaining and immunoblotting of muscle tissue may lead to a specific diagnosis. In general, the differential of MD includes inflammatory

TABLE 72

GRADING OF MUSCLE STRENGTH

Grade	Strength
0	No perceptible contraction.
1	Trace contraction is observed, but no movement is achieved.
2	Movement is achieved in horizontal plane but not against gravity.
3	Movement is achieved against gravity but not against additional resistance.
4−	Movement is achieved against slight resistance.
4	Movement is achieved against moderate resistance.
4+	Movement is achieved against large resistance but is less than expected, given patient age and fitness.
5	Intact strength.

From Aids to the examination of the peripheral nerves, ed 3, East Sussex, Balliere Tindall, 1986.

M

MUSCULAR DYSTROPHY

myopathy and spinal muscular atrophy. In the case of a distal presentation of MD, neuropathies such as Charcot-Marie-Tooth disease may be considered.

MUSCLE DYSTROPHIES

Dystrophinopathies

I. *Inheritance/genetic factors*. X-linked recessive inherited muscular dystrophies are related to quantitative or functional dystrophin deficiency. Dystrophin is an important protein linking the intracellular cytoskeleton with extracellular matrix. Dystrophin is a part of a large, tightly associated glycoprotein complex containing many other proteins. The dystrophin-associated protein complex results in stabilization of cell membranes; in the muscles, this allows the membrane to withstand contraction and relaxation. Dystrophin is ubiquitous in many cell types. In males with Duchenne muscular dystrophy (DMD), dystrophin is entirely absent, or is present in very low quantity. Becker muscular dystrophy (BMD) presents with a milder phenotype and results when there is a partial deficiency of dystrophin. Other dystrophinopathy phenotypes include X-linked cardiomyopathy, isolated quadriceps myopathy, muscle cramps with myoglobinuria, isolated hyper-CKemia, and DMD/BMD manifesting female carriers. The dystrophin gene is enormous; deletions occur in 65% of patients with DMD/BMD, with

TABLE 73

CHARACTERISTICS OF MUSCLE FIBER TYPES

Characteristic	Type 1	Type 2a	Type 2b
Speed	Slow	Fast	Fast
Metabolism	Oxidative	Oxidative-glycolytic	Glycolytic
Fatigue resistance	+	+	−

TABLE 74

SYNDROMIC CLASSIFICATION OF MUSCLE DISEASE

I. Acute (evolving in days) or subacute (weeks) paretic or paralytic disorders of muscle
  A. Rarely fulminant myasthenia gravis or myasthenic syndrome from a "mycin" antibiotic or hypokalemia
  B. Idiopathic polymyositis and dermatomyositis
  C. Viral polymyositis
  D. Acute paroxysmal myoglobinuria
  E. "Alcoholic" polymyopathy
  F. Familial (malignant) hyperpyrexia precipitated by anesthetic agents
  G. Neuroleptic malignant syndrome
  H. First attack of episodic weakness may enter into differential diagnosis (see below)
  I. Botulism
  J. Organophosphate poisoning
II. Chronic (i.e., months to years) weakness or paralysis of muscle, usually with severe atrophy
  A. Progressive muscular dystrophy
    1. Sex-linked recessive
      a. Duchenne
      b. Becker
      c. Benign with early contractures (Dreifuss-Emery)
      d. Scapuloperoneal
    2. Autosomal recessive
      a. Scapulohumeral (limb-girdle)
      b. Autosomal recessive dystrophy of childhood (Erb)
      c. Congenital.
  B. Normokalemic or hyperkalemic familial periodic paralysis
  C. Paramyotonia congenita (von Eulenberg)
  D. Nonfamilial hyperkalemic and hypokalemic periodic paralysis (including primary hyperaldosteronism)
  E. Acute thyrotoxic myopathy (also thyrotoxic periodic paralysis)

3. Autosomal dominant
  a. Facioscapulohumeral (Landouzy-Dejerine)
  b. Scapuloperoneal
  c. Late-onset recessive (Erb)
  d. Distal—adult onset
  e. Distal—childhood onset
  f. Ocular (Hutchinson-Fachs)
  g. Oculopharyngeal (Victor-Hayes-Adams)
  h. Myotonic dystrophy
  B. Chronic polymyositis or dermatomyositis (may be subacute)
    1. Idiopathic
    2. With connective tissue disease
    3. With occult neoplasm
    4. Inclusion body myositis
  C. Chronic thyrotoxic and other endocrine myopathies
  D. Chronic, slowly progressive, or relatively stationary polymyopathies
    1. Central core and multicore diseases
    2. Rod-body and related polymyopathies
    3. Mitochondrial and centronuclear polymyopathies
    4. Other congenital myopathies (reducing-body, fingerprint, zebra-body, fiber-type atrophies, and disproportions)
    5. Glycogen storage disease
    6. Lipid myopathies (carnitine deficiency myopathy and undefined lipid myopathies)
III. Episodic weakness of muscle
  A. Familial (hypokalemic) periodic paralysis
  B. Myopathy resulting from myophosphorylase deficiency (McArdle's disease), phosphofructokinase deficiency, and other forms of contracture
  C. Contracture with Addison's disease
  D. Idiopathic cramp syndromes
  E. Myokymia and syndromes of continuous muscle activity

TABLE 74

SYNDROMIC CLASSIFICATION OF MUSCLE DISEASE—*cont'd*

F. Conditions in which weakness fluctuates
 1. Myasthenia gravis, immunologic type
 2. Myasthenia associated with
  a. Lupus erythematosus
  b. Polymyositis
  c. Rheumatoid arthritis
  d. Nonthymic carcinoma
 3. Familial and sporadic nonimmunologic types of myasthenia
 4. Myasthenia resulting from antibiotics and other drugs
 5. Lambert-Eaton syndrome

G. Exercise intolerance
 1. Myoadenylate deaminase deficiency
 2. Ca-adenosine triphosphate deficiency.
 3. Hypothyroidism
 4. "Fibromyositis" syndrome
 5. Hypoparathyroidism
 6. Glycogenosis (debranching enzyme deficiency)

IV. Disorders of muscle presenting with myotonia, stiffness, spasm, and cramp

A. Myotonic dystrophy, congenital myotonia (Thomsen's disease), paramyotonia congenita, and Schwartz-Jampel syndrome.

B. Hypothyroidism with pseudomyotonia (Debré-Sémélaigne and Hoffman syndromes)

C. Tetany

D. Tetanus

E. Black window spider bite

V. Myalgic states

A. Connective tissue diseases (rheumatoid arthritis, mixed connective tissue disease, Sjögren's syndrome, lupus erythematosus, polyarteritis nodosa, scleroderma, polymyositis)

B. Localized multifocal fibrositis (myogelosis)

C. Trichinosis

D. Myopathy of myoglobinuria and McArdle's disease

E. Myopathy with hypoglycemia

F. Bornholm disease and other forms of viral polymyositis

G. Anterior tibial syndrome

H. Other
 1. Hypophosphatemia
 2. Hypothyroidism
 3. Psychiatric illness (hysteria, depression)

VI. Localized muscle mass(es)

A. Rupture of a muscle

B. Muscle hemorrhage

C. Muscle tumor
 1. Rhabdomyosarcoma
 2. Desmoid
 3. Angioma
 4. Metastatic nodules

D. Monomyositis multiplex
 1. Eosinophilic type
 2. Other

E. Localized and generalized myositis ossificans

F. Fibrositis (fibromyalgia)

G. Granulomatous infections
 1. Sarcoidosis
 2. Tuberculosis
 3. Wegener's granulomatosis

H. Pyogenic abscess

I. Infarction of muscle in the diabetic

From Adams RA, Victor M: *Principles of neurology,* ed 5, New York, McGraw-Hill, 1993.

TABLE 75

POSSIBLE DIAGNOSES OF MUSCLE WEAKNESS

Predominant Weakness Location	Differential Diagnosis
Ocular	Brainstem and motor cranial nerve pathology including Horner's syndrome, oculopharyngeal muscular dystrophy, Kearns-Sayre syndrome, Graves' disease, congenital myasthenia
Bulbar	Brainstem and multiple cranial nerve pathology, motor neuron disease, obstructive lesion of the nasal and oropharynx
Lateralized limb weakness	Stroke, peripheral nerve or root lesion
Distal extremity	
Arm	Distal myopathies
Leg	Peroneal neuropathy or L5 radiculopathy
Isolated respiratory	Acid maltase deficiency, myotonic dystrophy, polymyositis, motor neuron disease, Lambert-Eaton myasthenic syndrome,
Isolated neck	Motor neuron disease, inflammatory myopathy, paraspinous myopathy

Adapted from Kaminski H, Myasthenia gravis, in Katirji B et al, ed: *Neuromuscular diseases in clinical practice*, Boston, Butterworth-Heinemann, 2002.

point mutations somewhere in the gene causing most remaining cases. Deletions are detected with high sensitivity by the current genetic testing PCR techniques, but point mutations are not.

II. *Clinical presentation*. The incidence of DMD is approximately 1:3500 male births. Weakness manifests between 3 and 6 years of age, with difficulty walking. Affected boys develop a waddling gait with exaggerated lumbar lordosis. The characteristic maneuver performed by affected boys is the *Gower sign*. In attempting to rise from the floor, the boys roll into the prone position, kneel, elevate the hips, and use the hands to "climb up" the thighs. Pseudohypertrophy of the calves is present. Contractures of the heel cords and hip joints occur by age 6 in most patients, resulting in toe walking and limited hip flexion. By approximately 10 years of age, patients no longer climb stairs or rise from the floor independently. By 12 years, most are confined to a wheelchair. Once in a wheelchair, contractures progress and scoliosis develops. Cardiomyopathy is common. Involvement of other organ systems may include intestinal hypomotility and some impairment of intellectual functioning. *Death usually occurs in the third decade due to respiratory insufficiency or cardiomyopathy*. The immediate cause of death may not be apparent.

III. *Evaluation*. CK levels are as high as 15,000 to 20,000 U/L. Myoglobin may be present. Serum CK levels are also elevated in 50% to 70% of female carriers and may be spuriously low during pregnancy. ECG abnormalities are present in 80%. When DMD or BMD are suspected, DNA analysis is the first step in evaluation. Unfortunately, routine PCR amplification and sequencing will pick up only large deletions, which are found in approximately 60% of DMD patients and carriers. Testing for the point mutations found in the remainder of DMD patients is performed by only some laboratories. If DNA testing for deletions is negative, muscle biopsy may be necessary to make the diagnosis. Typical findings include marked variability of fiber size, scattered hypercontracted muscle fibers, and proliferation of endomysial connective tissue. Muscle immunostaining with antibodies to dystrophin will show the absence or paucity of dystrophin-positive fibers. The testing of possible female carriers poses problems due to the relatively low sensitivity of the routine PCR deletion testing. Female carriers are definitely at risk for cardiomyopathy and limb-girdle muscle weakness.

Becker muscular dystrophy presents in a manner quite similar to that of DMD, but with later onset, less severe disease, and prolonged survival. Most patients walk until at least 16 years of age. Intellectual impairment is less common than in DMD. Scoliosis and contractures are not as frequent or severe. Serum CK is elevated in all patients. ECG is abnormal in 30% to 40%. Muscle biopsy reveals findings similar to those of DMD; immunohistochemistry reveals decreased amounts of dystrophin staining.

IV. *Treatment*. Treatment involves physical therapy including appropriate stretching exercises to help prevent contracture. Night splints and bracing may delay contracture and prolong the ability to stand. Achilles tendon release may be indicated. In the teenage years the surgical correction of scoliosis may be necessary. Later in the course aggressive pulmonary care is important. Prednisone (0.75 mg/kg/day) has been demonstrated to significantly improve strength in DMD by increasing muscle mass and slowing muscle degradation, with major benefit in prolonging the independent ambulation time when given early in the course. Treatment with steroids should be offered to all patients. The weight gain associated with steroids is unfortunately a major problem.

Facioscapulohumeral Dystrophy

I. *Inheritance/genetic factors*. This autosomal dominant condition has strong penetrance but variable expression. Between 70% and 90% of patients inherit the disorder from an affected parent, and 10% to 30% of cases arise from de novo mutations. In almost all patients FSHD results from a large deletion of repeats (D4Z4) near the telomere of chromosome 4q in a noncoding region. The current consensus mechanism is that chromatin structure is altered, changing the expression of genes closer to the centromere.

Scapuloperoneal MD is an obsolete descriptive term that included a heterogeneous group of disorders. This is essentially now an obsolete classification. Patients with a scapuloperoneal distribution of weakness should be tested for FSHD, as facial weakness is not always prominent in FSHD.

II. *Clinical presentation*. The disease typically presents before age 20 with a characteristic pattern of weakness of the face and scapular stabilizer muscles. The course is slowly progressive. Facial weakness is absent in up to 15% of patients. Arm atrophy and weakness are characteristically worst in the biceps and triceps muscles, relatively sparing the deltoid, resulting in a characteristic "Popeye" appearance to the arm. A prominent axillary crease may be present due to pectoral muscle wasting. Asymmetrical weakness is common. Intellect is normal. The cardiovascular system is rarely involved. Life expectancy is normal. Severity is highly variable, and approximately 20% of patients eventually require a wheelchair. In patients with early onset, a largely asymptomatic retinal vasculopathy and mild hearing loss are common.

III. *Evaluation.* Serum CK is mildly elevated in 75% of patients. EMG is important in establishing that the disease is myopathic in origin. Muscle biopsy shows inflammatory changes in up to 30% of patients. Molecular genetic testing is 95% sensitive for FSHD.

IV. *Treatment.* There is no specific treatment for FSHD. Conservative treatment with nonsteroid anti-inflammatory drugs, range of motion exercises, and gentle stretching exercises may help with discomfort and pain in the shoulder and back. In carefully selected patients with relatively good deltoid function, surgical fixation of the scapula to the rib cage can improve arm function and enable the patient to carry or lift objects. The procedure is usually done unilaterally.

Emery-Dreifuss Muscular Dystrophy

I. *Inheritance/genetic factors.* The well-known mutation is in the coding region of the emerin protein on the X chromosome (EDMD1). More recently, a second disorder inherited in an autosomal dominant manner has been described (EDMD2). The emerin protein is a ubiquitous protein located in the nuclear membrane of many cells, including cardiac and skeletal muscle. The protein extends into the nucleoplasm. The altered gene in EDMD2 is lamin A/C, which codes for lamins A and C by alternate splicing. Lamins make up the nuclear lamina, located between the inner nuclear membrane and chromatin. The functions of both emerin and the lamins may be to stabilize the nuclear membrane.

II. *Clinical presentation.* This form is characterized by slowly progressive muscle weakness in a humero-peroneal distribution with contractures, or occasionally, cardiac onset with sudden death. Onset of contractures and muscle weakness typically begins in the first decade of life, but contractures progress during adolescence. Typically the biceps and the posterior leg muscles shorten resulting in elbow flexion contractures and equinus deformities of the feet. Rigid spine may result from contractures of the low back. Elbow flexion and finger extension are selectively weak compared to the scapular muscles. Facial muscles may be mildly involved. Unfortunately, cardiomyopathy is not correlated with the degree of muscle weakness. Sudden death may occur in up to 40% of patients, frequently without antecedent symptoms. The cardiac muscle is replaced with fibrous and fatty tissue. The atria are more affected than the ventricles. *Complete atrial standstill is the hallmark cardiac disturbance found in this condition.* Unfortunately, although muscle weakness and contractures are not a major issue in female carriers, these women are at risk for atrial standstill and sudden death.

III. *Diagnosis.* Early flexion contractures at the neck, elbows and ankles, the characteristic pattern of weakness, and cardiac involvement are suggestive of EDMD diagnosis. CK may be elevated as high as 10 times the upper limit of normal. EDMD1 may be diagnosed by analysis of emerin expression in skin biopsy or buccal smears, as the protein is ubiquitous. In EDMD2 genetic analysis is necessary.

IV. *Treatment.* The disease has no specific treatment. Early contractures can be managed by physical therapy and surgical release. All patients should be seen by a cardiologist, and annual cardiac evaluation (ECG, Holter monitor) is required. A cardiac pacemaker should be placed when indicated as the risk of sudden death is high. Female carriers should also be followed by a cardiologist.

Limb-Girdle Muscular Dystrophy

I. *Inheritance/genetic factors.* LGMD is a descriptive term for patients with genetically determined proximal hip girdle and shoulder weakness and atrophy. There has been an explosion of work on the genetics of LGMD. *Autosomal recessive LGMDs* include sarcoglycanopathies (alpha, beta, gamma, delta), calpainopathy and dysferlinopathy. *Autosomal dominant LGMDs* include caveolinopathy and lamin A/C mutations (overlapping with EDMD2, see above).

A. Sarcoglycanopathies (AR) often present in a manner similar to DMD or BMD, except that heart involvement is less severe and intelligence is normal. An individual with a DMD-like presentation with pseudohypertrophy of muscles but normal dystrophin studies is likely to have a sarcoglycan gene mutation. Sarcoglycan mutations account for only 10% of mild LGMDs presenting in adolescence or adulthood. CK levels are widely variable. All four sarcoglycans are associated with the dystroglycan complex. Deficiency of one sarcoglycan causes a functional deficiency of all, and immunostaining usually cannot resolve which of the sarcoglycan proteins is absent.

B. Calpainopathy (Reunion Island myopathy) is the cause of 10% to 30% of all AR LGMD in the general population, although in some inbred populations it is the cause of 90% of LGMD. Calpain is a calcium-sensitive protease and its function in muscle is not well understood. Weakness first presents as toe-walking and later is *more prominent in the gluteus maximus and hip adductors than in the iliopsoas and hip abductors, a feature that is helpful in clinically* differentiating from other LGMDs. Scapular winging is usually prominent, and usually begins after weakness of the hip extensors. Contractures may begin at an early age, as may scoliosis. *Cardiac disease is uncommon* and intelligence is normal. CK levels are typically 5 to 80 times normal. A different phenotype of isolated hyper-CKemia and no clinical weakness has been found in association with calpain mutations. Genetic testing for calpainopathies is currently on a research basis only. Immunoblotting of muscle may show absence of calpain 3; however, the test has low specificity.

C. Dysferlinopathy (AR) may present either as Myoshi distal myopathy or as an LGMD. Patients with the distal presentation have prominent gastrocnemius and soleus atrophy with initial preservation of the anterior compartment muscles. CK is strikingly elevated in the range of 20 to 150 times normal. The LGMD presentation is dominated by pelvic and shoulder girdle weakness with CK levels greater than 100 times normal. There is slow progression with onset in the teenage years or adulthood. Muscle biopsy of dysferlinopathy may notoriously show inflammation, but no rimmed vacuoles are present. Immunoblotting of muscle is the most sensitive test for dysferlinopathy.

A review of the AD LGMDs and other less common AR LGMDs is beyond the scope of this review.

II. *Differential diagnosis*. Differential diagnosis includes dystrophinopathies, and every male patient should first be tested for dystrophinopathy prior to testing for LGMDs. A female patient with MD is nearly as likely to have a dystrophin mutation and be a manifesting carrier as to have a form of LGMD.

Oculopharyngeal Muscular Dystrophy

I. *Inheritance/genetic factors*. Triplet repeat disorder caused by a small GCG expansion in the poly(A)-binding protein 2 gene (*PABPN1*) from a normal of 6 repeats to between 8 and 13. The full expansion of GCG to 8 to 13 repeats causes an autosomal dominant disorder. The 7 repeat expansion may act as an autosomal recessive disorder, manifesting in patients with 2 copies of the $(GCG)_7$ expansion. The repeat size is stable from generation to generation and OPMD does not show the phenomenon of anticipation. The PABPN1 protein regulates the length of the poly(A) tail added to messenger RNA transcripts. The mechanism by which this results in OPMD is not clear. OPMD has a worldwide distribution, and is more prevalent in the French-Canadian population (1:1000) and in Bukhara Jews (1:600). In the United States, there are numerous ethnic groups in which OPMD has been identified, including descendants of Spanish, British, and Jewish immigrants as well as the Cajun population.

II. *Clinical presentation*. OPMD is a very unusual MD in that it presents late in life. Onset almost always occurs after 50 years of age, and the seventh decade of life is the most common time of presentation. Ptosis with eventually some involvement of the extraocular muscles and dysphagia dominate the clinical picture. Proximal leg weakness and dysphonia eventually occur in most patients. Facial weakness and tongue atrophy are common.

III. *Diagnosis*. In the past, diagnosis was exclusively made by muscle biopsy. The specific histologic marker on electron microscopy is the presence of filamentous intranuclear inclusions. These inclusions consist of tubular filaments; 4% to 5% of nuclei in the deltoid muscle will show these inclusions in OPMD patients. More recently, DNA testing with PCR with identification of GCG repeat size became available. DNA testing has replaced muscle biopsy, except in confusing presentations, as when mitochondrial myopathy is a consideration.

IV. *Differential diagnosis*. Differential diagnosis includes myotonic dystrophy, mitochondrial myopathies including the Kearns-Sayre syndrome, myasthenia gravis, and isolated familial ptosis without dysphagia.

V. *Treatment*. There is no specific therapy for this condition. Surgical treatments are used to correct ptosis and relieve dysphagia in moderate to severely affected patients. Resection of the levator palpebrae aponeurosis and frontal suspension of the eyelids correct ptosis. Cricopharyngeal myotomy is useful for dysphagia; however, dysphagia will slowly reappear in most patients. As treatment is only symptomatic, there is no clear role for DNA presymptomatic screening, but such screening may be performed with adequate genetic counseling.

Distal Myopathies

Distal myopathies are characterized exclusively or predominantly by distal weakness. Currently, they are best categorized by age of onset, pattern of muscle involvement, and mode of inheritance.

I. Early adult onset distal myopathies

A. *Nonaka myopathy* is AR and has been linked to chromosome 9p12-q11, as have familial inclusion body myopathy and quadriceps sparing myopathy. These disorders are all presumed to be allelic.

1. *Clinically*, Nonaka myopathy presents with bilateral footdrop and a steppage gait resulting from weakness of the ankle dorsiflexors. Proximal weakness may eventually occur, but the quadriceps are always spared.

2. *Diagnosis:* CK is usually not more than five times normal. Muscle biopsy reveals dystrophic features accompanied by rimmed vacuoles containing basophilic granular material. Filaments associated with the vacuoles may be seen on electron microscopy (EM). These are the same histologic findings seen in familial inclusion body myopathy and quadriceps sparing myopathy.

B. *Miyoshi distal myopathy* is an AR dysferlinopathy and is allelic to LGMD2b (see previously).

1. *Clinically*, weakness characteristically begins in the posterior compartment of the legs with gastrocnemius muscle weakness

and atrophy. Progression is extremely variable, but patients may eventually require a wheelchair.

2. *Diagnosis:* CK is markedly elevated, ranging from 20 to 150 times normal. Muscle biopsy may show inflammatory changes, and immunoblotting for dysferlin is the most sensitive testing available.

C. *Laing myopathy* has only been reported in one family, and has been linked to chromosome 14q1.

II. Late adult onset distal myopathies

A. *Welander myopathy* is an AD disorder linked to chromosome 2p13, as are Miyoshi myopathy and LGMD2. Welander myopathy may in fact be a dysferlinopathy. Clinically, weakness begins in the distal upper extremities. Weakness of the ankle dorsiflexors may develop later. Onset is after the age of 30 and progression is slow. CK is normal. Fibrillation potentials may be present on EMG. Rimmed vacuoles may be present on muscle biopsy with nuclear filaments on EM.

B. *Udd myopathy* is an AD condition linked to chromosome 2q31.

1. *Clinically*, footdrop is typically the first symptom followed by variable involvement of the finger and wrist extensors. Onset is after age 40.

2. *Laboratory tests:* CK is normal. Muscle biopsy shows prominent vacuoles but no filaments.

3. *Differential diagnosis* includes unusual presentation of a typically proximal myopathy, congenital myopathies (nemaline rod, central core, centronuclear congenital myopathy), and metabolic myopathies.

Congenital Muscular Dystrophies

I. *Inheritance/genetic factors:* Mutations in multiple genes have been described. 50% of CMD is caused by laminin α_2 deficiency (merosin deficiency). Laminin α_2 is involved with the dystroglycan complex.

II. *Clinical presentation:* CMD are rare disorders with weakness present at birth with an abnormal muscle biopsy in infancy. Weakness tends to stabilize over time; however, complications of the weakness increase with age.

III. *Evaluation:* Testing should be guided by clinical presentation. MRI of the brain should be performed in all cases to assess for abnormalities of the central nervous system: (1) abnormal white matter signal, commonly found in merosin deficiency, or (2) brain structural abnormalities consistent with a syndromic CMD subtype. In patients with myopathy and brain structural anomalies, muscle biopsy may be avoided by testing for the genetic causes of syndromic CMD, specifically the *Walker-Warburg syndrome, Muscle-eye-brain disease, and Fukuyama CMD*. These conditions are caused by mutations in the *POMT1, POMGNT1,* and *Fukutin* genes, respectively. Syndromic CMD generally has a poor prognosis. If major brain structural anomalies are not found on MRI, nonsyndromic CMD is suspected. This category is divided into merosin-deficient and merosin-positive CMD. If MRI reveals diffuse white matter hypodensity and hypomyelination, this finding is highly suggestive of merosin-deficient CMD. The characteristic MRI white matter findings are not always present at birth, but develop in all cases of merosin-deficient nonsyndromic CMD by 6 months of age. The MRI in merosin-positive nonsyndromic CMD is usually normal. If a nonsyndromic CMD is suspected, usually a muscle biopsy with immunostaining for laminin α_2 must be performed, as genetic blood testing for laminin α_2 is not clinically available. Merosin-deficient CMD clinically results in severe disability and frequently death from respiratory failure; however, the children are usually cognitively normal. Merosin-positive CMD is clinically much milder and children usually learn to walk. There is no cognitive impairment.

Myotonic Dystrophy

Myotonic dystrophy is the most common muscular dystrophy, and is discussed fully in the section on myotonia.

REFERENCES

Greenberg SA, Walsh RJ: *Muscle Nerve* 31:431–451, 2005.
Katirji B et al: *Neuromuscular disorders in clinical practice*, Boston, Butterworth-Heinemann, 2002.
Mathews KD: *Continuum* 11(2):95–114, 2005.
www.genetests.org. Information regarding genetic testing can be obtained from this NIH-funded Web site with regularly updated gene reviews. Please refer to this site for the most recent information as this area changes rapidly.

MYASTHENIA GRAVIS

Myasthenia gravis (MG) is a disease affecting the neuromuscular junction (NMJ), characterized by muscle fatigue and fluctuating weakness. There are both congenital and acquired forms of MG.

Congenital myasthenic syndromes are classified by the pattern of inheritance or the site of defect, which can be presynaptic or postsynaptic. Patients with congenital myasthenia present in infancy or early childhood with fatigable weakness involving ocular, bulbar, and limb muscles and positive family history.

The acquired form of myasthenia gravis is more common and results from autoantibodies directed against the postsynaptic acetylcholine receptor. MG may begin at any age. Neonatal myasthenia affects newborns of mothers with MG. Females are more commonly affected than males and tend to develop the disease at an earlier age, with peak incidence between ages of 10 and 40 years; in males, the peak age is from 50 to 70 years. Acquired MG has an incidence of 2 to 10/100,000 and a prevalence of 4/100,000.

CLINICAL FEATURES

MG classically presents with muscle fatigue and weakness. Degree of weakness varies from day to day. Weakness tends to improve after rest or in the morning and worsen as the day proceeds. Ocular muscles and bulbar muscles are predisposed to weakness in MG. Weakness of ocular muscle is the initial manifestation of the disease in about half of the cases and is eventually involved in 90% of the cases. Ocular myasthenia with isolated ocular muscle weakness occurs in approximately 15% of the patients, although later on the patient can progress to have generalized myasthenia. Weakness of bulbar muscles, including muscles of facial expression, mastication, swallowing, and speech, is also common. Examination reveals weakness of the involved muscles, which worsens after sustained or repeated activity and improves after a brief rest. There is no muscle atrophy, and deep tendon reflexes are intact. Fatigability can be demonstrated by having patients look up for several minutes to determine the presence of ptosis or repetitively testing the proximal limb or neck muscles. Cooling of the frontalis muscles and eyelids (ice-pack test) can result in improvement in the ptosis.

DIAGNOSIS

Diagnosis is made on clinical grounds, with confirmation by the following diagnostic investigations:

I. *Tensilon test*. Edrophonium (Tensilon) is an ultra short-acting cholinesterase inhibitor. IV injection of Tensilon causes immediate improvement of the weak muscle. The usual dose of Tensilon given in the test is 10 mg. Initially a 2-mg dose is given IV to observe for side effects such as bradycardia, hypotension, or other arrhythmias. If tolerated, the other 8 mg is given in 2- to 3-mg increments over the next 2 to 3 minutes. Atropine sulfate 1 mg should be immediately available as an antidote for cardiac side effects. To maximize sensitivity and specificity, an objectively weak muscle should be selected for testing. Ptosis and major ocular muscle limitation are easily evaluated, but diplopia is subjective and not easily evaluated; limb weakness changes are harder to evaluate. False-positive findings can occur.

II. *EMG examination*. Routine nerve conduction studies and needle EMG examination are normal in MG, which will help to differentiate MG from other conditions such as myopathy. Ten percent or more decrement in compound muscle action potential (CMAP) amplitude is observed in response to slow repetitive stimulation in 50% to 70% of the patients with generalized myasthenia but may be normal in ocular myasthenia. The diagnostic yield is increased by stimulation of the proximal nerves (e.g., spinal accessory or facial nerve).

III. *Serum anti-acetylcholine receptor antibody titers*. Sensitivity is as high as 90%.

IV. *Single-fiber EMG*. This test demonstrates abnormal *jitter* (variation in time interval between the firing of adjacent single muscle fibers from the same motor unit, which primarily reflects variation in NMJ transmission time) in 95% to 99% of the patients with generalized MG. However, although single-fiber EMG is very sensitive, it is not specific. Single-fiber EMG can also be abnormal in several other neuropathic and myopathic diseases. Interpretation of single-fiber EMG needs to be used in combination with clinical presentation and routine EMG examination.

Other useful laboratory investigations are chest x-ray and CT of the chest to evaluate for thymoma. Tests of thyroid function, erythrocyte sedimentation rate, antinuclear antibody (ANA) titers, and vitamin B_{12} level can be helpful in looking for evidence of other autoimmune diseases. Baseline pulmonary function testing is also helpful.

TREATMENT

I. *Anticholinesterase agents* increase the amount of acetylcholine available at the neuromuscular junction, resulting in higher possibility for acetylcholine to bind to the acetylcholine receptor at the postsynaptic neuromuscular junction. Pyridostigmine (Mestinon) is started at 30 to 60 mg every 3 to 4 hours. Dosage ranges from 60 to 240 mg every 3 to 6 hours. It is available as a 60-mg tablet, a 12 mg/mL syrup, and an 180-mg sustained-release preparation for bedtime use. Side effects are due to the muscarinic acetylcholine receptor binding and include excess salivation, abdominal cramping, and secretory diarrhea. Diarrhea can be controlled with anticholinergic medications. Cholinergic crises due to medication excess should be suspected in patients with respiratory failure who have been on high dosage of Mestinon with miosis, sialorrhea, diarrhea, bronchorrhea, cramps, and fasciculations. Treatment consists of withdrawal of anticholinesterases.

II. *Thymectomy* is mandatory if thymoma is present and usually indicated in young patients with severe MG. Thymectomy has been shown in some studies to induce remission when done early on in younger patients. The patient's status should be optimized by plasma exchange before thymectomy.

III. *Immune-modulating agents* such as corticosteroids may be used before thymectomy, although some authorities recommend reserving steroids for when thymectomy fails. They are not recommended for ocular myasthenia except in extreme circumstances. Weakness may occur early on before improvement when starting prednisone. Steroids can be started at lower doses and slowly increased up to 1 to 1.5 mg/kg/day. This dose should be maintained until remission is induced, then switched to alternate-day dosing. Anticholinesterases should be tapered first to verify remission. Steroids are then tapered over 6 to 12 months. If the patient relapses, tapering is stopped and the dose-response optimized.

Azathioprine and cyclosporine have been used in conjunction with steroids for their steroid-sparing effect and they have been used alone. There may be a 6-month lag before they become effective.

Plasmapheresis and intravenous immunoglobulin are used in myasthenic crisis. Patients with severe weakness and symptoms and signs of respiratory compromise need to be hospitalized, and their respiratory status should be closely monitored. In the patients who are on high-dose anticholinesterase, the possibility of cholinergic crisis, which sometimes is difficult to differentiate clinically from myasthenic crisis, needs to be considered. Precipitating causes of myasthenic crisis such as infection and medications that interfere with neuromuscular transmission should be searched for and treated. These include muscle relaxants such as quinine and curare; antiarrhythmic drugs such as quinidine, procainamide, and propranolol; certain antibiotics; trimethadione; penicillamine; and fever.

Ocular MG might best be treated by merely patching an eye if the patient has double vision (provided the other eye has good motility), but it is reasonable to try a small dose of pyridostigmine. If the therapeutic effect is still suboptimal, further increases are not indicated when the weakness is limited to the eyes. Often, pyridostigmine will relieve a unilateral ptosis, only to unmask diplopia. In addition, it might make a large-angle diplopia into a more disconcerting small degree of diplopia. If diplopia is the problem and a low dose is ineffectual, the patient should be patched. If bilateral ptosis is the problem, ptosis crutches attached to spectacles by an optician may be helpful. Steroids are beneficial in treating ocular myasthenia, but, because of risk-versus-benefit considerations, steroids should be reserved for extreme severe cases such as bilateral ophthalmoplegia with frozen eyes, severe bilateral ptosis that renders the patient functionally blind, and strong insistence by the patient despite being warned of the risk of long-term steroid therapy. Thymectomy, immunosuppression, and plasmapheresis usually are not necessary in pure ocular myasthenia gravis, considering the risk-benefit ratio.

REFERENCES

Drachman DB: *N Engl J Med* 330:1797–1810, 1994.
Engel A, Franzini Armstrong C, eds: *Myology*, New York, McGraw Hill, 1994, pp 1798–1835.
Kaminski J, ed: *Myasthenia gravis and related disorders*, Totowa, NJ, 2002.
Lindstrom JM: *Muscle Nerve* 23:453–477, 2000.

MYELOGRAPHY

Traditionally, myelography was an imaging technique that combined conventional x-ray of the spine with injection of contrast into the subarachnoid space with indications including spinal cord and root compression. Currently, CT myelography is performed after conventional plane films have been obtained. Despite the use of CT along with conventional plain films, MRI has largely supplanted the role previously played by myelography. However, in cases in which MRI is equivocal, especially in assessing the nerve roots or in determining if a fluid collection communicates with the CSF, CT myelography is still useful. In addition, when MRI of the spine is contraindicated such as with a pacemaker or other MRI-incompatible metallic device, CT myelography would be the next best diagnostic tool.

REFERENCE

Miller GM, Krauss WE: *AJNR Am J Neuroradiol* 24(3):298, 2003.

MYOCLONUS

Myoclonus is defined as brief arrhythmic or repetitive muscular contractions of cortical, reticular, or spinal origin; the contractions are irregular in amplitude and frequency, asynchronous, and asymmetrical in distribution. Clonus refers to monophasic rhythmic contractions and relaxations of a group of muscles (compare with Tremors).

M

MYOCLONUS

CLINICAL PRESENTATION

The clinical presentation falls into four categories: (1) physiologic, (2) essential, (3) epileptic, and (4) symptomatic. Myoclonus is usually symptomatic and related to *posthypoxia, toxic-metabolic disorders, reactions to drugs, storage disease, and neurodegenerative disorders.* The assessment of myoclonus includes an initial screening for those causes that are common or easily corrected.

Precipitants of myoclonus include sensory stimuli, physical contact, and anxiety, which may modulate the intensity of the myoclonus.

Origin of myoclonus: Segmental and focal myoclonus can be rhythmic or arrhythmic, involving *somatotopic* areas such as head and neck (without palatal myoclonus) or limbs and torso *(spinal myoclonus).* It is associated with myelopathies resulting from infection, degenerative disease, osteoarthritis, neoplasm (especially colon carcinoma), and demyelination.

Palatal myoclonus: Rhythmic, synchronous contractions of the palate at an average rate of 120 to 130/minute can be either bilateral or unilateral and may be associated with contractions of extraocular muscles, larynx, neck, diaphragm, trunk, or limb. Palatal myoclonus persists during sleep. There is hypertrophic degeneration of the contralateral inferior olivary nucleus if the myoclonus is unilateral. The lesion can be anywhere within the *Guillain-Mollaret triangle*—red nucleus, inferior olivary nucleus, and contralateral dentate nucleus—and the connecting pathways (central tegmental tract and crossing dentato-olivary pathway). The movements disappear after damage to the pathways of corticobulbar or corticospinal motor neurons. Palatal myoclonus is seen in cerebrovascular disease, multiple sclerosis, and encephalitis, and occasionally it is idiopathic.

CLASSIFICATION

I. Physiologic (in persons with normal health)
   A. Sleep jerks (hypnic jerks)
   B. Anxiety induced

    C. Exercise induced

    D. Hiccough (singultus)

    E. Benign infantile myoclonus with feeding

II. Essential myoclonus (no known cause and no other gross neurologic deficit)

    A. Hereditary (autosomal dominant)

    B. Sporadic

III. Epileptic myoclonus (seizures predominate, and encephalopathy is absent, at least initially)

    A. Fragments of epilepsy

        1. Isolated epileptic myoclonic jerks

        2. Epilepsia partialis continua

        3. Idiopathic stimulus-sensitive myoclonus

        4. Photosensitive myoclonus

        5. Myoclonic absences in petit mal

    B. Childhood myoclonic epilepsies

        1. Infantile spasms (West syndrome)

        2. Myoclonic astatic epilepsy (Lennox-Gastaut syndrome)

        3. Juvenile myoclonic epilepsy (Janz)

    C. Benign familial myoclonic epilepsy

    D. Progressive myoclonus epilepsy

        1. Baltic myoclonus (Unverricht-Lundborg)

        2. Lafora's disease

        3. Myoclonic epilepsy with ragged red fibers (MERRF)

IV. Symptomatic myoclonus (progressive or static encephalopathy dominates)

    A. Storage diseases

        1. Lipidoses (such as GM2 gangliosidosis, Tay-Sachs disease, and Krabbe's disease)

        2. Ceroid lipofuscinosis (Batten disease and Kufs' disease)

        3. Sialidosis

    B. Spinocerebellar degenerations

        1. Ramsay-Hunt syndrome

        2. Friedreich's ataxia

        3. Ataxia-telangiectasia

    C. Basal ganglia degenerations

        1. Wilson's disease

        2. Torsion dystonia

        3. Hallervorden-Spatz disease

        4. Progressive supranuclear palsy

        5. Huntington's disease

        6. Parkinson's disease

    D. Dementias

        1. Creutzfeldt-Jakob disease

        2. Alzheimer's disease

    E. Viral encephalitides

    1. Subacute sclerosing panencephalitis
    2. Encephalitis lethargica
    3. Arboviral encephalitis
    4. Herpes simplex encephalitis
V. Postinfectious encephalomyelitis
   F. Metabolic
      1. Hepatic failure
      2. Renal failure
      3. Dialysis syndrome
      4. Hypoglycemia
      5. Infantile myoclonic encephalopathy (polymyoclonus) (with or without neuroblastoma)
      6. Nonketotic hyperglycemia
      7. Multiple carboxylase deficiency
      8. Biotin deficiency
      9. MERRF
   G. Toxic encephalopathies
      1. Bismuth
      2. Heavy metal poisonings
      3. Methyl bromide and DDT
      4. Drugs (levodopa, penicillin, amitriptyline, imipramine, morphine, meperidine, L-tryptophan plus monoamine oxidase inhibitor, lithium, and phenytoin)
   H. Physical encephalopathies
      1. After hypoxia (Lance-Adams syndrome)
      2. Posttraumatic
      3. Heat stroke
      4. Electric shock
      5. Decompression injury
   I. Focal CNS damage
      1. After stroke
      2. After thalamotomy
      3. Tumor
      4. Trauma
      5. Palatal myoclonus

M

MYOCLONUS

TREATMENT

Treatment of myoclonus depends on the underlying pathology; however, the degree of disability determines whether treatment is warranted. The following drugs have been helpful, especially in segmental or focal myoclonus:

  I. Treat or remove the underlying cause (drug, etc.).
 II. Clonazepam 1 to 1.5 mg/day is given in divided doses, with a gradual increase if necessary.
III. Valproic acid is the drug of choice for many of the myoclonic epilepsies but is also used to treat essential myoclonus, posthypoxic myoclonus, and other secondary myoclonic conditions such as Huntington's disease

with myoclonus. Initial dosage is 250 mg/day, increasing up to a usual therapeutic dosage of 1200 to 1400 mg/day.
IV. 5-Hydroxytryptophan 100 mg/day is given in divided doses, increasing by 200 mg every 2 to 3 days up to a total of 1000 to 4000 mg/day; carbidopa, 75 to 150 mg/day, may be given to prevent extracerebral decarboxylation of 5-hydroxytryptophan to serotonin. This regimen is reported to help many patients with posthypoxic myoclonus and some with progressive myoclonic epilepsy.
V. Many other medications have been used, mostly anecdotally, including alcohol, estrogens, botulinum toxin (palatal myoclonus), tetrabenazine, trihexyphenidyl, and benztropine.

REFERENCES

Caviness JN, Brown P: *Lancet Neurol* 3(10):598–607, 2004.
Fahn S, Marsden CD, Van Woert MH: In Fahn S, Marsden CD, Van Woert MH, eds: *Advances in neurology*, vol 43, New York, Raven, 1986.

MYOGLOBINURIA, RHABDOMYOLYSIS, CREATINE KINASE

Myoglobin in the urine is due to rhabdomyolysis that occurs within several hours of acute muscle necrosis.

CLASSIFICATION

I. Hereditary myoglobinuria
   A. Enzyme deficiency known
      1. Phosphorylase deficiency (McArdle's disease)
      2. Phosphofructokinase deficiency (Tarui disease)
      3. Carnitine palmityltransferase deficiency (DiMauro)
   B. Incompletely characterized syndromes
      1. Excess lactate production (Larsson syndrome)
   C. Uncharacterized
      1. Familial, no clear biochemical abnormality
      2. Familial susceptibility to succinylcholine or general anesthesia ("malignant hyperthermia")
      3. Repeated attacks in an individual; no known biochemical abnormality
II. Sporadic myoglobinuria
   A. Exertional myoglobinuria in untrained individuals
      1. Squat-jump and related syndromes, including "march myoglobinuria"
      2. Anterior tibial syndrome
      3. Convulsions, high-voltage electric shock
   B. Crush syndrome
      1. Compression by fallen weights
      2. Compression in prolonged coma
   C. Ischemic myoglobinuria
      1. Arterial occlusion
      2. Ischemic element in compression and anterior tibial syndrome

D. Metabolic abnormalities
  1. Metabolic depression
     a. Barbiturate, carbon monoxide, narcotic coma
     b. Diabetic acidosis
     c. General anesthesia
     d. Hypothermia
  2. Exogenous toxins and drugs
     a. Haff disease
     b. Heroin, cocaine
     c. Alcoholism
     d. Toluene
     e. Malayan sea-snake bite poison
     f. Malignant neuroleptic syndrome
     g. Plasmocid
     h. Fluphenazine
     i. Succinylcholine, halothane
     j. Glycyrrhizate, carbenoxolone, amphotericin B
  3. Other disorders
     a. Chronic hypokalemia
     b. Heat stroke
     c. Toxic shock syndrome
E. Myoglobinuria with progressive muscle disease
F. Myoglobinuria resulting from unknown cause

DIAGNOSIS

Diagnosis depends on further characterization of pigmenturia (myoglobin, hemoglobin, porphyrins) by spectrophotometry, electrophoresis, or immunoprecipitation. Myalgia or fever and malaise, or both, may be present. Serum muscle enzyme levels are elevated. Complications include acute tubular necrosis with oliguria and azotemia, hyperkalemia, hypercalcemia, hyperuricemia, and uncommonly, respiratory failure.

TREATMENT

Myoglobinuria is life-threatening only if there is renal injury, which should be treated with mannitol or alkalinizing agents or both.

CREATINE KINASE

Creatine kinase (CK) is an enzyme located on the inner mitochondrial membrane, on myofibrils, and in the muscle cytoplasm that catalyses the reversible conversion of ADP and phosphocreatine into ATP and creatine. It is the most sensitive indicator of muscle injury, and is the best measure of the course of muscle injury. CK is a dimer molecule and occurs in three distinct isoenzyme forms, termed MM, MB, and BB. Normal skeletal muscle CK is more than 99% MM with small amounts of MB. Serum CK level of more than 1000 U/L helps to distinguish muscle disease from neurogenic causes of weakness.

Causes of Elevation in Creatine Kinase

I. Diseases affecting muscle or causing excessive muscle breakdown.
   A. Inflammatory myopathies
      1. CK can approach 100 times the normal value.
      2. In dermatomyositis or polymyositis CK generally normalizes 4 to 6 weeks after the initiation of corticosteroid therapy. Failure to respond suggests an alternative diagnosis. CK is used to monitor for relapse of disease.
   B. Inclusion body myositis: CK may be normal but usually elevated two- to five-fold. CK elevations (<10 times normal) occur in about 80% of patients. CK does not normalize with steroids.
   C. Connective tissue diseases: CK is reported to be low in 39% of patients with rheumatologic disease. An inverse correlation has also been reported between the level of inflammation and the level of CK. CK elevation may suggest a subclinical myositis, drug-induced myopathy (chloroquine), or an overlap syndrome with polymyositis/dermatomyositis.
   D. Dystrophinopathies: CK levels are elevated in Duchenne and Becker muscular dystrophy from the newborn period, reaching levels that are 50 to 100 times normal. A child or adult with a CK level within normal reference range does not have a dystrophinopathy.
   E. Limb-girdle dystrophies: CK is usually 4 to 25 times the normal range in dominantly inherited types and higher (10–80 times the normal range) in the recessively inherited types.
   F. Other inherited/metabolic myopathies
      1. Acid maltase, carnitine palmitoyltransferase (CPT), and muscle phosphorylase deficiency present with episodic muscle damage severe enough to cause rhabdomyolysis.
      2. Miyoshi distal myopathy also may present with CK elevation more than 100 times the normal range.
   G. Rhabdomyolysis: An acute rise in CK level more than five times the normal range is due to a long list of hereditary and acquired causes. CK level may exceed 1000 times the normal range. CK level above 1600 IU/dL predicts renal failure in around 60% of patients with rhabdomyolysis. With adequate treatment, CK should normalize within 1 week (half-life of 1 to 3 days) unless there is an underlying or ongoing muscle injury.
   H. Medication-induced myopathy: Elevated CK is seen with colchicine, antimalarials, statins, gemfibrozil, nicotinic acid, clofibrate, cocaine, alcohol, nondepolarizing muscle blocking agents, and high-dose corticosteroids. Drug-induced myopathies often unmask a preexisting muscle abnormality.
   I. Infectious myopathies: HIV, other viruses (HTLV1, coxsackie, influenza), bacteria (TB, Lyme disease), fungi, and parasites

(trypanosomiasis, cysticercosis) can cause myositis with CK reaching 1000 times the normal range.

   J. Malignant hyperthermia: Fever, generalized muscular contraction and rigidity, metabolic acidosis, and rhabdomyolysis (with CK rising to 100 times normal) may occur in susceptible individuals and may be familial. CK may be elevated at baseline when asymptomatic.

II. Elevated muscle enzyme in the absence of muscle disease
   A. Exercise: Serum CK concentrations reach peak levels at 8 to 24 hours after exercise, begin to decrease by 24 to 48 hours, and return to baseline levels by 72 hours.
   B. Iatrogenic muscle injury: Intramuscular injection (phenothiazine injection), major surgery, electromyography, and muscle biopsy are among the possible causes.
   C. Motor neuron disease: Mild elevations in serum CK may occur in 75% of cases of amyotrophic lateral sclerosis, particularly in the early phases of the disease. No elevation of CK is noted in other neuropathies.
   D. Endocrine causes
     1. Hypothyroidism and hypoparathyroidism can cause small elevation in CK.
     2. Cushing's disease can cause a myopathy, but CK level is usually normal.
   E. Idiopathic: Idiopathic myopathy occurs more frequently in blacks (>whites) and males (>females).
   F. CK-immunoglobulin complexes: Macro CK-1 is a complex formed between the creatine kinase dimer, CK-BB, and IgG and is detected on electrophoresis. It is present in 1% to 2% of the normal healthy population.

III. Low serum CK levels are seen in chronic end-stage diseases in which muscle mass is reduced, corticosteroid treatment, hyperthyroidism, and rheumatologic diseases.

REFERENCES

Font J, Ramos-Casals M: *Clin Exp Rheumatol* 20:837–840, 2002.
Galassi, G, Rowland, LP: *Muscle Nerve* 10:346, 1987.
Gerami P, Schope JM: *J Am Acad Dermatol* 54:597, 2006.
Lotz BP, Engel AG: *Brain* 112(3):727–747, 1989.
Rowland LP: *Can J Neurol Sci* 11:1–13, 1984.

MYOPATHY

CLASSIFICATION

  I. Inflammatory
  II. Endocrine
  III. Metabolic
  IV. Toxic
  V. Congenital
  VI. Muscular dystrophies (see Muscular Dystrophy)

VII. Myotonic disorders (see Myotonia)

VIII. Periodic paralysis (see Periodic Paralysis)

INFLAMMATORY MYOPATHIES

I. *Polymyositis* (PM) and *dermatomyositis* (DM) are inflammatory, usually sporadic, myopathies (Table 76). Age distribution is bimodal, with peaks at 5 to 15 years of age and 50 to 60 years. Clinical presentation includes symmetrical, painless, proximal greater than distal limb weakness that progresses over weeks to months. Dysphagia or respiratory muscle weakness can occur, more commonly with DM. There may be spontaneous exacerbations and remissions. On examination muscle wasting is absent until late in the course, and reflexes are normal. The typical "heliotrope" rash of DM consists of a lavender discoloration of the eyelids and malar areas. A scaly red rash appears over the metacarpophalangeal and proximal interphalangeal joints (Gottron's sign). In group IV there is a generalized necrotizing vasculitis that may produce multiple infarctions of the GI tract, lungs, skin, nerves, and brain. In group V the associated collagen vascular disorders include scleroderma, systemic lupus erythematosus, rheumatoid arthritis, polyarteritis nodosa, and Sjögren's syndrome. The level of creatine kinase (CK) is usually elevated. ECG results may be abnormal, usually with a conduction block. EMG results show increased insertional activity, fibrillations, and short, low-amplitude polyphasic motor unit potentials. Muscle biopsy specimens demonstrate interstitial and perivascular inflammation, muscular fiber atrophy, necrosis, regeneration, and characteristic "ghost fibers." Occult malignancy should be excluded in older patients with PM or DM. Treatment begins with the administration of prednisone, 60 to 100 mg/day until weakness resolves (1 to 4 months), followed by a slow taper. Fifty percent of patients respond to corticosteroid therapy. Cyclosporine, azathioprine, methotrexate, IV immunoglobulin, and plasmapheresis have benefited some patients.

II. *Inclusion body myositis* consists of slowly progressive, painless, distal greater than proximal muscle weakness and wasting. Onset is after the

TABLE 76	
CLASSIFICATION OF POLYMYOSITIS/DERMATOMYOSITIS	
Group	**Description**
Group I	Primary, idiopathic polymyositis (PM)
Group II	Primary, idiopathic dermatomyositis (DM)
Group III	DM or PM associated with carcinoma
Group IV	Childhood DM or PM associated with a vasculitis
Group V	DM or PM with another associated collagen vascular disease (overlap syndrome)

Adapted from Bohan A, Peter JB: *N Engl J Med* 292:344, 1975.

age of 50 years. Men are affected twice as often as women. The level of CK is normal or mildly elevated; EMG findings resemble those in PM and DM. In addition to the inflammatory changes seen in PM and DM, muscle biopsy specimens show characteristic basophilic rimmed vacuoles and nuclear and cytoplasmic eosinophilic inclusions. No treatment is available. This condition may mimic spinal muscular atrophy on clinical examination.

III. *Sarcoid myopathy* is characterized by noncaseating granulomata in muscle as well as other organs. About 50% of sarcoid patients have muscle involvement on biopsy, and most of those are asymptomatic. Chronic, proximal myopathy is the most common clinical muscle presentation. Women are affected four times as often as men. Corticosteroid therapy is the treatment of choice.

IV. *Polymyalgia rheumatica* is characterized by muscle pain and stiffness that worsen with rest and abate with continued exercise. There is no muscle weakness. Onset is after the age of 55 years, and twice as many women as men are affected. Shoulder muscles are most commonly involved. Temporal arteritis may develop in 55% to 75% of patients. Erythrocyte sedimentation rate (ESR) is elevated, and anemia is often present. The level of CK, the EMG results, and the muscle biopsy specimens are usually normal. Treat with prednisone 30 to 50 mg/day for 2 months, then taper. Clinical response and ESR must be followed up during the taper.

ENDOCRINE MYOPATHIES

From 50% to 80% of patients with *Cushing's disease* and 2% to 21% of patients with chronic corticosteroid use have weakness. The distribution is proximal greater than distal, and legs are more involved than arms. Biopsy specimens show type 2 atrophy. To treat, decrease the steroid dose, change to alternate-day dosing, or change to a nonfluorinated steroid.

I. *Adrenal insufficiency (Addison's disease).* Twenty-five percent to 50% of patients have general weakness, muscle cramps, and fatigue that resolve with corticosteroid replacement. The results of EMG are usually normal, and the biopsy specimen is unremarkable. Hyperkalemic periodic paralysis (see Periodic Paralysis) can develop in patients with adrenal insufficiency.

II. *Thyrotoxic myopathy* develops in approximately 60% of thyrotoxic patients. There are weakness and wasting proximally or myalgias, or both; bulbar muscles are usually spared. Serum muscle enzyme levels are normal to low. Treat by restoring the euthyroid state. Thyrotoxic periodic paralysis resembles familial hypokalemic periodic paralysis (see Periodic Paralysis, Thyroid).

III. *Hypothyroidism* causes proximal weakness, fatigue, exertional pain, myalgias and stiffness, cramps, and occasionally, myoedema and muscle enlargement. Deep tendon reflex relaxation time is prolonged. Women are affected 10 times as often as men. The level of CK may be elevated. Treat by restoring the euthyroid state (see Thyroid).

M

MYOPATHY

IV. *Acromegaly (increased growth hormone)*: Fifty percent have paroxysmal muscle weakness, decreased exercise tolerance, and slight enlargement of muscles.

V. *Hypopituitarism* in adults causes severe weakness and fatigability with disproportionate preservation of muscle mass.

VI. *Hyperparathyroidism*: Of these patients 25% have fatigue, proximal muscle weakness and atrophy, myalgias, and stiffness. Bulbar muscles are spared. Deep tendon reflexes are brisk. Levels of CK and aldolase are normal. Alkaline phosphatase and calcium levels are elevated, and the phosphorus level is low.

VII. *Hypoparathyroidism* is usually not associated with significant weakness, but muscle cramping and tetany are common. Tapping the facial nerve causes muscular contraction (Chvostek's sign), and occluding venous return of the arm causes carpopedal spasm (Trousseau's sign).

VIII. *Osteomalacia*: In 50% of patients proximal muscle weakness, wasting, myalgias, and characteristic bony changes develop.

METABOLIC MYOPATHY

Metabolic myopathy refers to muscle disease caused by abnormalities of glycogen or lipid metabolism or a defect of the respiratory chain. Intramuscular glycogen provides energy for short-term, strenuous exercise, whereas fatty acids provide energy for endurance exercise. Thus glycogenoses usually become evident as weakness or cramps, or both, on heavy or intense short-term exercise, whereas lipidoses become evident as poor endurance (Figs. 32 and 33).

Glycogenoses

Glycogenoses are most often autosomal recessive. Muscle biopsy specimen shows abnormal accumulation of glycogen. The specific enzyme abnormality is diagnosed by biochemical analysis of the affected tissue (muscle, leukocytes, skin, and the like). Glycogenoses in general show blunted or no rise in venous lactate levels with ischemic forearm exercise testing. Acid maltase deficiency is the exception.

I. *Myophosphorylase deficiency (McArdle's disease)* and *phosphofructokinase deficiency (PFK)* cause early exercise intolerance. Strenuous exercise results in muscle pain, contractures, and myoglobinuria.

II. *Phosphoglycerate kinase deficiency* resembles McArdle's disease and PFK deficiency on clinical study but is distinguished by lack of increased glycogen on biopsy and X-linked transmission.

III. *Lactate dehydrogenase (LDH) deficiency* and *phosphoglycerate mutase deficiency*, both autosomal recessive, also resemble McArdle's disease and PFK deficiency on clinical study. In distinction, both give a rise (although blunted) of lactate level with forearm exercise testing, during which LDH deficiency also has a rise in pyruvate level.

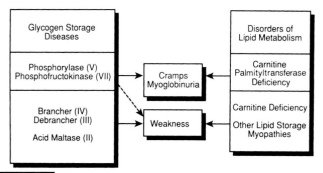

FIGURE 32

The two clinical syndromes associated with disorders of muscle glycogen and lipid metabolism. *Dotted line* represents less common clinical variant of phosphorylase and phosphofructokinase dificiencies. (Courtesy of the Continuing Professional Education Center, Princeton, NJ.)

IV. *Acid maltase deficiency (Pompe's disease)* results in generalized deposition of glycogen in all tissues. Quadriparesis in these patients is due to muscle, peripheral nerve, and CNS involvement. In the infantile type, death occurs by 1 year of age. In the adult type, there is proximal limb-girdle weakness with prominent respiratory involvement. Results of EMG may show myotonia. Life expectancy is normal or slightly decreased. Inheritance is autosomal recessive.

V. *Debranching enzyme deficiency (Forbes-Cori disease)*, also autosomal recessive, is characterized by abnormal glycogen accumulation in the heart, liver, spleen, and muscle. There is muscle wasting and weakness. Onset may be in infancy or adulthood.

VI. *Brancher enzyme deficiency* is probably autosomal recessive. Amylopectin accumulates in the liver, spleen, and nervous system. The deficiency is associated with cirrhosis, hypotonia, areflexia, and muscle wasting and is fatal by age 5 years.

Lipid Metabolism Myopathies

I. *Primary carnitine deficiency* occurs in two forms, myopathic and systemic. Both begin with progressive weakness during childhood or later. In the systemic form, in addition to weakness, there are recurrent episodes of hepatic encephalopathy. Muscle biopsy specimens and studies of histochemistry in both forms show abnormal lipid accumulation; biochemical analysis of muscle shows decreased carnitine content. Serum concentration of carnitine is normal in the myopathic form and decreased in the systemic form. EMG shows myopathic features. Prognosis in the systemic form is poor: death occurs in the late teens or early 20s. Most of the cases are sporadic, but there is evidence of autosomal recessive

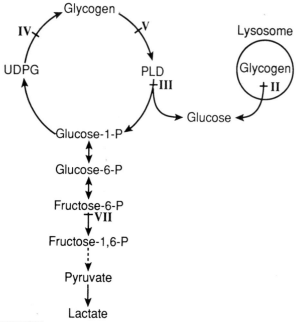

Scheme of glycogen metabolism and glycolysis, indicating the metabolic blocks in the five glycogenoses affecting muscle: II, acid maltase deficiency; III, debrancher deficiency; IV brancher deficiency; V, phosphorylase deficiency; VII, phosphofructokinase deficiency. PLD, phosphorylase-limit dextrin; UPDG, uridine-diphosphate-glucose. (Courtesy of the Continuing Professional Education Center, Princeton, NJ.)

inheritance in some cases. Treatment with high-dose oral carnitine or prednisone may be effective. Secondary carnitine deficiency may occur in cirrhosis, renal dialysis, dystrophies, organic acidemia, mitochondrial myopathies, chronic illness, and parenteral nutrition.

II. *Carnitine palmityltransferase (CPT) deficiency*. Symptoms begin in childhood with weakness, myoglobinuria, and painful cramps (contractures) in response to prolonged exercise or fasting, or both. Strength between episodes is normal. CK level rises during attacks. Forearm ischemic exercise testing shows normal rise in lactate level. Biochemical analysis of muscle and leukocytes shows markedly decreased CPT activity. Glycogen metabolism is normal; therefore, the ability to perform intense exercise of short duration is not impaired. The deficiency is more common in males. Treatment with high-carbohydrate, low-fat diet may reduce the frequency of attacks.

III. *Acyl coenzyme A (acyl-CoA) dehydrogenase deficiencies* are lipid myopathies with variable proximal muscle weakness, metabolic acidoses, and episodic hypoglycemia with minimal ketonuria. Biopsy specimen shows lipid myopathy. One variety becomes evident in early childhood with the preceding symptoms, as well as cardiomegaly, hepatomegaly, and hypotonia.

IV. *Multisystem triglyceride storage disorder* consists of congenital ichthyosis, hepatosplenomegaly, vacuolized granulocytes, and lipid myopathy. There may be nystagmus, retinal dysfunction, cataracts, corneal opacities, and sensorineural hearing loss.

Mitochondrial Disorders

Abnormal mitochondrial function results in disorders of the CNS or muscle, or both. Defects of oxidative metabolism may involve pyruvate metabolism, Krebs cycle, or the respiratory chain. These defects typically result in lactic acidosis in blood and CSF. When the defect involves mitochondrial DNA, the muscle biopsy specimen usually contains abnormal mitochondria that are seen as ragged red fibers on trichrome stains.

Mitochondrial myopathies result in weakness and exercise intolerance. In severe forms patients have profuse sweating and heat intolerance at rest without hyperthyroidism. The mitochondrial encephalomyopathies are primarily CNS disorders. They include the three clinical syndromes described in the next paragraph, whose common features include short stature, weakness, spongy degeneration of brain, dementia, and sensoneural hearing loss (Table 77).

TABLE 77

MITOCHONDRIAL SYNDROMES
KSS
Ophthalmoplegia
Retinal degeneration
Heart block
CSF protein increase
Ataxia
MELAS
Vomiting
Strokelike episodes
Seizures
Positive family history
MERRF
Myoclonic epilepsy
Ataxia
Central hypoventilation
Positive family history

KSS, Kearns-Sayre syndrome; MELAS, mitochondrial encephalopathy with lactic acidosis and strokelike episodes; MERRF, myoclonic epilepsy with ragged red fibers.

M

MYOPATHY

Kearns-Sayre syndrome (KSS) becomes evident before 20 years of age with ophthalmoplegia, retinal degeneration, heart block, and weakness. The defect is a mitochondrial DNA deletion. Mitochondrial encephalopathy with lactic acidosis and stroke-like episodes (MELAS) becomes evident in the first decade of life with episodic vomiting, recurrent hemiparesis or hemianopia, and seizures. The defect is in complex I of the respiratory chain and is maternally inherited. Myoclonic epilepsy with ragged red fibers (MERRF) becomes evident before 20 years of age with myoclonus, seizures, and ataxia. These patients have a maternally inherited defect in complex IV of the respiratory chain.

Treatment consists of avoiding conditions that increase the body's energy demands (fasting, infection, overexertion, and extreme temperatures) as well as medications that inhibit respiratory chain function (phenytoin and barbiturates) and medications inhibiting mitochondrial protein synthesis (tetracycline and chloramphenicol). The administration of coenzyme Q may benefit some patients with KSS.

Adenylate Deaminase Deficiency
Adenylate deaminase deficiency affects 1% to 2% of the population. It is probably not a true myopathy but becomes evident with cramps.

TOXIC MYOPATHIES
Alcohol myopathy takes two forms. There may be an acute attack of muscle pain, tenderness, swelling, weakness, and myoglobinuria after "binge" drinking. Thigh muscles are most commonly involved. The second form consists of a chronic, slowly progressive, proximal muscle weakness. The level of CK is slightly elevated. Results of biopsy are nonspecific.

Table 78 lists recognized toxins that cause a myopathy classified according to presence or absence of neuropathy or cardiomyopathy.

CONGENITAL MYOPATHIES
Symptoms are usually present from birth and include a "floppy infant" with hypotonia, decreased deep tendon reflexes, decreased spontaneous movement, muscular weakness, and often an abnormal consistency of muscle on palpation. Associated anomalies are variable and include scoliosis, high-arched palate, elongated facies, ophthalmoplegia, and pectus excavatum. Symptoms are nonprogressive or slowly progressive. The level of CK is often normal. Results of EMG show small-amplitude, polyphasic motor units. It is usually not possible to discern the specific types of myopathy on clinical basis alone; biopsy of a muscle specimen is necessary for classification.

I. *Central core disease* becomes evident as hypotonia, proximal weakness, delayed motor milestones; bulbar musculature is relatively spared. Biopsy specimens show a well-circumscribed circular region in the center of muscle fibers and a predominance of type I fibers.
II. *Nemaline myopathy* is usually associated with dysmorphic features and bulbar involvement (poor suck-and-swallow reflexes with a weak cry).

TABLE 78

RECOGNIZED TOXINS THAT CAUSE MYOPATHY

MYOPATHY WITH NEUROPATHY

Aminodarone (Cordarone)
Chloroquine (Aralen)
Clofibrate (Atromid)
Colchicine
Doxorubicin (Adriamycin)
Ethanol
Hydroxychloroquine (Plaquenil)
Organophosphates
Vincristine (Oncovin)

MYOPATHY WITH CARDIOMYOPATHY

Chloroquine (Aralen)
Clofibrate (Atromid)
Colchicine
Doxorubicin (Adriamycin)
Emetine, ipecac
Ethanol
Hydroxychloroquine (Plaquenil)
Metronidazole (Flagyl)

M

MYOTOMES

   The severe congenital type can result in respiratory failure and death.
   Biopsy specimens show a predominance of type I fibers and dark-
   staining rods originating from Z lines.
III. There are many other, less common congenital myopathies with
   specific abnormalities on biopsy, including myotubular myopathy,
   congenital fiber-type disproportion, multicore disease, fingerprint body
   myopathy, and sarcotubular myopathy.

REFERENCES

Banker BQ: In Engel AG, Banker BQ, eds: *Myology*, New York, McGraw Hill, 1986.
Bodensteiner J: *Neurol Clin* 6:499–518, 1988.
Carroll JE: *Neurol Clin* 6(3):563–574, 1988.
Dalakos MC: *N Engl J Med* 325:1487, 1991.
DeVivo DC, DiMauro S: *Int Pediatr* 5:112–120, 1990.
Harris JB, Blain PG: In *Baillière's clinical endocrinology and metabolism*, 4:665–686,
   1990.
Kuncl RW, Wiggins WW: *Neurol Clin* 6:593–621, 1988.
Ruff R, Weissman J: *Neurol Clin* 6(3):575–592, 1988.
Servidei S, DiMauro S: *Neurol Clin* 7(1):159–178, 1989.
Tritschler HJ, Medori R: *Neurology* 43:280–288, 1993.
Urbano-Marquez A et al: *N Engl J Med* 320:409–415, 1989.
Walton J: *J Neurol Neurosurg Psychiatry* 54:285, 1991.

MYOTOMES

Myotomes are discussed in Table 79.

REFERENCE

Aids to the examination of the peripheral nervous system, ed 4, St. Louis, Elsevier, 2005.

TABLE 79

MYOTOMES

Muscle	Nerve	Root	How to Test
Trapezius	Spinal accessory, C3, 4	C3, 4	Elevation of shoulder AR
Teres mayor	Subscapular	C5, 6, 7	Adduction of elevated upper arm AR
Levator scapulae	C3, 4, and dorsal scapular	C3, 4, 5	
Rhomboids (major and minor)	Dorsal scapular	C4, 5	Resting the palms of the hand on the back and pushing the shoulder AR
Supraspinatus	Suprascapular	C5, 6	First 30° of shoulder abduction
Infraspinatus	Suprascapular	C5, 6	External rotation of upper arm to shoulder AR
Deltoid	Axillary	C5, 6	Abduction of upper arm at 90° AR
Biceps brachii	Musculocutaneous	C5, 6	Flexion of supinated forearm AR
Brachioradialis	Radial	C5, 6	Flexion of forearm AR between pronation and supination
Supinator	Radial	C5, 6	Supination of forearm AR with forearm extended
Flexor carpi radialis	Median	C6, 7	Flexion and abduction of hand (at the wrist) AR
Pronator teres	Median	C6, 7	Pronation of forearm AR
Serratus anterior	Long thoracic	C5, 6, 7	Push against the wall with the palms of the outstretched hands.
Latissimus dorsi	Thoracodorsal	C6, 7, 8	Adduction AR with upper arm horizontal
Pectoralis major Clavicular head	Lateral pectoral	C5, 6	Push forward AR with upper arm above horizontal
Sternal head	Medial pectoral	C6, 7, 8	Adduction of upper arm AR
Triceps brachii	Radial	C6, 7, 8	Extension of forearm (at the elbow) AR
Extensor carpi radialis longus	Radial	C5, 6, 7	Extension and abduction of the hand (at the wrist) AR
Anconeus	Radial	C7, 8	Elbow extension AR
Extensor digitorum	Radial	C7, 8	Extension of metacarpophalangeal joints AR
Extensor carpi ulnari	Radial	C7, 8	Extension and adduction of the hand (at the wrist) AR

TABLE 79

MYOTOMES—cont'd

Muscle	Nerve	Root	How to Test
Extensor indicis propius	Radial	C7, 8	Extension of the index finger AR
Palmaris longus	Median	C7, 8, T1	
Flexor pollicis longus	Median	C7, 8, T1	Flexion of distal IP joint of thumb against resistance with proximal phalanx fixed
Flexor carpi ulnaris	Median	C7, 8, T1	Abduction of little finger AR: flexion and adduction of the hand (at the wrist) AR
Flexor digitorum sublimis	Median	C7, 8	Flexion of proximal IP joint AR with proximal phalanx fixed
Flexor digitorum profundus	I and II: median III and IV: ulnar	C7, 8, T1	Flexion of distal IP joint AR with middle phalanx fixed
Pronator quadratus	Median	C8, T1	Pronation of forearm AR
Abductor pollicis brevis	Median	C8, T1	Abduction of thumb to palm AR
Opponens pollicis	Median	C8, T1	Touch base of little finger with thumb AR
Flexor pollicis brevis	Median	C8, T1	
Lumbricals I and II	Median	C8, T1	Extension of IP joint AR with MCP joint hyperextended and fixed
First dorsal interosseous	Ulnar	C8, T1	Abduction of index finger AR
Abductor digit minimi	Ulnar	C8, T1	Abduction of little finger AR
Iliopsoas	Femoral	L2, 3, 4	Flexion of thigh at hip AR with knee and hip flexed
Adductor longus	Obturator	L2, 3, 4	Adduction of limb AR with knee extended
Gracilis	Obturator	L2, 3, 4	Adduction of limb with knee extended
Quadriceps femoris	Femoral	L2, 3, 4	Extension of leg AR with hip and knee flexed
Anterior tibial	Deep peroneal	L4, 5	Dosiflexioh of foot AR
Extensor hallucis longus	Deep peroneal	L4, 5	Dorsiflexion of distal IP joint of big toe AR
Extensor digitorum longus	Deep peroneal	L4, 5	Dorsiflexion of toes AR
Extensor digitorum brevis	Deep peroneal	L4, 5, S1	Dorsiflexion of proximal IP joint of toes AR

M

MYOTOMES

cont'd

TABLE 79

MYOTOMES—*cont'd*

Muscle	Nerve	Root	How to Test
Peroneus longus	Superficial peroneal	L5, S1	Foot eversion AR
Internal hamstrings	Sciatic	L4, 5, S1	Lying on back, flexion of knee AR with hip flexed
External hamstrings	Sciatic	L5, S1	Lying on face, flexion of knee AR
Gluteus medius	Superior gluteal	L4, 5, S1	Internal rotation of thigh AR with limb, knee, and hip flexed
Gluteus maximus	Inferior gluteal	L5, S1, 2	Extension of limb at hip AR with knee extended
Posterior tibial	Tibial	L5, S1	Foot inversion AR
Flexor digitorum longus	Tibial	L5, S1	Flexion of toes AR
Abductor hallucis brevis	Tibial (medial plantar)	L5, S1, 2	Usually not tested
Abductor digiti pedis	Tibial (lateral plantar)	S1, 2	Usually not tested
Gastrocnemius lateral	Tibial	L5, S1, 2	Usually not tested
Gastrocnemius medial	Tibial	S1, 2	Plantar flexion of foot AR with leg extended
Soleus	Tibial	S1, 2	Plantar flexion of foot AR with hip and knee flexed

AR, against resistance; IP, interphalangeal; MCP, metacarpophalangeal.

MYOTONIA, MYOTONIC DYSTROPHY

MYOTONIA

Myotonia is the repetitive firing of muscle action potential causing prolonged muscle contractions even after mechanical stimulation to the muscle has ceased. This results in a delay in muscle relaxation demonstrated after voluntary action (such as hand grip or forced eye closure) or percussion of a muscle such as the thenar or wrist extensor muscles (*percussion myotonia*). Results of EMG show repetitive discharges with waxing and waning amplitude and frequency, giving a characteristic "dive bomber" sound. In common myotonic disorders, myotonia results from hyperexcitability of muscle membrane caused by different channelopathies: I, reduced Cl conductance in muscle membrane, and II, abnormal inactivation of Na channel.

The following diseases present with myotonia:

   I. Myotonic dystrophy type 1 (dystrophia myotonica type 1, DM1)

  II. Myotonic dystrophy type 2 (DM2)

 III. Myotonia congenita (Thomsen's disease) – autosomal dominant

 IV. Autosomal recessive generalized myotonia (Becker's type)

V. Paramyotonia congenita (Eulenberg's disease)

VI. Hyperkalemic periodic paralysis (adynamia episodica hereditaria)

VII. Myotonia fluctuans

VIII. Pompe's disease (glycogen storage disease type II), pathophysiology unclear

IX. Chondrodystrophic myotonia (Schwartz-Jampel syndrome), abnormality of the neuromuscular junction and not a channelopathy

Diagnostic steps when evaluating a patient with myotonia are as follows:

I. Confirm myotonia by evaluating for grip myotonia or percussion myotonia.

II. Evaluate for presence of muscle atrophy or weakness, which is indicative of DM1 or DM2; these are absent in other myotonic disorders.

III. Evaluate for paramyotonia – myotonia occurring in cold environment or with exercise.

IV. Needle EMG may show insertion myotonia (bursts of action potentials elicited by needle electrode insertion).

V. Slit lamp examination for cataract. Check fasting blood sugar, hemoglobin A_{1c}, immunoglobulin levels, CK if DM1or DM2 is suspected.

VI. Consider appropriate genetic studies.

Myotonia can be treated with membrane-stabilizing drugs such as quinine, procainamide, phenytoin, or tocainamide. If potassium sensitivity is demonstrated, acetazolamide may be used. These medications treat myotonia with variable success but are often unable to improve associated weakness.

MYOTONIC DYSTROPHY

Myotonic dystrophy is the most common adult-onset muscular dystrophy (1:7500 persons). DM1 is more common than DM2 (Table 80A). Inheritance is autosomal dominant. "Anticipation," or earlier onset of more severe disease in successive generations, has been linked to an increasing number of repetitions of an unstable DNA sequence on chromosome 19 found in offspring of patients. Linkage analysis has been used for genetic counseling.

Weakness occurs in excess of myotonia, particularly involving the face and distal limbs. Atrophy of the temporalis and masseter muscles causes the jaw to hang open, producing a characteristic "hatchet-head" and "fish-mouth" appearance. Frontal balding, ptosis, and neck muscle atrophy add to this appearance. Muscle biopsy shows internalized nuclei, type I fiber atrophy, and ring fibers.

Neurologic features include hypersomnia, dysarthria, dysphagia with nasal regurgitation, and cognitive dysfunction.

Systemic features include cardiac conduction defects, impaired gastric motility, testicular atrophy, insulin resistance, hypoadrenalism, hypothyroidism, early subcapsular cataracts, hypogammaglobulinemia (particularly IgG and IgM), and increased risk associated with general anesthesia.

TABLE 80A

CLINICAL AND GENETIC ABNORMALITIES OF MYOTONIC DYSTROPHY 1 (DM1) VERSUS MYOTONIC DYSTROPHY 2 (DM2)

	Myotonic Dystrophy 1 (DM1)	Myotonic Dystrophy 2 (DM2)
Myotonia	+	+
Cataract	+	+
Muscle weakness	+ (distal muscles)	+ (proximal muscles)
Muscle pain	−	+
Cardiac arrhythmia	++	++
Muscle enzyme elevation	+	+
Cognitive dysfunction	+	+
Inheritance	Autosomal dominant	Autosomal dominant
Chromosome locus	19q 13.3	3q 21.3
Genetic abnormality	(CTG)n expansion	(CCTG)n expansion

The course is slowly progressive; death typically occurs in the sixth decade of life as a result of cardiac or respiratory complications.

Management revolves around managing the weakness, myotonia, and systemic manifestations. Physical and occupational therapy can help preserve or increase strength and flexibility in muscles and provide techniques to compensate for loss of strength and dexterity. Systemic management includes ophthalmology referral for cataracts and ptosis (upper lid blepharoplasty), cardiology referral for pacemaker placement if there is an infranodal conduction delay with H-V interval greater than 70 ms, metformin for diabetes, thyroid function tests and oral thyroxin if needed, hormone replacement for hypogonadism, modafinil for excessive daytime sleepiness, and CPAP for sleep apnea.

Congenital myotonic dystrophy is a rare disorder in which myotonia is a late feature. It is associated with maternal inheritance and presents with hypotonia and bulbar and respiratory weakness as a newborn. Affected children have "shark mouth" and club feet, and 70% have mental retardation. Treatment is symptomatic for adult and congenital forms of disease.

Myotonia congenita (*Thomsen's disease* is the autosomal dominant form; *Becker's disease* is the autosomal recessive form) patients typically complain of diffuse muscle stiffness after resting (due to mytonia), which relaxes with exercise.

In *paramyotonia congenita* (Eulenberg's disease) the stiffness is often induced by cold and worsened by exercise. Muscles of the face and distal upper extremities are most often involved.

Table 80B delineates the clinical features of the myotonias and myotonic dystrophies.

TABLE 80B
CHARACTERISTIC OF THE MYOTONIAS

| Feature | Myotonic Dystrophy | Myotonia Congenita | | Paramyotonia Congenita | Hyperkalemic Periodic Paralysis |
		Thomsen's Disease	Becker's Disease		
Inheritance	Autosomal dominant	Autosomal dominant	Autosomal recessive	Autosomal dominant	Autosomal dominant
Defect	Protein kinase	Chloride channel	Chloride channel	Sodium channel	Sodium channel
Gene locus	19q	7q	7q	17q	17q
Age of onset	Teens to twenties	Infancy to childhood	Childhood	Infancy	Childhood
Course	Slowly progressive	Nonprogressive	Rarely progressive	Variable weakness	Variable weakness
Presenting complaint	Distal weakness Systemic features	Diffuse stiffness	Diffuse stiffness, weakness	Cold-induced stiffness	Episodic weakness
Other features	Typical facies	Absence of type II fibers	± Muscle hypertrophy; absence of type II fibers	Paradoxic myotonia	May have cardiac arrhythmia

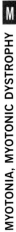

M

MYOTONIA, MYOTONIC DYSTROPHY

REFERENCES
Kurihara T: *Intern Med* 44(10):1027–1032, 2005.
Machuca-Tzili L, Brook D: *Muscle Nerve* 32:1–18, 2005.
Ptacek LJ, Johnson KJ, Griggs RC: *N Engl J Med* 323(7):482–489, 1993.

NEGLECT

Neglect is the failure to report, respond to, or orient to novel and meaningful stimuli presented to the side opposite a brain lesion when this failure cannot be attributed to either sensory or motor dysfunction. Components of neglect include inattention or sensory neglect, motor neglect, spatial neglect, personal neglect, allesthesia (hallucination of perception in response to a stimulus), and anosognosia. Bedside tests for neglect include visual confrontation, double simultaneous stimulation, letter or figure cancellation, figure drawing, and line bisection. Lesions associated with neglect correlate with the type of neglect syndrome. Attention system defects with sensory neglect are associated with right parietal lobe lesions. Motor neglect with varying degrees of akinesia and motor impersistence can be seen in frontal lesions. Defects in the representational system are often associated with right hemisphere lesions because the right hemisphere is important as an attention system for left and right hemispace, whereas the left hemisphere is primarily important only for attention to right hemispace. Another explanation posits a bihemispheric network of attention systems, which is overrepresented in the right hemisphere.

REFERENCE
Heilman KH, Valenstein E, eds, *Clinical neuropsychology*, ed 4, New York, Oxford University Press, 2003.

NEUROCUTANEOUS SYNDROMES

Neurocutaneous syndromes, or phakomatoses (Greek *phakos* = lens shaped, mole, freckle), represent disordered development early in embryogenesis, which produces defects in multiple organ systems roughly according to germ cell layers. They may be divided into disorders affecting ectodermal derivatives (neural and cutaneous tissue) or those involving mesodermal tissue (vascular elements, widespread) or classified by mode of inheritance.

AUTOSOMAL DOMINANT INHERITANCE
Neurofibromatosis type 1 (NF-1, von Recklinghausen's disease) is a neuroectodermal disorder related to genetic abnormality on chromosome 17.

It occurs in approximately 1 in 3000 people. The diagnosis requires at least two of the following:

I. Six or more café au lait spots greater than 5 mm in diameter.

II. Axillary or inguinal freckles.

III. Two neurofibromas of any type or one or more plexiform neurofibromas. (Neurofibromas occur along peripheral nerves and are made from Schwann cells, fibroblasts, vascular elements, or pigmented cells. They are pedunculated, nodular, or diffuse but not encapsulated. A neurofibroma that extends into the surrounding tissue is a plexiform neurofibroma; these have a 5% lifetime risk of malignant transformation.)

IV. Optic nerve or chiasmatic glioma.

V. Two or more Lisch nodules (pigmented hamartomas of the iris, best seen with slit lamp examination of the iris and more common in older patients).

VI. First-degree relative with NF-I by foregoing criteria.

VII. Bony abnormalities such as thinning of cortical long bone or sphenoid dysplasia. Other associated features of NF-I include tumors (pheochromocytoma, Wilms' tumor, leukemia), pseudoarthroses of radius and tibia, kyphosis, and endocrine dysfunction secondary to hypothalamic and pituitary compression from an optic glioma.

Neurofibromatosis type 2 (NF-2) is due to a genetic abnormality on chromosome 22. It occurs in approximately 1 in 50,000 people. Symptoms usually develop in adolescence and early adulthood and include headache, dizziness, tinnitus, hearing loss, and facial weakness. The diagnostic criteria include the following:

I. Bilateral eighth nerve tumors (acoustic neuromas).

II. Unilateral eighth nerve tumor and a first-degree relative with NF-2.

III. A first-degree relative with NF-2 and two of the following: glioma, schwannoma, presenile posterior cataract, astrocytoma, neurofibroma of another type, plexiform neurofibroma, or retinal hamartoma.

Tuberous sclerosis (Bourneville's disease) has multiple manifestations, including generalized or partial complex seizures after 3 months of age, occasionally associated with mental retardation or hemiparesis. Neuroradiologic features are multiple subependymal nodular calcification, cortical tubers, and ventricular dilatation. Development of giant astrocytomas is relatively frequent. Cutaneous manifestations include facial angiofibroma (hamartomas of facial skin that usually appear after the age of 5), adenoma sebaceum depigmented nevi, subungual fibromas, or Shagreen patches (hamartomas in the dermis that appear like cobblestone pavement, commonly located in the posterior neck and lumbar back region). Other associated conditions include renal angiolipomas and cysts, cardiac rhabdomyomas, pulmonary cysts, and retinal hamartomas.

Von Hippel-Landau disease (VHD): Diagnostic criteria include hemangioblastoma of the CNS (most commonly found in the cerebellum, medulla, spinal cord, or cerebral hemispheres) or retina and one additional characteristic lesion or a direct relative with the disease. Characteristic lesions include hypernephroma, renal cell carcinoma, pheochromocytoma, renal, pancreatic, or epididymal cysts, and islet cell tumors. Secondary polycythemia may occur due to production of an erythropoietic factor produced by a cerebellar or renal tumor. Retinal hemangioma may be the earliest sign and can appear in the first decade of life. Exudate from the hemangioblastoma may accumulate under the retina, causing detachment and blindness. Therefore, people at risk for VHD should be examined periodically after age 6 to prevent blindness from retinal lesions. Treatment involves surgical removal of the hemangioblastoma or radiotherapy (if inoperable).

AUTOSOMAL RECESSIVE INHERITANCE

Xeroderma pigmentosa is a rare disorder resulting from a defect in cellular repair of damaged DNA. This results in accelerated aging in tissue exposed to solar light and degeneration of neurons. Skin and eye manifestations usually occur within the first months of life. Neurologic findings are not present in all patients but may include microcephaly, ataxia, spasticity, and choreoathetosis. Peripheral nerve involvement results in hyporeflexia occasionally progressing to areflexia. The diagnosis is made by family history and laboratory tests showing deficient DNA repair in fibroblasts.

Chédiak-Higashi syndrome is a disorder of lysosomal abnormality resulting in large granulations in leukocytes, neurons, pigment cells, and platelets. Cellular immunity is deficient, and recurrent pyogenic infections include otitis media, bronchitis, pharyngitis, cellulitis, and subcutaneous abscesses. Leukemias are frequent in this syndrome. Neurologic symptoms occur in approximately 50% of patients and include mental retardation, seizures, cerebellar ataxia, increased intracranial pressure, and a chronic polyneuropathy with a stocking-glove type of sensory loss, weakness, and atrophy. The diagnosis is made by finding large granulations in leukocytes in peripheral blood, marrow, or giant lysosomes in the cytoplasm of Schwann cells.

Ataxia-telangiectasia is an autosomal recessive (AR) disease caused by a defect in the repair mechanism of the damaged DNA. It presents with progressive cerebellar ataxia, oculomotor apraxia, and choreoathetosis beginning in childhood. Telangiectasias of the conjunctivae, ears, and flexor surfaces appear later. Systemic manifestations include decreased IgA and IgE, increased alpha-fetoprotein, recurrent pulmonary infections, and development of reticuloendothelial tumors.

NONHEREDITARY NEUROCUTANEOUS DISEASES

Neurocutaneous melanosis occurs predominantly in white patients and is characterized by   large pigmented nevi that are light to dark brown. Melanin-containing cells in the pia may develop into intracranial or intraspinal melanomas. Hydrocephalus may result secondary to obstruction of the arachnoid villi. Patients rarely live beyond 20 years of age.

Sturge-Weber syndrome (meningofacial angiomatosis with cerebral calcifications) is a sporadic congenital malformation of the cephalic venous microvasculature, resulting in neurologic, cutaneous, and optic symptoms. Pathologically, there are venous angiomas with tortuous vessels involving the face, leptomeninges, and choroid, in addition to calcification of layers 2 and 3 of the parietal-occipital cortex. Neurologic manifestations include unilateral seizures, cerebral hemiatrophy with hemiparesis, hemisensory deficits, visual field defects, and mental abnormalities. Cutaneous lesions vary in extent from a small "port wine nevus" on the upper eyelid to those involving the entire face and other parts of the body. Ocular manifestations include congenital glaucoma.

OTHER NEUROCUTANEOUS SYNDROMES
I. *Klippel-Trenaunay-Weber syndrome* (limb hypertrophy and hemangiomas)
II. *Osler-Weber-Rendu syndrome* (hemorrhagic telangiectasias)
III. *Wyburn-Mason syndrome* (facial angioma, retinal arteriovenous malformations, cerebrovascular anomalies, and seizures)
IV. *Incontinentia pigmenti* (bullous lesions of skin, micropolygyria, microcephaly, and mental retardation), hypomelanosis of Ito (skin whorls, mental retardation seizures, and ocular deficits)
V. *Fabry's disease* (papular eruption, painful sensory neuropathy, and stroke) and *linear nevus syndrome* (linear yellow papules, mental retardation, and seizures)

REFERENCES
Herron J et al: *Clin Radiol* 55:82–98, 2000.
Kerrison JB et al: *Neurosurg Clin North Am* 10:775–787, 1999.
King A et al: *Neurology* 54:4–5, 2000.

NEUROLEPTIC MALIGNANT SYNDROME

Neuroleptic malignant syndrome (NMS) is a clinical syndrome consisting of a tetrad of *r*igidity, *a*utonomic instability, *h*yperthermia, and *m*ental status change (RAHM) occurring in the setting of the use of dopamine-blocking agents or the withdrawal of dopamine-enhancing medications. It is related to the acute blockade of the nigrostriatal and hypothalamic dopamine pathways in the brain.

CLINICAL PRESENTATION
The motor symptoms consist most commonly of parkinsonian rigidity, but other symptoms include a tremor superimposed on the rigidity, akinesia, bradykinesia, and dystonias (e.g., blepharospasm, opisthotonus, oculogyric crises, trismus, and orobuccal dyskinesia). The altered mental status ranges from delirium to stupor or even coma. A fever is seen in almost all cases, usually greater than 38°C and often greater than 41°C. Arrhythmias, blood pressure fluctuations, and respiratory abnormalities constitute the main, potentially life-threatening autonomic features of NMS. Rare clinical manifestations include seizures, ataxia, and nystagmus. NMS usually evolves over 24 to 72 hours.

RISK FACTORS

NMS is clearly medication-related (Table 81). Occasionally there can be a slower progression, and in the case of depot neuroleptics (e.g., intramuscular form of fluphenazine) progression over a couple of weeks may occur. The clinical course lasts around 7 to 10 days, with a longer time for depot neuroleptics due to slower clearance. In individuals with Parkinson's disease (most often in advanced stages) who have been on dopamine agonists, NMS can occur in the setting of a sudden withdrawal of the agonist agent or a change of dosage or change to a different agonist altogether.

TABLE 81

MEDICATIONS ASSOCIATED WITH THE DEVELOPMENT OF NEUROLEPTIC MALIGNANT SYNDROME

DOPAMINERGIC/DOPAMINE-AGONISTS WITHDRAWAL

Levodopa
COMT inhibitors
    Tolcapone
    Entacapone
Dopamine agonists
    Bromocriptine
    Pergolide
    Ropinirole
    Pramipexole
    Cabergoline
    Apomorphine
Amantadine

DOPAMINE-ANTAGONIST/NEUROLEPTIC ADMINISTRATION

Neuroleptics
    Phenothiazines
    Butyrophenones
    Thiothixanes
Atypical antipsychotics:
    Clozapine
    Olanzapine
    Risperidone
    Quetiapine
Antiemetics:
    Metoclopromide
    Droperidol
    Prochlorperazine
    Promethazine
Others (rare)
    Reserpine
    Carbamazepine
    Tricyclic and SSRI antidepressants
    Loxapine
    Diatrizoate
    Lithium
    Cocaine
    Amphetamines

NMS may occur in these patients in the perioperative period due to alterations in serum levels (e.g., in the patient unable to take oral medication) or to metabolic alterations. For patients who have been on dopamine-blocking agents, such as haloperidol, NMS can occur even after initial exposure. Increased dosages of or changes in the particular agent or parenteral administration of the neuroleptic are risk factors for the development of NMS in this group of patients. Incidence of NMS is estimated at 0.1% to 2% of neuroleptic exposed individuals. There is a preponderance of young males with NMS, but this may be because of the increased frequency of schizophrenia and affective disorders in this group and the subsequent increased use of neuroleptics. Other risk factors may include neuroleptic-induced catatonia, dehydration or malnutrition as a precipitating cause, and a history of elevated serum creatinine kinase (CK) during psychotic episodes not in association with NMS.

Leukocytosis is in the range of 10,000 to 40,000 cells/µL and elevated CK is in the range of 200 to 10,000 IU/L.

DIFFERENTIAL DIAGNOSIS

Malignant hyperthermia, which may have a genetic basis, appears in the setting of exposure to certain anesthetic agents such as halothane, isoflurane, sevoflurane, and desflurane, and depolarizing muscle relaxants like succinylcholine. *Acute lethal catatonia* involves hyperthermia, akinesia, and rigidity, but this is usually preceded in the previous couple of weeks by behavioral changes. The *serotonin syndrome* occurs in the setting of an overexposure to selective serotonin reuptake inhibitors (SSRIs) or the combination use of SSRIs together with monoamine oxidase inhibitors, tricyclic antidepressants, or meperidine.

TREATMENT

Treatment involves first and foremost reversing the inciting cause—either discontinuing the responsible agent or reinstituting the dopaminergic therapy that may have been stopped. Supportive care is essential because the complications associated with NMS include renal failure induced by rhabdomyolysis, venous thromboembolism with or without pulmonary embolus, cardiac arrhythmias, and respiratory failure. Aggressive cooling, careful monitoring of cardiovascular functions, and high-volume IV fluid therapy necessitate intensive care hospitalization for all but the mild cases. Pharmacologic therapy includes bromocriptine or dantrolene in addition to supportive care. These two medications are used independently or together. Administration is started immediately and continued for 10 days after the resolution of symptoms. Pharmacotherapy shortens the clinical course of NMS. Electroconvulsive therapy has been reported to be beneficial in cases of NMS refractory to other therapies.

REFERENCES

Bhanushali MJ, Tuite PJ: *Neurol Clin North Am* 22:389–411, 2004.
Chan TC, Evans SD, Clark RF: *Crit Care Clin* 13:785–808, 1997.
Sachdev PS: *Psychiatry Clin North Am* 28:255–274, 2005.

N

NEUROLEPTIC MALIGNANT SYNDROME

NEUROLEPTICS

Neuroleptics include several classes of compounds whose primary common feature is blockade of dopamine receptors, although all of them have other effects at other receptors, such as anticholinergic activity. An exception is clozapine and other "atypical antipsychotics" (olanzapine, quetiapine), which block serotonin receptors and have little dopamine receptor blockade. The primary clinical use of neuroleptics is in the treatment of psychosis and agitation. Neuroleptics are also used for control of hyperkinetic movement disorders (chorea, tics, and dystonia), for suppressing nausea, for control of vertigo, neuralgic pain, and acute and refractory migraines, and for treating the abdominal pain of porphyric crises.

Aliphatic phenothiazines such as chlorpromazine (Thorazine) are strongly sedating. Potent α-adrenergic antagonism results in postural hypotension. Antiemetic and anticholinergic effects are significant. Extrapyramidal and dystonic symptoms occur with medium frequency.

Piperidine phenothiazines such as thioridazine (Mellaril) and mesoridazine (Serentil) have a relative potency similar to that of the aliphatic compounds. Sedative and α-adrenergic antagonism are less than with aliphatic compounds. Antiemetic effects are negligible. This class has a low incidence of extrapyramidal and dystonic side effects.

Piperazine phenothiazines, such as prochlorperazine (Compazine), trifluoperazine (Stelazine), perphenazine (Trilafon), and fluphenazine (Prolixin), have the highest relative potency and the strongest antiemetic effects. They also have the highest incidence of extrapyramidal and dystonic symptoms. Sedation and α-adrenergic antagonism are minimal.

The pharmacologic features of butyrophenones such as haloperidol (Haldol) closely resemble those of the piperazines. They have strong dopaminergic-blocking effects and a high incidence of extrapyramidal and dystonic symptoms. Relatively less orthostatic hypotension and sedation occur than with lower potency neuroleptics.

Pimozide (Orap), a diphenylbutylpiperidine, is similar in effect to haloperidol and is used in the United States primarily for the treatment of Tourette's syndrome.

The thioxanthenes resemble the phenothiazines. Thiothixene (Navane) resembles the piperazines, with greater dystonic and extrapyramidal side effects.

Atypical antipsychotics differ from typical psychotics in their "limbic-specific" dopamine type 2 (D2)-receptor binding and high ratio of serotonin type 2 (5-HT2)-receptor binding to D2 binding. These include clozapine, olanzapine, risperidone, quetiapine, and ziprasidone. Clozapine use has fallen due to agranulocytosis in 1% to 2% of patients and significant lowering of seizure threshold. Complete blood counts must be closely monitored if clozapine is used. These medications can be sedating and associated with weight gain and anticholinergic side effects.

EXTRAPYRAMIDAL SIDE EFFECTS

Dystonia may occur early (1 to 3 weeks) in the course of neuroleptic therapy or after a single parenteral injection. It may consist of generalized torsion dystonia, opisthotonos, torticollis, retrocollis, oculogyric crisis, trismus, or focal appendicular dystonia. Dystonia is more common in younger patients, especially children or adolescents, and in black males. It usually resolves spontaneously within 24 hours of stopping use of the drug but may be terminated within minutes with benztropine (Cogentin) 1 mg IM or IV or diphenhydramine (Benadryl) 50 mg IV; oral therapy may be continued for 24 to 48 hours.

Parkinsonian symptoms of stiffness, "cog-wheeling," tremor, and shuffling gait are dose related and may begin as early as a few days to 4 weeks after starting therapy. The neuroleptic dosage should be decreased or an anticholinergic agent may be added. Anticholinergic agents in use include benztropine 0.5 to 4.0 mg bid, biperiden (Akineton) 2.0 mg qd to tid, and trihexyphenidyl (Artane) 2 to 5 mg tid. Anticholinergics carry the risk of precipitating anticholinergic delirium, which may mimic psychotic symptoms; therefore, prophylactic use should be limited to patients at high risk for extrapyramidal symptoms.

Akathisia is a subjective sensation of motor restlessness with an urge to move around that generally occurs within several weeks of starting neuroleptic therapy. It improves on decreasing the dose of neuroleptic or adding beta blockers or benzodiazepines. Neuroleptic dose should not be increased to treat this form of "agitation," which may mimic the initial psychotic symptoms.

Tardive dyskinesia, consisting of oral-lingual-facial-buccal movements or other choreoathetoid or ballistic movements, may occur after prolonged neuroleptic therapy. Its incidence may be decreased by using neuroleptics only when indicated, keeping doses as low as possible and duration of therapy as short as possible, and early detection through careful monitoring. The more advanced the dyskinesia, the less likely is resolution. Primary treatment consists of tapering and withdrawing the neuroleptic. Treatment with reserpine 0.25 mg/day, increasing by 0.25 mg/day to 1 to 5 mg/day in divided doses, with care to avoid orthostatic hypotension, may help. Neuroleptics themselves have no role in the treatment of tardive dyskinesias.

A *withdrawal syndrome*, seen particularly in children and consisting of choreic movements, may occur when long-term administration of neuroleptics is suddenly stopped. The syndrome usually resolves within 6 to 12 weeks but can be avoided by restarting the drug therapy and tapering more slowly.

The *neuroleptic malignant syndrome* is rare but often (20% to 30%) fatal. Hyperthermia, hypertonia of skeletal muscles, fluctuating consciousness, and autonomic instability are characteristic. Laboratory findings include elevated creatine kinase level, leukocytosis, and liver function abnormalities. The differential diagnosis includes heat stroke (neuroleptics

N

NEUROLEPTICS

may potentiate by decreasing sweating), malignant hyperthermia associated with anesthesia, idiopathic acute lethal catatonia, drug interactions with monoamine oxidase inhibitors, and central anticholinergic syndromes. Treatment begins with discontinuing the neuroleptic and providing cooling blankets, antipyretics, and IV hydration. Dantrolene sodium 0.8 to 10 mg/kg/day IV has been used. Bromocriptine, 2.5 to 10 mg PO tid, amantadine, and levodopa with carbidopa have also been used effectively.

Neuroleptics lower the seizure threshold and may precipitate seizures. Their use in patients with epilepsy is not contraindicated unless seizure control is a significant problem.

REFERENCES

Kaplan HI, Sadock BJ, eds: *Synopsis of psychiatry*, ed 6, Baltimore, Williams & Wilkins, 1991.
Stip E: *J Psychiatry Neurosci* 25:137–153, 2000.

NEUROPATHY (See also AAN GUIDELINE SUMMARIES APPENDIX)

CLINICAL CLASSIFICATION OF NEUROPATHY

I. Polyneuropathies
  A. Acute predominantly motor neuropathy with variable sensory involvement
    1. Acute inflammatory demyelinating polyradiculoneuropathy (Guillain-Barré syndrome)
    2. Polyneuropathy associated with
      a. Diphtheria
      b. Porphyria
      c. AIDS
      d. Thallium
      e. Triorthocresyl phosphate, dapsone
  B. Acute motor neuropathy
    1. Diabetic multiple mononeuropathy (asymmetrical proximal diabetic neuropathy, diabetic amyotrophy)
  C. Acute asymmetrical sensorimotor polyneuropathy (multiple mononeuropathy or mononeuritis multiplex)
    1. Polyarteritis nodosa
    2. Wegener's granulomatosis
    3. Diabetes
    4. AIDS
    5. Other angiopathies, vasculitides
  D. Subacute symmetrical sensorimotor neuropathy
    1. Toxic
      a. Heavy metals—arsenic, mercury, thallium
      b. Drugs
        i. Antibiotics—clioquinol, ethambutol, isoniazid, nitrofurantoin, streptomycin

        ii. Antineoplastic—vinca alkaloids, cisplatin, chlorambucil, methotrexate, daunorubicin

        iii. Cardiovascular—clofibrate, disopyramide, hydralazine

        iv. Other—gold salts, colchicine, phenylbutazone, methaqualone, penicillamine, chloroquine, disulfiram, cyclosporine A

     c. Industrial chemicals—triorthocresyl phosphate, acrylamide, methyl bromide, *n*-hexane, methyl-*n*-butyl ketone

  2. Nutritional deficiency—vitamin B_{12}, niacin (pellagra), thiamine (beriberi), pyridoxine, vitamin E

  3. Uremia

  4. Chronic alcoholism (nutritional deficiency)

  5. Early chronic relapsing demyelinating polyneuropathy

E. Subacute to chronic, predominantly sensory neuropathy

  1. Diabetes

  2. Drugs—chlorambucil, metronidazole, ethambutol, pyridoxine, phenytoin (rare), propylthiouracil

  3. Sjögren's syndrome

  4. Leprosy

  5. Paraneoplastic disease

  6. AIDS

  7. Idiopathic nonmalignant inflammatory sensory polyganglionopathy

  8. Vitamin deficiency: vitamins B_{12} and E

F. Subacute to chronic, predominantly motor neuropathy

  1. Diabetes—proximal diabetic motor neuropathy ("amyotrophy")

  2. Lead

G. Chronic sensory motor neuropathy

  1. Diabetes—mixed sensorimotor-autonomic neuropathy

  2. Associated with multiple myeloma

  3. Other dysproteinemias—macroglobulinemia, cryoglobulinemia, ataxia-telangiectasia

  4. POEMS syndrome—*p*olyneuropathy, *o*rganomegaly (lymphadenopathy, splenomegaly, or hepatomegaly), *e*ndocrinopathy (usually hypogonadism or hypothyroidism), *m*onoclonal gammopathy, and *s*kin changes

  5. Paraneoplastic disease

  6. Uremia

  7. Leprosy

  8. Amyloidosis

  9. Chronic inflammatory demyelinating polyradiculoneuropathy (CIDP)

  10. Sarcoidosis

H. Hereditary motor and sensory neuropathies (HMSN), types I to IV

I. Hereditary sensory neuropathies (HSAN), types I to IV

J. Hereditary neuropathies with known or suspected metabolic defects

  1. Fabry's disease (alpha-galactosidase deficiency, X-linked)

  2. Metachromatic leukodystrophy (aryl sulfatase A deficiency, autosomal recessive)

N

NEUROPATHY

      3. Refsum's disease (phytanic oxidase deficiency, autosomal recessive)

      4. Adrenomyeloneuropathy (X-linked)

      5. Tangier's disease (hypo-alpha-lipoproteinemia, autosomal recessive)

      6. Krabbe's disease (globoid cell leukodystrophy, galactosyl ceramidase deficiency, autosomal recessive)

  K. Other hereditary neuropathies

      1. Familial amyloid neuropathy

      2. Hereditary predisposition to pressure palsies

      3. Giant axonal neuropathy

      4. Friedreich's ataxia

II. Mononeuropathies

  A. Trauma—fractures and dislocations, penetrating injuries, and pressure palsies

      1. Brachial plexus—fracture of clavicle or humerus, birth trauma, traction injuries

      2. Axillary nerve—as for brachial plexus, also IM injections, shoulder subluxation

      3. Radial nerve—fracture of head of humerus, compression at the radial groove ("Saturday palsy" and "bridegroom's palsy")

      4. Ulnar nerve—fracture of radius or ulna

      5. Median nerve—carpal tunnel syndrome, anterior interosseous syndrome

      6. Sciatic nerve—fracture of pelvis (sacroiliac joint), fracture of acetabulum, IM gluteal injections

      7. Femoral nerve—fracture of femur, lithotomy position, renal transplants

      8. Lateral femoral cutaneous nerve (meralgia paresthetica)

      9. Tibial nerve—fracture of tibia or fibula

     10. Common or superficial peroneal nerve—pressure palsy at fibular head from crossed legs or after weight loss

  B. Entrapment (see Carpal Tunnel Syndrome, Ulnar Neuropathy)

  C. Carcinomatous infiltration

  D. Vasculitis

  E. Leprosy

CLINICAL FEATURES OF SELECTED NEUROPATHIES
HMSN (Charcot-Marie-Tooth Disease), Types I to IV

Hereditary neuropathies are common and may occur in subtle forms. Family history taking and examination of family members (including foot examination for pes cavus and EMG) are important.

    Differential diagnosis of HMSN types includes Friedreich's ataxia, hereditary distal spinal muscular atrophy, and chronic inflammatory demyelinating polyneuropathy (CIDP), which has slight asymmetries in involvement of different peripheral nerves as opposed to the hereditary types, which demonstrate uniform involvement.

I. *CMT I: Hypertrophic form of CMT* (peroneal muscular atrophy, Roussy-Levy syndrome).

    A. *Inheritance:* Autosomal dominant with variable penetrance, rarely autosomal recessive.

    B. *Onset* is usually in the second decade but may be later. Many patients have subtle findings and are undiagnosed. There is slowly progressive distal weakness and atrophy with little sensory loss. The lower extremities are more involved than the upper. Palpably thickened nerves occur in 50% of cases. Total areflexia is common. Foot deformity (pes cavus, calluses, hammertoes) results from unopposed flexor action of the posterior compartment muscles and may be the only clinical finding.

    C. *Laboratory tests:* Nerve conduction velocities are decreased by 40% to 75%. EMG reveals dispersed compound muscle action potentials with low amplitude due to chronic denervation. EMG abnormalities may precede and be more extensive than clinical involvement. The CSF is usually normal.

    D. *Pathologically*, there are hypertrophic ("*onion bulb*") changes and myelinated axon loss due to chronic demyelination and remyelination. Genetic testing for subtypes of CMT I showed that CMT1-A subtype is linked to chromosome 17p11.2-12 duplication, and CMT1-B subtype is linked to chromosome 1q22-23 point mutations. The linkage of CMT1-C is still undetermined.

    E. *Prognosis:* Life span is usually normal, with only rare wheelchair confinement.

II. *CMT II: Neuronal form* (peroneal muscular atrophy).

    A. *Inheritance* is as in CMT I, except that onset is slightly later. CMT2-A subtype is linked to chromosome 1p36, CMT2-B subtype is linked to chromosome 3q-22, and CMT2-D subtype is linked to chromosome 7p14. The CMT2-C subtype linkage is undetermined. CMT II is distinguished from CMT I by the *absence of hypertrophic changes*, later age of onset, slower progression, less involvement of upper extremities, and greater involvement of lower extremities (atrophy of ankle flexors, inverted champagne bottle).

    B. *Laboratory tests:* Nerve conduction velocities are normal or slightly slowed, but amplitudes are severely diminished. EMG reveals spontaneous activity and denervation changes. CSF is usually normal.

    C. *Pathologically:* No hypertrophic changes are seen and demyelination is mild; axonal number is decreased in distal myelinated nerves.

III. *CMT III: Dejerine-Sottas disease* (hypertrophic neuropathy of childhood, congenital hypomyelination neuropathy). Inheritance is autosomal recessive. Onset is congenital or in infancy. The congenital form is more severe. Motor milestones are initially delayed and then lost. Walking occurs after 15 months and as late as 3 to 4 years. Best motor performance occurs late in the first or early in the second decade. Patients are confined to a wheelchair by the end of the second decade.

Severe progressive weakness and atrophy are initially distal, but eventually affect proximal muscles. There is severe sensory loss and sensory ataxia. Skeletal deformities (short stature, kyphoscoliosis, hand and foot deformities) are more severe and frequent than in CMT I or II. Motor nerve conduction velocities are extremely slow and sensory nerve action potentials are unrecordable. CSF protein is elevated.

Pathologically, in addition to hypertrophic changes, myelin sheaths are thin or absent. Linkage studies show that CMT3-A subtype is linked to chromosome 17p11.2-12 duplication, and CMT3-B subtype is linked to chromosome 1q22-23 point mutation.

IV. *CMT IV*

    A. *Inheritance* is autosomal recessive. CMT4 subtype is linked to chromosome 8q13-21.1.

    B. *Clinically:* Early onset occurs in childhood and progressive weakness leads to inability to walk in adolescence.

    C. *Laboratory tests:* NCS are slow and CSF protein is normal. Nerve biopsy shows loss of myelinated fibers, hypomyelination, and onion bulbs.

V. *X-linked CMT:* X-linked CMT is clinically similar to CMT type I, but shows an X-linked pattern of inheritance (chromosome Xq13.3 point mutation). There is no male-to-male transmission. Symptoms usually start between ages 5 and 15.

There are other complex, poorly characterized forms of CMT, which show pyramidal tract signs, optic atrophy, spinocerebellar degeneration, or deafness, in addition to neuropathy.

Hereditary Sensory and Autonomic Neuropathies, Types I to IV

I. *HSAN I:* Dominantly inherited sensory neuropathy (hereditary sensory neuropathy of Denny-Brown).

    A. *Inheritance* is autosomal dominant.

    B. *Clinically*, onset is in the second to third decade. There is progressive distal lower-extremity dissociated sensory loss; pain and temperature are relatively more involved. There is distal hyporeflexia. Autonomic function is normal, except for impaired distal sweating. Painless ulcerations and foot deformities may be present. Mild distal lower extremity weakness and atrophy are late findings. Upper extremity sensory loss is mild. Life expectancy is normal. NCS of the lower extremity reveal decreased sensory amplitudes and normal or mildly decreased sensory conduction velocities; motor nerve conduction studies are normal.

    C. *Pathologically*, axonal degeneration causes decreased numbers of small myelinated fibers and unmyelinated fibers. Differential diagnosis includes diabetic neuropathy, hereditary amyloidosis (prominent autonomic dysfunction), and syringomyelia.

II. *HSAN II:* Infantile and congenital sensory neuropathy (Morvan's disease).

    A. *Inheritance* is autosomal recessive.

    B. *Clinically* HSAN II is similar to HSAN I except that onset is in infancy, and involvement of all sensory modalities is equal, severe, and proximal as well as distal. The lips and tongue may be affected. Strength is normal. Painless ulcerations and fractures are common. There is distal areflexia.

C. *Laboratory tests:* Sensory nerve action potentials are unrecordable; motor nerve conduction studies are normal.

D. *Pathologically,* myelinated axons are severely decreased, with moderately decreased numbers of unmyelinated fibers and some segmental demyelination and remyelination.

III. *HSAN III:* Familial dysautonomia (Riley-Day syndrome).

A. *Inheritance* is autosomal recessive, and it occurs primarily in Ashkenazi Jews.

B. *Clinically,* onset of symptoms is usually shortly after birth, with episodic cyanosis, vomiting, unexplained fever, poor suck, and an increased susceptibility to infection. There is characteristic blotching of the skin and no fungiform papilla on the tongue. Autonomic symptoms include decreased lacrimation, hyperhidrosis, fluctuating body temperature, and episodic postural hypotension. There is a dissociated sensory loss with predominant involvement of pain and temperature, causing corneal ulcerations, painless skin lesions, and deformed joints. Areflexia is generalized. Strength, sweating, and sphincter function are normal. Intelligence is usually normal.

C. *Laboratory tests:* Sensory nerve action potentials are diminished; motor nerve conduction studies may be mildly abnormal. Peripheral nerves show marked depletion of unmyelinated fibers.

D. *Prognosis* is generally poor, but occasional individuals survive to middle age.

IV. *HSAN IV:* Congenital sensory neuropathy. *Inheritance* is autosomal recessive. This very rare disorder is characterized by congenital anhidrosis, generalized insensitivity to pain and temperature, mental retardation, and episodic pyrexia.

Diabetic Neuropathy

This clinical or subclinical disorder of the somatic or autonomic peripheral nervous system occurs in patients with diabetes mellitus without other causes for peripheral neuropathy. Proposed etiologic factors include localized endoneurial hypoxia, chronic hyperglycemia, episodic hypoglycemia, polyol accumulation, myoinositol deficiency, and impaired axonal transport. Microangiopathy and infarction have been proposed as the mechanism for diabetic multiple mononeuropathies. The following diabetic neuropathy syndromes are recognized:

I. Symmetrical polyneuropathies

A. Distal sensory polyneuropathy is the *most common*.

1. *Clinically,* onset is usually insidious, but may occur acutely following an episode of diabetic coma or hypoglycemia. Usually, clinical manifestations reflect involvement of all fiber types. However, occasionally a large or small fiber pattern is more prominent.

The *large fiber* pattern presents with paresthesias in the feet and loss of distal reflexes, position sensation, and vibratory sensation. The *small fiber* pattern is loss of thermal and pinprick sensation associated with burning pain. Autonomic neuropathy often accompanies the small fiber pattern.

2. *Laboratory tests:* NCS show reduced sensory action potential amplitude and variable slowing of motor nerve conduction velocity (related to degree of demyelination). EMG shows denervation, despite little or no weakness.

3. *Pathologically*, there is distal axonal loss with variable degrees of segmental demyelination.

B. Autonomic neuropathy. *Clinical features* include abnormal pupillary reaction, postural hypotension, abnormalities of heart rate, peripheral edema, anhidrosis, abnormalities of reflex vasoconstriction, abnormal gastrointestinal motility, diarrhea, atonic bladder, and impotence. Sudden death may occur from lack of reaction to hypoglycemia or cardiorespiratory arrest.

C. Symmetrical proximal lower extremity motor neuropathy ("amyotrophy")

1. *Clinically*, there is slowly progressive, symmetrical weakness, which is distinct from asymmetrical "amyotrophy," which is discussed under the focal diabetic neuropathies. Initial manifestations include lower back and proximal lower extremity pain, which is followed by progressive proximal weakness, loss of patellar reflexes, and atrophy. Sensation is spared, but a distal sensory polyneuropathy may coexist.

2. *Laboratory tests:* Initial EMG shows reduced motor unit recruitment, while evidence of denervation appears later.

3. *Prognosis* for recovery varies, but is generally worse with insidious onset of symptoms. Control of hyperglycemia may promote recovery.

II. Focal and multifocal diabetic neuropathies

A. *Trunk and limb mononeuropathy* (including mononeuropathy multiplex)

1. *Clinically*, disease occurs acutely, most often in the ulnar, median, radial, femoral, lateral cutaneous, thoracic, and peroneal nerves. These lesions often occur at the same sites as entrapment neuropathies. It is important to exclude other causes, such as radiculopathy. It may not be possible to distinguish between a diabetic mononeuropathy and an entrapment syndrome.

2. *Prognosis* for recovery is good.

B. *Cranial neuropathies* most commonly affect the extraocular muscles (see Ophthalmoplegia) and may be associated with facial pain or headache. Third nerve lesions show rapid onset and pupillary sparing, whereas aneurysmal compression typically has an unresponsive pupil.

C. *Asymmetrical proximal lower limb motor neuropathy* is the unilateral form of "amyotrophy." Onset of unilateral pain and proximal weakness is sudden, progressing over 1 to 2 weeks. The patellar reflex is lost, and proximal atrophy eventually develops. Although the cause remains uncertain, prognosis is good. There have been reports of successful treatment with steroids, plasma exchange, and intravenous gamma globulins.

Inflammatory Demyelinating Polyneuropathies

I. *Guillain-Barré syndrome* (GBS) (Guillain-Barré-Strohl syndrome, acute inflammatory demyelinating polyradiculoneuropathy [AIDP]) is probably immunologically mediated, involving both cellular and humoral responses, but no single autoantigen has been identified (see AAN Guideline Summaries).

A. *Clinical presentation:* Paresthesias in the distal extremities are followed by lower extremity weakness. The weakness then ascends to involve the arms and face. Bilateral sciatica is common. Initial examination shows symmetrical limb weakness, absent or greatly diminished deep tendon reflexes, and minimal sensory loss. Progression to involve respiration, eye movements, swallowing, and autonomic function occurs in severe cases. Weakness progresses for 1 to 3 weeks before stabilizing and then recovering. Severity of symptoms varies among individuals. In severe cases, complications of pneumonia, sepsis, adult respiratory distress syndrome, pulmonary embolus, and cardiac arrest are responsible for most severe illness and even death.

B. *Risk factors:* GBS is often preceded by an infection, usually viral. Important associated infections include human immunodeficiency virus (HIV), Epstein-Barr virus, cytomegalovirus, influenza virus, and *Campylobacter jejuni* enteritis. Underlying systemic diseases such as systemic lupus erythematosus (SLE), Hodgkin's disease, and sarcoidosis are very occasionally associated with GBS. Surgery and vaccinations may also precede GBS.

C. *Evaluation:* LP shows CSF protein greater than 55 mg/dL with little or no pleocytosis (*albuminocytologic dissociation*) starting about 1 week after onset of symptoms. CSF protein is often normal during the first few days of the illness. NCS show signs of demyelination early, before CSF protein changes, with loss of F and H waves and nerve conduction block (>50% loss of action potential).

D. *Differential diagnosis* includes spinal cord disease, myasthenia gravis, neoplastic meningitis, vasculitic neuropathy, paraneoplastic neuropathy, botulism, diphtheria, heavy-metal intoxication, poliomyelitis, and porphyria.

E. *GBS variants:* These share signs of diminished reflexes, demyelination pattern on nerve conduction studies, and elevated CSF protein. Variant syndromes include *Fisher syndrome* (ophthalmoplegia, ataxia, and areflexia with little associated weakness), weakness without paresthesias and sensory loss, pharyngeal-cervical-brachial weakness, paraparesis, pure sensory and pure ataxia.

N

NEUROPATHY

F. *Treatment:* Plasma exchange significantly alters the progression and severity of GBS, decreasing the need for mechanical ventilation by approximately 50%. The efficacy of intravenous immunoglobulin treatment (IVIG) is probably comparable with plasmapheresis. IVIG given daily at 0.4 g/kg for 1 week is the preferred treatment in unstable patients; recent literature suggests a better response for IVIG in anti-GM1b-positive GBS (axonal variant). Corticosteroids are not efficacious in GBS but may be used for pain control. Dysautonomia is a major cause of morbidity and should be treated aggressively with hydration, vasoactive drugs, and pacemakers if needed.

II. Chronic inflammatory demyelinating polyradiculoneuropathy (CIDP), or chronic relapsing dysimmune polyneuropathy

A. *Clinical presentation:* CIDP is similar to GBS but shows a protracted, often relapsing course, pronounced sensory involvement, response to corticosteroid treatment, and greater association with systemic disease. *Worsening of symptoms for longer than 2 months, with subacute onset and fluctuation of symptoms over years, is characteristic of CIDP.* Sensory involvement often accompanies proximal extremity and neck flexor weakness and diminished reflexes. Laboratory findings are similar to CSF and EMG findings of GBS, with more chronic changes on EMG and NCS.

B. *Differential diagnosis* includes monoclonal gammopathies, lymphoma, connective tissue disease (polyarteritis nodosa, cryoglobulinemia, SLE), anti-MAG-associated polyneuropathies, Lyme disease, HIV infection, and sarcoidosis.

C. *Treatment:* Prednisone 100 mg/day for 4 weeks, tapering gradually over 1 year to 10 to 20 mg qod. Plasma exchange is usually given in 3 to 5 exchanges over 1 to 2 weeks. Plasmapheresis with lower dose prednisone may be tried as initial therapy. IVIG given at 0.4 g/kg/day for 5 days is efficacious according to some but not all studies. Immunosuppressive drugs are used only in refractory cases.

GENERAL PRINCIPLES OF TREATMENT OF NEUROPATHIES

I. Patient education and counseling
II. Genetic counseling
III. Withdrawal of medications suspected of causing neuropathy
IV. Withdrawal from toxic exposure
V. Correction of nutritional and vitamin deficiencies
VI. Treatment of alcoholism
VII. Blood glucose control in diabetic neuropathies
VIII. Specific drug therapies
    A. Chelating agents in lead neuropathy
    B. Hematin infusions in acute intermittent porphyria
    C. Long-term prednisone or other immune-modifying regimens in CIDP
    D. Phytanic acid (reduced) diet in Refsum's disease
IX. Plasmapheresis in AIDP and other autoimmune disorders

X. Pain control
- A. Improve blood glucose control in diabetic neuropathies
- B. Simple analgesics—aspirin and acetaminophen
- C. Gabapentin, phenytoin, and carbamazepine—achieve anticonvulsant levels
- D. Tricyclic drugs—amitriptyline and imipramine
- E. Transcutaneous electrical nerve stimulation

XI. Meticulous foot care

XII. Orthotic devices and splints

XIII. Surgical correction of entrapment neuropathies

XIV. Physical and occupational therapy

REFERENCES

Dalakas MC: *Muscle Nerve* 22:1479–1497, 1999.
Dyck PJ et al: *Neurology* 47:10–17, 1996.
Yuki N et al: *Ann Neurol* 47:314–321, 2000.

N

NYSTAGMUS

NUTRITIONAL DEFICIENCY SYNDROMES

Table 82 discusses nutritional deficiency syndromes.

NYSTAGMUS

Nystagmus is a biphasic ocular oscillation in which at least one phase is slow. The nystagmus direction is defined as the direction of the fast component. The direction may be horizontal, vertical, diagonal, or rotational. There are two general types, jerk and pendular. If the second phase is a fast eye movement, the nystagmus is termed "jerk." If the second phase is a slow eye movement, the nystagmus is termed "pendular." Jerk nystagmus usually reflects acquired disease of the brainstem but may also occur congenitally. Pendular nystagmus may be acquired or congenital.

When examining a patient with nystagmus, observe changes in amplitude and frequency with change in gaze direction. Nystagmus may indicate dysfunction somewhere in the posterior fossa, that is, vestibular system (and end organ), brainstem, or cerebellum. Table 83 provides a clinical classification of nystagmus.

Congenital nystagmus is noted within 6 months of birth. Its waveform may be pendular, jerk, or a combination of both. It may be found in the presence of ophthalmic disorders that diminish vision (sensory form) or may be related to as an isolated manifestation (motor form). The principal causes of vision loss in the sensory form of congenital nystagmus are corneal and lens opacities, albinism, aniridia, achromatopsia, Leber's congenital amaurosis, and optic neuropathy.

The distinguishing features of congenital nystagmus can be remembered by using the mnemonic CONGENITAL: convergence and eye closure dampen

TABLE 82

NUTRITIONAL DEFICIENCY SYNDROMES

Type	Source	Etiology of Deficiency	Neurologic Manifestations	Symptoms	Diagnostic Testing	Treatment	Prognosis
Vitamin B₁ (thiamine)	Grains Rice (fortified) Cereals Pork Organ meats	Alcoholism Malnutrition Pregnancy Malignancy Hemodialysis Refeeding syndrome	1. *Beriberi* (sensorimotor, peripheral neuropathy, cardiomyopathy) 2. *Wernicke's syndrome* (encephalopathy, ophthalmoplegia, gait ataxia) 3. *Korsakoff's syndrome* (anterograde and retrograde amnesia, confabulation)	Paresthesias Distal muscle weakness with footdrop Pain in muscles Subacute confusion Ophthalmoplegia (esp. lateral recti) Nystagmus Truncal ataxia Profound memory impairment, usually after symptoms of Wernicke's subside	Usually a clinical diagnosis MRI may show T2 and FLAIR signal abnormalities in periaqueductal regions, medial thalami, and bilateral mamillary bodies; the lesions may contrast enhance Serum thiamine and RBC transketolase activity may be decreased	Immediate treatment with thiamine 100 mg IV should be given before D50 to avoid worsening of symptoms of Wernicke's syndrome Continue IV thiamine for about 5 days, then continue PO 50–100 mg daily, indefinitely	Sensorimotor neuropathy in beriberi gradually improves with thiamine over weeks to months; in severe cases, recovery is incomplete
Vitamin B₆ (pyridoxine)	Chicken, fish Fruits Vegetables Grains	Isoniazid therapy Hydralazine Penicillamine Alcoholism	1. Peripheral neuropathy (adults) 2. Intractable seizures (infants)	Paresthesias: burning and tingling usually feet first; may proceed proximally	Mainly a clinical diagnosis Urinary 4-pyridoxic acid Serum PLP (active form of	Discontinue offending medication 50 mg pyridoxine daily for	Variable Convulsions, respond to treatment Long-term functional outcome variable

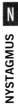

	Sources	Causes	Clinical Features	Diagnosis	Treatment	Prognosis
(pyridoxine, cont'd)		GI diseases End-stage renal disease on hemodialysis Malnutrition in infancy	Confusion Convulsions (infants) Exaggerated auditory startle (infants) Hyperirritability	pyridoxine RBC aspartate aminotransferase Clinical diagnosis (infants) by history of convulsions, response of seizures to pyridoxine	several weeks, then 2 mg daily In infants, 10 mg IV push to terminate seizures, then 75 mg daily for life	
Vitamin B$_{12}$	Meat Fish Legumes	Malabsorption Gastrectomy Pernicious anemia Small bowel resection Poor intake (rate)	1. *Peripheral neuropathy* (vibration and JPS especially) 2. *Myelopathy* 3. *Subacute combined degeneration* (posterior columns + corticospinal tract dysfunction) 4. *Dementia* 5. *Optic neuropathy* Paresthesias: mainly hands and feet Unsteady gait Weakness Mental slowing Depression Delusions GI symptoms Encephalopathy Dementia Lhermitte's sign Decreased vibration and JPS Variable reflexes Visual defects	Vitamin B$_{12}$ level, MMA homocysteine levels, folate CBC with peripheral smear (hypersegmented neutrophils) Parietal cell and intrinsic factor antibodies Schilling's test MRI brain and spinal cord (lateral and posterior columns) EMG/NCS (decreased sural in 80%)	Vitamin B$_{12}$: 1000 µg IM daily x 7 days, then 1000 µg IM weekly x 4 weeks, then 1000 µg IM monthly for life	At least partial improvement with treatment is likely; most in first 6 months, but can take up to a year Myelopathy is least likely to recover

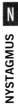

cont'd

NYSTAGMUS

TABLE 82

NUTRITIONAL DEFICIENCY SYNDROMES—cont'd

Type	Source	Etiology of Deficiency	Neurologic Manifestations	Symptoms	Diagnostic Testing	Treatment	Prognosis
Vitamin D	Milk (fortified) Fatty fish and fish oils	Hyperparathyroidism Hypophosphatemia Chronic renal failure Anticonvulsants Dietary deficiency Inadequate sunlight	1. Osteomalacia – bone weakness and proximal muscle weakness with waddling gait (pelvic girdle muscles weak) 2. Rickets	Muscle weakness Waddling gait Pain (bone fractures)	Elevated alkaline phosphatase Low or normal serum calcium and phosphorus Mildly elevated CK EMG may show myopathic pattern X-rays may show osteoporosis	Ergocalciferol 800–4000 IU daily for 8 weeks, then 400 IU/day until precipitating factor resolved Monitor serum calcium levels	Responsive to treatment over months
	Sunlight						
Vitamin E	Vegetable oils Nuts Green leafy vegetables Cereal (fortified)	GI disease (biliary atresia, chronic cholestasis, Crohn's disease, celiac disease) Cystic fibrosis Hereditary (abetalipoproteinemia)	1. *Spinocerebellar dysfunction* 2. *Peripheral neuropathy* (vibration and JPS) 3. *Retinopathy of prematurity*	Gait ataxia Areflexia Mild to moderate weakness Severely decreased vibration and JPS sense Ptosis Nystagmus Retinal pigmentation	Serum vitamin E level CBC with smear (acanthocytes) MRI spinal cord (posterior columns abnormal T_2 in some) NCS/EMG (mild axonal neuropathy)	For pure vitamin E deficiency: alpha-tocopherol 800–1200 mg daily For abetalipoproteinemia: alpha-tocopherol 5000–7000 mg daily	Variable

	Food	Causes	Clinical syndromes	Diagnosis	Treatment	Prognosis
Folate	Grains	Alcoholism, Small bowel disease (sprue, Crohn's, Ulcerative colitis, Pregnancy, Drugs: anticonvulsants, methotrexate, others)	1. Usually no symptoms 2. *Cognitive impairment* 3. *Subacute combined degeneration*	Mild cognitive impairment, Depression associated, Increased stroke risk (hyperhomocysteinemia)	RBC folate (better test than plasma folate) homocysteine, Vitamin B_{12} level (r/o B_{12} deficiency)	Folic acid 1 mg daily, May need to initially give parenterally, Adequate nutrition	Unclear
Nicotinic acid (niacin, vitamin B_3)	Bread	Dietary deficiency (underdeveloped populations where maize is a staple), Diarrhea, Cirrhosis, Alcoholism, Isoniazid therapy, Carcinoid tumor	1. *Pellagra* (endemic area) (dementia, diarrhea, dermatitis) 2. *Chronic unexplained encephalopathy* may resemble Wernicke's 3. *Spina bifida and neural tube defects* in fetal development	Neuropsychiatric (irritability, apathy, depression, memory loss), Stupor or coma, Spasticity, Babinski sign, Startle myoclonus, Gegenhalten	Mainly a clinical diagnosis, Decreased urinary NMN (nicN-methylnicotinamide) secretion	Parenteral nicotinic acid 100 mg IV daily x 5–7 days or Oral nicotinic acid 50 mg 10 times daily x 3 weeks	Excellent if treated appropriately

MMA, methylmalonic acid; JPS, joint position sense.

TABLE 83

CLINICAL CLASSIFICATION OF NYSTAGMUS

Types	Definition	Significance	Associated Condition
Optokinetic nystagmus	Composed of an initial slow pursuit eye movement and a compensatory fast eye movement (saccade, quick phase). Often can be elicited by looking at a spinning drum.	Physiologic response unless there is unequal or reduced amplitude in two eyes which would signify deep parietal lobe lesion or subtle internuclear ophthalmoplegia.	Internuclear ophthalmoplegia
Caloric nystagmus	Nystagmus induced by instilling either cold or warm water. Cold water results in fast phase beating away from irrigated side; warm water results in fast phase beating toward the irrigated side: COWS.	Physiologic response if vestibulo-ocular connection, cranial nerve III/VI and PPRF are intact.	Both structural and metabolic coma can result in diminished fast phase of nystagmus, and if severe, slow phase can also be eliminated
Nystagmus due to peripheral vestibular imbalance	Due to imbalance of the peripheral vestibular system, which will manifest as either purely horizontal or mixed - horizontal-torsional with the fast phase directed away from the side of the lesion.	Peripheral vestibulopathy.	Labyrinthitis or vestibular neuritis
Latent nystagmus	Congenital jerk nystagmus induced by monocular occlusion of either eye. Patient develops bilateral jerk nystagmus with the fast phase toward the open, fixating eye when one eye is closed.	Pathologic.	Often associated with infantile esotropia, amblyopia, or strabismus
Spasmus nutans	Triad of head tilt, head nodding, and nystagmus that is monocular or markedly asymmetrical. The nystagmus is pendular, rapid, and of small amplitude.	Often benign. Onset between ages 4 and 14 months and usually disappears by 5 years of age. However, it may be pathologic. MRI is indicated to rule out perichiasmal pathology.	May be associated with chiasmal glioma, third ventricular tumor, or degenerative disorder

Internuclear ophthalmoplegia	Nystagmus of the abduction eye.	Lesion at MLF.	Often associated with demyelinating disease such as multiple sclerosis
Downbeat nystagmus	Nystagmus in the primary position of gaze with the fast phase beating in a downward direction.	Often involved in cervicomedullary junction disorder. MRI is often indicated to examine cervicomedullary junction.	Arnold-Chiari malformation, spinocerebellar degeneration, anticonvulsant intoxication, magnesium deficiency, brainstem encephalitis, lithium use, alcoholic cerebellar degeneration
Upbeat nystagmus	Nystagmus in the primary position of gaze with the fast phase beating in an upward direction.	Always a sign of acquired disease of the brainstem, anywhere from midbrain to the medulla, or of the cerebellum. MRI is indicated to examine brainstem and cerebellar disease.	Tumors, stroke, intoxication, inflammation, and degeneration
Periodic alternating nystagmus	Horizontal jerk nystagmus which periodically changes direction. Usually consists of 90 sec of nystagmus in one direction and 10 to 15 sec of no nystagmus in primary position followed by nystagmus in the opposite direction.	May be congenital or may be due to craniocervical junction abnormalities or brainstem and cerebellar disease. MRI of the head is needed.	Arnold-Chiari malformation, multiple sclerosis, cerebellar pathology, brainstem infarction, and anticonvulsant use
Convergence-retraction nystagmus	Cocontraction of the extraocular muscles on attempted convergence or upgaze.	Often associated with papillary light-near dissociation and bilateral lid retraction. Lesion localized at dorsal rostral midbrain.	Pineal gland tumor in Parinaud syndrome

cont'd

NYSTAGMUS

TABLE 83

CLINICAL CLASSIFICATION OF NYSTAGMUS—*cont'd*

Types	Definition	Significance	Associated Condition
Seesaw nystagmus	Characterized by alternate elevation and depression of one eye accompanied by a similar movement in the other eye but in the opposite direction.	Often secondary to large parasellar lesion expanding into the third ventricle. Need to look for bitemporal hemianopia MRI of the brain with attention to parasellar area.	Pituitary tumor
Gaze-evoked nystagmus	Nystagmus induced by moving the eyes into an eccentric position.	Physiologic if it is unsustained. Pathologic if it is sustained and indicates dysfunctional neural integrator system.	Cerebral or brainstem process or a weak extraocular muscle if there is a paresis of gaze
Nystagmus in MG	Manifests as a gaze-evoked nystagmus in any direction with asymmetry between the two eyes especially after prolonged eccentric gaze.	Signifies fatigability of the ocular muscle. Also referred to as "pseudointernuclear ophthalmoplegia."	MG

COWS indicates for direction of fast nystagmus—cold water = opposite direction and warm water = same direction; MG, myasthenia gravis; MLF, medial longitudinal fasciculus; PPRF, paramedian pontine reticular formation.

the nystagmus; oscillopsia is usually absent; *n*ull zone is present; *g*aze position does not change the direction of nystagmus; *e*qual amplitude and frequency of nystagmus in each eye; *n*ear acuity is good (convergence dampens the nystagmus); *i*nversion of optokinetic nystagmus occurs; *t*urning of head or abnormal head posture to allow eyes to enter a null zone leads to better visual acuity; *a*bsent nystagmus during sleep; *l*atent nystagmus occurs.

ASSESSMENT OF NYSTAGMUS

First, one needs to determine whether nystagmus is congenital or acquired. In congenital nystagmus, visual loss often occurs early on and patients don't usually complain of oscillopsia. In acquired nystagmus, visual acuity is typically degraded but not severely affected. Second, the eye movement should be assessed in the following manner: (1) primary gaze position–esotropia, exotropia, or orthotropia; (2) perform pursued and saccade eye movement at extreme gaze and describe nystagmus in terms of its amplitude, frequency, and waveform; (3) complete other neurologic examinations to augment the localization of the lesion; (4) MRI of brain or cervical spine if necessary.

TREATMENT

Treatment of symptomatic nystagmus relies on physical and pharmacologic methods. Congenital nystagmus can be treated with prisms, surgery, and contact lenses. Baclofen may benefit acquired periodic alternating nystagmus. Gabapentin 900 mg/day may be useful for pendular nystagmus. GABAergic medications including clonazepam, valproate, isoniazid, and baclofen have been somewhat effective in treating downbeat nystagmus. Surgical decompression of Arnold-Chiari malformation may reduce downbeat nystagmus. Botulinum toxin A is still under investigation.

REFERENCES

Acheson JF, Sanders MD: *Eye movement abnormalities. Common problems in neuro-ophthalmology*, London, WB Saunders, 1997, p 152.

Leigh JR, Zee D, eds: *The neurology of eye movements*, ed 4, New York, Oxford University Press, 2006. Book and DVD.

OCCIPITAL LOBE

The occipital lobe extends from the parieto-occipital fissure on the medial surface of the brain to the lateral surface, where it merges with the parietal and temporal lobes. The calcarine sulcus divides occipital lobe into lingula and cuneus, and it marks the boundary of the primary visual area (Brodmann's area 17). The rest of the occipital lobe constitutes the visual association cortex (Brodmann's areas 18 and 19). Its function is mainly

O

OCCIPITAL LOBE

concerned with visual perception and interpretation. Clinical symptoms associated with occipital lesions include visual field defects, cortical blindness, visual agnosias, achromatopsia, metamorphopsias, illusions, and hallucinations. Visual symptoms occur commonly in migraine. Occipital lobe epilepsy may present with visual phenomena, and postictal blindness may also occur. Syndromes in occipital lobe lesion include the following:

Anton's syndrome (visual anosognosia or cortical blindness) includes lack of awareness of the defect and is associated with bilateral lesions.

Balint's syndrome, seen with bilateral occipital and parieto-occipital infarctions, consists of optic ataxia, paralysis of gaze and disturbance of visual attention, and simultanagnosia.

OCULAR OSCILLATIONS

The following abnormal oscillatory eye movements are distinct from nystagmus because of waveform differences (e.g., no distinct slow and fast phases):

I. *Ocular bobbing* consists of intermittent downward jerks of both eyes, followed by a slow drift to primary position. It is seen with destructive lesions of the pons but also occurs with pontine compression, obstructive hydrocephalus, and metabolic encephalopathy. Reflex eye movements are usually not brought out in this situation.

II. *Ocular dipping* is an inverse movement (slow downward, fast upward) with unreliable localization.

III. *Ping-pong gaze* denotes slow, horizontal, conjugate drift of the eyes that alternates every few seconds and is seen with *bilateral hemispheric dysfunction*.

IV. *Ocular myoclonus* refers to pendular vertical oscillations seen with brainstem lesions and often accompanied by rhythmic movements of the palate and other midline structures. It typically occurs with lesions between the *red nucleus*, *inferior olive*, and *dentate nucleus*.

The term *saccadic oscillation* includes several specific entities:

I. *Saccadic dysmetria* can produce oscillation when overshooting saccades are followed by one or more corrective saccades.

II. *Square-wave jerks* are seen most prominently in cerebellar disorders and progressive supranuclear palsy; saccades interrupt fixation with normal intersaccadic intervals.

III. *Macro square-wave jerks* are seen in multiple sclerosis and olivopontocerebellar atrophy.

IV. *Ocular flutter and opsoclonus* produce flurries of rapid eye movements without an intersaccadic interval; movements may be purely horizontal (*flutter*) or multidirectional (*opsoclonus*). Both can be secondary to viral infection, drug effects, tumor, or paraneoplastic syndromes such as neuroblastoma in children or with anti-Purkinje's cell antibodies in adults (mostly women with gynecologic tumors).

Superior oblique myokymia is a monocular torsional oscillation of small-amplitude, high-frequency contractions of a monocular superior oblique muscle. It causes oscillopsia, diplopia, or visual blurring. Although sometimes seen with brainstem disease, it is usually idiopathic and may respond to carbamazepine therapy.

Spasmus nutans is an ocular oscillation accompanied by head nodding and torticollis. It appears before 18 months of age and remits spontaneously, usually by age 3 years. The abnormal eye movements are usually dysconjugate and vary in direction. Although usually benign, this entity must not be confused with signs of intracranial tumor; the presence of poor feeding, optic atrophy, or raised intracranial pressure should be investigated by neuroimaging studies.

REFERENCES

Abel LA: In Daroff RB, Neetens A, eds: *Neurological organization of ocular movement*, Berkeley, Kugler, 1990.

Leigh JR, Zee D, eds: *The neurology of eye movements*, ed 4, New York, Oxford University Press, 2006. Book and DVD.

OLFACTION

The sense of smell is mediated by the first cranial nerve. *It is the only sensory modality without a thalamic relay.* Complaints may include anosmia, hyposmia, parosmia, or loss of appreciation of flavors in food. Smell is tested clinically using nonirritating, aromatic compounds such as oil of wintergreen, cloves, coffee, almond oil, or lemon oil. The stimulus is presented to one nostril with the other occluded. The ability to appreciate the presence of a substance, even if not properly identified, is evidence that anosmia is not present.

More detailed olfactory testing using the UPSIT (University of Pennsylvania Smell Identification Test) can distinguish hyposmia, anosmia, or malingering. Unilateral anosmia is more often due to a structural lesion rather than a diffuse process.

Causes of anosmia or hyposmia include the following:

I. Infection: rhinitis, sinusitis, basilar meningitis, frontal abscess, osteomyelitis (frontal, ethmoidal), viral hepatitis, syphilis, influenza

II. Toxic or metabolic disorders: pernicious anemia, zinc deficiency, lead and calcium intoxication, diabetes mellitus, hypothyroidism, medication effects

III. Neoplasms: frontal tumor, olfactory groove or sphenoid meningioma, radiation therapy

IV. Trauma to cribriform plate

V. Congenital: olfactory agenesis (Kallmann's syndrome) and septo-optic dysplasia (De Morsier's syndrome)

VI. Others: hydrocephalus, amphetamine and cocaine abuse, aging, smoking, trigeminal lesions (causing mucosal atrophy), anterior cerebral artery disease, nasal polyps, multiple sclerosis, Alzheimer's disease, sarcoidosis, Sheehan's syndrome, Parkinson's disease

Anosmia most commonly occurs secondary to head trauma, and may not be noticed until several weeks or months after the injury. A third of the cases spontaneously resolve within a year.

Hyperosmia is seen in hysteria, migraine, hyperemesis gravidarum, cystic fibrosis, Addison's disease, and strychnine poisoning.

Olfactory hallucinations can occur with neoplasms or vascular disease involving the inferomedial temporal lobe, near the hippocampus or uncus. They may also be seen in psychiatric disease (olfactory reference syndrome).

"Uncinate fits" are so called because of the presence of olfactory or gustatory hallucinations as part of complex partial or simple partial seizures; these seizures may be triggered or may even be arrested by olfactory stimulation. Anosmia is not present in such cases.

Multiple chemical sensitivities syndrome (MCS) is associated with unexplained odor sensitivity and excitability to multiple chemical and environmental stimuli. Sensitization by low levels of chemicals, fragrances, and perfumes is frequently associated with the reporting of MCS symptoms.

REFERENCES

Dawes PJ: *Clin Otolaryngol* 23:484–490, 1998.
Ross PM: *Prev Med* 28:467–480, 1999.

OPALSKI'S SYNDROME

Opalski's syndrome refers to lateral medullary syndrome (Wallenberg's syndrome) plus ipsilateral hemiplegia. Lesion is usually located lower than that in Wallenberg's syndrome, involving the corticospinal fibers caudal to the pyramidal decussation. The syndrome is usually caused by vertebral artery occlusion. A related syndrome is Babinski-Nageotte syndrome, with contralateral hemiparesis due to hemimedullary infarct before the pyramidal tract decussation.

REFERENCE

Kimura Y, Hashimoto H, Tagaya M et al: *J Neuroimag* 13:83–84, 2003.

OPHTHALMOPLEGIA

If extraocular muscle testing reveals misalignment of the visual axes, first determine whether this is due to nerve palsy or some other causes of impaired motility.

I. Causes of impaired ocular motility other than nerve palsy
  A. Concomitant strabismus
  B. Graves' ophthalmopathy
  C. Myasthenia gravis (and other pharmacologic or toxic causes of neuromuscular blockade)
  D. Convergence spasm
  E. Blowout fracture of the orbit with entrapment myopathy

F. Restrictive ophthalmopathy (*Brown's superior oblique tendon sheath syndrome*)
G. Orbital inflammatory disease (orbital pseudotumor)
H. Orbital masses, neoplasms
I. Orbital infections
J. Brainstem disorders causing abnormal prenuclear inputs (internuclear ophthalmoplegia, skew deviation)
K. Ocular myopathies
L. Chronic progressive external ophthalmoplegia (*Kearns-Sayre and related mitochondrial syndromes*)
M. Congenital syndromes

II. Causes of abducens nerve (CN VI) palsies
A. Nuclear (associated with ipsilateral horizontal gaze palsy)
    1. Developmental anomalies (Möbius, Duane's syndromes)
    2. Infarction
    3. Tumor (pontine glioma, cerebellar tumors)
    4. Wernicke-Korsakoff
B. Fascicular
    1. Infarction
    2. Demyelination
    3. Tumor
C. Subarachnoid space lesions
    1. Aneurysm or anomalous vessels (anterior inferior cerebellar artery, basilar artery)
    2. Subarachnoid hemorrhage
    3. Meningitis (infectious, neoplastic)
    4. Sarcoidosis
    5. Cerebellopontine angle tumor (acoustic neuroma, meningioma)
    6. Clivus tumor (chordoma, nasopharyngeal carcinoma)
    7. Trauma
    8. Surgical complication
    9. Postinfectious
D. Petrous
    1. Infection or inflammation of mastoid or petrous tip
    2. Trauma (petrous fracture)
    3. Thrombosis of inferior petrosal sinus
    4. Increased intracranial pressure (pseudotumor cerebri, supratentorial mass)
    5. Following lumbar puncture
    6. Aneurysm
    7. Persistent trigeminal artery
    8. Trigeminal schwannoma
E. Cavernous sinus and superior orbital fissure
    1. Aneurysm
    2. Cavernous sinus thrombosis
    3. Carotid cavernous fistula

    4. Dural arteriovenous malformation
    5. Tumor (pituitary adenoma, meningioma, nasopharyngeal carcinoma)
    6. Pituitary apoplexy
    7. Sphenoid sinusitis (mucormycosis)
    8. Herpes zoster
    9. Granulomatous inflammation (sarcoidosis, Tolosa-Hunt syndrome)
  F. Orbital
    1. Tumor
    2. Infection
    3. Trauma
  G. Uncertain localization
    1. Nerve infarction (diabetes, hypertension, arteritis)
    2. Migraine
III. Causes of trochlear nerve (CN IV) palsies
  A. Nuclear and fascicular
    1. Developmental anomalies
    2. Hemorrhage
    3. Infarction
    4. Trauma
    5. Demyelination
    6. Surgical complications
  B. Subarachnoid
    1. Trauma
    2. Tumor (pineal, tentorial meningioma, trochlear schwannoma, ependymoma, metastases)
    3. Surgical complication
    4. Meningitis (infectious, neoplastic)
    5. Mastoiditis
  C. Cavernous sinus and superior orbital fissure
    1. As for CN VI palsies
  D. Orbital
    1. Trauma
    2. Ethmoiditis
    3. Ethmoidectomy
  E. Uncertain localization
    1. Infarction (diabetes, hypertension, arteritis)
IV. Causes of oculomotor nerve (CN III) palsies
  A. Nuclear and fascicular
    1. Developmental anomaly
    2. Infarction
    3. Tumor
  B. Subarachnoid
    1. Aneurysm (posterior communicating artery)
    2. Meningitis (infectious, syphilitic, neoplastic)

3. Infarction
4. Tumor
5. Surgical complication

C. Tentorial edge
1. Increased intracranial pressure (uncal herniation, pseudotumor cerebri)
2. Trauma

D. Cavernous sinus and superior orbital fissure
1. As for CN VI palsies
2. Infarction

E. Orbital
1. Trauma
2. Tumor
3. Infection

F. Uncertain localization
1. Mononucleosis and other viral infections
2. Following immunization
3. Migraine
4. Cyclic oculomotor palsy of childhood
5. Guillain-Barré and Miller-Fisher syndromes
6. Sjögren's and Behçet's syndromes

Combined ophthalmoparesis (third, fourth, and sixth cranial nerve involvement) most commonly occurs with base of skull infiltrations, cavernous sinus or superior orbital fissure lesions, and generalized neuropathies. Proptosis, chemosis, and vascular engorgement suggest orbital or cavernous sinus involvement. Base of skull problems include extension of nasopharyngeal carcinoma, sarcoidosis, lymphoma, clivus chordoma, pituitary apoplexy, meningeal carcinoma, and cavernous sinus thrombosis.

Chronic progressive external ophthalmoplegia (CPEO) is a slowly progressive, painless, symmetrical ophthalmoplegia, without fluctuations or remissions. Saccades are slow, usually with no diplopia. Ptosis and orbicularis oculi weakness usually accompany the external ophthalmoplegia. The pupils are spared, and there are no orbital signs. Fibrotic changes of the extraocular muscles may occur over time, causing a superimposed restrictive ophthalmopathy. CPEO has multiple causes. *Kearns-Sayre syndrome* is one of the causes, due to a mitochondrial cytopathy. It has a childhood or adolescent onset without a family history (no male-to-male transmission), cerebellar ataxia, atypical retinal pigmentary degeneration, short stature, hearing loss, cardiac conduction defects often leading to Stokes-Adams attacks, increased CSF protein, spongiform changes of the cerebrum and brainstem, and muscle mitochondrial abnormalities. Both cardiac and endocrine complications may be life-threatening.

Painful ophthalmoplegias may be due to diabetes, aneurysm, tumors (primary and metastatic), *Tolosa-Hunt syndrome* (granulomatous inflammatory process affecting the cavernous sinus and surrounding structures), herpes zoster, cavernous sinus thrombosis, carotid cavernous fistula, ophthalmoplegic migraine, arteritis, carcinomatous meningitis, or fungal infection.

Internuclear ophthalmoplegia (INO) is characterized by (1) slow, incomplete adduction of the eye or complete inability to adduct past midline (*convergence movements may be preserved*) and (2) dissociated nystagmus of the opposite abducting eye. Skew deviation (hypertropia on the lesion site) is often present. INO is caused by a lesion of the medial longitudinal fasciculus (MLF) between mid-pons and the oculomotor nucleus ipsilateral to the side of impaired adduction. Subtle defects are best solicited by observing the fast phases of optokinetic nystagmus. In bilateral INOs, gaze-evoked vertical nystagmus, impaired vertical pursuit, and decreased vertical vestibular responses are often present. *The most frequent cause of INO in young adults (especially when bilateral) is multiple sclerosis.* Vascular causes tend to be more common in older patients. Other causes include intra- or extra-axial brainstem tumors, hydrocephalus, subdural hematoma, infection, nutritional and metabolic disorders, and drug intoxication. Myasthenia gravis and Miller-Fisher syndrome could cause similar appearing "pseudo-INO."

One-and-a-half syndrome refers to ipsilateral horizontal gaze palsy and INO (see Gaze palsy). This results from combined lesions of the MLF and the more ventral, ipsilateral abducens nucleus or paramedian pontine reticular formation (PPRF). The only intact horizontal movement is abduction of the contralateral eye. Acutely, the patient may appear exotropic, with nystagmus in the deviated eye. Vergence and vertical movements may be spared. Causes include brainstem ischemia (most common), multiple sclerosis, tumor, or hemorrhage. As with INO, myasthenia must be considered if there are no long tract or sensory signs. There is also a vertical one-and-a-half syndrome that has been described with a dorsal midbrain lesion.

REFERENCE

Leigh JR, Zee D, eds: *The neurology of eye movements*, ed 4, New York, Oxford University Press, 2006. Book and DVD.

OPTIC NERVE

The optic nerve (CN II) forms from the axons of the corresponding ipsilateral retinal ganglion cells, and transmits visual information posteriorly to the optic chiasm. Anatomically, the optic nerve has *four major portions*: (1) intraocular (1 mm); (2) intraorbital (~25 mm); (3) intracanalicular (~9 mm); and (4) intracranial (~16 mm). As each optic nerve contains information from the ipsilateral retina, an optic nerve lesion will produce a visual field defect referable to the retinal field of the affected eye.

The symptoms of optic nerve dysfunction may include blurry vision, a decreased sense of brightness, and color desaturation in the affected eye. Eye pain or headache may occur, depending on the cause.

The signs of optic nerve dysfunction include diminished visual acuity, color desaturation, and *characteristic visual field defects*—central, centrocecal, arcuate, or altitudinal scotomas. An afferent pupillary defect (APD) may be observed. This is demonstrated by the "swinging flashlight test" in which a light source is moved from one eye to the other, and the direct and consensual light responses on each side are observed. With a damaged optic nerve, the direct pupillary light response on the dysfunctional side will be abnormal owing to an impaired afferent limb (CN II). Consequently, swinging the light source from the normal eye to the affected eye will produce a paradoxic pupillary dilation due to the intact efferent limb (CN III) of the consensual response in the affected eye, in the face of a dysfunctional direct response. Funduscopic examination may reveal findings that may be helpful in diagnosing the optic nerve dysfunction including papilledema, papillitis, or optic atrophy:

I. *Papilledema* is disk swelling caused by increased intracranial pressure. The ICP is transmitted to the optic nerve causing stasis of axoplasmic transport resulting in intra-axonal edema. Initially, disk hyperemia and slightly blurred disk margins may be seen, as well as absent venous pulsations. This may develop into a grossly elevated optic disk with obliterated disk margins, venous congestion, peripapillary hemorrhages, exudates, and cotton-wool spots. Over months, the swelling resolves and the disk becomes gray or pale representing optic atrophy. Papilledema is usually bilateral. However, unilateral papilledema may be seen with some subfrontal masses such as meningioma in the *Foster-Kennedy syndrome* of anosmia, unilateral optic atrophy, and contralateral papilledema. Papilledema may not be seen acutely as it takes hours to days to develop. Furthermore, vision is usually not affected in the acute setting of papilledema, unless the inciting factor is directly injuring the optic nerve. A characteristic enlargement of the blind spot may occur in chronic elevated ICP. There may also be a constriction of visual fields due to selective involvement of damage to axons involving peripheral vision. Arcuate defects may be due to specific nerve fiber infarcts related to elevated ICP.

II. *Papillitis* refers to infarction or inflammation of the anteriormost region of the optic nerve. The differential diagnosis includes demyelinating disease, ischemia from branch or complete retinal artery occlusion, giant cell arteritis, syphilis, Lyme disease, systemic lupus erythematosus (SLE), and sarcoidosis.

III. *Retrobulbar neuritis* affects the intraorbital portion of the optic nerve and is usually the result of demyelinating disease. Idiopathic causes are more common here than in papillitis. The disk usually appears normal in the acute setting. Rapid loss of vision and pain on movement of the affected eye are typical in this case.

IV. *Optic atrophy* is a chronic finding seen in diseases that damage the axons of the optic nerve. Funduscopy shows that the optic disk appears pale. Atrophy may include part of or the entire disk, depending on the cause.

The differential diagnosis may include anterior ischemic optic neuropathy, nonischemic optic neuropathy, optic neuritis, trauma, and other inflammatory disorders (sarcoidosis, SLE, Lyme disease).

V. *Optic neuritis* is inflammation of the optic nerve. In two thirds of the patients the site of inflammation is *retrobulbar*. It is most common between 15 and 45 years of age, is seen more commonly in women, and presents as an acute unilateral visual loss, with increased periorbital pain with eye movement. Disk swelling occurs in 50% of affected adults. Visual acuity usually returns to near normal levels within several months. Most cases are idiopathic or associated with multiple sclerosis. About 60% of patients with an episode of idiopathic optic neuritis will be diagnosed with multiple sclerosis within 10 years. Other causes of optic neuritis include viral or postviral syndromes, sinusitis or meningitis, sarcoidosis, tuberculosis, syphilis, and paraneoplastic disease.

Treatment: One protocol that was successfully used in the Optic Neuritis Treatment Trial (ONTT) and was shown to hasten recovery in young patients (ages 18–46 years) with acute optic neuritis is the following: IV methylprednisolone 1 g/day for 3 days, followed by oral prednisone 1 mg/kg for 11 days. The risk of recurrent episodes of optic neuritis was lower in these patients than for patients treated with oral prednisone alone, but the long-term (5-year) risk of developing multiple sclerosis was not significantly different between the groups.

VI. *Anterior ischemic optic neuropathy* (AION) is caused by infarction of the optic nerve. AION usually presents as acute unilateral visual loss and is painless in about 90% of cases. It usually affects the papillae region, but the retrobulbar region is rarely affected. AION occurs more frequently in the elderly than optic neuritis. The recovery of vision is usually poor. Funduscopic examination may reveal disk swelling and pallor.

Treatment: The common "idiopathic" form is associated with hypertension and diabetes mellitus, a normal ESR, and steroid unresponsiveness. The rarer "arteritic" form is related to giant cell arteritis. Symptoms include headaches, weight loss, fever, arthralgias, myalgias, jaw claudication, scalp tenderness, an elevated ESR, and steroid responsiveness.

VII. *Toxic, nutritional, neoplastic, and infectious optic neuropathies* present as painless, slowly progressive bilateral visual deficits. They are usually retrobulbar. Pallor is more often in the temporal quadrant. Causes include drugs (e.g., ethambutol, isoniazid, chloramphenicol, and streptomycin), toxins (lead and methanol), and vitamin deficiencies (vitamin B_{12}, thiamine, niacin, and riboflavin). A *tobacco-alcohol amblyopia* is seen with heavy tobacco and alcohol abusers (thought to be nutritional). Optic neuropathy may be caused by *tumors* such as a compressive meningioma or astrocytoma, a primary optic nerve tumor (optic nerve gliomas, schwannomas), *infiltrative* tumors (such as lymphomas, plasmacytomas, histiocytomas), or carcinomatous meningitis. Other forms are *radiation induced* (may be delayed for years), *infectious* (Lyme disease, syphilis, and fungal infection), *inflammatory* (SLE, vasculitis, and sarcoidosis), or *hereditary* (Leber's hereditary optic neuropathy, mitochondrial mutation). *Trauma* may also lead to optic atrophy.

REFERENCE
Bradley WG, Daroff RB et al: *Neurology in clinical practice*, ed 4, Boston, Butterworth-Heinemann, 2004.

OPTOKINETIC NYSTAGMUS

The optokinetic system is an oculomotor subsystem that enhances the ability to stabilize images on the retina, thus allowing adequate visual acuity. When the head moves for an extended period, the vestibular response decays because of the mechanical properties of the labyrinthine sense organs. Only retinal information remains as the input resulting in compensatory eye movements. When the proper conditions are reproduced in the laboratory with movement of the entire visual surround, *optokinetic nystagmus* (OKN) is generated, consisting of slow components of nystagmus that match eye velocity with visual surround velocity and fast components that reset eye position.

At the bedside a true optokinetic stimulus is usually not possible. Stimulation with handheld moving stripes induces nystagmus, reflecting smooth-pursuit eye movement function (slow components) and saccadic system integrity (fast components). The examiner looks for the presence of both components of nystagmus and for symmetry in both horizontal and vertical directions. Some clinical conditions are well demonstrated by observation of the bedside OKN response, as follows:

I. Presence of optokinetic nystagmus proves that visual function is at least partially intact and is relevant in examining infants and in patients with suspected psychogenic blindness or complex visual impairment (parietal and occipital lesions).

II. Frontal lobe lesions often produce abnormalities of saccades but spare pursuit. The eyes tonically deviate in the direction of the moving target, and the fast phases may be absent or impaired when the target moves toward the side of the lesion.

III. Deep parietal lesions may impair pursuit toward the side of the lesion, causing an abnormal slow component of OKN when the target moves toward the side of the lesion. There may be an amplitude asymmetry between the two directions.

IV. Extensive hemispheric lesions may impair both pursuit and saccades. Movement of the target toward the side of the lesion may produce deficits in both slow and fast components.

V. Occipital or temporal lesions usually spare OKN. If the OKN response is asymmetrical, deep parietal involvement is probable.

VI. Moving the OKN target away from the field of action of an individual eye muscle prompts saccades in the appropriate direction and may help define a muscle paresis. Look for differences between paired muscles, for example, the left lateral rectus and the right medial rectus: the paretic eye moves more slowly and lags behind.

VII. Internuclear ophthalmoplegia may be demonstrated by horizontal movement of the target, resulting in dysconjugate saccades when fast components of OKN require action of the affected medial rectus muscle.

VIII. Downward movement of the OKN target may help demonstrate convergence retraction nystagmus (see Nystagmus).

IX. Congenital nystagmus may be accompanied by "inverted" OKN, in which the fast components are in the direction of target movement.

REFERENCE

Leigh JR, Zee D, eds: *The neurology of eye movements*, ed 4, New York, Oxford University Press, 2006. Book and DVD.

P

PAGET'S DISEASE

DEFINITION AND EPIDEMIOLOGY

Paget's disease of the bone, also known as *osteitis deformans*, is the most common bone disorder after osteoporosis. It affects about 3% of the population in the United States, has no gender preference, and increases in incidence after age 50.

PATHOPHYSIOLOGY

Abnormal osteoclastic, and later osteoblastic, activity results in sclerotic, trabecular bone remodeling, which weakens the skeleton, most commonly in axial locations. Etiology may be related to stimulation of the immune system via viral antigens, particularly measles, but family history is also present 40% of the time, suggesting a possible genetic predisposition.

CLINICAL PRESENTATION

Because pain is usually a late complication, many people, perhaps as high as 70%, may be asymptomatic. Bone pain typically increases with rest and weight bearing, as well as with limb warming and at night. The neurologic complications are usually the result of osseous overgrowth causing nerve compression, resulting in radiculopathy and spinal stenosis, as well as cranial neuropathy and brainstem compression. These are overshadowed however, by the potential for malignant transformation to osteosarcoma, and high-output cardiac heart failure due to hypervascularization of the bone marrow.

EVALUATION

X-ray findings are specific, showing early lytic or late sclerotic changes, but are not very sensitive. Bone scans can increase sensitivity, but are less specific. Biochemical markers including bone-specific alkaline phosphatase and urinary pyridinoline have replaced urinary hydroxyproline as a more accurate marker of disease activity and severity.

TREATMENT

Bisphosphonates or, less commonly, calcitonin is typically started on symptomatic patients, asymptomatic patients with involvement of weight-bearing regions, or when serum alkaline phosphatase levels rise above 125% of normal. Pain usually responds to nonsteroidal anti-inflammatory medications.

REFERENCE

Whyte MP: *N Engl J Med* 355:593–600, 2006.

P

PAIN

PAIN

Pain is produced by the stimulation of peripheral nocicepters or afferent nerve fibers. The perception of pain is modulated by many factors, including previous behavioral experiences, emotions, drugs, and hypnosis. This modulation suggests a neural mechanism that modifies either the transmission of pain or the emotional reaction to it, or both.

Cutaneous afferent nociceptive fibers enter the dorsal horn of the spinal cord, where they may ascend or descend one to two segments as Lissauer's tract. Primary afferents terminate in the superficial layers of the dorsal horn in an area known as the substantia gelatinosa. Second-order neurons decussate and ascend rostrally as the lateral and anterior spinothalamic tracts. The spinothalamic tract projects to the ventral posterolateral nucleus of the thalamus, which then sends its projections to other diencephalic structures, the brainstem reticular activating system, the limbic system, and the primary somatosensory cortex. In addition to the ascending pain system, there is a descending modulation system with origins in the brainstem periaqueductal gray and projections to the raphe nucleus. Projections from the raphe nucleus project directly to the ventral and dorsal horns of the spinal cord, including the substantia gelatinosa, and act to inhibit nociception. Serotonin is the main transmitter in this system. The locus ceruleus also acts as a descending modulating system, using norepinephrine as its transmitter. Prominent within the pain-modulating systems is the opiate receptor system and endogenous opioid peptides, which exist throughout the nervous system, particularly in the periaqueductal gray and raphe nucleus.

Acute pain follows an injury and generally resolves with healing. It has a well-defined temporal onset and is often associated with objective physical signs of autonomic activity such as tachycardia, hypertension, and diaphoresis.

Chronic pain persists beyond expected healing time and often cannot be related to a specific injury. It may not have a well-defined onset, does not respond to treatments aimed at the presumed origin or cause, and is not associated with signs of autonomic activity; the patients do not "look" like they are in pain.

Reflex sympathetic dystrophy (complex regional pain syndrome) and *phantom limb pain* are unique chronic pain syndromes. Reflex sympathetic dystrophy is characterized by burning pain, hyperesthesia, swelling, hyperhidrosis, and trophic skin and bone changes. It is treated with sympathetic denervation and aggressive physical therapy. Phantom limb pain differs from the usual nonpainful sensory illusion that the lost limb is still present. Phantom limb pain is refractory to most treatments, although local anesthetic injections have limited success.

Chronic (noncancer) pain requires an integrated multidisciplinary approach directed at both physical and psychological rehabilitation. The goal is to control the factors that increase pain. All therapies, especially drugs, should be given on a time-contingent basis, not as necessary (prn). The patient thus is not rewarded for having pain by getting medication. This approach serves to reduce the total amount of drug required daily. Each drug must be given an adequate trial. Start with simple analgesics, increase the dose or frequency before changing drugs, and when changing, use equianalgesic doses. Avoid excessive sedation.

Pharmacologic management of pain utilizes treatment directed at specific sites along the pain pathways. Peripherally, aspirin and nonsteroidal anti-inflammatory agents produce analgesia by preventing the formation of prostaglandin from arachidonic acid metabolism (inhibition of cyclooxygenase). Prostaglandin sensitizes tissues to the pain-producing effects of bradykinin and other substances resulting from tissue injury. These medications are effective in treatment of mild to moderate pain, especially bone pain. These substances also potentiate the effects of narcotic analgesics. Capsaicin, a derivative of hot peppers, acts by depleting nociceptors of substance P, rendering the skin insensitive to pain. A treatment trial requires 2 to 4 weeks of daily topical application, three to four times per day, to the affected area.

Tricyclic antidepressants (TCAs) act via influencing the biogenic amine system, affecting levels of serotonin, norepinephrine, and dopamine. Patients with pain are often locked into a pain-depression-insomnia cycle, and TCAs can affect each of these aspects of pain. The TCAs are effective in a variety of chronic pain conditions, including chronic low back pain, headache, neuropathy, and neuralgias. Anticonvulsants act to suppress spontaneous neuronal firing. They are useful in the management of chronic pain states such as trigeminal neuralgia, postherpetic neuralgia, diabetic neuropathy, and postamputation pain. Venlafaxine, which increases levels of both serotonin and norepinephrine, is emerging as a relatively nonsedating but effective medication for treating neuropathic pain.

Narcotic analgesics are used to treat severe, acute pain and chronic pain. When using narcotics, start with the lowest dose needed to obtain analgesia and titrate to pain relief or to the appearance of unacceptable side effects. Whereas prn dosing for several days allows for the determination of total daily dose, thereafter narcotic analgesics are given on a fixed dosing schedule. Add nonnarcotic drugs to increase analgesia. Tolerance to narcotics usually becomes evident as a reduction in duration of analgesia and the need for higher doses. Treat this situation by increasing the dose or by using an alternative drug (start with one half of the equianalgesic dose). The narcotic conversion nomograms can guide conversion between narcotics (Figs. 34 and 35). For example, 30 mg of oral methadone is equivalent to approximately 20 mg of parenteral morphine. Physical dependence occurs if the patient receives prolonged therapy in high doses, and patients experience withdrawal symptoms with abrupt narcotic cessation. Physical dependence is not to be confused with psychological dependence, which is a behavioral syndrome of drug craving.

Other pharmacologic interventions include the use of corticosteroids in the treatment of cancer, especially when cancer is due to bony metastasis;

P

PAIN

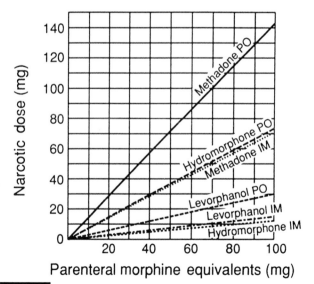

FIGURE 34

Narcotic conversion nomogram: high-potency narcotics. (From Grossman SA, Scheidler VR: *World Health Forum* 8:525, 1987.)

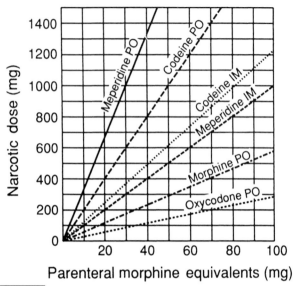

FIGURE 35

Narcotic conversion nomogram: low-potency narcotics. (From Grossman SA, Scheidler VR: *World Health Forum* 8:525, 1987.)

neuroleptics, venlafaxine, or gabapentin in dysesthetic pain; and dextroamphetamine for potentiating narcotic analgesia and reducing narcotic-induced sedation. Antihistamines (hydroxyzine) and neuroleptics can also be used to decrease nausea associated with narcotic use.

Other treatment modalities used in pain management include trigger-point injections; epidural, intrathecal, and sympathetic blockade; ganglionolysis; cordotomy; transcutaneous and percutaneous electrical stimulation; dorsal column stimulation; and relaxation techniques, including biofeedback and hypnosis.

REFERENCES

Bach S et al: *Pain* 33:297, 1988.
Portenoy RK: *CA Cancer J Clin* 38:327–392, 1988.
Schwartzmann RJ, McLellan TL: *Arch Neurol* 44:555, 1987.

PARANEOPLASTIC SYNDROMES

Paraneoplastic syndromes (PSs) are autoimmune remote effects of cancer that are not caused by metastatic complications of a systemic cancer.

TABLE 84

ANTINEURONAL ANTIBODY-ASSOCIATED PARANEOPLASTIC SYNDROMES

Antibody	Associated Cancer	Syndrome	Antigen	Onconeuronal Antigen
Anti-Hu	SCLC, neuroblastoma	Encephalomyelitis, sensory neuronopathy	All neuronal nuclei	HuD, HuC, and Hel-N1
Anti-Yo	Gynecologic, breast	Cerebellar degeneration	Cytoplasm Purkinje cells	CDR34, CDR62−1, and CDR62−2
Anti-Ri	Breast, gynecologic, SCLC	Cerebellar ataxia, opsoclonus	Neuronal nuclei CNS	NOVA1 and NOVA2
Anti-amphiphysin	Breast	Stiff-person, encephalomyelitis	Synaptic vesicles	Amphiphysin
Anti-VGCC	SCLC	LEMS	Presynaptic VGCC	A1-subunit
Anti-MYsB	SCLC	LEMS	Presynaptic VGCC	B-Subunit VGCC
Anti-Ma	Multiple	Cerebellar, brainstem dysfunction	Neuronal nuclei and cytoplasm	Ma1 and Ma2
Anti-Ta	Testicular	Limbic encephalitis, brainstem dysfunction	Neuronal nuclei and cytoplasm	Ma2
Anti-Tr	Hodgkin's lymphoma	Cerebellar degeneration	Cytoplasm neurons, Purkinje cells, spiny dendrites	In progress
Anti-CAR	SCLC, others	Photoreceptor degeneration	Retinal photoreceptor	Recoverin
Anti-CV2	SCLC, others	Encephalomyelitis, cerebellar degeneration	Glia	POP66

LEMS, Lambert-Eaton myasthenic syndrome; SCLC, small cell lung cancer; VGCC, voltage-gated calcium channels.

P

PARANEOPLASTIC SYNDROMES

Autoantibodies have been identified in several types of PS and are summarized in Table 84. Neurologic symptoms precede the identification of cancer in 50% of cases.

Clinical features that suggest a PS include (1) subacute onset, (2) severe neurologic disability, (3) inflammatory CSF with increased cells, elevated protein, and oligoclonal bands, (4) clinical syndrome that predominantly affects one specific portion of the nervous system, and (5) stereotypical presentation.

There are two main groups: (1) "classic" PSs, which strongly suggest an underlying cancer (Lambert-Eaton myasthenic syndromes [LEMS], subacute cerebellar degneration [SACD], opsoclonus/myoclonus in children), and (2) PSs that sometimes are associated with cancer but more often appear in the absence of a neoplasm (polymyositis, amyotrophic lateral sclerosis [ALS], polyneuropathy). Injury to the nervous system is mediated by the immune system, which directs a response at the tumor and against the shared antigens in the nervous system (onconeural antigens). This is the basis for antibody testing in PSs. The presence of autoantibodies helps to confirm the clinical diagnosis and to focus the search for an underlying malignancy. Furthermore, it is associated with a more indolent course than the same tumor in a patient without paraneoplastic syndrome. With the exception of myasthenia gravis, LEMS, neuromyotonia, dermatomyositis, carcinoid myopathy, and peripheral neuropathies associated with osteosclerotic myeloma, treatment of paraneoplastic syndromes is generally unsatisfactory. The PS may progress regardless of the underlying cancer, and only rarely does treatment of the primary disorder affect the course of the syndrome.

The paraneoplastic syndromes include the following:

I. *Brain and cranial nerves*: SACD, opsoclonus-myoclonus, limbic encephalitis and other dementias, brainstem encephalitis, optic neuritis, photoreceptor degeneration
II. *Spinal cord and dorsal root ganglia*: myelitis, necrotizing myelopathy, sensory neuronopathy, subacute motor neuronopathy, motor neuron disease
III. *Peripheral nerves*: subacute or chronic sensorimotor peripheral neuropathy, Guillian-Barré syndrome, mononeuritis-multiplex and vasculitic neuropathy, brachial neuritis, autonomic neuropathy, peripheral neuropathy with islet-cell tumors or paraproteinemias
IV. *Neuromuscular junction and muscle:* LEMS, myasthenia gravis, dermatomyositis or polymyositis, acute necrotizing myopathy, carcinoid myopathy, myotonia, cachectic myopathy, neuromyopathy
V. Multiple levels of central and peripheral nervous system or unknown site: encephalomyelitis, neuromyopathy, stiff-person syndrome

REFERENCES

Dalmau JO, Posner JB: *Arch Neurol* 56:405–408, 1999.
Posner JB, ed: *Neurologic complications of cancer*, ed 2, Philadelphia, FA Davis, 1995, pp 353–385.

PARIETAL LOBE

The parietal lobe consists of the postcentral gyrus, superior parietal lobule, and inferior parietal lobule, which includes the supramarginal gyrus and angular gyrus. The postcentral gyrus comprises the primary somatosensory and parietal association cortices (Brodmann's areas 3, 1, and 2) that deal with integration of multiple sensory modalities. It mainly receives fibers from the ventral posterior nucleus of the thalamus, but also contributes fibers to the corticospinal tracts (about 30%). Parietal lobe syndromes depend on the laterality of the lesion:

Hemisphere-independent parietal syndromes include contralateral cortical sensory loss, incongruent homonymous hemianopia, contralateral hemiparesis, impaired ipsilateral optokinetic saccades with compensatory nystagmus, sensory hallucinations, and simple sensory seizures.

Dominant parietal lobe syndromes include conduction aphasia, alexia, Gerstmann's syndrome (acalculia, agraphia, finger agnosia, and left-right disorientation), tactile agnosia, and apraxia (ideomotor and ideational).

Nondominant parietal lobe syndromes include neglect, anosognosia, topographic memory loss, constructional apraxia, "dressing apraxia," and acute confusional states.

Bilateral parietal lesions are associated with visual agnosia, Balint's syndrome, color agnosia, and catatonia.

PARKINSON'S DISEASE (See also AAN GUIDELINE SUMMARIES APPENDIX)

Parkinson's disease (PD) is the second most common neurodegenerative disorder.

CLINICAL FEATURES AND DIAGNOSIS

PD is age-related and occurs rarely before age 40. *The cardinal symptoms* are resting tremor (4 to 6 Hz, typically pill-rolling of the hands), bradykinesia (slowness, difficulty initiating or fatiguing of movement), rigidity (cogwheel or lead pipe), and, in the late stages, postural instability. *Classic signs* and symptoms include micrographia (small tapering writing), masked face, hypophonia, stooped posture, and shuffling gait accompanied by poor or absent arm swing. PD patients characteristically present with masked face and diminished blink rate (glabellar reflex) in the unmedicated state. Studies have found a correlation between central dopamine levels and spontaneous blink rate. Depression may precede the diagnosis of PD by several years, and cognitive deficit is commonly observed (30% to 60%).

Although the loss of multiple neurotransmitters is recognized in PD, the loss of dopaminergic pigmented neurons in the pars compacta of the substantia nigra evidenced in early pathologic studies predicted the therapeutic effects of L-dopa. L-dopa is the biochemical precursor to dopamine, which unlike dopamine, crosses the blood-brain barrier. Thus, dopamine replenishment therapy dominates the therapeutic strategies available for PD patients.

TREATMENT (See also AAN GUIDELINE SUMMARIES APPENDIX)

Dopaminergic agents: All anti-PD medications ameliorate symptoms, rather than change the course of the disease. Thus, dosage and intervals should be titrated to the individual patient's symptomatic need.

I. *Ergot-derived dopaminergic agonists* include bromocriptine (Parlodel) and pergolide (Permax), used as adjunct therapy for L-dopa or monotherapy in newly diagnosed patients. Effectiveness is assessed as a comparable level of anti-PD effects with a decrease in the "supplemental" L-dopa dosage required and a delay of the development of motor fluctuations. Cognitive deficit and hallucination tendencies may be exacerbated, and adverse GI symptoms and hypotension are not uncommon.

II. *Nonergot-derived dopaminergic agonists* include pramipexole (Mirapex) and ropinirole (Requip). These agents may be better tolerated than the ergot derivatives. A unique adverse effect of pramipexole is somnolence. Patients should be instructed to avoid driving immediately after a dose of pramipexole. As monotherapy, these agents are also effective in decreasing the required dose of L-dopa and delaying the adverse motor fluctuations. Some studies reveal these agents to be more effective than bromocriptine.

MAO inhibitors, such as selegiline (Eldepryl), inhibit monoamine oxidase B. Selegiline was found to delay and decrease the need for L-dopa in new patients. Controversy surrounds its use, secondary to the recognition of its metabolism to amphetamine and an early study that documented a higher mortality rate (later refuted). Avoid meperidine in patients taking selegiline because it may precipitate severe complications. Selective serotonin reuptake inhibitors or triptans may precipitate a hypertensive crisis if taken with selegiline.

COMT inhibitors include entacapone (Coptan) and tolcapone (Tasmar). These medications are recommended only as adjunctive therapy to L-dopa and should be given with each dose. They are primarily recommended in advanced PD patients who require greater than 600 mg of L-dopa daily. Adverse effects include worsening of L-dopa failure syndrome and liver failure.

Amantadine (Symmetrel) was discovered serendipitously to be an effective therapy in PD. It was subsequently found to have antiglutaminergic (NMDA antagonist) effects as well as dopamine reuptake inhibitory activity. It is occasionally effective in alleviating the severe dyskinetic symptoms of the L-dopa treatment. Adverse effects are predominantly cognitive (hallucinations), and thus lowering doses (to bid, last dose before 3 PM) is recommended in the elderly. Livedo reticularis can be a side effect.

Anticholinergic agents include benztropine (Cogentin) and trihexyphenidyl (Artane). Their usage in PD predates the administration of L-dopa. They are utilized mainly for refractory tremor and sialorrhea. The anticholinergic effects exacerbate cognitive symptoms and are therefore not recommended in the elderly or demented individuals or those with a predisposition to adverse cognitive effects.

L-dopa/carbidopa (Sinemet), and recently etilevodopa metabolized to L-dopa and EtOH for bypassing gastric emptying (no difference has been shown clinically), remains the standard therapy for progressive symptoms of PD. It has been found to be effective in bradykinesia, rigidity, and tremor (although the initial response may be exacerbation). It is less effective for akinetic symptoms involving gait and is ineffective and may exacerbate postural instability and gait freezing (this is true for all the dopaminergic agents). The levodopa failure syndrome is described as progressive symptoms of *on-off fluctuation, wearing off phenomenon, worsening hyperkinetic dyskinesia, and dystonia*. Patients with stable blood levels of L-dopa (i.e., undergoing intravenous infusion of L-dopa) do not experience these severe fluctuations. Thus, it has been hypothesized that the pulsatile concentrations of L-dopa exacerbate the motor fluctuation. Controlled release (CR) L-dopa/carbidopa preparations (50/200, 25/100, respectively) have been designed to prevent pulsatile stimulation of the receptors at the expense of reducing the bioavailability (by 30% to 70%); therefore, higher doses are required.

Stereotactic surgical intervention predates the discovery of L-dopa therapy. The resurgence of stereotactic surgery for PD followed the development of brain imaging systems, which allowed access to discrete basal ganglia nuclei. The increasing prevalence of L-dopa failure syndrome further promoted surgical interventions because dyskinesia, on-off fluctuation, and wearing off phenomenon are quite susceptible to stereotactic lesions:

I. *Posteroventral pallidotomy* is effective in alleviating symptoms of bradykinesia, akinesia, rigidity, and tremor, although it alleviates tremor to a lesser degree than thalamotomy or combined thalamotomy-pallidotomy. It is particularly effective in long-term improvement of dyskinesia, on-off fluctuation, and the wearing off phenomenon. Improvement in postural instability and gait disorders has been found, although reports on its durability are conflicting.

II. *Ventroinferomedial thalamotomy and thalamic stimulation* are effective in the attenuation of resting tremor, dyskinesia, dystonia, and rigidity. It is less effective for treating akinesia and may worsen it.

III. *Subthalamic nucleus stimulation or lesioning* is also effective in the akinetic symptoms of PD and the L-dopa failure syndrome. The advantage over pallidotomy appears to be in attenuation of L-dopa required by patient. Dyskinesia may continue to occur in patients despite stimulation requiring a decrement in L-dopa dose indicating less alleviation of dyskinesia than pallidotomy.

The following clinical guidelines are helpful in managing PD:

I. Most patients continue to require short-acting L-dopa for optimal therapeutic management, and shorter intervals (up to q 2 to 3 hr) are often effective in treating severe motor fluctuation. Concomitant intake of large amino acid loads (protein load particularly in dairy products) will competitively inhibit the transport of L-dopa into the brain.

II. Early morning dystonia usually can be treated with starting the L-dopa earlier.

III. Patients may also present with acute confusion and hallucinations. Recent changes or additions to medications should be investigated and discontinued. Anticholinergics, amantadine, the ergot agonists, and COMT inhibitors should be early suspects. The atypical antipsychotics utilized for patients with PD are olanzapine (Zyprexa), quetiapine (Seroquel), clozapine (Clozaril) (remember to check blood for dyscrasias), and risperidone (Risperdal). Recent studies suggest risperidone should be reserved as a last resort because it does precipitate extrapyramidal side effects.

IV. Patients who manifest significant dyskinetic symptoms should have their medication dosage decreased, and the interval between the doses decreased as well, to prevent motor fluctuation. *Peak dose dyskinesia* may be treated with reducing each dose of L-dopa or increasing the frequency, if decreasing the dose results in more wearing off. Slow release L-dopa or selegiline may be added. *Diphasic dyskinesia* is treated with increasing the dose of L-dopa or switching to a dopamine agonist with a lower dose of L-dopa. Amantadine may be helpful in alleviating dyskinesia. Over the long term, stereotactic surgical interventions may be most effective.

REFERENCES

Jankovic J, Tolosa E: *Parkinson's disease and movement disorders*, ed 4, Baltimore, Williams & Wilkins, 2002.

Koller WC: *Neurology* 58:79–86, 2002.

Olanow CW, Watts RL, Koller WC: *Neurology* 56:1–88, 2001.

PARKINSONISM

The cardinal symptoms of Parkinson's disease occur in other akinetic rigid syndromes. Parkinsonism disorders are distinguished from Parkinson's disease by the presence of additional neurologic symptoms, (supranuclear palsy, cerebellar signs, severe dementia, spasticity, symmetry, orthostatic hypotension, etc.) and are sometimes called "Parkinson's-plus syndromes." Parkinson's-plus syndromes have a transient or absent response to L-dopa, insidious onset, and rapidly progressive course to disability.

These syndromes include the following:

I. *Progressive supranuclear palsy* (PSP) is characterized by supranuclear ophthalmoplegia, pseudobulbar palsy, axial rigidity, and mild dementia.

Patients present with complaints of prominent postural instability and frequent falls within the first year (patients characteristically fall backward). Dysphagia and dysarthria are frequently noted by family and patient. Vertical slow saccades may be the earliest sign. Ophthalmoplegia is vertical in most patients at presentation and upward gaze is affected more than downward, although *downward gaze is much more specific* because upward gaze restriction is more common in the elderly. PSP has been linked to mutation of the tau gene on chromosome 17 (hence it is a *tauopathy*). PSP involves atrophy of the midbrain and pontine tegmentum, as well as of the basal ganglia and prefrontal cortex. Median survival time is about 5 to 6 years.

II. *Multiple system atrophy* (MSA) is an umbrella term for three separate disorders—sporadic olivopontocerebellar atrophy (OPCA), Shy-Drager syndrome (SDS), and striatonigral degeneration (SND)—which have considerable clinicopathologic overlap. Pathologically, varying degrees of neuronal loss and gliosis are found in the substantia nigra and striatum, as well as the olivopontocereballar pathways and intermediolateral cell columns of the spinal cord. Patients with MSA have a median survival of 6 years and are characterized by variable combinations of parkinsonism, dysautonomia, and cerebellar and corticospinal deficits. Patients usually have disabling dysautonomia, with prominent symptoms of postural hypotension, and other symptoms include erectile disturbances, bladder and bowel dysfunction, and hypohidrosis. Early postural and gait instability, dysarthria, and dysphagia are also indicative of MSA. Patients may manifest bradyphrenia, but dementia is not common. The ratio of heart to mediastinum uptake of ^{123}I using SPECT distinguishes PD from MSA. A hypointense putamen surrounded by a hyperintense rim on T_2-weighted images is a highly specific MRI sign for MSA but is only 60% sensitive. Patients with SND have predominantly akinetic rigid symptoms; a linear hyperintense signal can be seen on MRI between the claustrum and the putamen. Patients with the OPCA manifest cerebellar signs with prominent degeneration of cerebellum and pons on MRI.

III. *Corticobasal degeneration* (CBD) is distinguished from Parkinson's disease by the presence of asymmetrical cortical symptoms and signs. It is a rare disorder with asymmetrical bradykinesia, rigidity, limb dystonia, and postural instability. Other hallmarks include ideomotor apraxia, alien hand syndrome, gradual development of aphasia, and loss of cortical sensory functions. Pathologic findings include cortical frontoparietal atrophy, astrocytic gliosis, and neuronal loss in focal cortical regions and the substantia nigra. MRI reveals asymmetrical perirolandic frontotemporal atrophy. This disorder, similar to PSP, has also been linked to mutation of the tau gene on chromosome 17 and is therefore a tauopathy.

IV. *Vascular parkinsonism* accounts for 3% to 6% of cases of parkinsonism. These patients are more likely to present with gait difficulty than tremor, and are more likely to have an abrupt onset of symptoms, predominantly lower body involvement, postural instability, a history of falls, dementia, corticospinal findings, incontinence, or emotional lability.

V. *Medication-induced parkinsonism* occurs most often in patients who are treated with dopamine receptor antagonists (neuroleptic or antipsychotic agents and metoclopramide), MAO inhibitors (reserpine and tetrabenzine), and certain calcium channel blockers (cinnarizine and flunarizine). Other agents that can rarely induce parkinsonism include SSRIs, lithium, valproate, antiarrhythmics, and diazepam. Onset is usually abrupt, developing over weeks. Bradykinesia is typically symmetrical, and tremor and postural instability are less common. Symptoms are usually reversible over weeks or months if the causal agent is withdrawn.

VI. *Parkinsonism with dementia* includes dementia with Lewy body, Alzheimer's disease, and frontotemporal dementia with parkinsonism.

There are few current therapeutic options for the preceding syndromes. Patients do not respond well or for long term to anti-parkinsonian medications or surgical interventions. Symptomatic support of blood pressure in MSA and trial of dopaminergic agents are warranted, however, because a minority of patients may respond to dopamine therapy in the early stages.

Secondary parkinsonism refers to those disorders that are secondarily associated with an akinetic rigid syndrome, which includes the following: postencephalitis, hydrocephalus, hypoxia, trauma, metabolic imbalance (parathyroid), and toxins (manganese, carbon monoxide, MPTP, and cyanide). Treatment of secondary parkinsonism is mainly symptomatic and consists of elimination of the primary cause. Other neurologic diseases with parkinsonism include Hallervorden-Spatz disease, Huntington's disease, Lubag's disease, Wilson's disease, neuroacanthocytosis, and mitochondrial cytopathies with striatal necrosis.

REFERENCES

Christine CW, Aminoff MJ: *Am J Med* 117:412–419, 2004.
Gilman S, Low PA et al: *J Neurol Sci* 163:94–98, 1999.
Rowland LP: *Merritt's neurology*, Philadelphia, Lippincott Williams & Wilkins, 2000.

PERIODIC PARALYSIS (See MYOTONIA)

Periodic paralysis refers to remitting and relapsing episodes of flaccid, painless weakness traditionally categorized according to the serum potassium level during the attack. However, the episodes are better classified by sensitivity to potassium and changes in its level rather than by its absolute value. They can be primary familiar (autosomal dominant) forms or can result from other causes. Genetic forms of periodic paralysis associated with mutations in the α subunit of the skeletal muscle sodium channel protein include hyperkalemic periodic paralysis and paramyotonia congenita. Table 85 reviews clinical features of the primary familial kalemic periodic paralysis.

Secondary hypokalemic periodic paralysis occurs in illnesses with potassium depletion, including hyperaldosteronism, chronic diarrhea, or chronic use of potassium-depleting diuretics. A high incidence of hypokalemic periodic paralysis is associated with thyrotoxicosis in Oriental men.

Secondary hyperkalemic periodic paralysis is seen only with very high potassium levels, and cardiac abnormalities usually predominate. Causes include renal insufficiency, potassium-sparing diuretics, and adrenal insufficiency.

Normokalemic periodic paralysis has not been established as a distinct clinical entity. On clinical study it resembles hyperkalemic periodic paralysis and probably represents the approximately 20% of patients with normal potassium levels.

TABLE 85

PRIMARY FAMILIAL KALEMIC PERIODIC PARALYSIS

Characteristic	Hypokalemic	Hyperkalemic
Age of onset	10–20 yr, worse during third and fourth decades	Infancy/childhood
Inheritance	Autosomal dominant, 3 male:1 female, often not expressed in female	Autosomal dominant, male = female
Duration of attacks	Hours to days	Usually <1 hr
Frequency of attacks	Several per week to years between attacks	Several per day to months between attacks
Clinical signs	Often occurs in early morning, begins with hip weakness and spreads over 1 hr from proximal to distal; can totally paralyze patient, ↓ DTRs, spares face, eyes, and respiratory muscles	Proximal > distal weakness, spreads over minutes, associated with myotonia of face, eyes, hands; respiratory muscles may be involved
Laboratory findings	K^+ 1.5–3 mEq ECG changes of ↓ K^+ EMG silent during attack	K ↑ in 80%, ± ↑ CK ECG changes of ↑ K^+ EMG silent during attack
Precipitating factors	Heavy exercise followed by rest or sleep, cold, emotion, heavy meal, alcohol, trauma, epinephrine, corticosteroids	Rest after exercise, cold, anesthesia, sleep, pregnancy
Provocative tests	Glucose ± insulin	Oral KCl
Treatment	KCl, acetazolamide, spironolactone	Acetazolamide, calcium gluconate

P

PERIODIC PARALYSIS

All forms of periodic paralysis may respond to acetazolamide therapy. Its mode of action includes kaliuresis but it also induces metabolic acidosis, which may explain its benefit with hypokalemic periodic paralysis. Other kaliuretic diuretics (such as thiazides) may also be effective.

REFERENCE

Ebers GC et al: *Ann Neurol* 30:810–816, 1991.

PERIPHERAL NERVE DISEASE (See also NEUROPATHY)

This outline lists clinical clues that may be helpful in the diagnosis of focal peripheral nerve disease:

I. Upper extremity
   A. With marked differences in strength between biceps and brachioradialis (both innervated by C5-6 roots via *upper trunk*), think of:
      1. A lesion of the *lateral cord* or *musculocutaneous nerve* (if biceps is *weaker*).
      2. A lesion of the *posterior cord* or *radial nerve* (if brachioradialis is *weaker*).
   B. With marked differences in strength between biceps and deltoid, think of:
      1. A lesion of the *lateral cord* or *musculocutaneous nerve* (if biceps is *weaker*).
      2. A lesion of the *posterior cord* or *axillary nerve* (if deltoid is *weaker*).
   C. The *median nerve* sensory fibers to the hand pass via the upper brachial plexus, originating from:
      1. The C6 root to the thumb.
      2. The C6 and C7 roots to the index finger.
      3. The C7 root to the middle finger.
   D. It is not possible to differentiate C8 from T1 radioculopathy because all intrinsic muscles of the hand are innervated by C8 and T1 roots.
   E. With an *ulnar nerve* lesion of the arm, elbow, or upper forearm, sensory loss usually involves palmar and dorsal aspects of the little and ring fingers. With an *ulnar nerve lesion* of the distal forearm or wrist, sensory loss involves only the palmar aspect of these fingers (due to sparing of the *dorsal ulnar sensory branch* that arises 6 to 7 cm above the wrist).
   F. With *ulnar neuropathy*, sensory loss should not ascend above the wrist. With C8-T1 radiculopathy or *lower trunk plexopathy*, sensory loss can ascend to the entire medial aspect of the upper limb, following the distribution of the *medial cutaneous nerves* of the forearm and arm (both arising from the *lower trunk*).
   G. With weakness or atrophy of the thenar and hypothenar eminences, think of:
      1. C8-T1 radiculopathy.
      2. A *lower trunk* brachial plexopathy.

3. Concomitant *ulnar* and *median* mononeuropathy (e.g., carpal tunnel syndrome and ulnar neuropathy at the elbow). In this case, flexor pollicis longus should be intact (flexor of the distal phalanx of the thumb, located in the forearm, and innervated by the *anterior interosseus branch of the median nerve*).

H. If there is suspicion of a lower trunk brachial plexopathy or C8-T1 radiculopathy, the presence of a second-order-neuron Horner's syndrome is supportive evidence.

I. When evaluating wristdrop, correct the wrist angle to the neutral position before testing finger flexors and extensors:
   1. If the brachioradialis and triceps are spared, the lesion is an isolated *posterior interosseous* mononeuropathy. In such cases there is no sensory loss.
   2. If only the triceps is spared, the *radial nerve* lesion is at the spiral groove.
   3. If the triceps is weak, the *radial nerve* lesion is at the axilla.
   4. If, in addition to the triceps, the deltoid is weak, the lesion is not radial nerve, but rather a *posterior cord* brachial plexopathy (supplying *radial* and *axillary* nerves).

J. In the case of scapular winging, the winging is caused by:
   1. Serratus anterior weakness if:
      a. There is considerable winging at rest.
      b. There is medial translocation of the scapula (vertebral border closer to the midline).
      c. The shoulder appears lower on the affected side.
      d. Winging is accentuated by forward flexion of the humerus.
   2. Trapezius weakness if:
      a. There is less winging at rest.
      b. There is lateral translocation of the scapula.
      c. The shoulder is definitely lower on the affected side.
      d. Winging is decreased by forward flexion of the humerus.
      e. Winging is increased by abduction of the humerus.

II. Lower extremity

A. The *only L4-innervated* muscle below the knee is the tibialis anterior (L4-5, dorsiflexor of the ankle).

B. When evaluating footdrop (complete or incomplete), testing inversion of the ankle (tibialis posterior) and flexion of the toes (flexor digitorum longus) is very important. These muscles are innervated by L5 (and to a lesser extent S1) nerve roots via the *tibial nerve.* They are spared with *peroneal neuropathy* but are weak with L5 radiculopathy. Remember to correct the angle of the foot back to 90 degrees before testing eversion and inversion.

C. It is not possible to differentiate L2 from L3 radiculopathy because quadriceps, iliopsoas, and adductor muscles are innervated by L2 and L3 roots.

D. The testing of thigh adductors (L2-4, *obturator nerve*) is essential in differentiating "pure" *femoral neuropathy* from root or lumbar plexus involvement (thigh adductors are not involved in *femoral* neuropathy).

E. In proximal weakness of the lower extremity(ies), compare quadriceps and thigh adductors with thigh abductors (gluteus medius). If the weakness is significantly different, think of a selective root-plexus involvement rather than a myopathy (quadriceps and thigh adductors are L2-4 and gluteus medius is L5-S1).

Peripheral innervation is shown in Figures 36 to 43.

PET AND SPECT

Both positron emission tomography (PET) and single-photon emission computed tomography (SPECT) are based on cross-sectional reconstruction of images derived from the distribution of administered radionuclides. Spatial resolution is significantly lower than that obtained with CT or MRI. PET methodology provides both qualitative and quantitative data (the latter require an arterial line for serial blood sampling), whereas SPECT provides only qualitative data. Both methods are noninvasive, and actual radiation exposure is less than or equal to that received in many other routine radiologic procedures.

PET uses positron-emitting radionuclides such as oxygen-15, fluorine-18, carbon-11, and nitrogen-13, which are produced in a cyclotron. They have a short half-life, enabling administration of relatively high doses of radioactivity but remaining within safe limits of radiation exposure. These radionuclides can be incorporated into biologically active compounds to measure biochemical, pharmacologic, and metabolic processes. Deoxyglucose labeled with fluorine-18 (FDG) is used to measure brain glucose metabolism. Compounds labeled with oxygen-15 are used to measure regional cerebral blood flow and volume and cerebral metabolic rates. Specific receptors such as dopamine or serotonin can be targeted with positron-emitting analogues of those monoamines.

In clinical situations, PET has utility in the interictal evaluation of patients with refractory seizures of presumed focal origin. Detection of unilateral temporal hypometabolism using FDG is considered a highly specific procedure for localizing the epileptic focus. Gliomas can also be evaluated for malignant potential, with high-grade tumors demonstrating hypermetabolism and low-grade tumors demonstrating less activity. FDG uptake patterns can differentiate radiation necrosis (no or low activity) from tumor recurrence (increased activity). PET is also being used in ischemia and dementia. For evaluation of dementia, PET has been approved to differentiate Alzheimer's disease (hypometabolism in bilateral temporoparietal lobes) from frontotemporal dementia (hypometabolism in frontoparietal lobes). Other uses for PET have been limited to research

Text continiued on p. 397

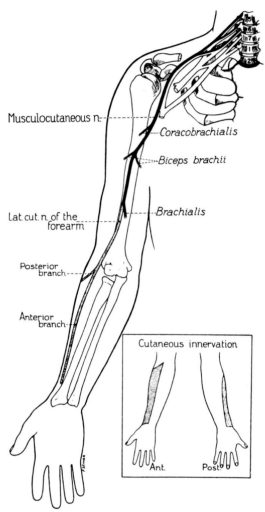

Musculocutaneous n.

Coracobrachialis

Biceps brachii

Brachialis

Lat. cut. n. of the forearm

Posterior branch

Anterior branch

Cutaneous innervation

Ant. Post.

FIGURE 36

Musculocutaneous nerve. (From Haymaker W, Woodhall B: *Peripheral nerve injuries: Principles of diagnosis*, Philadelphia, WB Saunders, 1953.)

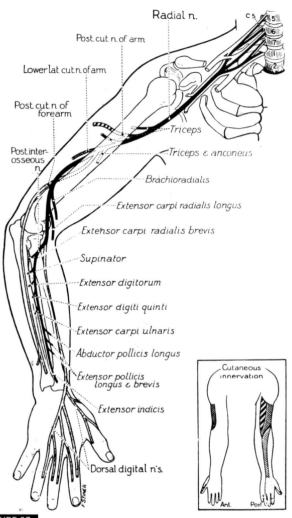

Radial n.

Post. cut. n. of arm

Lower lat. cut. n. of arm

Post. cut. n. of forearm

Post. inter-osseous n.

c 5

Triceps

Triceps & anconeus

Brachioradialis

Extensor carpi radialis longus

Extensor carpi radialis brevis

Supinator

Extensor digitorum

Extensor digiti quinti

Extensor carpi ulnaris

Abductor pollicis longus

Extensor pollicis longus & brevis

Extensor indicis

Dorsal digital n's.

Cutaneous innervation

Ant.   Post.

FIGURE 37

Radial nerve. (From Haymaker W, Woodhall B: *Peripheral nerve injuries: Principles of diagnosis*, Philadelphia, WB Saunders, 1953.)

P

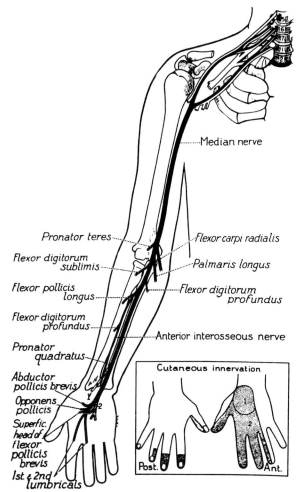

Median nerve

Pronator teres

Flexor digitorum sublimis

Flexor pollicis longus

Flexor digitorum profundus

Pronator quadratus

Abductor pollicis brevis

Opponens pollicis

Superfic. head of flexor pollicis brevis

Ist & 2nd lumbricals

Flexor carpi radialis

Palmaris longus

Flexor digitorum profundus

Anterior interosseous nerve

Cutaneous innervation

Post.   Ant.

FIGURE 38

Median nerve. (From Haymaker W, Woodhall B: *Peripheral nerve injuries: Principles of diagnosis*, Philadelphia, WB Saunders, 1953.)

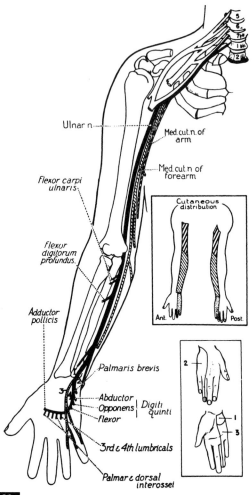

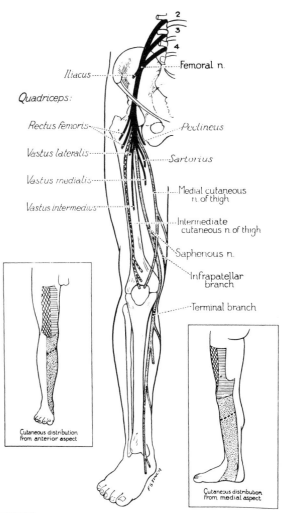

FIGURE 40

Femoral nerve. (From Haymaker W, Woodhall B: *Peripheral nerve injuries: Principles of diagnosis*, Philadelphia, WB Saunders, 1953.)

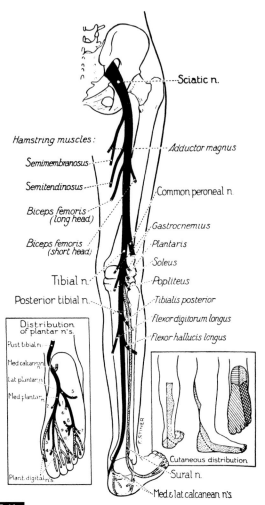

Sciatic, tibial, posterior tibial, and plantar nerves. (From Haymaker W, Woodhall B: *Peripheral nerve injuries: Principles of diagnosis*, Philadelphia, WB Saunders, 1953.)

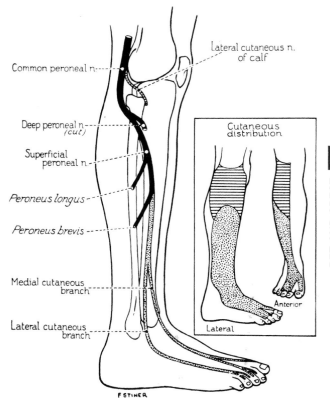

P

PET AND SPECT

FIGURE 42

Superficial peroneal nerve. (From Haymaker W, Woodhall B: *Peripheral nerve injuries: Principles of diagnosis*, Philadelphia, WB Saunders, 1953.)

studies by the high cost, invasiveness, and need for extremely sophisticated technology.

SPECT utilizes gamma emitters, such as iodine-123 or technetium-99, attached to highly lipophilic substances that easily pass the blood-brain barrier by simple diffusion. Thus, uptake, as measured by gamma camera, is proportional to regional blood flow. Gamma emitters have also been successfully labeled to various neurotransmitter analogues, allowing for localization and evaluation of receptor densities. Indications for studies are similar to those for PET. In contrast to PET, however, SPECT technology is widely available.

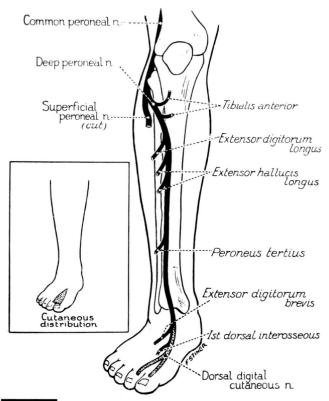

Common peroneal n.

Deep peroneal n.

Superficial peroneal n. *(cut)*

Tibialis anterior

Extensor digitorum longus

Extensor hallucis longus

Peroneus tertius

Extensor digitorum brevis

1st dorsal interosseous

Dorsal digital cutáneous n.

Cutaneous distribution

Deep peroneal nerve. (From Haymaker W, Woodhall B: *Peripheral nerve injuries: Principles of diagnosis*, Philadelphia, WB Saunders, 1953.)

REFERENCES

Alavi A, Hirsch LJ: *Semin Nucl Med* 21:58–81, 1991.
American Academy of Neurology: *Neurology* 41:163–167, 1991.
Silverman, DH: *J Nucl Med* 45:594–607, 2004.

PITUITARY ADENOMA, HYPO- AND HYPERPITUITARISM, APOPLEXY

The anterior pituitary gland produces thyrotropin, prolactin, corticotropin, growth hormone (GH), luteinizing hormone (LH), and follicle-stimulating hormone (FSH); it is supplied by the superior and inferior hypophysial arteries. The posterior pituitary gland produces vasopressin (antidiuretic hormone, ADH) and regulates oxytocin secretion; it is supplied by the inferior hypophysial arteries.

PITUITARY ADENOMAS

Pituitary adenomas may cause only endocrine symptoms if smaller than 10 mm (microadenoma). Larger tumors greater than 10 mm (macroadenomas) usually produce visual symptoms, headache, or both by mass effect. Adenomas are usually classified on histologic study on the basis of immunoperoxidase stains used to identify specific hormones.

I. Prolactinomas (27%)

Clinical presentation: Amenorrhea or galactorrhea, or both, in females and decreased libido and impotence in males. They may rapidly expand during pregnancy.

Differential diagnosis: Hypothalamic and infundibular lesions (loss of inhibitory control of prolactin secretion), renal failure, *Chiari-Frommel syndrome* (amenorrhea-galactorrhea syndrome following pregnancy), and drugs (phenothiazines, butyrophenones, benzodiazepines, reserpine, morphine, alpha-methyldopa, and isoniazid).

Diagnosis: Serum prolactin levels above 100 ng/mL (normal level, <15 ng/mL) are almost always due to tumor. Levels from 15 to 100 ng/mL may be due to tumor but are more commonly due to the other disorders listed previously, particularly drugs. MRI scan with gadolinium enhancement is the imaging test of choice. However, because microadenomas are sometimes undetected by MRI, endocrinologic testing is needed to confirm the diagnosis of small, hormone-secreting pituitary tumors if they are suspected on clinical examination.

Treatment: Symptomatic prolactinomas treatment often consists of bromocriptine (2.5–7.5 mg daily) because of the risk of tumor recurrence after surgical resection. Occasionally microadenomas resolve with medical treatment with optimal benefit from 2 to 6 months. Visual symptoms resulting from macroadenomas usually remit with bromocriptine use. Cabergoline (0.25–1 mg twice weekly) is a newer option for prolactinomas.

II. Glycoprotein hormone-secreting tumors

Clinical presentation: These tumors have considerable local mass effect and make up the majority of nonfunctioning adenomas.

III. Growth hormone–secreting (21%) and adrenocorticotropic hormone (ACTH)–secreting adenomas (8%)

Clinical presentation: These adenomas become evident as gigantism/acromegaly and Cushing's syndrome, respectively. Acromegaly may also be associated with entrapment neuropathies, such as carpal tunnel syndrome and diabetes. Cushing's syndrome may be associated with mental status changes, personality changes, and myopathy.

IV. Tumors secreting FSH, LH, and thyrotropin are rarely encountered.

V. Excess ADH in the posterior pituitary can cause SIADH leading to low serum sodium and high urine output of sodium.

Treatment: Tumor extension into brain parenchyma requires an intracranial approach. Corticosteroid coverage should be provided during surgery. Visual and endocrine function may improve after surgery and must be followed up regularly after surgery. Transsphenoidal microsurgical resection is the primary treatment in GH-secreting and ACTH-secreting tumors and in symptomatic glycoprotein hormone-secreting tumors. Postoperative *radiation therapy* is used only for macroadenomas that do not respond to medical or surgical management. Proton beam therapy and gamma knife are other options; however, risk of injury to the optic chiasm prevents regular use of these modalities.

SPECIAL SYNDROMES

I. *Hyperpituitarism* caused by any of the above adenomas may cause only endocrine symptoms if smaller than 10 mm (microadenoma). Larger tumors greater than 10 mm (macroadenomas) usually produce visual symptoms, headache, or both by mass effect. Endocrine abnormalities may or may not be present, including a hypopituitary variant.

II. *Hypopituitarism* from primary disease or as a complication of treatment requires supplementation of essential hormones. Growth hormone deficiency can lead to growth failure. Prolactin deficits can cause infertility and inability to breastfeed. LH/FSH problems cause delayed puberty, infertility, impotence, and amenorrhea. Hypothyroidism can be caused by thyrotropin deficits, and pro-opiomelanocortin (corticotropin) failure causes hypoadrenalism. Low ADH causes problems of fluid/electrolyte homeostasis in the form of diabetes insipidus (please see Diabetes Insipidus), while oxytocin is involved in lactation/labor difficulties. Critical hormones of ADH, TSH, and ACTH can be exogenously supplemented with DDAVP, L-thyroxine, and prednisone, respectively. Testosterone/estrogen (LH/FSH deficiency) and synthetic GH are also administered for their respective disorders. There is no current therapy for prolactin deficits. *Simmon's syndrome* is the eponym given to panhypopituitarism. *Sheehan's syndrome* is a pituitary infarction secondary to postpartum infarction.

III. *Pituitary apoplexy* refers to the sudden expansion of the pituitary gland, usually the result of hemorrhage into a preexisting adenoma. Sudden severe headache, variable ocular motor palsies, rapid loss of vision (chiasmal or optic nerve), evidence of hypopituitarism, and subarachnoid hemorrhage with associated changes in mental status including coma may be present. Features helpful in the difficult clinical distinction from aneurysmal subarachnoid hemorrhage are the presence of mixed oculomotor palsies or bilateral ophthalmoplegias and the presence of an afferent pupillary defect or chiasmal patterns of field loss. Diagnostic procedures include CT and MRI, which may show a pituitary mass containing blood; angiography to exclude an intracavernous aneurysm; and lumbar puncture. Baseline hormonal levels should be obtained before treatment for subsequent determination of endocrine dysfunction. Treatment includes immediate high-dose IV corticosteroid therapy and prompt transsphenoidal decompression to prevent further vision loss.

IV. Empty sella syndrome is the major cause of asymptomatic sellar enlargement. The subarachnoid space extends into the sella through an incompetent diaphragm with flattening of the gland inferiorly and posteriorly. Empty sella syndrome may also follow pseudotumor cerebri, spontaneous regressive changes of pituitary adenomas, and surgery. Although usually asymptomatic, symptoms may occur, including headache, occasional mild endocrine abnormalities, CSF rhinorrhea, and rarely, visual disturbances. If symptoms are present, pituitary tumor should be excluded with endocrine and neuro-ophthalmic evaluations and MRI. Differential diagnosis of an enlarged sella turcica in the absence of endocrinopathy includes nonsecreting adenoma, empty sella syndrome, and craniopharyngioma. Hypopituitarism, diabetes insipidus, and visual field defects are much less common in empty sella syndrome. A ballooned sella without erosion is more characteristic of craniopharyngioma.

V. Syndrome of inappropriate secretion of antidiuretic hormone (see SIADH and Cerebral Salt-Wasting Syndrome).

DIFFERENTIAL DIAGNOSIS OF SELLAR MASS LESION

1. Sellar masses: dermoids, teratomas, arachnoid cysts, and rare tumors of the neurohypophysis. Meningiomas, metastases, and cholesteatomas may occur in any location around the sella.
2. Suprasellar masses: craniopharyngiomas, optic gliomas, chondromas, hypothalamic gliomas, supraclinoid carotid artery aneurysms, choroid plexus papillomas, and colloid cysts of the third ventricle.
3. Parasellar lesions: cavernous carotid aneurysms, temporal lobe neoplasms, and gasserian ganglion neuromas.
4. Retrosellar region: chordomas and basilar artery aneurysms.
5. Infrasellar lesions: sphenoid sinus mucoceles, carcinomas, granulomas, and other nasopharyngeal tumors.

REFERENCES

Chung SM: *Neurosurg Clin North Am* 10:717–729, 1999.
Klibanski A, Zervas NT: *N Engl J Med* 324:822–831, 1991.

PORPHYRIA

The porphyrias are rare disorders of heme biosynthesis with neurologic, cutaneous, and other organ manifestations. They are classified as hepatic and erythropoietic. Neurologic symptoms occur in the *hepatic porphyrias:*

acute intermittent porphyria (AIP), variegate porphyria (VP), hereditary coproporphyria (HC), and Doss porphyria (DP). These disorders (except DP, which is inherited as an autosomal recessive) are autosomal dominant enzymatic defects of the pathways of heme biosynthesis in the liver, resulting in elevations and excess excretion of the porphyrins and the porphyrin precursors (Fig. 44). Although the enzymatic defects are well characterized, the pathogenesis of neurologic dysfunction is not known. It has been postulated that the delta-aminolevulinic acid (ALA) and porphobilinogen (PBG) are directly neurotoxic. Other possibilities include abnormalities of heme metabolism in neurons or interference with serotonergic metabolism.

The first step in the pathway catalyzed by ALA synthase results in the formation of ALA, and it is the rate-limiting step. Heme exerts control at this step via three different mechanisms: (1) repression of synthesis of new enzyme, (2) interference of transfer of the enzyme from cytosol to mitochondria, and (3) direct inhibition of enzyme activity. Processes that deplete the regulatory pool of heme by inducing cytochrome P450 or increasing the turnover of hemoglobin will drive the heme synthesis pathway. For example, phenytoin induces the cytochrome P450 system,

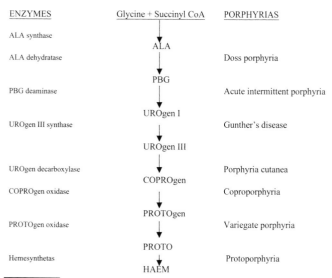

ENZYMES	Glycine + Succinyl CoA	PORPHYRIAS
ALA synthase	↓ ALA	
ALA dehydratase	↓ PBG	Doss porphyria
PBG deaminase	↓ UROgen I	Acute intermittent porphyria
UROgen III synthase	↓ UROgen III	Gunther's disease
UROgen decarboxylase	↓ COPROgen	Porphyria cutanea
COPROgen oxidase	↓ PROTOgen	Coproporphyria
PROTOgen oxidase	↓ PROTO	Variegate porphyria
Hemesynthetas	↓ HAEM	Protoporphyria

FIGURE 44

The Hemesynthetase pathway. Enzymes involved in porphyrias: ALA, delta aminolevulinic acid; COPROgen, coproporphyrinogen; PBG, porphobilinogen; PROTO, protoporphyrin; PROTOgen, protoporphyrinogen; URO, uroporphyrin; UROgen, uroporphyrinogen.

and starvation increases the turnover of hemoglobin. Both processes deplete the heme pool, thereby removing repression of ALA synthetase.

Depending on the specific enzyme deficiency, there will be an excess of intermediates from preceding steps in the pathway excreted in urine and stool; it is the pattern of porphyrin precursors in the urine, feces, and serum that characterizes the type of porphyria. Diagnosis is complicated by the variable intensity of porphyrin excretion in affected individuals and drug-induced porphyrinuria in some normal individuals leading to occasional false-positive results (Table 86). Lead poisoning can lead to elevation of ALA and porphyrins. Special handling of specimens obtained for porphyria is necessary. Twenty-four-hour urine collections should be kept refrigerated in a dark container. Twenty-four-hour stool collections must be kept frozen and in a light-free container.

The most common one of these rare disorders is AIP. Prevalence is estimated at 5 to 10 per 100,000 in the United States. Up to 90% of people with the enzyme deficiency (50% of normal activity) are asymptomatic. During the acute attacks, large amounts of PBG and ALA (20- to 200-fold elevated above normal levels) are excreted. About one third of clinically asymptomatic carriers show an abnormal excretion of PBG (two- to fivefold above the normal level), whereas the rest show normal excretion of this precursor. AIP lacks cutaneous manifestations; the PBG is not a porphyrin.

Variegate porphyria occurs mainly in South Africa but has occurred worldwide; hereditary coproporphyria and Doss porphyria are very rare. HC and VP have neurologic and cutaneous manifestations such as photosensitive skin and blistering with excessive sun exposure or mild trauma.

Clinical manifestations include the following:
I. Dysautonomia presenting as abdominal pain (95%) out of proportion to clinical findings, nausea, vomiting (90%), diarrhea or constipation (85%),

TABLE 86

HEPATIC PORPHYRIAS: BIOCHEMICAL FEATURES

Type of Porphyria	Enzyme Defect	Erythrocyte Porphyrins	Urine	Feces
Acute intermittent porphyria	PBG deaminase	None	↑ALA, PBG	None
Variegate porphyria	Protoporphyrinogen oxidase	None	↑ALA, PBG, COPRO	↑COPRO, PROTO
Hereditary coproporphyria	Coproporphyrinogen oxidase	None	↑↑COPRO	↑↑COPRO
ALA dehydratase deficiency	ALA dehydratase	Protoporphyrin	ALA	None

ALA, aminolevulinic acid; COPRO, coproporphyrin; PBG, porphobilinogen; PROTO, protoporphyrin tachycardia (70%), orthostatic hypotension, hypertension (36%), diaphoresis, and urinary retention.

II. A motor more than sensory polyneuropathy often occurs (50%); rare cases have mononeuritis multiplex as well as ascending flaccid paralysis (2%) resembling Guillain-Barré syndrome, which may result in fatal respiratory failure. Cranial nerves may be involved.

III. Headaches.

IV. Seizures in adults (15%) and in children (30%).

V. Psychiatric symptoms (25%): depression, delirium, psychosis, or agitation.

VI. Myalgia (72%).

Definitive diagnosis requires measuring PBG deaminase activity in erythrocytes. Screening for the porphyrias is accomplished by measuring stool porphyrins and urinary ALA and PBG concentration.

Treatment consists of avoiding precipitating factors, such as drugs that activate heme biosynthesis (Table 87), weight loss, or skipping meals.

TABLE 87

DRUGS AND ACUTE PORPHYRIA

DRUGS THAT MAY PRECIPITATE AN ATTACK OF ACUTE INTERMITTENT PORPHYRIA

Alcohol	Meprobamate
Barbiturates	Methsuximide
Carisoprodol	Methyldopa
Chloramphenicol	Methyprylon
Chlordiazepoxide	Pentazocine
Chloroquine	Phenylbutazone
Dichloralphenazone	Phenytoin
Ergots	Progesterones
Estrogens	Pyralones
Eucalyptol	Sulfonamides
Glutethimide	Sylfonal
Griseofulvin	Testosterones
Imipramine	Tolbutamide
	Trional

DRUGS THAT DO NOT EXACERBATE ACUTE INTERMITTENT PORPHYRIA

Ascorbic acid	Nitrofurantoin
Aspirin	Opiates
Atropine	Penicillins
B vitamins	Phenothiazines
Chloral hydrate	Promethazine
Corticosteroids	Propranolol
Digoxin	Rauwolfia alkaloids
Diphenhydramine	Scopolamine
Guanethidine	Streptomycin
Methenamine mandelate	Tetracyclines
Meclizine	Tetraethylammonium bromide
Neostigmine	

Other prophylactic measures include high carbohydrate diet and propranolol. Acute attacks are treated initially with IV glucose 10 to 20 g/hour; severe attacks may require IV hematin 3 to 4 mg/kg/24 hours, usually during the first 4 days. Urinary ALA and PBG decrease dramatically after 2 to 3 days of therapy. Hematin should not be used in conjunction with anticoagulant therapy because of its side effects, such as coagulopathy and phlebitis (the vein for infusion has to be changed each day). Women with cyclic perimenstrual acute attacks have benefited from luteinizing hormone releasing hormone (LHRH) agonists. Psychiatric symptoms may be treated with phenothiazines. Abdominal symptoms respond to chlorpromazine. Opiates are used for treatment of pain. Treatment of seizures is perplexing because many anticonvulsants are porphyrinogenic, although benzodiazepines may be less likely to induce porphyria. Gabapentin, which is not metabolized by the liver, may be useful in this clinical setting. The safety of other new antiepileptic drugs is unknown.

REFERENCES

Gordon N: *Brain Dev* 21:373–377, 1999.
Nordmanny: et al: *J Hepatol* 30:12–16, 1999.

PREGNANCY

A variety of neurologic disorders may begin during or be modified by pregnancy. Conversely, the course and outcome of pregnancy can be affected by the presence of a neurologic disorder. These situations are best considered by disease category, as follows:

I. Peripheral nerve disorders and muscle disease
    A. Mononeuropathies: Endometrial implants may occur along the cauda equina, roots, lumbosacral plexus, or sciatic nerve.
       1. *Bell's palsy:* Incidence increases threefold during pregnancy, with the majority of cases occurring in the third trimester and the first 2 puerperal weeks.
       2. *Carpal tunnel syndrome* may occur transiently during pregnancy, regressing after delivery. Weakness and wasting are unusual.
       3. *Meralgia paresthetica* is due to the entrapment of the lateral femoral cutaneous nerve of the thigh. It presents with mid-lateral thigh numbness, tingling, or stinging pain, which is exacerbated by extending the hip when standing and relieved by sitting down. Although self-limited, usually resolving 3 months after delivery, treatment is occasionally necessary. This includes avoidance of excessive weight gain and, if severe, local anesthetic infiltration; more recently, 5% lidocaine patch has been used.
    B. Plexopathies: *Recurrent brachial plexopathy* may be familial and presents as severe, persistent pain, and rapid onset of weakness in the arm and shoulder. As the pain diminishes, weakness increases

and wasting of the shoulder girdle ensues. Improvement begins in 4 to 8 weeks; functional recovery occurs in 90% of patients at 4 years.

C. Polyneuropathies
1. *Guillain-Barré syndrome:* Incidence and course are unaffected by pregnancy. Pregnancy is not complicated except possibly increased premature labor in third trimester in severe cases.
2. *Chronic inflammatory demyelinating polyradiculopathy* (CIDP) may begin during pregnancy; the relapse rate is three times greater during pregnancy, mostly occurring during the third trimester and postpartum period.
3. *Gestational distal polyneuropathy* is a symmetrical axonal neuropathy associated with malnutrition consequent to hyperemesis.
4. *Acute intermittent porphyria:* Pregnancy may induce crisis in some patients. Most relapses occur early; more serious are those (15%) that occur in the second and third trimester or are complicated by hypertension, hyperemesis, eclampsia, and preexisting renal disease. These cases are associated with prematurity and high fetal and maternal mortality.
5. *Charcot-Marie-Tooth disease* may worsen during pregnancy.

D. Obstetric palsies: Compression of a peripheral nerve or nerve trunk may be caused by the fetal head, forceps, trauma, hematoma during cesarean section, or improper positioning in leg holders. The most common maternal obstetric palsy is peroneal compression, followed by femoral neuropathy, obturator neuropathy, and rarely sciatic neuropathy or lumbosacral trunk compression. The risk of permanent weakness with recurrent maternal obstetric palsies is unknown, but requires recognition of underlying cephalopelvic disproportion and assessment of severity of the first neuropathy.

E. Myotonic dystrophy disability remains the same or worsens during pregnancy, especially the third trimester. *Regional anesthesia is preferred and depolarizing muscle relaxants are contraindicated.* Polyhydramnios suggests fetal myotonia.

II. Movement disorders
A. Chorea gravidarum occurs in slightly more than 1 in 100,000 pregnancies. Most chorea occurs during the first trimester and dramatically disappears after childbirth. It may recur with subsequent pregnancies. Approximately one third have had Sydenham's chorea in the past. Differential diagnosis includes acute rheumatic fever, Wilson's disease, lupus, polycythemia, hyperthyroidism, and idiopathic hypoparathyroidism.

B. Wilson's disease: These infants are healthy, although penicillamine may be hazardous to the fetus. Pyridoxine, 50 to 100 mg/day, is recommended, and a reduction in penicillamine dosage to 250 mg/day for the last 6 weeks of pregnancy is recommended if cesarean section is to be performed.

III. Autoimmune disorders
  A. Multiple sclerosis (MS): The course during pregnancy is variable. Gestation, labor, and delivery may be normal in MS. MS exacerbations tend to occur less during pregnancy; when they do occur, they tend to be mild. In the first 3 to 6 months post partum, 20% to 30% of women with MS will experience exacerbations and there is a two- to threefold increase in exacerbations compared to the prepregnancy year. Breastfeeding does not preclude the use of interferon-beta and glatiramer. Beta-interferon is contraindicated in pregnancy.
  B. Myasthenia gravis may improve, stabilize, or worsen in about equal proportions during pregnancy, but there is frequent immediate postpartum exacerbation. Pregnancy-associated exacerbation is less frequent following thymectomy. Myasthenia may present during pregnancy or the postpartum period. Magnesium sulfate, scopolamine, and large amounts of procaine are contraindicated. Care must be taken in the use of anesthesia and sedative drugs. Newborns should be observed carefully for 72 hours for neonatal myasthenia due to passive transfer of the acetylcholine receptor antibodies from the maternal circulation. There is no contraindication to breastfeeding because of anticholinesterase drugs or prednisone.
IV. *Cerebrovascular disease:* Age-adjusted relative risk of any hemorrhagic stroke is at least 2.5 times higher during pregnancy and increases to 28 times the nonpregnant risk in the first 6 weeks post partum.
  A. Subarachnoid hemorrhage incidence during pregnancy is estimated to range from 1 to 5 per 10,000 pregnancies. Cerebral arteriovenous malformations (AVMs) and aneurysms are the most common causes. Other causes include placental abruption, disseminated intravascular coagulation (DIC), anticoagulants, endocarditis and mycotic aneurysm, metastatic choriocarcinoma, eclampsia, postpartum cerebral phlebothrombosis, and spinal cord AVMs. AVMs tend to bleed during the second trimester and during childbirth. Aneurysms rupture most commonly during the third trimester, with the greatest risk of rebleeding occurring in the first few weeks after the initial hemorrhage or in the postpartum period. The decision to operate should be based on the same criteria used in nonpregnant patients. The natural history of both AVMs and aneurysms shows that both can rebleed during childbirth with fatal results. Hyperventilation, hypothermia, and steroids have been safely used during pregnancy, *but mannitol should be restricted.* An untreated aneurysm is a relative contraindication to future pregnancies.
  B. Cerebral ischemia: The relative risk of ischemic stroke is not increased during pregnancy but is almost nine times that of the nonpregnant state during the first 6 weeks post partum. Eclampsia is the most commonly identified cause of ischemic stroke in pregnancy. Arterial occlusion accounts for 60% to 80%, cerebral

P

PREGNANCY

venous thrombosis for 20% to 40% of strokes, and arterial dissection is less common. Mortality rate with cerebral venous thrombosis is around 30%, with residual disability varying with extent and site of the lesion. The assessment of the pregnant patient with transient ischemic attacks or stroke is the same as that of stroke in a young person. *Current guidelines suggest that no adverse fetal effects are associated with MRI.* At present, recombinant tissue plasminogen activator (rtPA) should be utilized during pregnancy only in women with significant neurologic deficits and with great caution. *Warfarin and aspirin are both contraindicated in pregnancy.*

C. Others: *Sheehan's syndrome* of postpartum hypopituitarism is secondary to pituitary infarction (usually the anterior pituitary) due to severe shock at the time of delivery. Failure to lactate is followed by amenorrhea, hypothyroidism, and hypoadrenocorticism. *Carotid cavernous sinus fistula* has also been reported during the second half of pregnancy. *Reversible segmental cerebral vasoconstriction* is a rare syndrome presenting with headache and focal deficits, frequently in the early postpartum period.

V. *Neoplasms:* Excluding pituitary tumors, primary intracranial tumors do not have an increased incidence during pregnancy. Most primary brain tumors will enlarge during pregnancy and shrink again post partum. This appears to be secondary to the intrapartum increase in intravascular volume or tumor hormone dependence. Therefore, symptoms or signs may be more apparent during the second half of pregnancy. Although slow-growing tumors can be resected post partum, *malignant gliomas and many posterior fossa tumors require prompt surgery.* Choriocarcinomas frequently metastasize (usually hemorrhagic) to the brain.

VI. *Headaches:* Headaches are frequent during pregnancy; extensive evaluation, including neuroimaging, is often required because aneurysms and AVMs may present during this period. Episodic or chronic tension headache is most common. *Migraines* may first manifest during pregnancy, usually during the first trimester. Approximately 75% of migraineurs will improve or be free of headaches during pregnancy, especially during the second and third trimester, with the remainder failing to improve or worsening. *Treatment* is limited to acetaminophen and avoidance of precipitants during pregnancy. Low-dose narcotics may be used, including demerol and morphine, but not nonsteroidal anti-inflammatory agents. Preventive therapy should be avoided. Biofeedback is a safe adjunctive therapy. *Pseudotumor cerebri* has the same incidence as in the nonpregnant, age-matched population. Symptoms will commonly begin in the first half of pregnancy.

VII. *Epilepsy:* It is estimated that 0.3% to 0.5% of all births involve women with epilepsy. Pregnant women during epilepsy can be divided into two subtypes.

A. Gestational epilepsy constitutes seizures occurring only during pregnancy. Half of these women will have epilepsy during their first pregnancy. Only 25% have recurrent seizures during subsequent pregnancies. Seizures tend to occur in the sixth or seventh month of gestation. Most patients have no identifiable lesions; a few have underlying pathology, such as tumors or vascular malformations.

B. In chronic seizure disorder, the onset of seizure is before pregnancy. Most women experience no change in seizure frequency. In 15% of women, the seizures are more frequent. Less than 1% of all epileptic women experience status epilepticus during pregnancy. Multiple factors are responsible for exacerbation of seizures, including decreased antiepileptic drug (AED) levels, hormonal changes, stress, sleep deprivation, and medication noncompliance.

Pregnant women with epilepsy have been reported to be at increased risk for a number of complications such as vaginal bleeding, premature labor or delivery, abruptio placentae, fetal loss, and premature eclampsia. The rate of spontaneous abortions is comparable to that of the general population. Perinatal mortality rate is increased 1.2- to 3-fold. A convulsive seizure occurs during labor in 1% to 2% of women with epilepsy and in another 1% to 2% within 24 hours post partum. Total AED concentration declines as pregnancy progresses due to dynamic changes in plasma protein binding. Therefore, *it is recommended to measure free AED concentration* and make appropriate dose adjustments on the basis of patient clinical condition, seizure frequency, and free AED concentration. The reversal of pregnancy-induced physiologic changes post partum may cause drug toxicity, so *drug levels should be checked periodically for at least the first 2 months after delivery*.

C. Epilepsy and birth defects: More than 90% of women with epilepsy who receive AEDs will deliver normal children free of birth defects. Major malformations and minor anomalies occur in a small but significant percentage of fetuses (6% to 8%) exposed in utero to AEDs. These children have been reported to be at increased risk for low birth weight, low Apgar scores, prematurity, microcephaly, prenatal and infant death, mental deficiency, development delay, and epilepsy. Risks to the fetus are probably higher when AEDs are used in combination and when there is a family history of birth defects. It is advisable to give *folate supplementation before conception and to treat with monotherapy* adjusted to the lowest effective level to avoid unnecessary fetal exposure.

VIII. *Eclampsia:* Unique to pregnancy, eclampsia is heralded by the onset of hypertension, proteinuria, and edema, occurring after 20 weeks' gestation, usually in a young primigravida. It may be complicated by oliguria or multiorgan failure. Eclampsia is also associated with chronic hypertension and renal disease. Maternal mortality rate ranges from 0% to 14%. There is now compelling scientific evidence in favor

P

PREGNANCY

of magnesium sulfate rather than diazepam or phenytoin for treating eclamptic seizures. Hypertension control and fluid management are required. Delivery of the fetus and placenta is the definitive treatment for eclampsia occurring prepartum or intrapartum.

REFERENCES

Abramsky O: *Ann Neurol* 36:S38–S41, 1994.
American Academy of Neurology, Quality Standards Subcommittee: *Neurology* 51:944–948, 1998.
Delgado-Escueta AV et al: *Neurology*, 42(suppl 5):8–11, 1992.
Donaldson JO: *Neurology of pregnancy*, Philadelphia, WB Saunders, 1989.
Goldstein PJ et al: *Neurological disorders of pregnancy*, Mount Kisco, Futura, 1992.
Hiilesmaa VK: *Neurology* 42(suppl 5):149–160, 1992.
Kittner SJ et al: *N Engl J Med* 335:768–774, 1996.

PSEUDOBULBAR PALSY

Most lower brainstem nuclei are bilaterally innervated. Unilateral involvement of supranuclear pathways, therefore, may not produce symptoms. Bilateral involvement of corticobulbar fibers and frontal efferents subserving emotional expression, which pass through the genu of the internal capsule and the medial cerebral peduncles, results in pseudobulbar palsy. This should be distinguished from nuclear involvement (see Bulbar Palsy). In pseudobulbar palsy, there is decreased voluntary movement and spastic hyperreflexia of the involved muscles. Thus, gag and jaw jerk reflexes may be hyperactive, even though the patient is unable to swallow or chew. Frequently, there is a spontaneous release of emotional responses such as crying or laughing with little or no provocation (*labile emotion*). Frontal release signs (grasp, palmomental, suck, snout, rooting, and glabellar reflexes) may be prominent. These should be interpreted with caution, because many normal elderly persons (over age 80 years) exhibit palmomental and snout reflexes. Dementia is frequently present in patients with pseudobulbar palsy, except those with motor neuron disease.

Although a variety of lesions (demyelinating disease, motor neuron disease) can interrupt the corticobulbar and anterior frontopontomedullary fibers, infarction is most common.

A syndrome similar to pseudobulbar palsy may occur with bilateral involvement of the opercular cortex, producing the anterior operculum syndrome (*Foix-Chavany-Marie syndrome*). It differs from classical pseudobulbar palsy in that emotional symptoms are rare, and there is loss of voluntary control of facial, pharyngeal, lingual, masticatory, or ocular muscles, with retention of reflexive and automatic movements in these muscle groups. This syndrome may be acquired or congenital as in *Worster-Drought syndrome*.

Successful treatment of pseudobulbar palsy, especially the emotional lability, has been reported with SSRIs, amitriptyline, levodopa, and amantadine.

REFERENCE

Christen HJ et al: *Dev Med Child Neurol* 42:122–132, 2000.

PSEUDOTUMOR CEREBRI

Pseudotumor cerebri (PTC) is characterized by clinical signs and symptoms of increased intracranial pressure (ICP) without evidence of intracranial mass, infection, hydrocephalus, or other apparent structural CNS pathology on neuroimaging studies and CSF examination.

Clinical features: More than 90% of PTC patients are obese and more than 90% are women. Mean age at diagnosis is about 30 years. Symptoms of PTC include increased ICP, headache (most frequent), nausea/vomiting, dizziness, tinnitus, "sounds in head," and also visual complaints and changes in visual acuity that may lead to total vision loss, diplopia, and pain on eye movements. Signs include optic disk swelling, CN VI palsy, contrast sensitivity deficits, color vision loss, constricted visual fields, and visual loss late in the course. Blind spot enlargement is always present with papilledema.

The *etiology* of PTC is unknown. Disorders associated with PTC are obesity and hypertension; rarely, PTC is associated with endocrinopathies, hyper/hypovitaminosis A, anemia, recent use of medications (tetracycline, indomethacin, nalidixic acid, nitrofurantoin, oral contraceptives, lithium), and prolonged use of corticosteroids. Systemic disorders linked with PTC include systemic lupus, hyperthyroidism, iron deficiency, and venous sinus thrombosis. An increased incidence of PTC is seen during pregnancy.

Diagnosis is made by exclusion of other causes of headache, papilledema, and increased ICP. This may require MRI and LP.

General principles of *management* include baseline and follow-up visual field and neuro-ophthalmologic evaluation for perimetry, optic disk stereophotographs, visual acuity testing, and contrast sensitivity testing. Initial treatment is often with acetazolamide (250 to 1000 mg PO qd to tid). This is generally well tolerated, but side effects include metabolic alkalosis, paresthesias of the extremities, liver dysfunction, and allergic reactions. Furosemide has also been used. Weight loss is also essential. Repeated LPs may provide relief, and some cases may provide remission, necessitating ventriculoperitoneal shunting in rapidly progressing visual loss. Steroids provide symptomatic relief but increase weight and are not often useful for prolonged treatment. Acute visual loss may also be treated by optic nerve sheath decompression in patients who have failed medical therapy.

REFERENCE

Friedman DI: *Neurosurg Clin North Am* 10:609–621, 1999.

PTOSIS

Ptosis is the drooping of the upper eyelid and may be caused by paralysis of the third cranial nerve or sympathetic innervation. The differential diagnosis of ptosis includes the following:

I. Congenital ptosis
   A. Isolated
   B. With double elevator palsy
   C. Anomalous synkinesis (including Gunn jaw winking)
   D. Lid or orbital tumor (hemangioma, dermoid)
   E. Neurofibromatosis
   F. Blepharophimosis syndromes
   G. First branchial arch syndromes (*Hallerman-Streiff, Treacher Collins*)
   H. Neonatal myasthenia

II. Ptosis resulting from myopathy neuromuscular junction disease
   A. Myasthenia gravis—ptosis may be variable and asymmetrical; may see Cogan's lid twitch sign; improves with edrophonium
   B. Myopathy restricted to levator palpebrae superioris or including external ophthalmoplegia
   C. Oculopharyngeal muscular dystrophy
   D. Myotonic dystrophy
   E. Polymyositis
   F. Aplastic levator muscle
   G. Dysthyroidism
   H. Chronic progressive external ophthalmoplegia
   I. Topical corticosteroid eye drops
   J. Levator dehiscence-disinsertion syndrome resulting from aging, inflammation, surgery, trauma, or ocular allergy

III. Ptosis resulting from sympathetic denervation (see Horner's syndrome)

IV. Ptosis resulting from third-nerve lesions
   A. Nuclear lesions involving the levator subnucleus produce severe bilateral ptosis, medial rectus weakness, skew deviation if the IV nerve is involved, or upgaze paresis and pupillary dilatation if entire third-nerve nucleus is involved.
   B. Peripheral third-nerve lesions produce unilateral ptosis with mydriasis and ophthalmoplegia; isolated ptosis is rare.

V. Pseudoptosis
   A. Trachoma
   B. Ptosis adiposis
   C. Blepharochalasis
   D. Plexiform neuroma
   E. Amyloid infiltration
   F. Inflammation resulting from allergy, chalazion, blepharitis, conjunctivitis
   G. Hemangioma
   H. Duane's retraction syndrome
   I. Microphthalmos phthisis bulbi
   J. Enopthalmos
   K. Pathologic lid retraction on opposite side
   L. Chronic Bell's palsy
   M. Hypertropia
   N. Decreased mental status
   O. Hysterical

REFERENCE

Glaser JS: *Neuro-ophthalmology*, Philadelphia, Lippincott, 1990.

PUPIL

Pupils are examined in both light and darkness, with attention to size, shape, and reactivity to light.

Bilateral dilation (mydriasis) may be produced by the following:

I. Drugs (Table 88)
II. Emotional state
III. Thyrotoxicosis
IV. Ciliospinal reflex
V. Bilateral blindness resulting from severe visual system involvement anterior to the chiasm
VI. Parinaud's syndrome
VII. Seizures
VIII. During rostrocaudal herniation caused by supratentorial mass lesions

Bilateral constriction (miosis) may be produced by the following:

I. Near triad (accommodation, convergence, miosis)
II. Old age
III. Drugs (see Table 88)
IV. Pontine lesions
V. Argyll Robertson pupils

Anisocoria, or unequal pupil size, can be an important localizing sign. A difference of less than 1 mm exists in approximately 20% of the normal population; more than 1 mm in as much as 5%. The asymmetry remains constant in light and dark. Drugs and toxins, including eye drops, may cause constriction or dilation of pupils, which is usually symmetrical unless agents are applied locally in one eye. Causes of significant anisocoria may be determined on a clinical and pharmacologic basis using Table 89.

Causes of *episodic anisocoria* include the following:

I. Parasympathetic paresis (incipient uncal herniation, seizure, migraine)
II. Parasympathetic hyperactivity (cyclic oculomotor paresis)
III. Sympathetic paresis (cluster headache [paratrigeminal neuralgia])
IV. Sympathetic hyperactivity (*Claude-Bernard syndrome* following neck trauma)
V. Sympathetic dysfunction with alternating anisocoria (cervical spinal cord lesions)
VI. Benign unilateral pupillary dilation (involved pupil has normal light and near responses)

Relative afferent pupillary defect (RAPD) (Fig. 45), also called *Marcus-Gunn pupil*, results from a lesion of the optic nerve. Resting pupil sizes are normal. Both direct and consensual pupillary responses are decreased with bright illumination of the involved side, whereas both responses are normal with illumination of the normal side. When alternately stimulating each eye

---

TABLE 88	

DRUG EFFECTS ON THE PUPILS

MIOTICS (CAUSE CONSTRICTION)	MIDRIATICS (CAUSE DILATION)
Systemic Effect	
Narcotics	Anticholinergics
Morphine and opium alkaloids	Atropine
Meperidine	Belladonna
Methadone	Scopolamine
Propoxyphene	Propantheline
Barbiturates	Jimsonweed
Diphenoxylate	Nightshade
Chloral hydrate	Tricyclic antidepressants
Phenoxybenzamine	Trihexyphenidyl
Dibenzyline	Benztropine
Phentolamine	Antihistamines
Tolazoline	Diphenydramine
Guanethidine	Chlorpheniramine
Bretylium	Phenothiazines
Reserpine	Glutethimide
Monoamine oxidase inhibitors	Amphetamines
Alpha-methyldopa	Cocaine
Bethanidine	Ephedrine
Thymoxamine	Epinephrine
Indoramin	Norepinephrine
Meprobamate	Ethanol
Cholinergics	Botulinum toxin
Edrophonium	Snake venom
Neostigmine	Barracuda poisoning
Pyridostigmine	Tyramine
Cholinesterase inhibitor pesticides	Hemicholinium
Phencyclidine	Magnesium compound
	(hypermagnesemia)
Thallium	Thiopental
Lidocaine and related agents	Lysergic acid diethylamide
Marijuana	Fenfluramine (patients receiving
Phenothiazines	reserpine)
Local Effect	
Pilocarpine	Phenylephrine
Carbachol	Hydroxyamphetamine
Methacholine	Epinephrine
Physostigmine	Cocaine
Neostigmine	Eucatropine
Isoflurophate	Atropine
Echothiophate	Homatropine
Demecarium	Scopolamine
Aceclidine	Cyclopentolate
	Tropicamide
	Oxyphenonium

Adapted from Thurston SE, Leigh RJ: In Henning RJ, Jackson DL, eds: *Handbook of critical care neurology and neurosurgery,* New York, Praeger, 1985.

TABLE 89

CHARACTERISTICS OF PUPILS ENCOUNTERED IN NEURO-OPHTHALMOLOGY

Condition	General Characteristics	Responses to Light and Near Stimuli	Room Condition in Which Anisocoria Is Greater	Response to Mydriatics	Response to Miotics	Response to Pharmacologic Agents
Essential anisocoria	Round, regular	Both brisk	No change	Dilates	Constricts	Normal and rarely needed
Horner's syndrome	Small, round, unilateral	Both brisk	Darkness	Dilates	Constricts	Cocaine 4%, poor dilation; paredrine 1%, no dilation if third-order neuron damage
Tonic pupil syndrome (Holmes-Adie syndrome)	Usually larger* in bright light; sector pupil palsy, vermiform movement; unilateral or, less often, bilateral	Absent to light, tonic to near; tonic redilation	Light	Dilates	Constricts	Pilocarpine 0.1% or 0.125%, constricts; mecholyl 2.5%, constricts
Argyll Robertson pupils	Small, irregular, bilateral	Poor to light, better to near	No change	Poor	Constricts	
Midbrain pupils	Mid-dilated; may be oval; bilateral	Poor to light, better to near (or fixed to both)	No change	Dilates	Constricts	
Pharmacologically dilated pupils	Very large,† round, unilateral	Fixed†	Light		No‡	Pilocarpine 1%, does not constrict
Oculomotor palsy (nonvascular)	Mid-dilated (6–7 mm), unilateral (rarely bilateral)	Fixed	Light	Dilates	Constricts	

*Tonic pupil may appear smaller following prolonged near-effort or in dim illumination; affected pupil is initially large, but with passing time gradually becomes smaller.
† Atropinized pupils have diameters of 8 to 9 mm. No tonic, midbrain, or oculomotor palsy pupil ever is this large.
‡ Pupils may be weakly reactive, depending on interim after instillation.
From Glaser JS: Neuro-ophthalmology, Philadelphia, Lippincott, 1989.

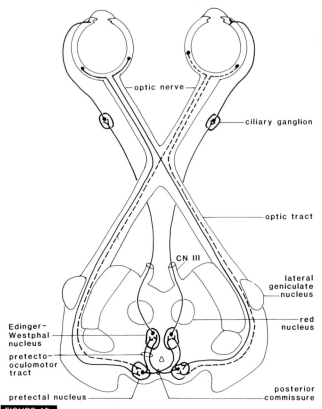

FIGURE 45

Pupillary light reflex pathways.

("swinging flashlight test"), both pupils dilate with stimulation on the abnormal side, and both constrict with the stimulation on the normal side.

The near reflex should be tested whenever pupils react poorly to light. Have the patient fixate a distant target, then quickly fixate his own fingertip held immediately in front of his nose.

Light-near dissociation may occur in the following:

I. Severe anterior visual dysfunction (such as severe glaucoma, bilateral optic neuropathy)

II. Neurosyphilis (*Argyll Robertson pupil*)

III. Adie's tonic pupil: *Holmes-Adie's syndrome* in which nearly 90% of the people have diminished deep tendon reflexes and orthostatic hypotension. Seventy percent are females. In 80% of patients, there is

unilateral involvement, although the second pupil may become
involved later.
  IV. Rostral dorsal midbrain syndrome (*Parinaud's syndrome*)
   V. Aberrant III nerve regeneration
  VI. Diabetes (out of proportion to any retinopathy)
 VII. Amyloidosis
VIII. Myotonic dystrophy

LESIONS OF THE MIDBRAIN

Efferent pupillary defects may occur with lesions involving the oculomotor
nucleus or the fascicles of the third nerve coursing ventrally to exit the
brainstem. Generally other signs of brainstem involvement or third-nerve
palsy will also be apparent.
  Three syndromes are clinically important:
  I. *Argyll Robertson pupil:* Some patients have tertiary syphilis involving
     the CNS. Affected patients have small irregular pupils, less than
     approximately 2 mm, which do not react to light with normal near
     response (light-near dissociation) and visual acuity. Similar pupils are
     seen in diabetes mellitus, chronic alcoholism, and encephalitis.
 II. *Parinaud dorsal midbrain syndrome:* This is seen in pineal tumors.
     Pupils are midposition with light-near dissociation. Afferent pupillary
     pathways in the pretectum are usually affected. Dorsal midbrain
     syndrome also causes paresis of conjugate upgaze (occasionally
     downgaze), convergence retraction nystagmus, lid lag, and *Collier's sign*
     (lid retraction).
III. *Pretectal afferent pupillary defects:* Occasionally a pretectal lesion will
     be predominantly unilateral and hence produce RAPD.

REFERENCE

Loewenfeld IE: *The pupil: Anatomy, physiology and clinical applications*, vol 1,
   Ames, Iowa State University, 1993.

R

RADIAL NERVE

ANATOMY

The radial nerve is formed by axons from C5 to T1 roots and is branched
off the lateral cord of the brachial plexus. Axons pass through several
structures including spiral groove of humerus, fibrous arch attachment of
triceps to humerus, lateral intermuscular septum below deltoid insertion,
and arcade of Froshe. Above the elbow, it branches off to innervate triceps,
anconeus, brachioradialis, extensor carpi radialis longus/brevis, and

RADIAL NERVE

posterior cutaneous nerves of arm and forearm. At or below the elbow, branches are divided so that they come off either before or after the arcade of Froshe. Branches that come off the radial nerve before the arcade of Froshe include the superficial radial nerve, which supplies sensory innervation to dorsolateral hand and the first $3\frac{1}{2}$ digits; and the posterior interosseus nerve, which innervates the extensor carpi radialis brevis and supinator. Branches below the arcade of Froshe are the terminal motor branch of posterior interosseus nerves, which innervate finger/thumb extensor, extensor carpi ulnaris, abductor pollicis longus, and articular branches to the wrist joint. Radial nerve injury is the least affected nerve among the three major nerves (median, ulnar, and radial) in the upper extremities. Radial nerve compression or injury may occur at any point along the anatomic course, ranging from proximally involving brachial plexus to distally involving the radial aspect of the wrist, and may have varied causes (Table 90). The most frequent site of compression is in the proximal forearm in the area of the supinator muscle and involves the posterior interosseous branch.

SYNDROMES

I. *Radial tunnel syndrome* is characterized by pain over the anterolateral proximal forearm in the region of the radial neck. This syndrome often appears in individuals whose work requires repetitive elbow extension or forearm rotation. It is sometimes mistakenly referred to as "resistant tennis elbow." The maximum tenderness is located 4 to 5 fingerbreadths distal to the lateral epicondyle, as compared with lateral epicondylitis (seen in tennis elbow) in which maximum tenderness is usually directly over the epicondyle. Symptoms are intensified by extending the elbow and pronating the forearm. In addition, resisted active supination and extension of the long finger cause pain. Weakness and numbness usually are not demonstrated.

TABLE 90

RADIAL NERVE LESION: LOCATION VS. ETIOLOGY

Location of Lesion	Etiology
Axilla	Pressure palsy; often occurs in sedated patient
Upper arm	Pressure,[*] fracture of humerus,[†] injection and neonatal
Posterior interosseus	Radial fracture, soft tissue mass, laceration, supinator syndrome[‡]
Superficial radial	Rupture, synovial effusion, compression, trauma, surgery, injection, and nerve tumor

[*] Pressure on medial arm compressing against humerus; often seen in sleep paralysis (Saturday night palsy), during anesthesia, and with tourniquet.

[†] Holstein-Lewis fracture, mid-third humerus fracture.

[‡] Related to repetitive pronation-supination movement. Sometimes mistakenly referred to as "resistant tennis elbow." Maximum tenderness located 4 to 5 cm distal to lateral epicondyle.

II. *Posterior interosseous syndrome:* The etiology of posterior interosseous nerve syndrome is similar to that of radial tunnel syndrome. Compression is thought to occur after takeoff of the branches to the radial wrist extensors and the sensory branches. After emerging from the supinator, the nerve may be compressed before it bifurcates into medial and lateral branches, causing a complete paralysis of the digital extensors and dorsoradial deviation of the wrist secondary to paralysis of the extensor carpi ulnaris. If compression occurs after the nerve bifurcates, selective paralysis of muscles occurs, depending on which branch is involved. Compression of the medial branch causes paralysis of the extensor carpi ulnaris, extensor digiti quinti, and extensor digitorum communis. Compression of the lateral branch causes paralysis of the abductor pollicis longus, extensor pollicis brevis, extensor pollicis longus, and extensor indicis proprius. Most commonly, entrapment occurs at the proximal edge of the supinator.

III. *Wartenberg syndrome:* Patients with the diagnosis of Wartenberg syndrome complain of pain over the distal radial forearm associated with paresthesia over the dorsal radial hand. They frequently report symptom magnification with wrist movement or when tightly pinching the thumb and index digit. These individuals demonstrate a positive Tinel sign over the radial sensory nerve (RSN) and local tenderness. Hyperpronation of the forearm can cause a positive Tinel sign. A high percentage of these patients reveal physical examination findings consistent with de Quervain tendovaginitis.

R

RADIAL NERVE

DIAGNOSIS

Plain x-ray can be obtained to rule out fracture, dislocation, bone tumor, and arthrosis. MRI can be used to look for soft tissue lipoma, ganglioma, aneurysm, and synovitis. EMG can also be really useful in determining the location, the timing (acute, subacute, or chronic), and the severity (demyelination or axon lost) of the nerve injury. However, EMG can be normal in the acute setting before wallerian degeneration occurs, which usually takes about 3 to 7 days.

TREATMENT

Conservative treatment varies according to the level and the cause of radial nerve neuropathy. A period of immobilization and anti-inflammatory medication may diminish swelling and improve symptoms. In addition, functional splints help prevent contracture and improve function as signs of nerve healing follow. Surgical approach especially for radial tunnel syndrome is highly controversial at this point. However, surgical approach would be warranted if the nerve injury is caused by structure compression (i.e., bone tumor, lipoma).

REFERENCE

Preston DC, Shapiro BE, eds, *Electromyography and neuromuscular disorder*, ed 2, Boston, Butterworth-Heinemann, 1998.

RADIATION INJURY

Injury to the nervous system occurs either as a result of treatment of CNS tumors or when nervous tissue falls into the field of treatment of another organ system. The five major manifestations of radiation injury are outlined as follows:

CEREBRAL INJURY

I. Acute encephalopathy

Presentation and diagnosis: It occurs during the first few days of radiotherapy with headache, fever, nausea, depressed sensorium, and worsening of previous focal deficit. It is more frequent and severe in patients with large brain masses or those receiving daily dose fractions higher than 300 cGy of whole-brain irradiation. It is probably caused by an increase in preexisting cerebral edema but may not be apparent on neuroimaging.

Treatment: It responds well to increased doses of dexamethasone or pretreatment with corticosteroid 24 to 72 hours before radiotherapy in large or multiple brain tumors.

II. Early delayed encephalopathy

Presentation and diagnosis: It occurs from *a few weeks up to 12 to 18 months* after irradiation and becomes evident as headache, somnolence, nausea, irritability, fever, and transient papilledema. It usually resolves after several weeks to months. Early delayed encephalopathy also occurs in 50% of children who receive prophylactic whole-brain irradiation for leukemia. It is more severe in children younger than 3 years old. MRI shows worsening edema and contrast enhancement in up to one third of patients with gliomas within a few months after fractionated radiation therapy, and in 5% to 20% of patients following stereotactic radiosurgery for brain metastases or meningioma.

Treatment: Corticosteroids may offer symptomatic relief and hasten recovery.

III. Focal cerebral necrosis

Presentation and diagnosis: This may develop several months to 10 years (peak onset of 15 to 18 months) after focal or whole-brain irradiation for brain tumors and head and neck cancers. It also occurs in patients who receive other forms of radiotherapy including brachytherapy, hyperfractionated radiation therapy, and stereotactic radiosurgery (gamma knife). Incidence is 3% to 10% after receiving 5000 cGy of daily fractionated radiation, 0% to 15% after stereotactic radiosurgery, and up to 50% of patients treated with interstitial brachytherapy. *Patients usually present with a subacute space-occupying lesion.* CT or MRI reveals edema and a patchy or ring-enhancing mass lesion. *PET, SPECT, and several MRI techniques including MR spectroscopy, perfusion-sensitive MRI, and diffusion-weighted imaging may help differentiate cerebral necrosis from tumor recurrence and may be useful for identification of a "hot spot" for a stereotactic biopsy.* Radiation necrosis occurs around the tumor and primarily involves the white matter, mostly sparing of cortex and deep gray structures, with demyelination, loss of oligodendrocytes, axonal injury, calcification, fibrillary gliosis, and mononuclear perivascular infiltrate. The most constant feature is fibrinoid vascular necrosis.

Treatment: Corticosteroids frequently cause improvement, albeit temporary. Hyperbaric oxygen treatment may be of benefit in some cases. A recent small randomized trial showed that high-dose vitamin E (2000 IU/day) improves cognitive function in patients who suffered from radiation necrosis in the temporal lobe from nasopharyngeal carcinoma treatment. Surgical debulking of necrotic lesions may be necessary in some patients.

IV. Diffuse cerebral injury

Presentation and diagnosis: This most frequent (2% to 19%) delayed effect of radiation therapy occurs in adults with primary brain tumors receiving 4000 to 6000 cGy of whole-brain irradiation and occurs in up to 50% of children with primary brain tumors following 2500 to 4000 cGy whole-brain radiation therapy. It becomes evident as moderate to severe cortical dysfunction, progressive dementia, and gait disturbance. Initial signs include memory, attentional, and visuospatial difficulties (especially in children younger than 4 or 5 years of age); ataxia; and focal motor deficits. Children with concomitant radiation therapy with methotrexate have higher risk of developing neurocognitive impairment. MRI may show enlarged ventricles, widening sulci, areas of calcification (especially basal ganglia), and diffuse hyperintense T_2 signal abnormalities. Pathologic study shows multifocal white matter destruction, especially in the centrum semiovale and periventricular white matter, dystrophic calcification of the lenticular nuclei, and mineralizing microangiopathy.

Treatment: Methylphenidate, acetylcholinesterase inhibitors, and other psychostimulants have been used in both children and adults with attention deficits from radiation treatment.

SPINAL CORD INJURY

I. Transient myelopathy

Presentation and diagnosis: The most common radiation-induced spinal injury, this usually occurs 1 to 30 months after radiotherapy, with peak at 4 to 6 months. It occurs in 10% to 15% of patients receiving mantle field radiation therapy for Hodgkin's disease. Lhermitte's sign (paresthesias radiating down the spine and limbs, precipitated by neck flexion) is often present, and myelopathic signs are usually absent. CT, MRI, and myelography results are normal.

Treatment: The syndrome resolves gradually over 1 to 9 months without risk of developing delayed, severe radiation myelopathy.

II. Delayed progressive myelopathy

Presentation and diagnosis: This has a peak time of onset of 9 to 18 months after radiotherapy with a frequency of 1% to 12%. Risk is correlated with the dose and schedule; risk is less than 5% with total doses of 4500 cGy in daily fractions of 180 cGy. Delayed progressive myelopathy usually begins with hypoesthesias or dysesthesias in lower extremities, then weakness and sphincter dysfunction. Pain is not a prominent symptom. The level of dysfunction ascends up to the area irradiated. Symptoms progress over weeks to months, with paraplegia or quadriplegia in about 50%. MRI may show focal or diffuse fusiform spinal cord enlargement with intrinsic cord signal abnormalities. CSF may show high levels of protein or white blood cells. Pathologic study shows coalescing foci of demyelination, axonal degeneration, and fibrinoid vascular necrosis.

Treatment: Patients may show improvement or stabilization of symptoms spontaneously or following corticosteroids, hyperbaric oxygen, or warfarin.

III. Motor neuron syndrome

Presentation and diagnosis: Beginning 4 to 14 months after radiotherapy, this rare lower motor neuron syndrome becomes evident as subacute, diffuse leg weakness, asymmetrical atrophy, fasciculations, depressed deep tendon reflexes, and flexor plantar responses without sensory or sphincter involvement. Symptoms gradually progress over several months, and then stabilize without improvement. EMG shows diffuse denervation in affected limb and lumbar paraspinal muscles. CSF may be normal or have increase in protein. This syndrome may result from damage to lumbosacral anterior horn cells, motor axons, or nerve roots.

Treatment: Therapy is supportive.

PERIPHERAL NERVE DAMAGE

Radiation plexopathy of the brachial or lumbosacral plexi must be distinguished from recurrent tumor. Radiation plexopathy tends to produce less pain but more weakness. Paresthesias and edema are common. EMG may show myokymic discharges. Contrast-enhanced CT, MRI, and PET often help in differentiating radiation plexopathy from other compressive lesions.

CEREBROVASCULAR DISEASE

Extracranial carotid disease, with transient ischemic attacks or strokes, may develop 6 months to 50 years (median, 10–20 years) after radiation therapy for head and neck cancers. Vascular studies show disease limited to the field of radiation, including such unusual sites as proximal common carotid artery and internal carotid artery distal to the common carotid bifurcation. Occlusive disease of the intracranial arteries follows irradiation of optic gliomas, pituitary, or suprasellar tumors (2 to 20 years later; median, 5 years). The most frequent finding on arteriography is narrowing or occlusion of the supraclinoid internal carotid artery and proximal middle cerebral artery.

Vasculopathy following radiation therapy in early childhood (usually for suprasellar tumors) frequently shows a "moyamoya" pattern. Radiation-induced stenosis is better treated with stenting than open surgery.

RADIATION-INDUCED TUMORS

In order of decreasing frequency, meningiomas, gliomas, and sarcomas may occur after radiation therapy. Meningiomas have a latency of 15 to 50 years (mean, 36 years) after irradiation, and gliomas may develop around 10 years after irradiation.

REFERENCES

Dropcho EJ: *Neurol Clin* 9:969–988, 1991.
Giglio P, Gilbert MR: *Neurologist* 9:180–188, 2003.

R

RADICULOPATHY

Radiculopathy is often the result of any process that affects the nerve at the level of the root. Processes include degenerative disk disease, spondylosis, avulsion, metastasis, epidural abscess, or any infiltrative diseases. Cervical and lumbosacral regions are the two most commonly involved areas.

CLINICAL PRESENTATION

Radioalopathy presents as radiating pain, weakness, loss of deep tendon reflexes, and sensory changes in a segmental distribution. Symptoms may be aggravated by sneezing, coughing, straining with defecation, or neck (sometimes known as Spurling's sign) or trunk movement. Moderate exercise and analgesics often offer relief. *Bed rest is no longer recommended, especially in lumbosacral radiculopathy, because it has been believed to decondition axial muscles and further cause worsening of the symptoms*. On examination, straight leg raising sign and Spurling's (pain to the side of neck rotation usually indicative of foraminal stenosis and nerve root irritation) sign may be present in cases of lumbar or cervical radiculopathy, respectively. Crossed straight leg raising usually indicates a larger lesion. An isolated root lesion may result in a smaller area of sensory disturbance than expected by standard dermatomal maps owing to cutaneous nerve overlap. Hyporeflexia is restricted to the involved root level (Table 91). Weaknesses may occur in the appropriate myotomal distribution and may indicate a larger lesion with greater anterior root involvement. Central lumbar lesions may result in a cauda equina syndrome or conus lesion (Table 92). Central disk herniation is relatively uncommon as a cause of radiculopathy.

Although herniated intervertebral disk material is the most common cause of radiculopathy, other mass lesions and structural abnormalities should be excluded. These may include tumors, epidural abscess, spondylosis, brachial or lumbar plexopathy, and peripheral neuropathy.

TABLE 91

SIGNS AND SYMPTOMS OF RADICULOPATHY

Root Lesion	Reflex Affected	Sensory Symptoms	Motor Symptoms
C5	Biceps	Pain and sensory loss in the shoulder and anterior and lateral arm	Proximal arm weakness (biceps, deltoid, infra- and supraspapular muscles[a]) Diaphragmatic paresis may occur rarely, owing to C5 fibers within the phrenic nerve[b]
C6		Pain radiating down the arm into thumb Sensory loss involving lateral arm and forearm	Proximal arm weakness, pronation[c] and finger/wrist extension
C7	Triceps	Pain radiating into third finger	Triceps[d] weakness and wrist extensor
C8	Finger flexor	Pain radiating into fourth and fifth fingers Sensory loss involving medial forearm	Weakness of intrinsic hand muscles
T1		Pain radiating down the medial aspect of the arm	Weakness of intrinsic hand muscles and possibly ipsilateral Horner's symdrome[e]
L4	Patella	Pain radiating from knee to medial malleolus. Pain elicited by "reverse straight-leg raising"	Weakness of knee extension and hip adduction
L5		Pain radiating down posterior aspect of leg into great toe	Weakness of ankle dorsiflexion[f]
S1	Achilles	Pain radiating down posterior aspect of leg and into lateral aspect of foot	Weakness of foot eversion

[a] Axillary nerve is solely innervated by C5 and solely involved in abduction above 45 degrees.
[b] Phrenic nerve usually composed of mostly C2, 3, 4, and occasionally C5.
[c] Pronator is innervated by C6 and C7.
[d] Triceps is almost solely innervated by C7.
[e] Sympathetic fibers descend from hypothalamus all the way to T1 or T2 before they exit to form sympathetic trunk. Symptoms include ptosis, miosis, and anhydrosis.
[f] Tibialis anterior is often predominantly innervated by L5.

TABLE 92

COMPARISON OF CAUDA EQUINA AND CONUS MEDULLARIS SYNDROME

Cauda Equina Syndrome	Conus Medullaris Syndrome
Asymmetrical sensory impairment	Symmetrical sensory impairment
Variable pain	Constant dull ache pain
Flaccid lower extremities with partially preserved sensation	Flaccid lower extremity paralysis
Knee and ankle jerks are absent	
Saddle anesthesia	Patellar reflexes are spared until very late
Loss of bowel, bladder, and sexual function	
Common causes are large, centrally herniated disks, severe spinal stenosis, metastatic diseases*	Loss of bladder and anal sphincter tone
	Common causes are ependymomas, dermoid cysts, lipomas, arteriovenous malformation, lymphomas, mestastatic disease

* Metastatic diseases include prostate cancer, leukemia, lymphoma, lung cancer, and pinealoma.

R

REFLEXES

EVALUATION

Plain x-rays with oblique views may be most helpful. Nerve conduction studies and EMG may identify evidence of denervation in a root distribution and exclude more peripheral lesions. Myelogram followed by CT is being supplanted in many centers by MRI, although MRI with contrast would be the best modality to look for epidural abscess.

TREATMENT

Initial treatment of disk disease should begin conservatively with traction, cervical collar, physical therapy for axial muscle strengthening exercise, and nonsteroidal anti-inflammatory agents provided there are no clinical myelopathic signs. *The majority of patients improve with time regardless of the type of intervention*. Surgical decompression is indicated when symptoms are unresponsive to conservative therapy, when there is progressive weakness, or when central herniation results in myelopathy or a cauda equina syndrome.

REFERENCES

Bradley WG, Daroff RB et al: *Neurology in clinical practice*, ed 4, Boston, Butterworth-Heinemann, 2004.

Brazis PW, Masdeu JC, Biller J: *Localization in clinical neurology*, Boston, Little Brown, 1996.

REFLEXES

Reflexes are evaluated for latency of response, degree of activity, and duration of the contraction. Reflexes should be both observed and palpated. Compare right and left sides. In general, reflexes are not pathologic if they are symmetrical unless they are absent or 4+ (see Table 93).

Hyporeflexia results from dysfunction of any part of the reflex arc. Conditions include neuropathy, radiculopathy, tabes dorsalis,

TABLE 93	
GRADING OF MUSCLE STRETCH REFLEXES	
Grade	Description
0	Absent, abnormal
1+	Diminished, may or may not be abnormal
2+	Normal
3+	Increased, may or may not be abnormal
4+	Markedly increased, abnormal; may be associated with clonus

syringomyelia, intramedullary tumors, and spinal motor neuron dysfunction. Bilateral hyporeflexia is the hallmark of neuropathies. Isolated, unilateral absent reflexes suggest radiculopathy. Hyporeflexia may occur in late stages of primary muscle diseases because of loss of muscle mass. Areflexia with rapidly progressive weakness and only mild sensory loss is the hallmark of Guillain-Barré syndrome. Hyporeflexia is seen transiently in acute upper motor neuron lesions such as cerebral infarction or spinal cord compression (spinal shock). Prolongation of both the contraction and relaxation times ("hung-up" reflex) is seen with hypothyroidism. This prolongation is most evident in the knee jerks. Areflexia may be a component of Adie's syndrome (see Pupil; see also Hypotonic Infant).

Hyperreflexia usually results from an upper motor neuron lesion with loss of corticospinal inhibition. The extrapyramidal system may also play a role. Involvement may occur anywhere from the cortical Betz cell to just proximal to the spinal cord motor neuron. Unilateral hyperreflexia results from a unilateral lesion anywhere along the corticospinal tract, most commonly in the cerebral hemispheres or brainstem. Bilateral hyperreflexia occurs more commonly with myelopathy but also occurs with bilateral cerebral hemisphere or brainstem involvement. Symmetrical, 3+ reflexes in the absence of clonus; Babinski's, Tromner's, or Hoffmann's signs; or weakness and with a normal result of neurologic examination is usually benign. Reflexes are variable (usually normal) with extrapyramidal system dysfunction. Reflexes are normal, slightly decreased, or pendular with cerebellar tract dysfunction (see also Rigidity, Spasticity).

"Pathologic reflexes" (pyramidal tract reflexes) indicate upper motor neuron dysfunction. The extensor plantar response (Babinski's sign) consists of dorsiflexion of the great toe and fanning of the remaining toes on stimulating the plantar surface of the foot. Hoffmann's and Tromner's signs are elicited by "flicking" the index or middle finger down or up, respectively, producing flexion of the thumb; they may be normal if present bilaterally, especially if reflexes are 3+ and symmetrical. Ankle clonus is the continuing rapid flexion and extension of the foot elicited by forcibly and quickly dorsiflexing the foot. Pyramidal tract reflexes are normally present in infants (see Child Neurology).

Segmental muscle stretch and cutaneous reflexes are listed in Table 94.

TABLE 94

SEGMENTAL MUSCLE STRETCH AND CUTANEOUS REFLEXES

Reflex	Level	Nerve
MUSCLE STRETCH (DEEP TENDON) REFLEXES		
Jaw (masseter and temporal muscle)	CN V	Mandibular branch
Biceps	C5, 6	Musculocutaneous
Brachioradialis	C5, 6	Radial
Pectoral major	C5, 6, 7	Lateral pectoral
Triceps	C6, 7, 8	Radial
Finger flexors	C8	Medial (ulnar)
Adductor	L2, 3, 4	Obturator
Quadriceps (patellar knee jerks)	L2, 3, 4	Femoral
Internal hamstring	L4, 5, S1	Sciatic
External hamstring	L5, S1	Sciatic
Gastrocnemius-soleus (Achilles, ankle jerks)	L5, S1, 2	Tibial
CUTANEOUS (SUPERFICIAL) REFLEXES		
Corneal	Pons	CN V (afferent), VII (efferent)
Pharyngeal gag reflex	Medulla	CN IX (afferent), X (efferent)
Upper abdominal	T6–9	
Middle abdominal	T9–11	
Lower abdominal	T11–L1	
Cremasteric	L1, 2	Femoral (afferent), genitofemoral (efferent)
Plantar	L5, S1, 2	Tibial
Anal	S3, 4, 5	Pudendal
Bulbocavernosus	S3, 4	Pudendal, pelvic autonomics

R

RESPIRATORY FAILURE

Respiratory failure is the failure of the lungs and muscles of respiration to maintain adequate respiration. Patients can have acute or chronic respiratory failure (Table 95).

   I. Acute respiratory failure (ARF)

      A. Two main forms of acute failure are hypoxic and hypercapnic respiratory failure.

      B. Hypoxic failure (type I ARF) is the failure of the respiratory system to maintain arterial oxygenation within or above the predicted normal range for a given patient's age (and ambient barometric pressure, assuming no baseline right-to-left shunting of blood)—usually an arterial oxygen content at or above 60 mm Hg.

      C. Hypercapnic failure (type II) is the failure to maintain arterial CO_2 below 50 mm Hg (not due to respiratory compensation of metabolic alkalosis).

NEUROLOGIC CAUSES OF RESPIRATORY FAILURE

Etiology	Prominent Clinical Manifestation
Neuromuscular disease (e.g., myasthenia gravis, Guillain-Barré syndrome)	Weakness of respiratory muscles
Myopathies and neuropathies (e.g., polymyositis, critical care myopathy and neuropathy, muscular dystrophy)	
Brainstem stroke	
High cervical spine injury	
Neuromuscular blocking agents (e.g., botulism, certain toxins or poisons)	
Brainstem strokes	Inability to protect airway
Bulbar palsy	
Massive ischemic or hemorrhagic strokes	
Diffuse cerebral edema (from any cause)	
Dysphagia/inability to clear secretions (from any cause)	
Sedating medications (e.g., opiates)	Decreased drive of respiration
Brainstem injuries (ischemic stroke, hemorrhage, tumors)	
Massive ischemic or hemorrhagic strokes	
Central hypoventilation (Ondine's curse)	

D. Type I ARF is usually seen in parenchymal pathologies within the lungs, such as pneumonia, pulmonary embolism, pulmonary edema, alveolar hemorrhage, or acute respiratory distress syndrome (ARDS).

E. Neurologic causes constitute a prominent etiologic portion for type II ARF, including myasthenia gravis, Guillain-Barré syndrome, brainstem stroke, amyotrophic lateral sclerosis, and some myopathies.

F. A decreased level of consciousness places a patient at significant risk for an inability to maintain a patent airway. Therefore, in addition to intubation of patients in acute respiratory failure, patients with a Glasgow Coma Scale (GCS) score below 8 are often intubated and placed on mechanical ventilation. This will include patients with a wide variety of neurologic and neurosurgical conditions.

II. Determination of respiratory failure (clinical and laboratory)

A. Patients in acute respiratory failure can develop paradoxical respiration (abdomen contracts as chest wall expands), rapid respiratory rate, and use of accessory respiratory muscles.

B. Measuring pulse oximetry will give an accurate measure of blood hypoxia, and arterial blood gas sampling will give an accurate measure of arterial CO_2 content.

C. For patients with progressive respiratory impairment, bedside measurements of ventilatory function are also useful in predicting impending respiratory failure. Most commonly in neurologic conditions, the negative inspiratory force (NIF) and the vital capacity (FVC, or simply VC) are measured. The normal NIF has an absolute value greater than 70 cm H_2O (NIF is measured as a negative pressure), and VC has a normal value of at least 60 mL/kg.

D. There is increased risk for developing respiratory failure when NIF is below 20 cm H_2O. At a VC below 25 mL/kg atelectasis develops and hypoxemia may begin. At 15 mL/kg there is shunting. At 5 to 10 mL/kg hypercapnia will develop. It is recommended that patients be electively intubated at 20 mL/kg, especially if there is a risk of further compromise of respiratory drive.

E. Other laboratory tests and investigations such as a chest x-ray are useful in elucidating causes of respiratory failure.

III. Treatment of respiratory failure

A. In general, treatment involves support of the respiratory system in such a way as to correct hypoxia or hypercapnia.

B. This can be done through either noninvasive positive pressure ventilation or—most commonly—endotracheal intubation with mechanical ventilation. The appropriate use of noninvasive ventilation is currently limited.

C. Mechanical ventilation has three main modes of respiratory support: AC (assist-control), SIMV (synchronized intermittent mandatory mode of ventilation), and CPAP (continuous positive airway pressure). There are other modes used in select circumstances. Generally, after endotracheal intubation with mechanical ventilation, patients are initially supported as fully as possible in their respirations, using the AC mode, in order to rest patients fully.

D. Recommended settings when initiating mechanical ventilation include a tidal volume of 6 mL/kg and a positive end-expiratory pressure (PEEP) of 5 cm H_2O.

E. The other two main modes of ventilation, SIMV and CPAP, require patient effort, and they are used as patients are weaned from mechanical ventilation. SIMV allows intubated patients to make some respiratory effort, while CPAP allows patients to breathe spontaneously. A 2-hour CPAP trial in intubated patients is often predictive of success in extubation.

IV. Medical aspects in patients with respiratory failure

A. Ensuring adequate nutrition

B. Prophylaxis of gastrointestinal hemorrhage

C. Prophylaxis of deep venous thrombosis

D. Monitoring of electrolytes and acid-base status

E. Prophylaxis against or treatment of ventilator-associated pneumonia (e.g., via chest physical therapy to prevent atelectasis)

R

RESPIRATORY FAILURE

REFERENCES

Acute Respiratory Distress Syndrome Network: *N Engl J Med* 342:1301–1308, 2000.

Esteban A et al: *N Engl J Med* 332:345–350, 1995.

Esteban A et al: *N Engl J Med* 350:2452–2460, 2004.

Pontoppidan H, Geffin B, Lowenstein E: *N Engl J Med* 287:743–752, 1972.

Suarez JI, ed: *Critical care neurology and neurosurgery*, Totowa, NJ, Humana Press, 2004.

The National Heart, Lung, and Blood Institute ARDS Clinical Trials Network: *N Engl J Med* 351:327–336, 2004.

Tobin MJ: *N Engl J Med* 344:1986–1996, 2001.

RESTLESS LEGS SYNDROME (EKBOM SYNDROME)

Restless legs syndrome is characterized by ill-defined, deep, "crawling" paresthesias in the lower legs, thighs, and occasionally, the arms; it is usually bilateral and occurs especially while at rest or during drowsiness, resulting in insomnia. There is a strong impulse to move or walk, to avoid the sensations. It is usually intermittent and lasts from minutes to hours. There is frequently an overlap between the restless legs syndrome and periodic movements of sleep (nocturnal myoclonic movements consisting of discrete, brief, repetitive flexion at the hips, knees, and thighs during light sleep). There may be a familial predisposition. Some similarities exist between this syndrome and growing pains in children.

A variety of conditions have been described in association with restless legs syndrome, including the following:

Uremia

Chronic obstructive pulmonary disease

Pregnancy

Carcinoma

Iron deficiency anemia

Diabetes

Exposure to cold

Acute intermittent porphyria

Parkinson's disease

Amyloidosis

Vitamin deficiencies

Caffeine

Hyperlipidemia

Barbiturate withdrawal

Prochlorperazine

Treatment involves correcting the underlying condition. Diazepam, clonazepam, baclofen, dopamine agonists (levodopa and bromocriptine), carbamazepine, propoxyphene, and amitriptyline have been used with varying success. Recently, pramipexole has been shown to be quite effective. Its tendency to cause paroxysmal sedation may be obviated if it is given only at bedtime.

REFERENCES

Ekbom KA: *Neurology* 10:388, 1960.

Mahowald MW, Ettinger MG: *J Clin Neurophysiol* 7:119–143, 1990.

Montplaisir J et al: *Neurology* 52(5):938–943, 1999.

Walters AS, Hening WA, Chokroverty S: *Mov Disord* 6:105–110, 1991.

RETINA AND UVEAL TRACT

I. Systemic and neurologic disorders associated with retinal pigmentary degeneration

A. Typical retinitis pigmentosa changes include early-onset nyctalopia, progressive visual loss, bone spicules, narrowing of retinal arterioles, and electroretinogram (ERG) changes. They may be associated with the following:

1. Myotonic dystrophy (rarely)
2. Leber's congenital amaurosis
3. Senear-Loken disease (Leber's congenital amaurosis + juvenile nephronophthisis)
4. Friedreich's ataxia (may also rarely be associated with optic atrophy and deafness)
5. Spielmeyer-Vogt disease
6. Neonatal and childhood adrenoleukodystrophy
7. Usher's syndrome (vestibulocochlear dysfunction, mutism)
8. Pelizaeus-Merzbacher disease (mental retardation, ataxia)
9. Hallgren's disease (mental retardation, ataxia, deafness)

B. Atypical central and peripheral retinal pigmentary changes occur with variable degrees of visual impairment. The presumed mechanism in storage diseases is disruption of pigment epithelial function by accumulated metabolic material with secondary retinal receptor degeneration. Primary rod or cone dystrophy may exist in the first four of the following syndromes:

1. Laurence-Moon-Biedl syndrome (hypogenitalism, mental retardation, polydactyly)
2. Biemond syndrome (hypogenitalism, mental retardation, iris coloboma)
3. Alström syndrome (hypogenitalism, deafness, diabetes mellitus)
4. Bassen-Kornzweig syndrome (abetalipoproteinemia, ataxia, acanthocytosis)
5. Refsum's disease (polyneuropathy, ataxia)
6. Sjögren-Larsson syndrome (ichthyosis, spastic paresis, mental retardation)
7. Amalric-Dialinos syndrome (deafness)
8. Cockayne's syndrome (dwarfism, neuropathy, deafness)
9. Hallervorden-Spatz syndrome (neuropathy, basal ganglia degeneration)
10. Alport's syndrome (nephritis, hearing loss)
11. Hurler's (mucopolysaccharidosis [MPS] I), Hunter's (MPS II), Sanfilippo's (MPS III), and Scheie's disease (MPS V)

C. Postinflammatory diseases

1. Congenital and acquired syphilis
2. Congenital rubella (German measles)—"salt and pepper fundus"
3. Congenital rubeola (measles)

D. Avitaminoses and vitamin metabolism disorders
  1. Pellagra
  2. Vitamin B_{12} metabolism disorder associated with aminoaciduria
E. Toxic
  1. Chlorpromazine
  2. Thioridazine
  3. Indomethacin

II. Hereditary cerebromacular dystrophies
  A. With cherry red spot of the macula
    1. Sphingolipidoses—Tay-Sachs disease, Niemann-Pick disease, Gaucher's disease, metachromatic leukodystrophy (infantile form), Sandhoff's disease
    2. Mucolipidoses—GM1 gangliosidosis, Farber's syndrome
    3. Mucolipidosis I
    4. Mucopolysaccharidoses—Hurler's syndrome (MPS I), MPS VII
    5. Goldberg's disease
  B. Without cherry red spot
    1. Ceroid lipofuscinoses—Jansky-Bielschowsky disease
    2. Batten-Mayou, Spielmeyer-Vogt disease
    3. Kufs-Hallervorden disease

III. CNS vasculitides: All vasculitides may involve the retinal circulation with variable manifestations (arterial occlusive retinopathy, hemorrhages, retinal infiltrates).

IV. Phakomatoses
  A. Vascular malformations of the choroid or retina and the CNS
    1. Von Hippel-Lindau syndrome (retinal angiomas and cerebellar hemangioblastomas)
    2. Sturge-Weber syndrome (choroidal hemangioma, parieto-occipital arteriovenous malformations [AVMs])
    3. Wyburn-Mason syndrome (AVMs in the retina and brainstem)
    4. Retinal cavernous hemangioma (unclassified phakomatosis, rarely associated with intracranial AVMs)
  B. Retinal and intracranial tumors
    1. Tuberous sclerosis
    2. Neurofibromatosis

V. Dystrophies of the uvea
  A. Angioid streaks (ruptures of Bruch's membrane) occur in the following diseases, which may be associated with neurologic dysfunction:
    1. Francois dyscephalic syndrome
    2. Paget's disease
    3. Acromegaly
    4. Sickle cell anemia
  B. Gillespie's syndrome (aniridia, ataxia, psychomotor retardation)

VI. Retinovitreal syndromes and vitreal involvement
  A. Wagner's vitreoretinopathy (rarely associated with encephaloceles)
  B. Dominant familial amyloidosis (diffuse vitreous opacification)

Table 96 summarizes the diseases that affect retinal and uveal tract and CNS.

TABLE 96

DISEASES THAT MAY INVOLVE THE UVEAL TRACT AND CENTRAL NERVOUS SYSTEM

BACTERIAL INFECTIONS

Meningococcosis
Syphilis
Tuberculosis
Whipple's disease
Brucellosis
Leptospirosis
Listeriosis
Lyme disease (*Borrelia*)

PARASITIC INFECTIONS

Trypanosomiasis
Toxoplasmosis
Ameliosis
Malaria

VIRAL INFECTIONS

Cytomegalovirus infection
Herpes simplex
Herpes zoster
Varicella
Mumps
Rubella
Rubeola
Subacute sclerosing panencephalitis
Variola

FUNGAL INFECTIONS

Aspergillosis
Candidiasis
Cryptococcosis
Histoplasmosis
Mucormycosis

GRANULOMATOUS DISEASE

Sarcoidosis
Wegener's granulomatosis

COLLAGEN VASCULAR DISEASE

Systemic lupus erythematosus
Temporal arteritis
Polyarteritis

NEOPLASMS

Leukemia
Metastatic carcinoma
Reticulum cell sarcoma

OTHER

Behçet's syndrome
Multiple sclerosis
Sympathetic ophthalmia

cont'd

DISEASES THAT MAY INVOLVE THE UVEAL TRACT AND CENTRAL NERVOUS
SYSTEM—*cont'd*

Trauma

Uveal effusion

Vogt-Koyanagi-Harada (uveomeningoencephalitic) syndrome

Bing's syndrome (chorioretinitis, ophthalmoplegia, macroglobulinemia)

Romberg's syndrome (posterior uveitis, ophthalmoplegia, trigeminal neuralgia,
seizures, unilateral facial atrophy)

Adapted from Finelli PF et al: *Ann Neurol* 1:247–252, 1977.

REFERENCE

Nussenblatt RB, Palestine AG: *Uveitis*, St. Louis, Mosby, 1989.

RHEUMATOID ARTHRITIS

Neurologic complications usually occur in patients with moderate to severe
rheumatoid arthritis (RA) and consist of neuropathy, myopathy,
myelopathy, and involvement of the brain and meninges; subclinical
involvement may occur earlier.

Peripheral neuropathy is the most frequent complication of RA and has
three main types:

I. Most common are entrapment neuropathies, resulting from
inflammation around the joints causing nerve compression. Carpal
tunnel syndrome is the most common. Other nerves involved include
ulnar (at wrist or elbow), posterior interosseous (at elbow), posterior
tibial (at popliteal fossa or tarsal tunnel), peroneal (at popliteal fossa),
and medial and lateral plantar nerves.

II. Distal sensory neuropathy may be asymptomatic or can cause
dysesthesias. Vibration is most frequently involved, but all sensory
modalities are affected. Segmental demyelination is the presumed cause.

III. Mononeuritis multiplex is usually of sudden onset from ischemic injury,
causing both demyelination and axonal loss. It may be severe and may
result in quadriparesis. Autonomic dysfunction can also occur.

Myelopathy from subluxation of the cervical spine is frequently observed
in severe RA. Atlantoaxial subluxation, separation of the anterior arch of the
atlas from the dens by greater than 3 mm, is most frequent. Lateral cervical
spine films during *active* flexion and extension are usually sufficient for
diagnosis. MRI, CT, myelography, and vertebral angiography may be needed
in selected cases. Vertical upward subluxation of the odontoid process from
lack of lateral support of the atlas usually occurs on the background of
atlantoaxial subluxation. Atlantoaxial subluxation may cause myelopathy,
headaches, or hydrocephalus, or lead to brainstem deficits from direct
medullary compression or vertebral artery involvement. Sensory loss in the
trigeminal and C2 distributions, nystagmus, and pyramidal tract signs can
result. Basilar invagination, the penetration of the odontoid through the
foramen magnum with compression of ventral medulla, is occasionally seen.

Complications affecting *muscle* include disuse atrophy, focal myositis (usually adjacent to actively involved joints), disseminated nodular myositis (non-necrotizing lymphocytic and plasma cell perivascular infiltrates), steroid myopathy, polymyositis (rare, more malignant course), and ischemia due to vasculitis.

CNS complications of RA include temporal arteritis, vasculitis (systemic vasculitis or isolated CNS angiitis), cranial neuropathies, infarction, hemorrhage, encephalopathy, dural nodules (often asymptomatic), rheumatoid pachymeningitis (seizures and encephalopathy), and hyperviscosity syndrome (rare).

Neurologic symptoms may also be caused by drugs used to treat RA, such as gold (myokymia and peripheral neuropathy with rapid onset suggestive of Guillain-Barré syndrome), steroids (myopathy), chloroquine (neuropathy, myopathy, or retinopathy), and penicillamine (reversible form of myasthenia gravis or inflammatory myopathy).

REFERENCES
Bekkelund SI et al: *J Rheumatol* 26:2348–2351, 1999.
Brick JE et al: *Neurol Clin* 7:629–639, 1989.
Dreyer SJ et al: *Clin Orthop* 366:98–106, 1999.

RIGIDITY

Rigidity is a form of increased muscle tone that is present throughout the range of motion of a limb and *is not dependent on velocity (compare to spasticity)*. When released, the rigid limb does not spring back to its original position. Rigidity is not associated with hyperreflexia. EMG reveals persistent motor unit activity during apparent relaxation.

Forms of rigidity include the following:
I. *Cogwheel rigidity* is increased resistance to passive movement, with a superimposed palpable tremor (extrapyramidal disease).
II. *Lead-pipe rigidity* is constant resistance to movement of a limb, which may maintain its position at the end of the displacement; this may also be seen in catatonia.
III. *Gegenhalten* or *paratonia* refers to increasing tone equal in response to increasing effort to move a limb passively throughout its range of motion (i.e., velocity and load-dependent resistance); this is seen in bilateral frontal lobe or mesial basal temporal lobe disease, encephalopathies, and dementias.

The following are not considered true rigidity:
I. *Voluntary rigidity*: Agonist-antagonist cocontraction is associated with heightened emotional states.
II. *Involuntary rigidity:* For example, an acute condition in the abdomen may cause rigidity.
III. *Reflex rigidity:* Spasms may occur in response to pain or cold.

IV. *Decorticate and decerebrate rigidity:* Decorticate posturing is a slow, stereotyped flexion of arm, wrist, and fingers with adduction at the shoulder and leg extension with plantar flexion of the foot. It occurs with supratentorial processes compressing the diencephalon. Decerebrate posturing is pronation of the arm with adduction and internal rotation of the leg, along with plantar flexion of the foot. It occurs with more caudal compression of the midbrain and rostral pons. Extension in the arms with flexion or flaccidity in the legs is associated with lesions of the pontine tegmentum (see also Herniation).

REFERENCE
Lee RG: *Eur Neurol* 29:S1–S13, 1989.

ROMBERG SIGN

A test comparing the stability of a person standing with both feet together and eyes open to that with eyes closed. A normal response is a slight increase in sway. A marked increase in sway indicates proprioceptive sensory loss. Increased sway may also indicate cerebellar ataxia, vestibulopathy, frontal lobe impairment, or other motor impairment. Patients with cerebellar or vestibular dysfunction tend to fall toward the side of the lesion.

S

SARCOIDOSIS

DEFINITION AND EPIDEMIOLOGY
Sarcoidosis is a multisystem disorder of unknown etiology characterized by noncaseating granulomas. Although the pulmonary system is most often affected, any organ system can be involved. Generally it affects young adults and is more common in North Americans of African descent. Most patients present with respiratory symptoms. Isolated neurosarcoidosis is rare with estimated incidence of less than 0.2 per 100,000. In 5% of patients, nervous system involvement is clinically apparent, and in a small minority this involvement can be the presenting sign. Bilateral hilar adenopathy, pulmonary infiltrate, uveitis, and skin lesion are usually the presenting signs. The most common neurologic symptoms are cranial nerve deficits (50%), headache (30%), and seizures (10%).

CLINICAL PRESENTATION
I. Neurologic manifestations of sarcoidosis
   A. Cranial neuropathies. The cranial nerves themselves are most commonly involved, but they can also be compressed by meningeal

involvement. Facial nerve is the most commonly affected, as facial motor paresis with or without dysgeusia becomes apparent at some point during the course in up to 50% of those with CNS sarcoidosis. The eighth nerve is the next most commonly affected, with either auditory or vestibular symptoms, which can be sudden in onset. Optic nerve is affected in about 15% of neurosarcoidosis cases, as optic neuropathy or papilledema. Ocular motor dysfunction is seen only occasionally (CN III, IV, or VI), as is facial sensory (CN V) involvement; other cranial nerves are very rarely affected.

B. Meningitis is quite common (up to 100% in some studies), but may be clinically inapparent. Typically it is most prominent in the basal cisterns. Meningitis manifests as cranial nerve symptoms, obstructive hydrocephalus, or rarely as mass effect on the cerebral cortex when large swellings of meninges result.

C. Neuroendocrine dysfunction. Granulomas in the hypothalamus or pituitary can produce secondary hypothyroidism, hypogonadism, adrenal insufficiency, SIADH or diabetes insipidus, or disruption of vegetative functions such as appetite or sleep.

D. Brain parenchymal lesions present either as focal cerebral dysfunction, or as hydrocephalus if occluding CSF pathways, or as diffusely raised intracranial pressure if in noneloquent cortex and sufficiently large. These lesions may produce a diffuse cerebral vasculitis or encephalitis, manifesting as encephalopathy or seizures. They may also mimic tumors, especially meningioma, necessitating biopsy.

E. Spinal cord and myelopathy. Extra- or intradural (60%) or even extramedullary or intramedullary (1%) granuloma may cause compression and spinal block. Arachnoiditis can occur.

F. Neuropathies. The most common neuropathy is chronic axonal peripheral polyneuropathy; neuropathies can present in multiple ways, however, including polyradiculopathies, individual focal mononeuropathies, or mononeuritis multiplex. They can even, rarely, present similarly to Guillain-Barré syndrome.

G. Myopathy, although pathologically common, is rarely clinically manifest.

H. Opportunistic infection. Because treatment is immunosuppression, an important part of the differential diagnosis of CNS involvement in a patient with known systemic sarcoidosis is the various viral, fungal, and mycobacterial infections that can result from such treatment.

II. Most common systemic manifestations

A. Pulmonary involvement is seen at some point in 90% of patients. Any combination of parenchymal inflammation and hilar lymphadenopathy may be seen.

B. Peripheral lymphadenopathy.

C. Skin. Dermal or epidermal granulomas, or erythema nodosum.

D. Eye. Inflammation of any portion of the orbit (conjunctivae, anterior chamber/iris, vitreous, or retina) can lead to visual impairment.

DIAGNOSIS

Definitive diagnosis is based on biopsy demonstration of noncaseating granulomas; otherwise, the diagnosis is based on the pattern of clinical organ involvement and imaging evidence of inflammatory involvement of typical tissues. CT or preferably MRI may be helpful in localizing lesion(s) in the CNS. Spectrum of MRI findings includes nodular or diffuse leptomeningeal enhancement (40%), periventricular white matter lesion (40%), multiple intraparenchymal lesions (35%), solitary intra-axial mass (10%), and solitary extra-axial mass (5%). CSF may show high protein level (40–70%), lymphocytic pleocytosis (50–70%), and low glucose level. High IgG index and oligoclonal bands may be present (70%). Serum angiotensin-converting enzyme (ACE) levels may be elevated, but have a sensitivity of only 56% to 86%, and very low specificity; CSF ACE level is far less sensitive, but more specific if CNS structures are involved.

High erythrocyte sedimentation rate and high calcium in serum/urine may be noted. Ophthalmologic examination, conjunctival biopsy, gallium scan, chest radiograph, and bronchoscopy may help in the diagnosis of systemic sarcoidosis.

TREATMENT

Prednisone, 0.5 to 1 mg/kg daily, is the mainstay of treatment. In acute severe cases, 1 g/day of IV methylprednisolone may be administered over 3 to 5 days. If steroids are not sufficient or cannot be tapered, other immunosuppressive agents such as cyclophosphamide, azathioprine, methotrexate, or cyclosporine may be added. Most patients respond to treatment but one third relapse when treatment is discontinued. Long-term treatment with corticosteroids is usually required, particularly in those with involvement of basal leptomeninges or diffuse parenchymal lesions. Radiation therapy with 20 Gy should be considered in medical refractory cases.

PROGNOSIS

Unfortunately, neurologic involvement is itself a poor prognostic sign. Peripheral nerve involvement and muscle involvement are often fairly benign. Cranial neuropathy and aseptic meningitis are the least poor prognostic central manifestations, with 90% of patients improving or recovering; those with symptomatic brain or spinal cord lesions, by contrast, very frequently have a progressive course.

REFERENCES

Gullapalli D, Phillips LH: *Curr Neurol Neurosci Rep* 4:441–447, 2004.
Gullipalli D, Phillips LH: *Neurol Clin* 20:59–83, 2002.
Krumholz A, Stern BJ: In Aminoff MJ, ed: *Neurology and general medicine*, ed 3, New York, Churchill Livingstone, 2001.

SCIATIC NERVE, SCIATICA

SCIATIC NERVE ANATOMY

The sciatic nerve is the largest and longest single nerve in the human body. The nerve originates in the lower spine as nerve roots exit the spinal cord, and extends all the way down the back of the leg to the toes. It is formed on the right and left side of the lower spine by the combination of the fourth and fifth lumbar nerves and the first three nerves in the sacral spine. The five nerves group together on the front surface of the piriformis muscle and become one large nerve: the sciatic nerve. This nerve then travels down the back of each leg, branching out to innervate specific regions of the leg and foot. Above the back of the knee, the sciatic nerve divides into two nerves, the tibial and peroneal nerves, which innervate different parts of the lower leg: The peroneal nerves travel laterally along the outer aspect of the knee to the upper foot. The tibial nerves continue to travel downward toward the feet and innervate the heel and sole of the foot. The sciatic nerve supplies sensation and strength to the leg as well as the reflexes of the leg. It connects the spinal cord with the outside of the thigh, the hamstring muscles in the back of the thighs, and muscles in the lower leg and feet. Sciatic nerve injury can lead to muscle weakness in the leg and numbness or tingling.

SCIATICA

Sciatica commonly refers to pain that radiates along the sciatic nerve and is typically felt in the buttock, down the back of the leg, and possibly to the foot. Sciatica is one of the most common forms of pain caused by compression of the spinal nerves, and the leg pain often feels much worse than the back pain. Is this a form of compressive neuropathy? Most often, sciatica pain is caused when the L5 or S1 nerve root in the lower spine is irritated by a herniated disk. When this happens, pain radiates into the buttocks and back of the thigh and calf, and occasionally may extend down to the foot. Numbness, tingling, burning, and prickling sensation are also common symptoms. Degenerative disk disease may also irritate the nerve root and cause sciatica, while conditions that mimic sciatica include piriformis syndrome and sacroiliac joint dysfunction. Sciatica may also be felt if the nerve is actually mechanically compressed, such as from spondylolisthesis, spinal stenosis, or arthritis in the spine. Most cases of sciatica are caused by a simple irritation to the nerve and will get better with time and conservative care.

SEPSIS

Sepsis is the constellation of active infection and changes in respiratory rate, pulse, and fever. Neurologic complications most frequently include obtundation (up to 70%) and less commonly include paratonic rigidity, seizures, and asterixis. It is important to distinguish septic encephalopathy from disorders producing primary neurologic disease (e.g., meningitis, stroke, brain abscess), other metabolic encephalopathies (e.g., hypoxia, hypo- and hyperglycemia, thyrotoxicosis, adrenal failure, Reye's syndrome), drug reactions, hematologic conditions (such as hyperviscosity syndromes, primary disseminated intravascular coagulation, leukemia, sickle cell crises), and other disorders of thermoregulation.

Neuromuscular complications of sepsis include critical illness polyneuropathy, a pure axonal sensorimotor polyneuropathy presenting as respiratory failure, distal weakness, and reduced reflexes with relative sparing of cranial musculature. This condition has been associated with the use of high-dose corticosteroids, particularly in combination with neuromuscular blocking agents having a steroid structure (e.g., pancuronium). Prognosis for recovery is often poor.

Other syndromes include disuse atrophy and myositis. These conditions need to be distinguished from Guillain-Barré syndrome, nutritional deficiency neuropathies, paraneoplastic syndromes, and neuromuscular blockade from some antibiotics (such as aminoglycosides).

REFERENCES
Bolton CF et al: *Ann Neurol* 33:94–100, 1993.
Vincent JL: *Lancet* 351:922–923, 1998.
Wanze RP et al: *Clin Infect Dis* 22:407–412, 1996.

SHUNTS, THIRD VENTRICULOSTOMY

I. *Ventriculoperitoneal (VP) shunts* are utilized primarily for the treatment of hydrocephalus. They are favored in infants and growing children because extra tubing can be left in the peritoneal cavity, allowing for growth and extending the time between shunt revisions.

II. *Ventriculojugular (VJ) shunts and ventriculoatrial shunts* are also used for the treatment of hydrocephalus and may be used after major growth is completed. Complications (thrombi, endocarditis, septic or tubing emboli, and arrhythmias) are more frequent and serious than with VP shunts and thus these shunts are less utilized.

III. *Endoscopic third ventriculostomy* is a newer method of approaching noncommunicating hydrocephalus affecting the third ventricle, particularly in the treatment of colloid cysts. This procedure utilizes an endoscope from a frontal burr hole to traverse the lateral ventricle and foramen of Monro, and then enter the third ventricle to create a fistula between the third ventricle and the subarachnoid space.

IV. *Lumboperitoneal (LP) shunts* are useful in communicating hydrocephalus, particularly normal-pressure hydrocephalus. Similarly, a *lumbar drain* can be utilized for temporary, constant relief of CSF pressure for the treatment of acute surgical complications. An *intrathecal pump*, as in the chronic administration of baclofen, can be placed in the spinal canal for more direct and efficacious treatment of spasticity.

V. *External ventriculostomy (external ventricular drains, or EVDs)* temporary shunts placed in the lateral ventricles are useful immediately after cranial surgical procedures, when CSF protein level is very high, or when there is debris in the CSF as well as to measure and control ICP in traumas or acute ICH.

VI. *Ventricular access devices (Ommaya reservoir)* are also available to monitor ICP, to provide CNS antimicrobial treatment access, and to directly treat CNS cancers with chemotherapy. They directly access the lateral ventricle from a frontal burr hole.

Complication rates for VP shunts range from 4% to 30% in the literature, while endoscopic ventriculostomy yields a complication rate as high as 40%.

SHUNT MALFUNCTION

Classic symptoms of shunt dysfunction in older children and adults are headache, lethargy, nausea, and vomiting. Gradual shunt malfunction may come to medical attention as impaired school performance, irritability, or personality change. Infants may have irritability, poor feeding, vomiting, and an abnormal shrill cry. Children with repeated episodes of shunt malfunction generally come to medical attention in a similar manner with each episode.

I. *Mechanical malfunction* can be due to disconnection, breakage, or obstruction: ventricular catheter plugged with glia or choroid plexus; valve plugged with high-protein CSF or debris; distal catheter plugged with thrombus (VJ) or omentum (VP).

Evaluation includes several steps: (1) Pump the valve. Difficulty with compression of the valve ("pumps hard") suggests distal obstruction; slow refill suggests proximal obstruction or slit ventricles. Even if the shunt pumps, it may not be working properly. (2) Palpate the shunt tubing for any interruption. (3) Obtain a shunt series. Obtain plain x-rays of the entire shunt system (reservoirs and pumps may be radiolucent) to look for interruption and a noncontrasted head CT scan to assess ventricular size (old films are invaluable for comparing ventricular size). (4) Tap the shunt (Huber needle only) for CSF pressure (if obstructed proximal to reservoir, measured pressure will not be elevated) and CSF examination. Over 90% of shunt failures occur in the first 3 months. In uncomplicated shunt placements, 6- to 12-month postoperative CT should be scheduled.

II. *Shunt infection:* A shunt tap is not always necessary when a fever develops in a child with a shunt. Upper respiratory infection, otitis media, pharyngitis, urinary tract infection, and gastroenteritis are frequent causes of febrile illness in any child, including those with shunts. *A tap should be performed if the child is lethargic, unusually irritable, photophobic, or has neck stiffness. A shunt tap should also be* considered if there is a history of similar presentation with a previous shunt infection or if there is unexplained fever or leukocytosis. *Staphylococcus epidermidis* and *S. aureus* are the two most common types of infective agents. Although intrathecal antibiotics may be successful, removal of an infected shunt is usually necessary for effective treatment.

III. *Other CNS complications* of shunts include meningitis, seizures, hematomas, and hygromas. Asymptomatic bilateral subdural effusions are common (30%) in VP shunts and can occur secondary to a siphoning effect of the shunt causing excess CSF to be drained. Programmable valves lessen this complication. Peritoneal complications include ascites and cyst formation, perforation of viscus or abdominal wall, infection with obstruction of the distal end of the catheter, and peritoneal metastases from CNS tumors (e.g., medulloblastoma). Other complications include soft tissue infection along the shunt tract and pressure necrosis of the skin.

Figure 46 shows the major components of typical shunt systems.

REFERENCE

Pople IK: *J Neurol Neurosurg Psychiatry* 73:i17–i22, 2002.

SICKLE CELL DISEASE

Sickle cell *anemia* is a homozygous state (HbSS) with a genetic defect of the beta-hemoglobin chain, creating hemoglobin S (HbS). This leads to red blood cells that are rigid and easily damaged under deoxygenated conditions and results in a hemolytic anemia. However, sickle cell *disease* often results from a heterozygous state with inheritance of HbS and one sickle cell gene mutation of a HbC gene (heterozygous HbSC disease). Sickle cell *trait* (HbAS) is unlikely to produce neurologic manifestations.

Neurologic manifestations are seen in one third of patients with sickle cell disease and may be the presenting sign. The frequency of neurologic manifestations is proportional to the propensity for sickling: 6% to 35% in SS disease, 6% to 24% in SC disease, and 0% to 6% in sickle cell trait (AS).

I. Stroke. In a population-based study, sickle cell disease is the most common cause of childhood stroke (39%). The lifetime risk of stroke is 25% to 30%. The infarct prevalence on MRI is 17%. The highest incidence of first infarct occurs between the ages of 2 and 5 years with the incidence decreasing between the ages of 20 and 29 years; another increase in ischemic stroke occurs between the ages of 35 and 45 years. The recurrence rate of infarction in patients who have had a prior clinical stroke is as high as 67%, with a mean interstroke interval of 28 months. Eighty percent of recurrences occur within 36 months of the initial infarct. *Risk factors for cerebral infarction include prior TIAs, anemia, recent acute chest syndrome, increased incidents of acute chest syndrome in the preceding 2 years,*

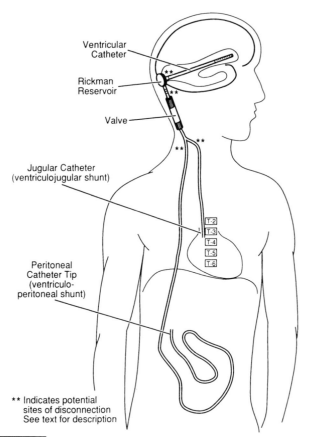

Ventricular
Catheter

Rickman
Reservoir

Valve

Jugular Catheter
(ventriculojugular shunt)

Peritoneal
Catheter Tip
(ventriculo-
peritoneal shunt)

** Indicates potential
sites of disconnection
See text for description

FIGURE 46

Typical shunt system (many variations exist).

*hypertension, silent infarcts, and high transcranial Doppler velocity
(>200 cm/second) in middle cerebral or intracranial carotid arteries
(40% stroke risk over 3 years).* Intracranial hemorrhage occurs in 3%
of sickle cell patients at a mean age of 25 years. Risk factors for
cerebral hemorrhage include history of prior infarcts, anemia, and high
leukocyte counts. Hemorrhages are more often subarachnoid in
children and intraparenchymal in adults. They may occur in
association with aneurysms, rupture of dilated vessels, hemorrhage
into infarcted tissue, or moyamoya disease. *Angiography can
precipitate sickling but may be safely performed after abnormal
hemoglobin is reduced to less than 20% by transfusions.* MRA may

serve as an alternative vascular evaluation with 85% accuracy compared to conventional angiography.

Patients with SS disease have a higher stroke rate than patients with SC disease. The level of fetal hemoglobin (HbF) correlates inversely with stroke incidence. Three intrinsic mechanisms contribute to ischemia in sickle cell disease. (1) There is large vessel endothelial injury because of the sickled cells, resulting in activation of inflammatory and thrombogenic cascades, intimal hyperplasia, and vessel occlusion. Particularly common are middle cerebral artery infarcts and watershed infarcts. (2) There is evidence of small vessel sludging and a relative deficiency of nitric oxide in these vessels, causing ischemia in small vessel distribution. (3) The chronic anemia leads to chronically increased cerebral perfusion and vasodilation and lack of cerebral autoregulatory reserve in meeting regional cerebral metabolic demands, causing a relative perfusion insufficiency. In addition, other unknown genetic (mutation resulting in thrombogenesis) and environmental (hypoxia and inflammation) factors may contribute to stroke risk in patients with sickle cell disease.

Treatment should be directed at improving the anemia with normalization of cerebral blood flow. It is recommended as a result of the STOP study to perform transfusions in all patients with elevated transcranial Doppler velocity (>200 cm/second). Transfusions decrease the stroke risk by 90%. Exchange transfusions are also recommended in patients with acute stroke to exchange HbA for HbS without increasing cerebral blood volume. Recurrence of ischemic stroke may be prevented by chronic intermittent exchange transfusion aimed at keeping HbS fraction below 30%. There are no established data of exchange transfusions after a cerebral hemorrhage. The role of bone marrow transplantation in preventing stroke recurrence is unclear. Hydroxyurea and short-chain fatty acids may offer some benefits by increasing production of fetal hemoglobin and decreasing sickling. Encephaloduroarteriosynangiosis procedures in conjunction with chronic intermittent transfusion may improve collateral circulation in patients with moyamoya-like syndrome.

II. Acute or chronic encephalopathy may occur and possibly represents a manifestation of cerebrovascular disease. Posterior reversible encephalopathy syndrome (PRES) has been reported in sickle cell patients with acute chest crisis. Cognitive dysfunctions are common in patients with silent and clinically evident infarcts.

III. Seizures occur in 8% to 12% of patients and are usually generalized tonic-clonic. In SS disease, they can occur in the absence of recognized cerebrovascular disease or intercurrent illness, although there may be precipitating factors such as medications, surgery, anesthesia, and acute chest syndrome. In SC disease intercurrent illness is frequently responsible. Patients undergoing bone marrow transplantation may develop seizures, particularly those patients with history of prior stroke.

Busulfan also increases the risk of seizures during the myeloablative phase.

IV. CNS infections with encapsulated organisms (such as *Streptococcus pneumoniae*) occur in patients with SS disease as a result of decreased phagocytic ability of the reticuloendothelial system (autosplenectomy).

V. Pain during sickle crisis is often severe and localizes to the affected organ. It is commonly treated with opiate analgesics. Headache is common and may be related to anemia and increased cerebral blood flow. It often improves after transfusion.

VI. Myelopathy resulting from vertebral body infarction, extramedullary hematopoiesis, and spinal cord infarction has been reported.

VII. Visual disturbances are much more frequent in SC than in SS disease. About one third of patients with SC disease first seek medical attention for visual impairment. Visual complications include vitreous, retinal, and subretinal hemorrhages; central retinal artery and vein occlusions; proliferative retinopathy; and other retinal vascular changes.

REFERENCES

Adams RJ, McKie VC et al: *N Engl J Med* 339:5–11, 1998.
Prengler M, Pavlakis SG et al: *Ann Neurol* 51:543–552, 2002.

SLEEP DISORDERS

The four major categories of sleep disorders are dyssomnias, parasomnias, medical-psychiatric disorders, and proposed sleep disorders.

I. Dyssomnias are disorders of initiating and maintaining sleep and are characterized by insomnia, excessive sleepiness, or abnormal circadian cycle.

A. Intrinsic dyssomnias arise from an endogenous source. These disorders include insomnias (details later), narcolepsy (details later), recurrent and idiopathic hypersomnias, obstructive sleep apnea (OSA), central sleep and hypoventilation apneas, periodic limb movements (PLMs), and restless legs syndrome (RLS).

B. Extrinsic dyssomnias arise from an external source such as sleep restriction or medications. These include sleep hygiene and insufficient sleep disorders, nocturnal eating syndrome, and drug-induced or dependent syndromes.

C. Circadian rhythm sleep disorders are common causes of excessive daytime sleepiness (EDS) and insomnias of varied forms, including time zone change (jet lag) and shift work syndromes and delayed/advanced sleep phase syndromes.

II. Parasomnias are abnormal physiologic or behavioral events occurring in sleep or its transitions of behavioral states.

A. Arousal disorders include sleepwalking, confusional arousals, and sleep terrors; they occur in non-REM sleep (versus nightmares, which occur during REM sleep).

B. Sleep-wake transition disorders are triggered by state changes and include rhythmic movement, sleep starts, and sleep talking disorders as well as nocturnal leg cramps.

C. Parasomnias are usually associated with REM sleep and include nightmares, sleep paralysis, REM sleep behavior disorder, and sleep-related painful erections.

D. Other parasomnias include sleep enuresis and bruxism, nocturnal paroxysmal dystonia, sudden infant death syndrome (SIDS), primary snoring, benign neonatal myoclonus, and sleep-related abnormal swallowing disorder.

III. Sleep disorders associated with mental, neurologic, or other medical disorders may be associated with the following:

A. Mental disorders, including psychosis, mood and panic anxiety disorders, and alcoholism

B. Neurologic disorders, including degenerative and dementing disorders, parkinsonism, fatal familial insomnia, status epilepticus of sleep, and sleep-related headaches

C. Other medical disorders, including sleep sickness, nocturnal cardiac ischemia, sleep-related breathing disorders, reflux and ulcer disease, and fibrositis syndrome

IV. Proposed sleep disorders include short and long sleepers and others, but insufficient information is available to verify their key features.

V. *Insomnia* is the most common sleep disorder.

Treatment: Associated medical or psychiatric conditions should be treated. General management of insomnia includes optimizing the patient's "sleep hygiene" as follows: Wake and retire at the same time each day (including weekends); use the bed only for sleep and sex; leave the bed if not asleep within 10 minutes of retiring; avoid heavy exercise or large meals just before bedtime; avoid daytime napping; make sure the bedroom is not too warm or cold; exercise regularly; and discontinue use of alcohol, caffeine, cigarettes, and psychoactive drugs. Other treatments include biofeedback and sleep restriction therapy. Short-acting benzodiazepines may offer temporary adjunctive benefit, but their long-term use is not recommended. Other sedatives, including chloral hydrate, zolpidem, and diphenhydramine, may be used judiciously.

VI. *Narcolepsy* is characterized by EDS or sudden muscle weakness, recurrent daytime naps or sleep lapses for more than 3 months, cataplexy, associated features of sleep paralysis and hypnogogic hallucinations, and abnormal multiple sleep latency tests (MSLTs) on polysomnogram (PSG). HLA DQ1B *0602 or DR2 positive.

Treatment is with stimulants and sodium oxybate.

REFERENCES

Gillin JC, Byerley WF: *N Engl J Med* 322:239–248, 1990.

American Academy of Sleep Medicine: *International classification of sleep disorders revised— Diagnostic and coding manual,* 2000.

SPASTICITY

Spasticity is a *velocity-dependent increase in muscle tone*. That is, more resistance will occur with rapid stretching of a muscle than with slow stretching. The underlying mechanism is a *hyperactive stretch reflex.* It results from damage to various descending pathways, most notably the dorsal and medial reticulospinal tract and the vestibulospinal tract.

Treatment: Overall, no medication is particularly useful in relieving the disabling spasticity of cerebral lesions (tightly flexed and adducted upper extremities, extended and adducted lower extremities). Painful flexor spasms can be markedly reduced by administration of baclofen or diazepam. Dantrolene may be helpful but causes mild to moderate muscle weakness, sedation, and dizziness. Combinations may be more effective, with fewer side effects.

I. *Baclofen* is a gamma-aminobutyric acid (GABA) agonist and also interferes with the release of excitatory transmitters. Starting dosage is 5 mg tid, increased by 5 mg per dose every 3 days to therapeutic effect. Maximum dosage is 80 mg/day in divided doses. Adverse effects include drowsiness, dizziness, weakness, nausea, mood changes, hallucinations, gastrointestinal symptoms, hypotension, changes in accommodation and ocular motor function, and deterioration of seizure control. Care should be used if renal disease is present; avoid abrupt withdrawal of the drug. Continuous infusion of intrathecal baclofen by means of an implanted infusion pump at a rate of 15 to 450 μg/day is useful in spasticity caused by spinal cord lesions or demyelinating disease and may be useful in spasticity of cerebral origin in cerebral palsy.

II. *Diazepam* facilitates GABA-mediated presynaptic and postsynaptic inhibition. Starting dosage is 2 mg bid, increased slowly to a maximum dosage of 60 mg/day in divided doses. Side effects are habituation and sedation.

III. *Dantrolene* sodium interferes with excitation-contraction coupling by decreasing the release of calcium at the sarcoplasmic reticulum. Starting dosage is 25 mg every day, increased by 25 mg every week to a maximum dosage of 100 mg qid. Side effects are hepatotoxicity (monitor liver enzymes) and diarrhea.

Drugs that bind to α_2-adrenergic receptors and decrease sympathetic outflow along with inhibiting afferent inputs into the spinal reflex arc can be used to treat spasticity.

I. *Tizanidine* should be started at 2 mg bid and increased by 2 to 4 mg with each dose until therapeutic effect is reached. Maximum dose is 12 mg tid. It is generally well tolerated but may cause increased fatigue or sedation.

II. *Clonidine* 0.2 to 1 mg/day in divided doses has similar effects but may cause sedation, orthostatic hypotension, and rebound hypertension.

III. *Chlorpromazine* (25 to 75 mg/day) causes α-adrenergic blockade and has been used to reduce spasticity, but sedation and fear of tardive dyskinesia have limited its use.

Others treatment includes the following:

Phenytoin (100 to 400 mg/day) and carbamazepine (600 to 1200 mg/day) act on the Ia afferent muscle spindle to reduce spontaneous and stretch-evoked discharges.

Surgical intervention with selective posterior rhizotomy has been used in patients with cerebral palsy and severe spasticity. Longitudinal myelotomy has been used to control severe flexor spasms. Spinal cord and cerebellar stimulation act by stimulating inhibitory pathways.

Botulinum toxin can be used to manage spasticity locally regardless of etiology (cerebral palsy, multiple sclerosis, stroke, etc.). Side effects include flaccidity, development of neutralizing antibodies, and rare systemic weakness. Doses take effect several days after injection and may last up to 3 months.

REFERENCES

Gormley ME, O'Brien CF, Yablon SA: *Muscle Nerve* Suppl 6:S14–20, 1997.
Satkunam LE: *CMAJ* 169:1173–1179, 2003.

SPINAL CORD

The relationships of the spinal cord segments and roots to the vertebral column are depicted in Figure 47. Cross-sectional anatomy of the cervical cord is shown in Figure 48.

SPINAL CORD SYNDROMES

Spinal shock is seen in the acute period after a spinal cord injury. It is a syndrome of paralysis, areflexia, anesthesia, and bowel or bladder dysfunction below the level of the lesion. *Spinal shock may last weeks*, after which the chronic symptoms of spinal cord injury appear: spasticity, exaggerated tendon and withdrawal reflexes, and positive Babinski's sign.

Anterior cord syndrome is characterized by paresis and impaired pain perception; proprioception is preserved below the lesion. The syndrome is usually caused by spinal cord compression or anterior spinal artery occlusion/infarction.

Posterior cord syndrome consists of pain and paresthesias out of proportion to motor impairment that are referable to the affected segments; the syndrome is commonly associated with demyelinating lesions.

Central cord syndrome, often seen with hyperextension injuries in the neck, results in patchy sensory loss, urinary retention, and weakness disproportionately affecting the legs.

Spinal cord hemisection produces the "*Brown-Sequard syndrome*," consisting of (1) ipsilateral spastic paresis; (2) ipsilateral loss of touch and vibratory and joint position sense; and (3) contralateral loss of pain and temperature sensation below the level of the lesion.

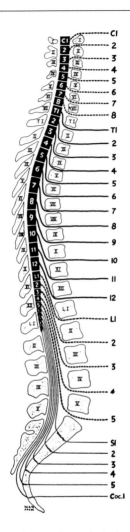

FIGURE 47

Relation of spinal segments and roots to the vertebral column. (From Haymaker W, Woodhall B: *Peripheral nerve injuries: Principles of diagnosis*, Philadelphia, WB Saunders, 1953.)

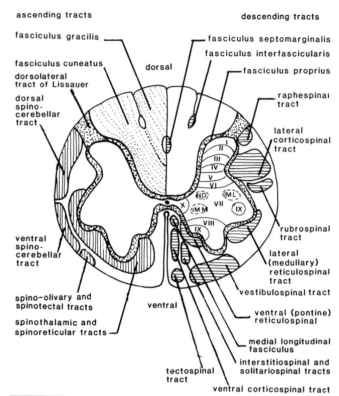

ascending tracts   descending tracts

fasciculus gracilis

fasciculus cuneatus
dorsolateral
tract of Lissauer
dorsal
spino-
cerebellar
tract

dorsal

fasciculus septomarginalis
fasciculus interfascicularis
fasciculus proprius

raphespinal
tract

lateral
corticospinal
tract

ventral
spino-
cerebellar
tract

spino-olivary and
spinotectal tracts

spinothalamic and
spinoreticular tracts

ventral

rubrospinal
tract

lateral
(medullary)
reticulospinal
tract

vestibulospinal tract

ventral (pontine)
reticulospinal

medial longitudinal
fasciculus

interstitiospinal and
solitariospinal tracts

tectospinal
tract

ventral corticospinal tract

FIGURE 48

Cervical spinal cord (cross section). Gray matter columns: *I–X*, Rexed's laminae:
IML, interomedial column; ND, nucleus dorsalis (Clark's column); PM, posteromedial
column.

CAUSES OF MYELOPATHY

I. *Congenital or developmental:* spinal dysraphism (see Developmental
Malformations), craniocervical junction abnormalities, syringomyelia,
congenital cervical spinal stenosis, tethered-cord syndromes,
diastatomyelia

II. *Degenerative:* spondylosis, motor neuron disease, spinocerebellar
degeneration, hereditary spastic paraplegia

III. *Demyelinating:* multiple sclerosis, neuromyelitis optica (*Devic's disease*)

IV. *Infectious:* poliomyelitis, herpes zoster, rabies, viral encephalomyelitis,
bacterial meningitis, epidural or subdural abscess, syphilis,
tuberculosis, typhus, spotted fever, fungal infections, trichinosis,

schistosomiasis, HTLV-1, human immunodeficiency virus (HIV), cytomegalovirus

V. *Inflammatory or immune response:* postinfectious, postvaccination, arachnoiditis, sarcoidosis, lupus erythematosus

VI. *Metabolic or nutritional:* pernicious anemia (vitamin B_{12} deficiency), pellagra, chronic liver disease

VII. *Neoplastic:* extramedullary or intramedullary tumors, meningeal carcinomatosis, paraneoplastic tumors

VIII. *Toxic:* ethanol (direct effect and through hepatic cirrhosis and portacaval shunting), arsenic, cyanide, lathyrism, clioquinol, intrathecal contrast or chemotherapeutic agents

IX. *Traumatic* (see later discussion): vertebral subluxation or fracture, transection, contusion, concussion, hemorrhage, birth injury (particularly breech delivery), electrical injury

X. *Vascular* (see later): arterial and venous infarction, hemorrhage (epidural, subdural, intraparenchymal), vasculitis, vascular malformations, aneurysms, effects of radiation therapy (see Radiation)

DEGENERATIVE JOINT DISEASE

Degenerative joint disease of the spine occurs as a result of changes in the intervertebral disks (spondylosis) with aging. Spondylosis leads to osteophyte formation, meningeal fibrosis, and disk herniation.

Spondylosis in the cervical spine can cause progressive myelopathy, radiculopathy, or both. Thoracic lesions become evident mainly as paraparesis. Lumbar lesions cause radiculopathies, neurogenic claudication, or back pain syndromes. Neurogenic claudication, like vascular claudication, causes exertional pain, but it differs from vascular claudication as follows: (1) the pain may be felt in buttock or thigh with prolonged standing or walking; (2) the pulses are normal; (3) reflexes may be decreased while at peak pain; and (4) the pain is relieved with waist flexion or rest but generally takes several minutes or more to resolve.

Syringomyelia describes a condition in which there is an abnormal cavity or cyst in the spinal cord. Syrinxes are usually cervical but may extend rostrally (syringobulbia) or caudally. They are frequently associated with developmental malformations of the craniocervical junction (Arnold-Chiari malformations, platybasia), myelomeningocele, kyphoscoliosis, intramedullary tumors, vascular malformations, or trauma. Hand numbness is the usual initial complaint with cervical syrinxes. Loss of pain and temperature sensation in a capelike (suspended) distribution with sparing of vibratory and joint position sense (dissociated sensory loss) is due to destruction of crossing pain fibers at the lesion level. Segmental weakness, atrophy, fasciculations, spasticity, incontinence, and hyperreflexia occur frequently. The course is usually slowly progressive; a sudden decline may indicate development of hematomyelia or progression of an underlying condition. Management includes cyst drainage and scrupulous hand care to prevent painless cuts and wound infections.

TRAUMA (See also SPINAL CORD TRAUMA)

Initial management of spinal cord trauma should include maintenance of airway, breathing, and circulation; immobilization (spine board, collars); bladder catheterization; nasogastric intubation; and serial neurologic examinations. Radiographic studies are directed to the area of interest but generally include cross-table lateral and AP cervical views (all seven cervical vertebrae must be seen) and films of the thoracic and lumbar spine. An open-mouth odontoid film may be obtained in conscious patients. CT is sensitive for identification of fractures. Myelography or MRI can identify acute compressive lesions such as hematomas. High-dose IV corticosteroids are commonly given, but their use is controversial. The NASCIS clinical trials, which have been criticized for their design flaws, fail to show conclusive evidence of the efficacy of corticosteroids in spinal cord injury. If given, methylprednisolone must be started in the first 8 hours after injury, as a bolus of 30 mg/kg, followed by an infusion of 5.4 mg/kg for 23 (first study) or 48 (second) hours.

VASCULAR SYNDROMES

I. *Anterior spinal artery infarctions* typically affect the midthoracic region, causing severe local, radicular, and deep pain; paraparesis; sphincter disturbance; and dissociated distal sensory loss (pain and temperature sensation more affected than vibration, touch, and joint position sense). Sacral sensation may remain intact. Causes include systemic hypotension, aortic dissection, vasculitis, embolism, sickle cell disease, and extrinsic arterial compression by tumor, bone, or disk material.

II. *Posterior spinal artery infarction* is less common and produces pain, loss of proprioception, and variable involvement of corticospinal and spinocerebellar tracts.

III. *Spinal subdural and epidural hemorrhage* most commonly occurs after trauma, lumbar puncture, or spinal or epidural anesthesia. Other causes include anticoagulant use, blood dyscrasias, thrombocytopenia, neoplasm, and vascular malformation. The initial symptom is severe back pain at the level of the bleed. Myelopathy or cauda equina syndrome with symptoms dependent on lesion level develop over hours to days. MRI is especially useful in determining lesion location. Laminectomy with clot evacuation should be performed as soon as possible because prognosis for recovery is better when surgery is performed early and the preoperative deficits are not severe.

IV. *Spinal subarachnoid hemorrhage* most commonly results from aneurysm rupture but may occur with vascular malformations. Other causes include aortic coarctation, spinal artery rupture, mycotic aneurysms, polyarteritis nodosa, spinal tumors, lumbar puncture, blood dyscrasias, and anticoagulants. Severe back pain followed by signs of meningeal irritation is usually the first manifestation. Multiple radiculopathies and myelopathy may develop. Headache, cranial neuropathies, and obtundation are associated with diffusion of blood above the foramen magnum. CSF is bloody and intracranial pressure may be elevated; treatment is directed at the underlying cause.

V. *Hematomyelia*: Intramedullary spinal hemorrhage is rare but occurs after trauma, spinal arteriovenous malformation rupture, hemorrhage into tumor or syrinx, or venous infarction or with clotting or bleeding disorders. Emergency surgical decompression is often indicated.

See also Spinal Cord Trauma, Spinal Cord Compression, and Tumors. See also Spinal Cord Injury in the Neurologic Emergency appendix for treatment of traumatic spinal cord compression.

REFERENCES

Bracken MB et al: *JAMA* 277(20):1597–1604, 1997.
Delamarter RB, Coyle J: *J Am Acad Orthop Surg* 7:166–175, 1999.
Derwenskus J, Zaidat OO: In Suarez JI, ed: *Critical care neurology and neurosurgery*, Totowa, NJ, Humana Press, 2004.

SPINAL CORD COMPRESSION (See also SPINAL CORD TRAUMA, SPINAL CORD INJURY IN NEUROLOGIC EMERGENCY APPENDIX)

CLINICAL PRESENTATION

Unlike cord trauma, spinal cord compression tends to develop more subacutely. Occasionally osteoporotic compression fractures and pathologic fractures from metastatic disease can produce more acute loss of function. However, the more common causes of cord compression such as metastatic tumors, hemorrhage, and abscess tend to progress slowly over a period of days to weeks. Clinically, these patients tend to present with progressive paraparesis or quadriparesis, though ataxia and altered sensory complaints may also present early depending on the location of the compressive lesion. Ventral lesions tend to produce motor symptoms early due to the ventrolateral position of the corticospinal tracts and less commonly due to involvement of the anterior spinal artery. More laterally placed lesions can cause the classic "crossed" sensory findings in which pain and temperature are lost below and contralateral to the lesion and vibration and proprioception are lost below and ipsilateral to the side of the lesion.

EVALUATION

Imaging with either CT or MRI forms the basis of diagnosis and should be obtained emergently to distinguish between demyelinating conditions and cord compression, as the outcome of compression is dependent on the time to decompression.

TREATMENT

Rapid decompressive surgery is the definitive therapy; however, IV steroids (see Spinal Cord Trauma for dosing) are also typically given at the time of presentation. Metastatic compression may be treated with large doses of dexamethasone (Decadron) 25 mg q 6 hr initially, then tapered down, and possibly radiation therapy.

REFERENCES

Derwenskus J, Zaidat OO: In Suarez JI, ed: *Critical care neurology and neurosurgery*, Totowa, NJ, Humana Press, 2004.

SPINAL CORD TRAUMA (See also SPINAL CORD COMPRESSION AND NEUROLOGIC EMERGENCIES APPENDIX)

Epidemiology: Spinal cord injury (SCI) is a leading cause of morbidity in the United States with an annual incidence of 10,000 cases per year. The most frequently affected group is young males with an average age of 30, and some 60% of cases affect males 16 to 30 years of age.

Causes: The most common causes of cord trauma are motor vehicle accident (37%), violence (26%), falls (22%), sports (7%), and other causes (8%).

Treatment: Short-term management involves quick recognition and stabilization of the spine along with rapid assessment for other life-threatening injuries. Prompt administration of IV methylprednisolone at 30 mg/kg over 1 hour followed by 5.4 mg/kg/hour for the next 23 hours has been shown to improve outcomes when started within 8 hours of injury. Placement of a Foley to prevent urinary retention and initiation of DVT (deep vein thrombosis) prophylaxis are also indicated. Long-term care is multidisciplinary and includes spinal cord medicine physicians and nurses, neurosurgeons or orthopedic surgeons, and urologists.

Prognosis: Although a devastating injury, with appropriate treatment survival is greater than 90% for isolated SCI. Overall outcome and functionality are primarily determined by the level of injury. Initial FIM and ASIA scores may predict disability and outcome.

REFERENCES

Derwenskus J, Zaidat OO: In Suarez JI, ed: *Critical care neurology and neurosurgery*, Totowa, NJ, Humana Press, 2004.

SPINAL EPIDURAL ABSCESSES

Anatomy: Below the foramen magnum there is a true epidural space in the lateral and posterior aspect of the spinal foramen that extends all the way down the length of the canal. This space is filled with fat, arteries, and venous plexus. Anterior to the cord the space is only virtual because the dura is adherent to the vertebral bodies from the foramen magnum to L1. As result, the majority of spinal epidural abscesses (SEAs) are posterior; when anterior, they are usually below L1.

Infectious routes: In one third of cases no source is identified. The other two thirds are most commonly associated with skin and soft tissue infections or complications of spinal surgery and spinal procedures, including epidural catheters. The spread is usually hematogenous but it may be contiguous from psoas, paraspinal, or retropharyngeal abscesses.

Risk factors:

I. *Compromised immunity*: diabetes (most common), steroid or immunosuppressive therapy, malignancy, pregnancy, cirrhosis, alcoholism, and HIV infection

II. *Disruption of the spinal column integrity*: trauma, spinal surgery, and spinal instrumentation

III. *Source of infection*: active urinary, respiratory, or skin infection; patients with indwelling catheters or epidural catheters, and IV drug use

Pathogenesis: Most SEAs begin as focal pyogenic diskitis. Inflammation and pus extend longitudinally to the epidural space, causing damage to the spinal cord at several levels by direct compression, thrombosis, and thrombophlebitis of nearby veins, interruption of arterial blood supply with ischemia, focal vasculitis, bacterial toxins, and local inflammatory process.

Microbiology: Staphylococcus aureus 63%, gram-negative bacilli 16%, streptococci 9%, coagulase-negative staphylococci 3%, anaerobes 2%, unknown 6%. In specific settings with more subacute clinical presentation *Mycobacterium tuberculosis* still represents 25% of SEAs.

Clinical presentation: The classic triad of back pain + fever + neurologic deficit is seen in only 13% of cases. Usually fever appears first followed by focal and severe back pain and possibly meningismus in cervical SEA. Root pain (shooting and electric pain) progresses over hours to days to progressive myelopathy with bladder/bowel incontinence. Once paraplegia-tetraplegia occurs, it quickly becomes irreversible.

Diagnosis: For clinically suspicious SEA an immediate MRI of spine with and without contrast (CT with contrast as alternative) is ordered. Also needed are ESR, blood cultures (×2), urinalysis for reflux, chest x-ray, and sputum cultures (for possible organism identification).

Differential diagnosis includes disc and bony disease, metastatic tumors, vertebral diskitis and osteomyelitis, meningitis, and herpes zoster before the skin lesions appear.

Treatment: Early decompression and drainage and prolonged antibiotic treatment remain the cornerstone treatment. Prompt infectious disease and neurosurgery consult is mandatory. Empiric Abx: vancomycin 1 g q 12 hr IV, metronidazol 500 mg q 6 hr IV, cefotaxime 2 g q 12 hr IV, or cefepime 2 g q 24 hr.

Prognosis: Mortality rate is 10% to 16%, and degree of recovery is related to the duration of neurologic deficits; absence of neurologic symptoms for less than 36 hours conveys better outcomes.

REFERENCES

Durack DT, Sexton DJ: *Up to Date,* 2006.
Grewal S, Hocking G, Wildsmith JA: *Br J Anaesth* 96(3):292–302, 2006.

SPINOCEREBELLAR ATAXIA (See also ATAXIA)

The spinocerebellar ataxias (SCAs) are a group of autosomal dominant disorders that are mostly triplet repeats. The number of repeats tends to be greater than 40 in diseased individuals, but varies between diseases. Many of these diseases have been identified, and most are merely numbered from 1 to 23 (i.e., SCA1, SCA2, etc.). The most common is Machado Joseph disease (MJD), also called SCA3. The episodic ataxias and dentatorubropallidoluysian atrophy are also included in the list. They usually begin in middle age. There is much clinical overlap in the syndromes, and genetic testing is required to identify the type. SCA5 through SCA7 are purely ataxic; SCA1 through SCA3 (MJD) and SCA4 have ophthalmologic, extrapyramidal, and cognitive involvement; and SCA7 has macular pigmentation. Research is ongoing about the mechanisms of these diseases. Most diseases show evidence of anticipation (worsening with later generations). Supportive care should be provided for most patients, including physical therapy, speech therapy, and social organization. Genetic counseling is recommended for all patients of reproductive age.

REFERENCE

Bradley WG, Daroff RB et al: *Neurology in clinical practice*, ed 4, Boston, Butterworth-Heinemann, 2004.

SPINOCEREBELLAR DEGENERATION

Spinocerebellar degeneration is a general term used to describe a heterogeneous group of inherited, acquired, or idiopathic disorders in which ataxia is a prominent manifestation.

STATUS EPILEPTICUS (See also EPILEPSY NCC AND NEUROLOGIC EMERGENCIES APPENDIX)

Status epilepticus represents one of the most common neurologic emergencies, with an incidence of around 150,000 cases annually. Generally, seizure activity that continues for more than 5 minutes or two or more seizures without a return to baseline mentation constitutes status epilepticus. The term status epilepticus can refer to several forms of ongoing seizure activity. The patient can be in convulsive status epilepticus, which is the classic continuous generalized tonic-clonic activity, or the patient can be in focal or partial status epilepticus, which may involve only a single part of the body such as the face or hand. Another type, which is much more difficult to diagnose, is nonconvulsive status epilepticus in which the patient is altered or comatose and has generalized seizure activity electrographically, but does not exhibit generalized tonic-clonic motor activity. Regardless of the type, all forms of status epilepticus should be treated promptly using the protocol given in the Neurologic Emergencies Appendix or some similar protocol. It has been shown that as many as 50% of cases of treated status epilepticus continue to show electrographic seizures on continuous EEG. Thus, an anticonvulsant should be IV loaded even if seizures appear to have stopped with administration of a benzodiazepine.

REFERENCE

Chen JWY, Wasterlain CG: *Lancet Neurol* 5:246–256, 2006.

SUBDURAL HEMATOMA

A subdural hematoma (SDH) is a collection of blood that develops from the extravasation of venous blood into the subdural space underneath the dura mater surrounding the brain (and rarely, the spinal cord). The cause varies with location, age of the patient, and whether the SDH is acute or chronic. The clinical presentation depends upon the size, location, and acuity of the SDH. Although subdural hematoma may be suspected clinically, diagnosis is made by CT or MRI as described later under Imaging.

ACUTE SUBDURAL HEMATOMA

In almost all cases of acute SDH, the cause is head trauma. In comatose patients with traumatic brain injuries, 20% to 25% will have a SDH. SDH is theorized to develop from injury to the bridging veins between the brain surface and adjacent dural venous sinuses or from disruption of major venous sinuses. Acceleration or deceleration injuries cause tearing or shearing of these bridging veins in the parasagittal or sylvian areas. When trauma causes parenchymal contusions or cortical lacerations, direct damage to the overlying veins can lead to SDH. The anatomic location of these kinds of SDH typically is along cerebral convexities, above the orbital roofs, or the temporal poles. In rare cases an acute SDH can develop following a lumbar puncture, and SDH can occur with spontaneous intracranial hypotension. On rare occasions SDH may develop acutely in patients with a bleeding diathesis.

In acute SDH the clot tends to develop quickly, and venous bleeding may stop as the intracranial pressure rises. Typical clinical features of acute SDH include headache (usually ipsilateral to the SDH), decreased alertness or confusion but with fluctuating mentation, and hemiparesis—if the SDH is located over the appropriate cortical areas. Hemiparesis is usually less pronounced than a lesion within the cortical parenchyma itself. If the SDH is large enough to cause compression of the contralateral cerebral peduncle against the free edge of the tentorium (Kernohan's notch), the hemiparesis may in fact be ipsilateral. Some language dysfunction (aphasia) may be observed for SDH appropriately located. Hemianopia is rare because of the deep anatomic location of the visual pathways.

CHRONIC SUBDURAL HEMATOMA

Chronic SDH is usually noted after the fact—when patients come in for workup of nonspecific, subacute or chronic symptoms, such as headaches, lightheadedness, psychomotor slowing, apathy, drowsiness, and less commonly a seizure. Patients tend to be elderly or on anticoagulation therapy, and a history of trauma may be unclear or remote from the time of clinical presentation.

IMAGING

Head CT imaging is the first choice of a diagnostic modality for cranial SDH, with sensitivity for hematomas having a thickness greater than 5 mm exceeding 90%. Acute SDH has a hyperdense appearance on CT, consistent with the appearance of acute intracranial bleeding. The shape is often crescentic because of the spread of the SDH over the hemispheric convexities. A thin border separating the clot from the cortex is often visible. After about a week, an acute SDH changes appearance to being isodense with brain tissue. Over the succeeding 2 to 6 weeks, the SDH evolves heterogeneously toward a hypodense appearance. MRI imaging makes a similar progression over time, beginning in the acute phase as hyperintense on T_1-weighted imaging and hypointense on T_2-weighted imaging. Over time the imaging qualities show chronicity of the SDH, with hypointensity of T_1-weighted images and hyperintensity of T_2-weighted images. The chronic SDH may form a vascular capsule after several weeks, which can enhance on MRI imaging. A majority of SDHs will liquefy within the capsule and may then enlarge actually. For uncertain reasons a minority (less than half) of SDHs remain stable in size and do not liquefy. In spinal SDH the preferred modality is spinal MRI for accurate diagnosis and delineation of the hematoma.

TREATMENT

Treatment of SDH depends upon its location, size, and acuity. Large or neurologically devastating SDHs require emergent drainage, usually with large craniotomies. Sometimes, burr holes are drilled in the hyperacute setting, when head imaging may be delayed or when there is rapid deterioration in the setting of severe head trauma. Posterior fossa SDH carries a high risk of brainstem compression and usually requires rapid surgical evacuation. SDHs that cause minor deficits or negligible midline shifts (commonly defined as less than 3–5 mm) may still need emergent evacuation, if acute, because there is a significant chance of enlargement within the acute period. Such patients are appropriately admitted for observation over several days (e.g., 2–3 days) to observe for clot enlargement. For chronic SDHs that are large or causing neurologic deficits, burr hole drainage may suffice if the clot has liquefied sufficiently.

PROGNOSIS

Patients who are rapidly treated and had good surgical results may do well. Comatose patients with acute SDH uniformly tend to have poor outcomes. Treatment of spinal SDH is less uniform because of its infrequency and therefore depends upon surgeon experience.

SDH in infants who do not present with an obvious history of head trauma (e.g., fall or vehicular accident) needs to be investigated for child abuse (e.g., shaken baby syndrome), particularly when there is an interhemispheric SDH and retinal hemorrhages, raising suspicion of abuse.

REFERENCES

Hung KS, Lui CC et al: *Spine* 27:E534–538, 2002.
Kemp AM: *Arch Dis Child* 86:98–102, 2002.
Stieg PE, Kase CS: *Neurol Clin* 16:373–390, 1998.

SYNCOPE

Syncope is brief loss of consciousness and postural tone resulting from decreased cerebral perfusion.

CLINICAL PRESENTATION

Syncope may occur after prodromal features, such as diaphoresis, pallor, nausea, and visual changes (blurring, dimming, constriction), or it may occur suddenly without prodrome; the generalization that the latter situation is more suggestive of an arrhythmogenic source does not preclude that an arrhythmia can also produce a prodrome. If cerebral hypoperfusion persists, as when the subject is held upright in a procedure chair, tonic-clonic jerks and urinary incontinence (convulsive syncope) may result. After a syncopal spell, some patients have transient generalized weakness, but confusion, headache, and drowsiness are uncommon.

Syncope can be classified by pathophysiologic mechanism as follows.

I. *Vasovagal* (vasodepressor, neurocardiogenic) syncope occurs either spontaneously or in response to stimuli that include prolonged standing, hot conditions, stress, pain, fear, or other strong emotional stimuli (such as the sight of blood). This common type of syncope is thought to be mediated by the Bezold-Jarisch reflex: venous pooling in the lower extremities results in reduced cardiac output and blood pressure, thus activating aortic arch and carotid sinus baroreceptors with a resultant increase in sympathetic outflow that causes the poorly filled ventricle to contract vigorously. Mechanoreceptors (C-fibers) in the heart chambers and pulmonary artery are activated in some individuals; via projections to the dorsal vagal nucleus of the medulla, the mechanoreceptors produce an increase in vagal tone and a withdrawal of peripheral sympathetic tone, resulting in bradycardia, vasodilation, and consequently loss of consciousness. Vasovagal syncope is particularly common in young adults.

II. *Impaired splanchnic and visceral vasoconstriction* results in a defective vasopressor response to postural changes. Causes include medications (antihypertensives, tricyclic antidepressants, phenothiazines, levodopa, lithium), autonomic neuropathy (diabetes, amyloidosis, porphyria, Guillain-Barré syndrome, Riley-Day syndrome), idiopathic orthostatic hypotension, central dysautonomias, sympathectomy, and prolonged bed rest.

III. *Hypovolemia* occurs in the context of dehydration (as from strenuous exercise, hot environment, vomiting, diarrhea, or inadequate oral intake), hemorrhage, or another source of blood loss (hemodialysis, phlebotomy). In contrast to "benign" conditions such as vasovagal syncope, here loss of consciousness may indicate that the patient is going into circulatory shock and requires volume resuscitation.

IV. *Reflex syncope* is an inappropriate response to vagal stimuli. Syncope may thus occur in the context of micturition (mostly in men), the postprandial state (or after ingesting cold liquids), vagal irritation by esophageal diverticula or mediastinal masses, carotid sinus stimulation (by a tight collar, head turning, or shaving), Valsalva maneuver (weightlifting, strain, defecation), coughing (classically in overweight smokers), or glossopharyngeal neuralgia.

V. *Cardiac syncope* is generally unrelated to posture and may be classified as follows:

A. Arrhythmias that diminish cardiac output: long QT syndrome, third-degree atrioventricular (AV) block (Stokes-Adams attack), sick-sinus syndrome, profound sinus bradycardia and other bradyarrhythmias, supraventricular tachycardias, ventricular tachycardia and fibrillation, and pacemaker failure

B. Outflow obstruction: aortic stenosis, hypertrophic obstructive cardiomyopathy, pulmonary stenosis, pulmonary embolism, pulmonary hypertension, tetralogy of Fallot

C. Pump failure: myocardial infarction, cardiac tamponade, severe congestive heart failure

VI. *Cerebrovascular disease* is a very uncommon cause of syncope, but vertebrobasilar insufficiency and the subclavian steal syndrome have been associated with syncopal episodes. A history of acute severe headache preceding the loss of consciousness should prompt evaluation for subarachnoid hemorrhage.

VII. *Metabolic derangement* such as hypoxia, hypocapnia, and hypoglycemia frequently produces lightheadedness, but rarely syncope.

Conditions that may mimic syncope include atonic seizures, cataplexy, acute vertigo, and conversion and factitious disorders. True syncope should not produce postictal confusion, and neither vertigo nor cataplexy is associated with loss of consciousness.

DIAGNOSIS

The most useful tools for evaluation of syncope are the *clinical history* (ask about precipitants, body position, prodrome, prior episodes, orientation on awakening, family history, seizure risk factors, cardiac and cerebrovascular disease, autonomic and neuropathic symptoms, and medications); *physical examination* (orthostatic vital signs, estimate of volume status, cardiac and cervical auscultation, and peripheral nerve and autonomic examination); and *ECG* (always check the corrected QT interval). More sophisticated (but lower yield) evaluation can be undertaken with prolonged ambulatory ECG monitoring and head-upright tilt test (the gold standard test for diagnosis of vasovagal syncope, with an estimated specificity of 90% in the absence of provocative agents such as isoproterenol). EEG, carotid ultrasound, MRA, and head CT have low diagnostic yield with unremarkable history and examination.

TREATMENT

Treatment of vasovagal syncope (Table 97) may proceed in a stepwise fashion. First, patients are educated to avoid precipitants, and dietary sodium intake is liberalized. Medications that may cause or exacerbate orthostasis or volume depletion are discontinued if possible. If these measures fail, beta-blockers are employed as first-line therapy. Should beta-blockers fail or be contraindicated, the patient may be tried on fludrocortisone or midodrine. If pharmacologic measures fail, pacemaker placement may be considered.

REFERENCES

Atiga WL et al: *J Cardiovasc Electrophysiol* 10:874–888, 1999.
Getchell WS et al: *J Gen Intern Med* 14:677–687, 1999.
Grubb BP: *N Engl J Med* 352:1004–1010, 2005.

TABLE 97

GENERAL MANAGEMENT OF SYNCOPE*

Management Approach	Dose	Comments
Lifestyle changes		
Fluid intake	About 2 L/day	Poor compliance, frequent urination
Salt intake	2 g/day	Edema, gastrointestinal upset
Physical maneuvers	Isometric arm contraction; leg crossing	Unable to use in absence of prodrome
Tilt training	10–30 min/day of standing	Poor compliance
High thigh stocking		
Drugs		
Midodrine	2.5–10 mg tid	Nausea, scalp pruritus, hypertension
Fludrocortisone	0.1–0.2 mg daily	Bloating, hypokalemia, headache
Beta-blockers	Drugs such as metoprolol (50 mg qd to bid)	Prosyncope, fatigue, bradycardia
Selective serotonin reuptake inhibitors	Drugs such as paroxetine (20 mg daily) or escitalopram (10 mg daily)	Nausea, diarrhea, insomnia, agitation

*Adjust management measures according to the underlying cause and comorbid conditions.

S

SYNCOPE

SYNDROME OF INAPPROPRIATE SECRETION OF ANTIDIURETIC HORMONE

SIADH is due to nonphysiologic stimulation of antidiuretic hormone (ADH) secretion, resulting in hypotonic (serum osmolality < 280 mOsm/L) hyponatremia (Na < 134 mEq/L) with concentrated urine (osmolality > 300 mmol/kg) and urine sodium excretion (>20 mEq/L).

Diagnosis: The diagnostic criteria are (1) *euvolemia/hypervolemia*; (2) normal adrenal, renal, and thyroid function; (3) absence of an iatrogenic cause of ADH release.

Etiology: Neurologic causes include stroke, subdural hematoma, subarachnoid hemorrhage, head trauma, intracranial surgery, tumors, basal skull fractures, cerebral atrophy, acute encephalitis, tuberculous or purulent meningitis, Guillain-Barré syndrome, acute intermittent porphyria, CNS lupus erythematosus, and sarcoidosis. Nonneurologic causes include bronchogenic carcinoma, tuberculosis, pulmonary aspergillosis, anemia, stress, severe pain, hypotension, acute intermittent porphyria, and drugs such as chlorpropamide, oxytocin, thiazide diuretics, and carbamazepine. This syndrome must be differentiated from cerebral salt-wasting (CSW) syndrome, which can occur in similar intracranial disorders as SIADH. In CSW, patients are usually hypovolemic, with increased plasma albumin, BUN/creatinine ratio, and high hematocrit.

Manifestations are due to the hyponatremia and include mental status changes, behavioral changes, weakness, anorexia, nausea, vomiting, muscle cramps, and extrapyramidal signs. Seizures, coma, and death may occur with severe hyponatremia.

Therapy involves treatment of the underlying cause and fluid restriction to 800 to 1000 mL daily. If hyponatremia is severe or the patient is symptomatic, correction with hypertonic saline is recommended. The rate of infusion should be no faster than 0.5 mEq/hour to avoid the possibility of inducing central pontine myelinolysis.

REFERENCES
Adrogue HJ, Madias NE: *N Engl J Med* 342:1581–1589, 2000.
Palmer BF: *Trends Endocrinol Metab* 14:182–187, 2003.

SYPHILIS

Neurosyphilis results from meningeal invasion by *Treponema pallidum*; parenchymal involvement occurs in later stages (i.e., general paresis and tabes dorsalis). Symptomatic neurosyphilis develops in only 4% to 9% of patients with syphilis who do not receive treatment. Clinical syndromes include the following:

I. *Asymptomatic neurosyphilis* refers to the presence of CSF abnormalities in the absence of neurologic signs and symptoms. The highest rate of abnormalities occurs early, 13 to 18 months after initial infection; the diagnosis is made on the basis of positive results of serum or CSF serologic tests and abnormal CSF, usually with a mildly increased level of protein (40 to 200 mg/dL); a normal glucose level; and a mild lymphocytic pleocytosis (50 to 400 cells/mm^3). The level of CSF gamma globulins may be increased. Normal CSF 5 years after infection reduces the risk of CNS syphilis to 1%. Ten percent to 25% of patients with asymptomatic neurosyphilis who do not receive treatment become symptomatic. Lumbar puncture, therefore, should be performed in all patients in whom a diagnosis of syphilis is made beyond the primary stage or in whom the dating of primary infection cannot be established.

II. *Acute syphilitic meningitis* usually occurs within the initial 2 years of infection and becomes evident as headache, nuchal rigidity, confusion, and cranial nerve palsies (especially CN II, III, VI, and VIII).

III. *Meningovascular syphilis* usually occurs within 4 to 7 years after initial infection and results from an endarteritis, most commonly of the middle cerebral artery. Meningovascular syphilis becomes evident as a focal CNS ischemia that evolves acutely or over days and is often associated with a prodrome (weeks to months) of headache, dizziness, and psychiatric disturbances.

IV. *General paresis (meningoencephalitis)* usually occurs 15 to 20 years after initial infection as a result of spirochete invasion of the cortex. Dementia is the initial manifestation. Seizures may occur. Untreated, the condition is fatal within 4 years.

V. *Tabes dorsalis* occurs 20 to 25 years after infection and results from inflammation of the posterior roots and posterior columns. Classic presentation includes triads of symptoms (lightning pain, dysuria, and ataxia) and signs (Argyll-Robertson pupils, areflexia, and proprioceptive loss). Later involvement includes visceral crises, optic atrophy, ocular motor palsies, Charcot joints, and foot ulcers. Early treatment usually arrests the progression and may reverse some of the symptoms.

VI. Less common manifestations include optic neuropathy, eighth nerve neuropathy, spinal neurosyphilis (e.g., meningomyelitis and meningovascular), and gumma (granulomatous mass lesions in brain or spinal cord).

VII. Patients coinfected with HIV have a higher rate of early neurosyphilis (meningitis or meningovascular) and may be at an increased risk for neurologic relapse after treatment of primary and secondary syphilis with IM benzathine penicillin. This may indicate that the CNS is a "sheltered" site from which relapse may proceed.

Diagnosis depends on clinical findings, serum serologic results, and CSF examination. Serum treponemal serologic tests (VDRL and RPR) become nonreactive with treatment and therefore can be used to assess therapeutic efficacy. However, their titers progressively decline, even during the course of untreated disease, becoming nonreactive in 25% of patients with late syphilis (neurosyphilis). Serum treponemal tests (FTA-ABS, MHA-TP) are usually unaffected by treatment, their titers remaining elevated indefinitely. Therefore, a nonreactive FTA-ABS result excludes neurosyphilis.

S

SYPHILIS

The CSF in neurosyphilis usually shows elevated protein level, normal glucose level, and lymphocytic pleocytosis (10 to 400 cells/mm^3). The CSF VDRL has very high specificity but low sensitivity (30% to 70%). Thus, nonreactive CSF VDRL does not exclude neurosyphilis. The CSF FTA-ABS test has a high false-positive rate, and its role in diagnosis is unclear. As with all CSF serologic studies, a traumatic spinal fluid sample may also give misleading results.

Treatment of neurosyphilis consists of a regimen of aqueous penicillin G, 2 to 4 million units IV q 4 hr for 10 to 14 days. An alternative treatment is penicillin G procaine 2 to 4 million units IM qd with probenecid 500 mg PO qid for 10 to 14 days. In cases of penicillin allergy, treatment options include penicillin desensitization followed by standard penicillin therapy; other regimens, such as tetracycline hydrochloride 500 mg PO qid for 30 days, erythromycin 500 mg PO qid for 30 days, or ceftriaxone 250 mg IM qd, are recommended for primary, secondary, or latent syphilis but are of unproven value for tertiary neurosyphilis.

Follow-up CSF examination should be performed at 6 and 12 months. The CSF cell count is the earliest indicator of response and relapse and should normalize within 6 months. CSF protein level declines more slowly, taking as long as 2 years to normalize. CSF VDRL titers are the last to decline and may remain mildly elevated despite adequate treatment. Repeat treatment is indicated if the CSF pleocytosis persists after 6 months or is abnormal 2 years after treatment. Because CSF protein level and VDRL titers take much longer to normalize, treatment cannot be considered inadequate unless these values unequivocally increase.

REFERENCES

Hook EW, Marra CM: *N Engl J Med* 326:1060–1069, 1992.
Katz DA, Berger JR, Duncan RC: *Arch Neurol* 50:234–249, 1993.
Simon RP: *Arch Neurol* 42:606–613, 1985.

TASTE

Taste buds containing receptor cells are located in the anteroposterior aspect of the tongue, soft palate, pharynx, epiglottis, and proximal one third of the esophagus. The facial, glossopharyngeal, and vagus nerves mediate taste sensation. Facial nerve afferents mediate taste from the anterior two thirds of the tongue, and the greater superficial petrosal branch of the facial nerve carries taste from the soft palate. The lingual, tonsillar, and pharyngeal branches of the glossopharyngeal nerve carry taste from the posterior one third of the tongue and pharynx. The superior laryngeal branch of the vagus nerve carries taste from the esophagus and epiglottis. All afferent taste fibers project to the solitary tract nucleus. Fibers then project to the thalamus, ventral forebrain, lateral hypothalamus, and amygdala. From the thalamus, fibers mediating taste sensation project to the insular cortex.

Loss of taste sensation (ageusia or hypogeusia) can be due to a variety of focal and metabolic causes. Complete ageusia is rare. Loss of olfactory sensation is the most common cause of loss of "taste." Tobacco smoking, loss of salivary function (e.g., Sjögren's syndrome), head and neck surgery, postirradiation, amyloidosis, Kallmann's syndrome, vitamin B_{12} deficiency, inner or middle ear inflammation, viral infections of the upper respiratory tract, and medications such as sulfa-containing drugs, calcium channel blockers, and chemotherapeutic drugs (e.g., doxorubicin) are associated with hypogeusia. Proximal lesions of the facial nerve between the pons and facial canal where the chorda tympani joins the facial nerve result in the unilateral loss of taste. Cerebellopontine angle tumors occasionally cause a loss of taste. Gustatory hallucinations may occur as an aura of partial epilepsy or in delirium and are usually associated with olfactory hallucinations.

Spontaneous dysgeusia or glossodynia is more complex to evaluate. Differential diagnosis is similar to the preceding list, but may also include entities such as diabetic neuropathy, fibromyalgia, and gastroesophageal reflux disease. The burning tongue or burning mouth syndrome is often responsive to clonazepam, but may also respond to topical steroids, paroxetine, clotrimazole, or olanzapine.

Taste testing for the primary modalities of salty, sweet, sour, and bitter is accomplished with the use of a cotton applicator. Ideally, the patient should not speak but should point to cards with the words sweet, salty, bitter, and sour written on them. More sophisticated testing with electrogustometry or filter paper disks with progressive dilutions are sometimes clinically useful, particularly in cases of mild disease or sensory loss.

REFERENCE

Pribitkin E, Rosenthal MD, Cowart BJ: *Ann Otol Rhinol Laryngol* 112(11):971–978, 2003.

TEMPORAL LOBE

The temporal lobe is bordered superiorly by the sylvian fissure and merges with the parietal and occipital lobes. It consists of superior, middle, inferior, and transverse temporal gyri. The transverse temporal gyrus hiding within the lateral fissure contains the primary auditory cortex (Brodmann's area 41) and secondary auditory cortex (Brodmann's area 42). The superior temporal gyrus contains Wernicke's area on the dominant hemisphere. Other functionally important structures such as the amygdala, hippocampus, and olfactory and entorhinal cortices also harbor in the temporal lobe. Symptoms of temporal lobe dysfunction include partial complex seizures, memory difficulties (especially bilateral hippocampal involvement, but nonverbal memory may be impaired with nondominant hippocampal damage and verbal with dominant hemisphere lesions), Wernicke's aphasia with dominant temporal lesion, auditory agnosias, visual field defects (superior quadrantanopias), and behavioral and emotional disturbances. The *Klüver-Bucy syndrome* of placidity, apathy, hypersexuality, hyperorality, and visual and auditory agnosia occurs with bilateral anterior temporal lobe injury such as brain trauma, encephalitis, stroke, tumors, or degenerative dementias.

THYROID

Both hyperthyroidism and hypothyroidism can have neurologic manifestations. Prompt recognition and treatment can result in good clinical outcomes.

HYPERTHYROIDISM

I. *Thyrotoxic crisis* is a medical emergency. It initially manifests as high fever, tachycardia, hypotension, vomiting, diarrhea, and delirium and may progress to coma and death if not treated promptly. Crisis may be precipitated by infection or inadequate preparation for thyroid surgery.

   Treatment involves thiourea agents, sodium iodide, adrenergic blockers, corticosteroids, sedatives, body cooling, and fluid/electrolyte maintenance.

   Prognosis: Mortality rate is as high as 30%.

II. *Acute thyrotoxic encephalomyelopathy* may occur, presenting as an acute bulbar palsy with associated encephalopathy. Brain swelling and focal hemorrhages are seen pathologically. Symptoms may resolve with achievement of a euthyroid state. Seizures, usually generalized, may develop or be exacerbated during thyrotoxicosis. EEG abnormalities (generalized slowing and increased alpha activity) are seen in 60% of patients with hyperthyroidism.

III. *Psychological manifestations:* Psychosis is also associated with hyperthyroidism. "Apathetic hyperthyroidism" is common in the elderly and may manifest as dementia with apathy and depression.

IV. *Tremor:* An accentuation of physiologic tremor, due to increased sensitivity to sympathetic input, is very common in hyperthyroid patients and involves primarily the upper extremities. Treatment consists of correcting the thyroid abnormality; propranolol is also useful.

V. *Other CNS syndromes:* Chorea, resulting from hypersensitivity of dopaminergic receptors, responds to neuroleptics. Stroke results from cerebral embolism in thyrotoxic atrial fibrillation. Acute anticoagulation may be appropriate.

VI. *Peripheral nervous system abnormalities* associated with thyroid disease include a rare *chronic thyrotoxic myopathy*; however, complaints of nonspecific weakness are common. Creatine kinase (CK) is normal or decreased. EMG reveals short-duration polyphasic motor unit potentials. Muscle power normalizes as the patient becomes euthyroid. Thyrotoxic periodic paralysis that resembles hypokalemic periodic paralysis also occurs. Myasthenia gravis has an increased incidence in patients with hypo- or hyperthyroidism and hypo- or hyperthyroidism has an increased incidence in myasthenic patients. *Neuropathy* is very uncommon.

HYPOTHYROIDISM

Hypothyroidism may present in infancy with mental retardation and growth abnormalities, resulting in cretinism. Fortunately, this is now rare, because many countries have instituted neonatal screening programs.

I. CNS manifestations

Clinical presentation: In the elderly, hypothyroidism may present with *cognitive dysfunction*, sometimes confused with a primary degenerative dementia. Associated signs of systemic hypothyroidism are variable and psychosis may occur. All new-onset dementia patients must be screened for hypothyroidism. *Coma* occurs rarely, usually in chronic, severe, undiagnosed disease. Seizures may occur.

Laboratory tests: EEG changes include slowing of alpha activity and decreased driving response with high-frequency photic stimulation. Markedly reduced background amplitude may be seen in hypothermic states. CSF protein is elevated in 40% to 90% of hypothyroid patients, occasionally greater than 100 mg/dL. Gamma globulin may also be increased in both CSF and serum for unknown reasons.

Treatment: Emergency management consists of thyroid replacement (PO or IV); corticosteroids; treatment of hypoglycemia, fluid/electrolyte abnormalities, and hypothermia; and ventilatory support as needed. Cerebellar ataxia with impaired tandem gait and limb incoordination but often without nystagmus or dysarthria has also been reported.

II. *Peripheral manifestations* occur in a variety of forms. *Hypothyroid myopathy* has weakness (proximal > distal), cramps, pain, and stiffness as common complaints, but objective weakness is less common. Creatine phosphokinase (CPK) is often elevated. EMG findings are nonspecific. *Myoedema*, a percussion-induced local mounding of contracted muscle that relaxes slowly, may be elicited, but can also occur in emaciated patients and some normal subjects. The contraction is electrically silent on EMG. Muscle hypertrophy, known as *Hoffman's syndrome* in adults and *Kocher-Debre-Semelaigne syndrome* in children, is rare. Patients complain of stiffness and painful muscle cramps, and the movements are slow and weak. The muscles are large and firm. *Pseudomyotonia*, or delayed muscle relaxation after handshake or percussion, may be present and is differentiated from myotonia by its electrical silence on EMG.

Peripheral neuropathies are mostly entrapment neuropathies (carpal tunnel), resulting from mucoid infiltration of the nerve and the surrounding tissue. Eighty percent of patients complain of distal paresthesias. Polyneuropathies are less frequent. Deep tendon reflexes have slowed relaxation time and are also seen in hypothermia, leg edema, diabetes, parkinsonism, drugs, and normal aging.

REFERENCES

Anagnos A, Ruff RL, Kaminski HJ: *Neurol Clin* 15:673–696, 1997.
Horak HA et al: *Neurol Clin* 18:203–213, 2000.

TOURETTE'S SYNDROME (GILLES DE LA TOURETTE'S SYNDROME)

Tics are sudden, intermittent, stereotypical involuntary movements. The DSM-IV defines this syndrome as characterized by the following:

I. Both multiple motor tics and one or more vocal tics present at some time during the illness, although not necessarily concurrently.

II. Tics occur many times a day (usually in bouts), nearly every day, or intermittently for more than 1 year, without a tic-free interval of more than 3 consecutive months.

III. Anatomic location, number, frequency, complexity, and severity of tics change over time.

IV. Onset occurs before 18 years of age.

V. It does not occur exclusively during psychoactive substance intoxication or known CNS disease.

VI. Social, academic, or occupational functioning is impaired.

HISTORY

The onset of tics is most commonly between ages 3 and 8 years. Boys are affected three to four times more than girls. Tourette's syndrome typically waxes and wanes in severity, with many patients having a dramatic reduction in tics in their 20s. Obsessive compulsive disorder (OCD) and attention deficit hyperactivity disorder (ADHD) occur in 25% to 35% of these patients and have a profound impact on both an academic and a social scale.

PHYSICAL EXAMINATION

Motor tics may be simple, like eye blinking, or complex, like facial gestures, grooming behaviors, jumping, or obscene gestures *(copropraxia)*. Vocal tics include sniffing, snorting, throat clearing, or barking. More complex vocal tics include *coprolalia* (utterance of obscenities), *echolalia*, and *palilalia*. In contrast to public perception, coprolalia is quite rare. Tics may be exacerbated by anger or stress, may be diminished during sleep, and become attenuated during some absorbing activity. They may be voluntarily suppressed for minutes to hours.

PATHOGENESIS

Pathogenesis is still unclear. Recent theories have focused on genetics and autoimmune causes, particularly following streptococcal infection. The term PANDAS refers to pediatric autoimmune neuropsychiatric disorder, and this entity is somewhat controversial. Other possible risk factors include maternal caffeine, tobacco, cocaine, and alcohol use, transient perinatal hypoxia, and low Apgar scores.

TREATMENT

Treatment should be reserved for those cases in which the child's self-esteem or social interactions are affected. It is not uncommon for the parents to be more troubled about the tics than the patient.

A multidisciplinary therapeutic program must be established, in close collaboration with the parents, child, and school. Frequently, these patients will have special talents (athletic or music skills), which should be encouraged. When treatment is initiated, it is often difficult to gauge efficacy because of the natural waxing and waning severity of the disorder. Thus, drastic changes in dose or medications should be avoided, especially during exacerbations. *Clonidine,* an α_2-adrenergic agonist, has often been used as a first choice in an attempt to delay use of neuroleptic agents. This medication is beneficial in treating the associated hyperactivity as well, and warrants first-line consideration based on its efficacy in controlled trials. *Dopamine receptor antagonists* are the mainstay in treatment. Traditionally, haloperidol and pimozide had been used for treatment, but because of side effects, transition to the "atypical" antipsychotics (fluphenazine, olanzapine, risperidone, quetiapine, and ziprasidone) has been recommended. *Risperidone and olanzapine* have been found to be efficacious, but their use may be limited in children because of associated weight gain. The associated comorbid conditions of ADHD and OCD are often more disabling and should be treated prior to treating tics as these conditions produce stress, which can often make tics worse. *Stimulant medications have been accused of exacerbating tics*, but this is not supported by randomized trials. These medications should be used in patients who have ADHD. OCD should be treated with selective serotonin reuptake inhibitors. Early treatment of tics does not alter the natural history.

REFERENCES

Leckman JF: *Brain Devel* 25(Suppl 1):S24–S28, 2003.
Sandor P: *J Pyschosomatic Res* 55:41–48, 2003.

TOURETTE'S SYNDROME

TRANSCRANIAL DOPPLER ULTRASOUND (See also AAN GUIDELINE SUMMARIES APPENDIX)

Transcranial Doppler ultrasound (TCD) is becoming increasingly used in clinical neurology and in the neurocritical care unit. Doppler ultrasound scanning measures blood flowing through the carotid arteries or the arteries at the base of the brain. TCD is used to evaluate ischemic and hemorrhagic stroke, Patent Foramen Ovale (PFO), and right-to-left shunt with quantification of the high-intensity signals transits (HITS) when performed with saline bubbles and contrast medium, sickle cell disease, brain death evaluation, intraoperative cardiac and carotid surgery monitoring, and other physiologic testing of cerebrovascular reserves.

The four types of Doppler ultrasound are as follows:

I. Continuous wave Doppler measures how continuous sound waves change in pitch as they encounter blood flow. This type of ultrasound can be done at the bedside to provide a quick estimate of the disease.

II. Duplex Doppler produces a picture of a blood vessel and surrounding tissue. A computer converts the Doppler sounds into a graph that provides information about the speed and direction of blood flow through the blood vessel being examined.

III. Color Doppler uses a computer to convert the Doppler sounds into colors that are overlaid on the image of a blood vessel. The colors represent the speed and direction of flow through the vessel.

IV. Power Doppler is a new technique being developed that is up to five times more sensitive than color Doppler. Power Doppler can get pictures that are difficult or impossible to obtain standard color Doppler.

TCD is performed by insonating the major cerebral arteries through different bone/skull "windows." Depending on the window, depth and direction of the waveform away or toward the probe, and sound pitch the vessels insonated will be identified. The following windows are commonly utilized:

I. The transtemporal window: The intracranial vessels are insonated through the thinnest portion of the squamous component of the temporal bone.

II. The transorbital window: The carotid siphon and the ophthalmic artery can be directly insonated by having the ultrasound beam cross the contents of the orbit. In some cases, cross-insonation of the contralateral half of the circle of Willis is also possible.

III. The suboccipital or transforaminal window: Insonation of the vertebral and the basilar arteries can be accomplished by taking advantage of the space between the atlas and the base of the skull, as well as passing the ultrasound beam through the foramen magnum.

The mean cerebral blood flow velocities (MCBFVs) are obtained and sampled for each vessel at various depths. Normal values vary for each laboratory and generally are below 100 m/second in all insonated vessels. MCBFVs increased in vasospasm secondary to SAH to more than 150 m/second and in intracranial stenosis, sickle cell disease, and severe anemia. The ratio of the middle cerebral artery (MCA) MCBFV to the extracranial internal carotid artery (ICA) MCBFV is called Lindegaard ratio (MCA/ICA), which correlates very well with real increase in the velocity and presence of vasospasm in SAH when it is more than 3. Asymmetry in MCBFVs is another indication of disease. Elevated pulsatility indices indicate increase in downstream pressure that can be seen in brain death, cerebral edema, and hydrocephalus and other causes of increased ICP.

REFERENCE

Babikian VL, Wechsler LR, eds: *Transcranial Doppler ultrasonography*, ed 2, Boston, Butterworth-Heinemann, 1999.

TRANSPLANTATION

ORGAN HARVEST

Death determination prior to organ harvest is based on neurologic criteria. At present, most jurisdictions require absence of function of the entire brain (see Brain Death).

CLINICAL SYNDROMES IN ORGAN RECIPIENTS

Following organ transplantation, 30% to 60% of patients develop neurologic complications. Some of the syndromes are due to preexisting deficits due to underlying illness; others can be classified as complications during surgery, metabolic encephalopathies, neurotoxicity of immunosuppressant agents, opportunistic CNS infections, and secondary malignancies as a direct side effect of immunosuppression and other specific neurologic complications seen mostly after certain organ transplantations.

Specific clinical syndromes are outlined in the following:

I. Procedure-related complications
  A. Femoral or lateral cutaneous nerve injuries after kidney transplantation
  B. Mononeuropathies after traumatic cannulation of catheters
II. Encephalopathy
  A. Post-transplantation delirium is seen in orthotopic liver transplantation (particularly for alcoholic liver disease), calcineurin inhibitors (cyclosporine and tacrolimus), opioid antagonists, beta-blockers, high-dose corticosteroids, and Wernicke's encephalopathy due to total parenteral nutrition.
  B. Post-transplantation stupor or coma is seen in central pontine myelinolysis (liver transplantation), intracerebral hematoma (not uncommonly due to *Aspergillus* infection), hemolytic-uremic syndrome (bone marrow transplantation), acute organ rejection, bilateral cerebral or brainstem infarctions, prolonged intraoperative hypotension causing hypoxic-ischemic encephalopathy, nonconvulsive status epilepticus, and accumulation of anesthetic

and sedative agents due to different pharmacokinetics in transplantation recipients.

III. Peripheral nervous system complications
  A. Neuropathy: drugs (interferon-alfa, colchicine, tacrolimus, cyclosporine, and etoposide), critical illness neuropathy, Guillain-Barré syndrome, and CIDP
  B. Neuromuscular junction disorders: prolonged neuromuscular blockade, myasthenia gravis as a rare manifestation of a graft-versus-host disease
  C. Myopathy: critical illness myopathy (with IV corticosteroids), polymyositis (in bone marrow transplantation), cyclosporine, cholesterol-lowering agents, and colchicine

IV. Effect of immunosuppressant agents
  A. Calcineurin inhibitors (cyclosporine and tacrolimus)
    1. *Cyclosporine* can cause postural and intention tremor, headache, visual hallucination to cortical blindness, seizures, and language-motor dysfunctions.
    2. *Tacrolimus* (FK506) produces neurologic complications that are similar to those from cyclosporine, but less frequent.
    3. Risk factors for developing toxicity include high drug level, IV administration, hypomagnesemia, hyperlipidemia, high blood pressure, and concurrent high-dose steroid therapy. MRI may show reversible posterior leukoencephalopathy findings.
  B. *Corticosteroids* can cause proximal myopathy, anxiety and dysthymia, psychosis (3%), "steroid pseudorheumatism," headache, fever, lethargy on withdrawal.
  C. *OKT3 monoclonal antibody* may produce transient flu-like symptoms, aseptic meningitis (2% to 14%), encephalopathy (1% to 10%).
  D. *Busulfan* can cause seizures.
  E. *Methotrexate* can cause leukoencephalopathy.
  F. *Ifosfamide* can cause hallucinations, mutism, and coma.

V. Opportunistic CNS infection occurs in up to 10% of recipients and carries a high mortality rate:
  A. First month after transplantation: Infections are usually due to gram-negative bacteria or staphylococci from the surgical procedure itself, the hospitalization, or the presence of indwelling catheters. Bone marrow transplant patients are at risk for reactivation of a latent CNS viral infection (HSV-1, VZV, HHV-6, and EBV) in the immediate period after transplantation.
  B. Two to 6 months after transplantation: Recipients are at greatest risk for the classic CNS infections associated with transplantation. Infections are mostly due to viruses (CMV, HSV-1, HSV-2, HHV-6, VZV, and West Nile) and various opportunistic organisms (*Aspergillus* spp., *Nocardia asteroides*, *Toxoplasma gondii*, *Candida* spp., and *Listeria monocytogenes*).

C. Beyond 6 months after transplantation, infections are due to lingering effects of previously acquired infections.
1. Fungi: *Cryptococcus* is the most common pathogen, and infection usually presents after 6 months of immune suppression. *Aspergillus* infection often presents as vasculitis or encephalopathy. *Candida* causes fungemia and meningitis; it is the most common invasive fungal infection in liver transplantation patients. Neutropenia is the most significant risk factor. *Rhinocerebral mucormycosis* is seen in diabetic recipients.
2. Bacteria: *Listeria* is the most common bacterium, usually causing meningitis. *Nocardia* usually causes abscess. *Tuberculosis* is uncommon.
3. Parasites: *Toxoplasmosis* may result from receiving an actively infected organ or from reactivation of latent disease.
4. Viruses: *Cytomegalovirus* may cause chorioretinitis, meningoencephalitis, and polyradiculomyelitis. *Varicella-zoster* virus in a new infection may cause encephalitis with high morbidity; reactivation produces shingles, either diffusely or in dermatomal distribution. Human herpesvirus 6 (*HHV-6*) causes a unique syndrome of limbic encephalitis, particularly in patients with allogeneic bone marrow transplantation. HHV-6 PCR in CSF is sensitive for the diagnosis. *HTLV-I* causes myelopathy after blood transfusion in heart, bone marrow, and kidney recipients. *JC virus* can cause progressive multifocal leukoencephalopathy (see Encephalitis).
VI. Post-transplant lymphoproliferative disorders (PTLDs) are invariably EBV-driven expansions of B lymphocytes in organ transplantation patients. Intense immunosuppression has emerged as a risk factor. Two forms of PTLD are early, with onset 0.5 year after transplantation and median survival of 37 months, and late, with onset 5 years after transplantation and median survival of 1 month. MRI often shows necrotic, ring-enhancing lesion(s), resembling findings in AIDS-associated primary CNS lymphoma. Treatments include modifying immunosuppressive agents and methotrexate-based chemotherapy with or without radiotherapy. Prognosis is generally poor.
VII. Other neurologic syndromes include the following:
A. *Akinetic mutism:* OKT3 and cyclosporine
B. *Cerebellar dysfunction:* dysarthria, ataxia due to neurotoxicity of several immunosuppressants
C. *Creutzfeldt-Jakob disease:* increased risk for patients receiving cadaveric dura transplantation
D. *Hearing loss:* due to cyclosporine-mediated thromboembolic process or antibiotic toxicity
E. *Language disorders:* reversible, due to cyclosporine or tacrolimus neurotoxicity
F. *Metabolic acidosis:* can cause coma in kidney recipients

G. *Migraine:* in bone marrow recipients, due to cyclosporine or hypothesized defect in donor-derived platelets

H. *Movement disorder:* chorea due to cyclosporine in liver transplantation for Wilson's disease; tremor in calcineurin inhibitors

I. *Neuromyotonia:* antibody-mediated channelopathy, seen in patients after bone marrow transplantation

J. *Neurocardiogenic symptoms:* angina and vasovagal syncope seen in heart recipients, presumably due to reinnervation

K. *Pain:* due to varicella-zoster virus; local effects at operative sites; musculoskeletal pain, cyclosporine effects in kidney recipients; oral mucositis in bone marrow recipients

L. *Seizures:* generalized tonic-clonic seizures with a regimen of busulfan, cyclophosphamide, cyclosporine; seen in severe cases of tacrolimus-associated neurotoxicity

M. *Sleep disorder:* somnolence syndrome related to radiation in bone marrow recipient

N. *Stroke and cerebral ischemia:* 44% to 59% of all neurologic complications of post-transplantation patients. Prolonged intraoperative hypotension can cause watershed infarcts. Cardioembolic sources should be considered in heart-lung transplantation. Angioinvasive fungal parasites such as *Aspergillus* can cause hemorrhagic infarction, particularly in liver transplantation patients.

O. *Taste disturbance:* in bone marrow recipients

REFERENCES

Liguori R: *Neurology* 54:1390–1391, 2000.
Nakamura Y et al: *Neurology* 53:218–220, 1999.
Roos KL et al: *Continuum* 10(2):9–61, 2004.

TREMORS (See also THERAPEUTIC APPENDIX)

DEFINITION

Tremors are regular, rhythmic oscillations produced by alternating contraction of agonist and antagonist muscles. They usually affect the distal extremities (especially fingers and hands), head, tongue, jaw, and only rarely the trunk. Tremors disappear during sleep. The frequency is usually consistent in all the affected parts, regardless of the size of muscles involved. It is important to observe the amplitude, frequency, and rhythm of the tremor, as well as the effects of physiologic (posture, limb movement, diurnal variation, and so forth) and psychological factors. It is the most common movement disorder.

CLASSIFICATION

I. *Action or postural tremor:* Present when the limbs and trunk are held in certain positions or during active movements.

A. *Physiologic tremor:* Small-amplitude, high-frequency (6 to 12 Hz) tremor seen in normal individuals; exaggerated by stress, endocrine disorders (hyperthyroidism, hypoglycemia, and pheochromocytoma), drugs (such as lithium, tricyclics, phenothiazines, epinephrine, theophylline, amphetamines, thyroid hormones, isoproterenol, corticosteroids, valproate, levodopa, and butyrophenones), and toxins (such as mercury, lead, arsenic, bismuth, and carbon monoxide). Dietary factors (caffeine, monosodium glutamate, and ethanol withdrawal) may contribute.

Treatment: Management depends on the cause; relaxation methods and stress reduction may help if psychological factors are involved. Beta-blockers have been used with some success, particularly in performers with "stage fright."

B. *Essential tremor:* A postural tremor that often increases with action or intention. It has a frequency of 4 to 11 Hz and usually consists of flexion-extension of the fingers and hands initially, but may progress proximally; the head and neck, jaw, tongue, or voice may be involved. It is exacerbated by emotional and physical stress and diminished with rest, relaxation, and use of ethanol. It may be familial (dominant inheritance), sporadic, or associated with other movement disorders (Parkinson's disease, torsion dystonia, or torticollis).

Treatment: Propranolol is the drug of choice but is contraindicated in patients with asthma or diabetes and in older patients with heart failure. Start with doses of 10 to 20 mg tid or qid, increasing dosage if necessary. Primidone therapy is also useful, starting at 25 to 50 mg. It may be increased up to 250 mg tid as tolerated. Sedation or GI complaints may limit its use. Benzodiazepines are also useful in treating essential tremor.

C. *Primary writing tremor:* Occurs only during writing. Electrophysiologic studies suggest that it may be a form of dystonia.

Treatment: It may respond to anticholinergic therapy or botulinum toxin.

D. *Rubral tremor:* A coarse tremor is present at rest, increasing with postural maintenance and even more with movement. This tremor suggests ipsilateral cerebellar outflow lesion.

II. *Rest tremors:* Present when limbs are at rest.

Parkinsonian tremor has a frequency of 4 to 6 Hz with variable amplitude, sometimes asymmetrical. It occurs at rest and disappears with movement and during sleep. It is prominent in the hands, with flexion-extension or adduction-abduction of the fingers. There is also pronation-supination of the hands. Movements of the feet, jaw, and lips may be present.

Treatment consists of anticholinergic therapy or dopaminergic drugs.

III. Intention tremor.

Cerebellar tremor is a tremor of 3 to 5 Hz occurring during the performance of an exact, projected movement and worsening as the action continues. There may be tremors of the head or trunk (titubation). The oscillation begins proximally and occurs perpendicular to the line of movement. Causes include lesions of cerebellar pathways, cerebellar degeneration, Wilson's disease, and drugs or toxins (such as phenytoin, barbiturates, lithium, ethanol, mercury, and fluorouracil).

IV. *Other tremors.*
   A. *Orthostatic tremor*, a tremor of the legs, is present only when standing and disappears with walking. As such, it may be considered a task-specific tremor.
      Treatment: It responds to clonazepam therapy, 4 to 6 mg/day.
   B. *Hysterical tremor* may be a symptom of conversion disorder. The tremor is often irregular in frequency and may diminish or disappear with distraction.
   C. *Dystonic tremor:* Treatment is now mainly botulinum toxin (Botox).

REFERENCES
Findley LJ, Koller WC: *Neurology* 37:1194–1197, 1987.
Louis ED: *N Engl J Med* 345:887, 2001.

TRIGEMINAL NEURALGIA (TIC DOULOUREUX)

CLINICAL PRESENTATION
Trigeminal neuralgia is characterized by paroxysmal, shooting facial pain in a unilateral distribution of one or more branches of the trigeminal nerve (most commonly the second and third divisions). Paroxysms tend to occur in clusters and last from a few seconds up to 2 minutes. Trigger points are set off by touching, chewing, talking, or swallowing due to stimulation of the skin, mucosa, or teeth innervated by the ipsilateral trigeminal nerve. The historical term "tic douloureux" describes the reactionary tic-like grimace reaction at the onset of pain. Onset is after age 40 in 90% of patients and is more common in women (male-female ratio of 2:3). There is a right (61%) greater than left predominance with a very rare bilateral presentation (4%). Pain does not cross at the midline. Neurologic examination may show sensory loss in up to one fourth of patients, but otherwise is unremarkable.

ETIOLOGY
The cause is unknown, but theories include peripheral and central mechanisms. Demyelination (multiple sclerosis), compression (cerebellopontine angle tumors and schwannomas), and vascular compromise account for small proportion of cases and should be suspected with onset before age 40, with trigeminal sensory or motor abnormalities on examination or with any other findings referable to the base of the skull or posterior fossa.

DIFFERENTIAL DIAGNOSIS

Posterior fossa mass lesions such as tumor (meningioma, acoustic neuroma, trigeminal neuroma), aneurysm, or arteriovenous malformations (AVMs) may produce trigeminal neuralgia. Trigeminal neuralgia pain may be seen in multiple sclerosis, brainstem infarction, and syringobulbia. Evaluation should include MRI with gadolinium, MRA, and evoked potentials for patients with sensory anomalies.

TREATMENT

Treat the underlying cause if trigeminal neuralgia is secondary. Idiopathic trigeminal neuralgia is treated medically and surgically in refractory cases. Medications that are commonly used are as follows:

I. Carbamazepine is the drug of choice and is effective in 75% to 80%. Start at 50 to 100 mg/day and increase gradually as tolerated to 1 to 1.2 g/day in divided doses. Serum levels of 8 to 12 mg/dL should be achieved.

II. Imipramine or amitriptyline is started at 25 to 50 mg orally at bedtime and gradually increased to 150 mg.

III. Phenytoin 300 to 500 mg/day may achieve therapeutic levels.

IV. Baclofen is started at 5 mg orally tid and increased gradually to 20 mg orally qid.

V. Clonazepam is started at 0.5 mg orally bid and increased to 0.5 to 10 mg/day in two or three divided doses.

VI. Valproic acid and pimozide as well as more recent medications such as oxcarbamazepine, gabapentin, lamotrigine, and topiramate are other options. There is much speculation for neuropathic pain control with two new drugs: duloxetine and pregabulin.

VII. Combination approaches have utilized phenytoin with carbamazepine or imipramine. Baclofen has also been used with phenytoin or carbamazepine.

When pain has been controlled, medications should be tapered periodically because spontaneous remissions can occur.

Surgical therapy is reserved for intractable pain unresponsive to drug treatment and includes the following:

I. Local neurolysis and nerve block is associated with a risk of painful anesthesia and persistent paresthesias as well as recurrence.

II. Percutaneous radiofrequency thermocoagulation of the trigeminal ganglion can be done under local anesthesia. Painful anesthesia and recurrences are less common.

III. Trigeminal rhizotomy is used less often than previously.

IV. Microsurgical vascular decompression of the trigeminal root entry zone has been performed.

V. Several new procedures have shown promise in patients with refractory cases. These procedures include percutaneous trigeminal nerve compression and stereotactic radiosurgery with the gamma knife.

REFERENCE

Dalessio D, Silberstein S, Lipton R: *Wolfe's headache and other facial pain*, ed 7, New York, Oxford Univ. Press, 2001, pp 509–520.

TRINUCLEOTIDE REPEAT EXPANSION

Triplet repeat expansion diseases result from the amplification of CAG, CTG, CGG, CCG, or GAA motifs embedded within the coding and noncoding regions of specific genes. Expansion of triplet repeats increases in offspring of affected individuals, and this increase generally results in progressive severity of the disease or earlier age of onset, providing the molecular basis of the clinical phenomenon called "anticipation." Since the original discovery of triplet repeat expansion as the responsible mechanism for fragile X syndrome in 1991, it has proved to be a general phenomenon responsible for a growing number of neurologic disorders (Table 98).

REFERENCE

Siyanova EY: *Molec Biol* 35(2):168–182, 2001.

TUMOR EMBOLIZATION

Preoperative embolization of highly vascular tumors such as meningioma, pericytoma, hemangioblastoma, and renal cell or thyroid carcinoma spine metastasis may markedly reduce intraoperative blood loss.

Meningiomas primarily derive their blood supply from dural branches of the external and, to a lesser extent, internal carotid arteries. Pial arteries may supply the tumor periphery. Besides identifying the arterial supply to the tumor, angiography also evaluates arterial encasement or displacement by the tumor, and possible dural sinus invasion by adjacent tumor. Particle embolization (polyvinyl alcohol, PVA) is performed through ECA branches; ICA embolization is avoided because particle reflux into the parent artery may lead to stroke. Surgery should be undertaken within 2 to 4 days, because recanalization of remaining viable tumor may occur. Studies have demonstrated upward of a 60% decrease in intraoperative blood loss following embolization. Tumor necrosis may also convert a firm, fibrous tumor into a much softer consistency, markedly decreasing operative time as well as traction on adjacent brain parenchyma. Complications are rare, although the presence of dangerous ECA-ICA anastomoses must be sought prior to embolization. These anastomoses include anterior middle meningeal artery (MMA) or internal maxillary artery (Imax) to ophthalmic, occipital to vertebral arteries, and anterior pharyngeal to vertebral arteries. The MMA at the level of the foramen spinosum also supplies CN IX to XII; embolization in this region risks lower cranial nerve dysfunction. Scalp necrosis may occur with distal embolization of small (45-150 μm) particles.

Hemangioblastomas are uncommon, highly vascular tumors, typically originating in the posterior fossa. Their arterial supply is primary from the

TABLE 98

TRINUCLEOTIDE REPEAT DISORDERS

Disorder	Inheritance	Gene/Chromosome	Protein	Normal No. of Repeats	No. of Repeats in Mutant Protein
Fragile X syndrome	XD	FMR1 / Xq27.3	FMR1	(CGG)<50	(CGG)>200
Fragile XE mental retardation	X	FMR2 / Xq28	FMR2	(CCG)<35	(CCG)>200
Myotonic dystrophy	AD	DMPK / 19q13	MD protein kinase	(CTG)<35	(CTG)>50
Huntington's disease	AD	HD/IT15 / 4p16	Huntingtin	(CAG)<40	(CAG)>40
Spinal and bulbar muscular atrophy (Kennedy's disease)	XR	AR / Xq11-q12	Androgen receptor	(CAG)<30	(CAG)>40
SCA1	AD	SCA1 / 6p22-p23	Ataxin 1	(CAG)<40	(CAG)>40
SCA2	AD	SCA2 / 12q24.1	Ataxin 2	(CAG)<30	(CAG)>35
SCA3/MJD (Machado-Joseph disease)	AD	MJD1 / SCA3 / 14q24.3-q31	Ataxin 3	(CAG)<40	(CAG)>40
SCA6	AD	CACNL1A4 / 19p13.1-p13.2	α–1A voltage dependent calcium channel	(CAG)<20	(CAG)>20
SCA7	AD	SCA7 / 3p14-p21.1	Ataxin 7	(CAG)<20	(CAG)>40
SCA8	AD	SCA8 / 13q21	?	(CTG)<40	(CTG)>110
Friedreich's Ataxia	AR	FRDA / X25 / 9q13	Frataxin	(GAA)<35	(GAA)>100
Dentatorubro-pallidoluysian atrophy (DRPLA)/Haw-River syndrome	AD	DRPLA / 12p13	Atrophin 1	(CAG)<35	(CAG)>50
Progressive myoclonus epilepsy type	AR	CSTB / 21q22.3	Cystatin B	(C4GC4GCG)<3	(C4GC4GCG)>60

SCA, spinocerebellar ataxia.

communicating arteries (AICA, PICA, SCA), and the meningeal branches of the cerebral arteries (ICA and VA) and of posterior circulation (AICA, PICA, SCA). These arteries are typically dilated, with easily accessible branches terminating directly in the tumor.

Resection of spinal metastases is associated with high blood loss, especially hypervascular renal cell and thryroid carcinoma metastasis. Preoperative embolization may reduce operative blood from 3500 to 300 mL. Identification of the artery of Adamkiewicz is mandatory prior to embolization to avoid anterior spinal cord infarction. PVA particles are typically used, and surgery should be performed within 2 to 4 days. Periprocedural steroids should be administered to minimize peritumoral edema with spinal cord/nerve root compression following embolization.

Embolization may also be effective for the control of intractable bone pain secondary to spinal metastasis. Vertebral body collapse may occur several weeks after embolization in this population, necessitating long-term spinal bracing.

REFERENCE

Dowd CF, Halbach VH, Higashida RT: *Neurosurg Focus* 15(1):1–4, 2003.

TUMORS (See also PARANEOPLASTIC SYNDROMES, RADIATION INJURY, SPINAL CORD)

The presence of tumor within the nervous system is often suspected by the development of *subacute or acute progressive focal symptoms*. Some tumors, metastases, or carcinomatous meningitis may result in multifocal signs (see Table 99 and Fig. 49).

BRAIN

I. *Epidemiology:* Although primary brain tumors occur about five times more often in adults than in children, the CNS is the second most common site for childhood malignancies. Ionizing radiation is the only unequivocal risk factor for glial and meningeal tumors. Metastases account for the majority of CNS tumors in adults. Approximately 20% of all patients with systemic cancer have CNS involvement during their course of illness.

II. *Clinical presentation:* Symptoms and signs of CNS neoplasm may be generalized and nonlocalizing, usually as a result of diffuse edema, hydrocephalus, or increased intracranial pressure. Headache occurs in about half of all patients with brain tumors. It is classically diffuse, but when it is unilateral it accurately indicates the hemisphere in which the tumor is located. *Headache is usually worse in the morning and, even without treatment, resolves within a few hours.* Seizures occur more often with slow-growing tumors (65–95% in low-grade glioma versus 15–25% in malignant glioma) and with tumors in the frontal and parietal lobes. Vomiting occurs most consistently with posterior fossa tumors. Localizing symptoms and signs depend on tumor location.

TABLE 99

HISTOLOGIC CLASSIFICATION OF NEUROLOGIC TUMORS

Neuroepithelial tumors
  Astrocytic tumors:
    Diffuse astrocytoma
    Astrocytoma
    Anaplastic astrocytoma
    Glioblastoma multiforme
    Juvenile pilocytic astrocytoma
    Subependymal giant cell astrocytoma
  Oligodendroglial tumors:
    Oligodendroglioma
    Anaplastic oligodendroglioma
  Ependymal tumors:
    Ependymoma
    Myxopapillary ependymoma
    Anaplastic ependymoma
    Subependymoma
  Choroid plexus tumors:
    Choroid plexus papilloma
    Choroid plexus carcinoma
  Neuronal tumors:
    Ganglioglioma
    Gangliocytoma
  Primitive neuroectodermal tumors:
    Medulloblastoma
    Pineoblastoma
    Neuroblastoma
Meningeal tumors
  Meningioma
  Papillary meningioma
  Anaplastic meningioma

Nerve sheath tumors:
  Schwannoma (neurilemmoma)
  Neurofibroma
  Neurofibrosarcoma
Tumors of blood vessel origin:
  Hemangioblastoma
  Hemangiopericytoma
Germ cell tumors:
  Germinoma
  Embryonal carcinoma
  Choriocarcinoma
  Teratoma
Malignant lymphomas:
  Hodgkin's disease
  Non-Hodgkin's lymphoma
Malformative tumors:
  Craniopharyngioma
  Epidermoid cyst
  Dermoid cyst
  Neuroepithelial (colloid) cyst
  Lipoma
Regional tumors:
  Chordoma
  Glomus jugulare tumor
  Chondroma
Metastatic tumors:
  Carcinoma
  Sarcoma
  Lymphoma

From Cohen ME: In Bradley WG, Baroff RB, Fenichel GM, Marsden CD, eds: *Neurology in clinical practice*, Boston, Butterworth-Heinemann, 1991.

T

TUMORS

Frontal lobe masses may be silent or, if anterior and midline, may produce changes in personality and memory. *Pineal region tumors* often produce dorsal midbrain syndrome and aqueductal obstruction leading to hydrocephalus. *Brainstem tumors* produce cranial neuropathies, long-tract signs, and hydrocephalus resulting from compression of the cerebral aqueduct.

III. *Diagnosis:* MRI with gadolinium contrast is the imaging technique of choice. Hemorrhage occurs most often with glioblastoma multiforme and metastatic tumors, especially renal cell carcinoma, melanoma, and choriocarcinoma. Calcification occurs more commonly with oligodendroglioma and meningioma. Skull x-rays or CT with bone windows is useful in evaluating bony metastasis, while angiography helps define vascular anatomy. MR spectroscopy (elevated choline:NAA ratio) and PET scan may be helpful in the diagnosis of some cases. In primary CNS lymphoma, lumbar puncture for CSF cytology and ophthalmologic examination should be considered; 25% of patients have lymphoma in the CSF and 20% of patients have lymphomatous infiltration of the eye.

IV. *Treatment:* Available treatment modalities include surgery, radiation therapy including stereotactic radiosurgery, chemotherapy, and combinations. Dexamethasone is the mainstay for symptomatic treatment and is usually started at 4 mg PO/IV every 4 to 6 hours.

LOW-GRADE GLIOMAS

I. Biopsy to confirm diagnosis and to rule out high-grade gliomas.
II. If there are no other symptoms than well-controlled seizures, defer treatment until progression.
III. Progressive symptoms require resection with or without chemotherapy; consider radiation therapy only in refractory cases.

HIGH-GRADE GLIOMAS (ANAPLASTIC ASTROCYTOMA AND GLIOBLASTOMA MULTIFORME)

I. Resection (good prognosis with gross total resection).
II. Radiation therapy with concurrent daily temozolomide for 6 weeks.
III. After resection and radiation, consider adjuvant chemotherapy or refer patients for clinical trial enrollment.

Oligodendroglioma (particularly with loss of heterozygosity of chromosome 1p and 19q) is more sensitive to chemotherapy treatment and has favorable prognosis.

PRIMARY CNS LYMPHOMA

Chemotherapy is the treatment of choice with methotrexate-based regimens (complete response rates of 50–80%). Temozolomide has been shown to be effective as well. Radiation therapy is generally considered in refractory cases.

SPINAL CORD

I. *Epidemiology:* Tumors of the spinal cord and its coverings account for approximately 15% of all CNS tumors. Extradural cord tumors arise from the vertebral bodies and epidural tissues or are metastatic lesions to the epidural space.
II. *Location:* Intradural tumors are either intramedullary (arising within the substance of the cord) or extramedullary (arising from the leptomeninges or nerve roots).
III. *Clinical presentation:* Local back or radicular pain, myelopathy, weakness, sensory complaints, and sphincter dysfunction.

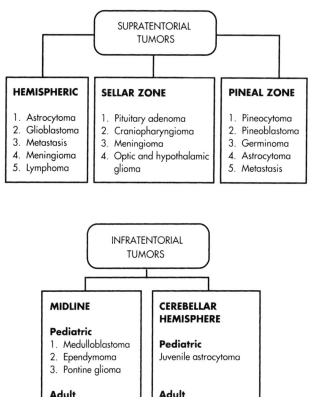

Tumors by location. (From AAN: *Contemporary neuropathology*, vol 6, *Basic neurosciences*, AAN Courses 1993; courtesy of JC Goodman.)

Figure continued on following page

IV. *Diagnosis:* On plain radiographs these masses may produce widening of the interpeduncular distance or of the neural foramina, as well as scalloping of the vertebral bodies. The loss of a pedicle and signs of bone destruction are associated with malignant extradural lesions.

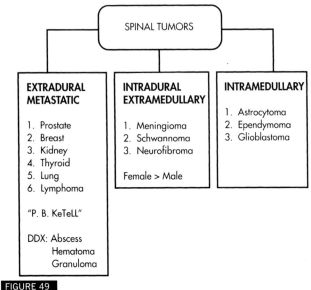

FIGURE 49
cont'd

MRI is the imaging technique of choice, and myelography with CT scanning has been the traditional procedure in the evaluation of spinal cord masses and allows for the simultaneous collection of spinal fluid. Myelography with CT can demonstrate the presence of spinal block, but the upper extent of that may require a second spinal puncture (e.g., cervical tap).

V. *Treatment:* The majority of spinal tumors are benign, producing symptoms by compression rather than by invasion; therefore, surgery is the treatment of choice for most masses. Steroid therapy is adjunctive, and radiation is used for patients who are not candidates for surgery due to life expectancy.

METASTATIC DISEASE

I. *Epidemiology:* Metastases to the brain parenchyma are often found at the gray-white matter junction with 20% single lesion and 80% multiple lesions at presentation. They are typically well demarcated with a zone of surrounding edema. They are usually carcinomas rather than sarcomas or lymphomas. Cancers most commonly associated with metastases vary according to site as follows:

A. Skull: breast, prostate, multiple myeloma
B. Brain parenchyma: lung, breast, colorectal, renal, melanoma

C. Leptomeninges: breast, lung, melanoma, colorectal, lymphoma, leukemia

D. Epidural (spinal cord): lung, breast, prostate, lymphoma, sarcoma, renal

II. *Treatment:*

A. Single lesion: surgical resection or stereotactic radiosurgery + whole-brain radiation therapy (median survival: 24–43 weeks)

B. Multiple lesions: whole-brain radiation therapy alone; may consider stereotactic radiosurgery after recurrence following whole-brain radiation therapy

EPIDURAL SPINAL CORD COMPRESSION

I. *Epidemiology:* Spinal cord compression represents a neurologic emergency. Thoracic spines are the most common site for epidural metastasis; and 17% to 30% of patients present with two or more lesions. *The diagnosis should be suspected in anyone with a known cancer and back pain who seeks medical attention with leg weakness or myelopathic signs.* Sensory loss may not be prominent at presentation.

II. *Diagnosis:* Diagnosis can be suspected from the presence of bony destruction if present on plain radiographic films; confirmation should be obtained by MRI, CT myelography, or occasionally, bone scan. The entire spinal cord should be imaged.

III. *Treatment:* Any patient suspected to have an epidural spinal cord compression should be treated immediately with high-dose IV dexamethasone 10 to 100 mg, even prior to the emergent MRI. Once the diagnosis is confirmed by imaging, treatment usually consists of radiotherapy and high-dose oral or IV dexamethasone 16 to 100 mg/day. Peptic ulcer prophylaxis with H_2 blocker or proton pump inhibitors should be considered. Chemotherapy may be of benefit in chemosensitive tumors such as lymphomas.

Indications for possible surgery include the following:

I. Failure during or after prior radiation therapy

II. Spinal instability; pathologic fracture or dislocation

III. Bony compression of neural structures

IV. Rapid (<72 hours) clinical deterioration (plegia), despite administration of high-dose corticosteroids

V. Intractable pain

VI. The need for biopsy when the diagnosis is unclear

VII. Recent data showed that surgical resection followed by radiation therapy in solitary epidural metastasis of relatively radioresistant tumors may offer an improved outcome (functional scores and continence) over radiation therapy alone.

REFERENCES

Behin A, Hoang-Xuan K et al: *Lancet* 361:323–331, 2003.

DeAngelis LM: *N Engl J Med* 344:114–123, 2001.

Zaidat OO, Ruff RL: *Neurology* 58:1360–1366, 2002.

T

TUMORS

ULNAR NERVE (See also PERIPHERAL NERVE)

Entrapment at the elbow results from compression of the ulnar nerve as it courses in the elbow joint under the aponeurosis connecting the two heads of the flexor carpi ulnaris. It commonly results from extrinsic compression, from leaning on the elbow (especially in patients with a shallow ulnar groove) or from malpositioning of the arms on operating room tables or the arm rests of wheelchairs. "Tardy ulnar palsy" occurs following an elbow fracture or in association with arthritis, ganglion cysts, lipomas, or neuropathic (Charcot) joints. Symptoms include elbow pain, sensory loss and paresthesias of the fifth and ulnar half of the fourth digits and ulnar aspect of the hand, and wasting of the hypothenar and intrinsic hand muscles. There may be a claw-hand deformity. Marked weakness of the flexor carpi ulnaris suggests that the lesion is above the elbow. There may be tenderness or enlargement of the ulnar nerve (palpable in the epicondylar groove); Tinel's sign may be present at the elbow.

Differential diagnosis includes C8 or T1 radiculopathy, syringomyelia, amyotrophic lateral sclerosis, lower trunk brachial plexopathy (Pancoast syndrome), and peripheral polyneuropathy. Nerve conduction studies may show conduction block or slowing across the elbow; EMG may show denervation.

Treatment involves removing exacerbating factors by padding the elbow or armchair rests. If this fails, or if motor involvement is found on physical examination or EMG, surgical decompression may be indicated. There is no clear advantage of more complex procedures (such as ulnar nerve transposition) over simple slitting of the aponeurosis of the flexor carpi ulnaris. However, transposition may be indicated in patients with fibrosis from joint disease.

Entrapment at the wrist or hand (Guyon's canal) consists of variable involvement of the deep and superficial branches of the ulnar nerve to the hand, with sparing of the dorsal cutaneous branch that supplies sensation to the dorsal ulnar sensory distribution. The same etiologic factors as for the elbow apply. The EMG and nerve conduction studies should demonstrate involvement of the hand ulnar motor fibers with sparing of sensory function to the dorsal hand.

ULTRASONOGRAPHY

The carotid and vertebral arteries and their branches can be evaluated with ultrasound, that is, sound with frequency higher than 20,000 Hz. *B-mode* (brightness modulation) is based on the transmission of ultrasound through tissues and reflection from tissue interfaces. This imaging technique produces a real-time two-dimensional picture of examined extracranial vessels in longitudinal or transverse view. It allows measurement of vessel diameter and reveals the presence of stenosis or occlusion. High-resolution scans can also determine plaque morphology, such as ulceration, calcification, or hemorrhage. In *Doppler ultrasonography*, the ultrasound is reflected off moving targets (erythrocytes). Increased blood flow velocity in a narrowed segment of arterial lumen (stenosis) is associated with higher frequency shift, which correlates with flow velocities. The best result in vascular ultrasonography can be obtained by combination of these two techniques in *duplex ultrasonography*, which combines the advantages of B-mode with exact sampling of the site, and systolic, diastolic, and mean velocities measured in Doppler mode. Carotid duplex ultrasonography has an excellent accuracy for detection of stenotic process compared with angiography. For arteries with more than 50% stenosis, sensitivity is approximately 94% to 100%; for occlusions, sensitivity is 80% to 96% and specificity is 95%. However, these results vary considerably with the experience of the ultrasonographer. Examination of vertebral arteries allows determination of flow direction (for example, subclavian steal syndrome), but morphologic evaluation is not always possible.

Blood flow velocities in the major intracranial arteries can be examined by *transcranial doppler* (TCD). TCD has established value in detection of stenosis greater than 65% in the major basal intracranial arteries, assessing collateral flow, evaluating and monitoring vasospasm after subarachnoid hemorrhage, detecting arteriovascular malformations, and assessing patients with brain death. The accuracy of TCD also depends highly on operator skill and experience. TCD may also be used for intraoperative monitoring during carotid endarterectomy and cardiac surgery and in testing cerebrovascular reactivity and hemodynamic reserve.

REFERENCES

Babikian VL et al: *J Neuroimaging* 10:101–115, 2000.
Beletsky VY, Kelley RE: *J La State Med Soc* 148:467–473, 1996.

UREMIA

Uremia refers to the constellation of signs and symptoms associated with renal failure, regardless of the cause. The presentation varies from patient to patient, depending upon the remaining renal function and the rapidity at which the function is lost. With glomerular filtration rate about 20% to 35% of normal, azotemia occurs. The likely toxins are byproducts of protein and amino acid metabolism such as urea, guanidine compounds, aliphatic amines, tyrosine, and phenylalanine.

I. Uremic encephalopathy correlates with *rate of progression of uremia*, as opposed to the absolute blood urea nitrogen and creatinine levels.

A. *Clinically*, clouding of consciousness may be associated with hallucinations, increased reflexes, and increased tone (may be asymmetrical). Asterixis, myoclonus and chorea, stupor, seizures, and coma are signs of terminal uremia.

B. *EEG* is characterized by low voltage slowing early; later there may be a generalized paroxysmal slowing. Triphasic waves or epileptiform activity is not uncommon. CSF protein level may be elevated, and aseptic meningitis may occur, accompanied by stiff neck and marked pleocytosis.

C. Management consists of dialysis, supportive care, and antiepileptic drugs.

II. Seizures in renal failure are usually generalized but may be focal. They may occur in the setting of uremic encephalopathy, hypertensive crisis, coexistent electrolyte disturbance, or drug toxicity. Purely uremic seizures often respond to dialysis. When anticonvulsants are required, dosage must be adjusted for glomerular filtration rate. *Diminished renal clearance requires decreased dosages of carbamazepine, phenobarbital, and gabapentin.* Changes in clearance and protein binding lead to decreased total phenytoin levels with an increased unbound fraction. These changes necessitate *free-fraction monitoring for optimal control.* Anticonvulsants with low protein binding affinity are sometimes preferable in patients on hemodialysis.

III. Peripheral neuropathy (distal, symmetrical sensorimotor polyneuropathy type) is common in advanced renal failure and can result in flaccid paralysis. It is often painful and may be associated with restless leg syndrome. Abnormal nerve conduction studies may precede clinical symptoms and signs. The neuropathy stabilizes or improves with hemodialysis. The greatest improvement seems to occur with renal transplantation. Tricyclics or anticonvulsants may alleviate pain.

IV. Myopathy: Patients with chronic renal failure often have symmetrical proximal weakness with atrophy and painful stiffness. Serum creatine kinase (CK) and aldolase levels are usually normal, but EMG shows myopathic changes, sometimes due to secondary hyperparathyroidism. Rarely, ischemic myopathy occurs with elevated levels of serum CK, severe weakness, and gangrenous skin lesions.

V. Tetany that does not respond to calcium may occur.

REFERENCES

Bachman D et al: *Seizure* 5:239–542, 1996.
Burn DJ et al: *J Neurol Neurosurg Psychiatry* 65:810–821, 1998.
Fraser CL, Arieff AL: *Ann Intern Med* 109:143, 1988.
Ruff RL et al: *Neurol Clin* 6:575, 1988.

V

VASCULITIS

DEFINITION
Vasculitis refers to a clinicopathologic process characterized by inflammation of the blood vessels. Vasculitides can be primary (idiopathic) or secondary, which is related to the known cause (Table 100). Angiographic beading is common (Fig. 50).

ISOLATED ANGIITIS OF THE CNS
I. *Clinical presentation:* This rare disease has nonspecific symptoms, including recurrent headaches, confusion, or focal signs such as hemiparesis or aphasia. Systemic symptoms are generally absent.
II. *Diagnosis:* CSF shows mild lymphocytic pleocytosis and elevated protein. Erythrocyte sedimentation rate (ESR) is mildly elevated. Angiography has low sensitivity and specificity. Biopsy of the nondominant frontal or temporal pole with leptomeninges is recommended before treatment.
III. *Treatment* consists of high-dose prednisone plus cyclophosphamide.

TEMPORAL ARTERITIS (GIANT CELL ARTERITIS)
I. *Clinical presentation:* Patients are older than 55 years. It mainly affects the extracranial arteries and tends to spare the intracranial vessels. The superficial temporal and the ophthalmic arteries are commonly involved. The most common symptoms are headaches and constitutional complaints. Jaw claudication is seen in 40% of the patients and is due to ischemia of the muscles. Amaurosis fugax is seen in 10% of patients and is likely to progress to blindness if left untreated. More than half of the patients with temporal arteritis have polymyalgia rheumatica.
II. *Physical examination* often shows erythematous, tender, tortuous, thickened, and pulseless temporal arteries.
III. *Diagnosis:* ESR is high in almost all cases. Angiography can demonstrate luminal irregularities and alternating stenosis and dilatation. Histologic confirmation should be obtained.
IV. *Treatment* should be initiated immediately on the basis of the clinical suspicion with high-dose prednisone for 1 month and a subsequent slow taper. The ESR can be used to monitor the disease activity.

TAKAYASU'S ARTERITIS (THE PULSELESS DISEASE)
I. *Clinical presentation:* It affects young women of Asian and South American descent. It involves the tunica media of the aortic arch and its proximal branches. The carotids are more affected than the vertebral arteries. The intracranial arteries are typically spared. Constitutional symptoms such as malaise, fever, weight loss, night sweats, myalgia, and arthralgia may be the presenting symptoms. Visual changes,

TABLE 100

COMMON KEY MANIFESTATIONS AND EVALUATION OF VASCULITIS

Vasculitis Type	Key Clinical Feature	Diagnostic Tests
Giant cell arteritis		
Temporal arteritis	Blindness, jaw claudication, high ESR	ESR, temporal artery biopsy
Takayasu's arteritis	Pulseless disease, pulse deficit	ESR, angiography
Systemic necrotizing arteritis		
Polyarteritis nodosa	Painful mononeuritis multiplex + kidney involvement	Inflammatory markers, angiography and tissue biopsy
Churg-Strauss syndrome	Granuloma, eosinophilia, mononeuritis multiplex + severe asthma	Inflammatory markers and tissue biopsy
Wegener's granulomatosis	Peripheral and cranial neuropathy + upper and lower respiratory tract and kidney involvement	c-ANCA specific and sensitive, biopsy
Connective tissue disease vasculitis		
Systemic lupus erythematosus	Neuropsychiatric lupus, seizure, stroke, optic neuritis, myelitis, systemic involvement	ds- and ss-DNA, ANA titers, angiography, biopsy
Sjögren's syndrome	Headaches, aseptic meningitis, myelopathy, mononeuritis + dry mouth and eyes	Schirmer's test, salivary gland biopsy, inflammatory markers
Rheumatoid arthritis	Atlantoaxial subluxation with myelopathy + deforming arthritis	RF, plain x-rays, other inflammatory markers
Cogan's disease	Encephalomyelitis, polyneuropathy, vestibular and auditory + interstitial keratitis	Inflammatory markers, typical clinical features, biopsy
Behçet's disease	Meningitic syndrome, and multiple sclerosis–like picture + recurrent oral and genital ulcers + uveitis	Typical clinical features and inflammatory markers
Hypersensitivity vasculitis		
Hypocomplementemia	Encephalomyelitis + peripheral nerve involvement + systemic response	Hepatitis C, complements panel
Cryoglobulinemia	Encephalomyelitis + peripheral nerve involvement + systemic response	Hepatitis C, cryoglobulin levels

cont'd

TABLE 100

COMMON KEY MANIFESTATIONS AND EVALUATION OF VASCULITIS—*cont'd*

Vasculitis Type	Key Clinical Feature	Diagnostic Tests
Infectious vasculitis		
Herpes zoster	Eye and ear involvement + contralateral weakness (stroke)	Typical clinical features with viral titers, PCR
Lyme disease	Encephalomyelitis, polyradiculitis, peripheral nerve involvement + erythema migrans	Lyme titers, exposure to tick bite, CSF analysis
HIV infection	AIDS features, dementia, encephalitis, peripheral nerve involvement	Viral titers, typical clinical features, imaging findings
Drug-induced vasculitis	History of exposure to drugs and cold medicine	Positive toxicology titers, negative inflammatory markers, angiogram
Sympathomimetics (amphetamine, cocaine, phenylproponalimine, pseudophedrine)		

vertigo, syncope, recurrent headache, focal neurologic deficits such as hemiparesis or aphasia, and seizures are common neurologic symptoms.
II. *Physical examination* reveals pulse deficits and multiple vascular bruits in most cases.
III. *Diagnosis:* High ESR and angiography are essential for the diagnosis.

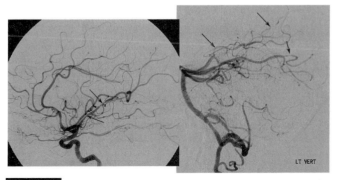

FIGURE 50
Angiographic beading.

IV. *Treatment:* High-dose oral steroids. If response to the steroids is poor, then methotrexate or cyclophosphamide can be considered. The ESR is not as reliable a parameter to follow as it is with temporal arteritis. Aggressive surgical or angioplastic treatment may improve prognosis significantly in certain cases.

POLYARTERITIS NODOSA

I. *Clinical presentation:* It usually develops in the fifth or sixth decade of life and affects *men almost twice as often as women*. This chronic disease causes patchy necrosis in the walls of medium-sized and small arteries. Kidney, heart, and liver are the most frequently affected organs. *CNS involvement* presents with headache, changes in mental status, seizures, visual change, or hemiparesis. The peripheral nervous system is affected in 50% to 60% of the patients. Painful mononeuritis multiplex is common, but polyneuropathies, plexopathies, and radiculopathies can also occur.

II. *Diagnosis:* The diagnosis is based on angiography or tissue biopsy. Many of the patients are seropositive for hepatitis B or C.

III. *Treatment:* Steroids combined with cyclophosphamide are the treatment of choice.

WEGENER'S GRANULOMATOSIS

I. *Clinical presentation:* Granulomatous, necrotizing vasculitis involves the small arteries and veins in the upper and lower respiratory tract, kidney (glomerulonephritis), skin or eye (50%), CNS, and PNS. Besides the constitutional symptoms, the most common neurologic manifestations are peripheral and cranial neuropathies. Strokes and seizures are less common. The c-ANCA titers are sensitive and specific for active Wegener's. ESR is usually markedly elevated.

II. *Diagnosis:* Biopsy of respiratory tract or renal tissues provides the diagnosis.

III. *Treatment* consists of prednisone combined with cyclophosphamide. Azathioprine can be used in those who cannot tolerate cyclophosphamide.

CHURG-STRAUSS SYNDROME

I. *Clinical presentation:* Granulomatous vasculitis affects mainly the lungs. There is a strong association with severe asthma and peripheral eosinophilia. Mononeuritis multiplex may occur, but it is not common.

II. *Treatment* consists of steroids, and cyclophosphamide may be added.

SYSTEMIC LUPUS ERYTHEMATOSUS

I. *Clinical presentation:* SLE is a disease involving multiple organs and mainly affecting women. Besides systemic symptoms, neurologic involvement in SLE is common and includes headaches, cognitive and behavioral changes, psychosis, depression, seizure, cerebral ischemia, myelitis, optic neuritis, cranial and peripheral neuropathies, and movement disorders.

II. *Diagnosis:* Markers, angiography, and biopsy (noninflammatory vasculopathy) provide the diagnosis.

III. *Treatment:* For severe CNS manifestations, high-dose IV steroids are given and then slowly tapered to an oral dosage. Cyclophosphamide or azathioprine can be used if steroids fail. IVIG and plasmapheresis trial was also reported in the literature.

SJÖGREN'S SYNDROME

I. *Clinical presentation:* This chronic inflammatory and autoimmune disorder affects lacrimal and salivary glands and causes dry mouth (xerostomia) and dry eyes (xerophthalmia). Neurologic symptoms include headaches, aseptic meningitis, myelopathy, mononeuritis multiplex, and focal deficits.

II. *Treatment* is supportive, but steroid and immunosuppressive agents are used in life-threatening conditions.

RHEUMATOID ARTHRITIS

Clinical presentation: Systemic arthritis can be seen in up to 25% of adult patients, but the CNS is rarely involved. Myelopathy, brainstem, or cranial nerve deficits and headache can occur due to atlantoaxial subluxation. Peripheral nerve involvement is relatively common, including distal sensory or sensorimotor neuropathy, mononeuropathy multiplex and entrapment, or compression neuropathy.

COGAN'S DISEASE

This is a rare disease of the young. It presents with interstitial keratitis, vestibular and auditory dysfunction, encephalomyelitis, and polyneuropathy.

Treatment: Steroid or immunosuppressive agents may be the treatment of choice.

BEHÇET'S DISEASE

I. *Clinical presentation:* Recurrent oral and genital ulcers, uveitis, and nondeforming arthritis are seen. It affects mostly young patients and is more common in eastern Mediterranean countries and in Japan. Neurologic symptoms (10%) are headache, meningitic syndrome, dementia, psychosis, and a multiple sclerosis–like picture.

II. *Treatment:* Uveitis and CNS involvement require high-dose prednisone in conjunction with azathioprine or cyclosporine.

HERPES ZOSTER OPHTHALMICUS HEMIPLEGIA

I. *Clinical presentation:* This form presents weeks or months after herpes zoster ophthalmicus in an older adult. Involvement of the ipsilateral anterior and middle cerebral arteries causes contralateral hemiparesis.

II. *Treatment:* Acyclovir and steroids provides treatment.

REFERENCES

Bradley WG, Daroff RB, Fenichel GM et al: *Neurology in clinical practice*, ed 4, Boston, Butterworth-Heinemann, 2004, pp 1079–1083, 1103–1106, 1323–1326.

Younger DS: *Curr Opin Neurol* 17:317–336, 2004.

VEIN OF GALEN MALFORMATION

DEFINITION

Vein of Galen malformation (VGM) is a congenital midline arteriovenous fistula with aneurysmal dilatation of the vein of Galen. It may be defined as direct arteriovenous fistulas between choroidal or quadrigeminal arteries and an overlying single median venous sac. This sac could be the embryonic median prosencephalic vein of Markowski or the vein of Galen. The frequent concurrent venous abnormalities are (1) retention of fetal anatomic features and (2) frequent occlusions of the dural sinuses of the posterior fossa, especially the sigmoid sinuses.

CLINICAL PRESENTATION

The most common presenting symptoms are congestive cardiac failure, raised intracranial pressure secondary to hydrocephalus, cranial bruit, focal neurologic deficit, seizures, and hemorrhage. The most characteristic vascular supply to the midline fistula involves multiple bilateral vessels, although bilateral posterior cerebral and unilateral posterior cerebral supply are relatively common.

DIAGNOSIS

Ultrasound, MRI and MRA, and angiogram provide the diagnosis.

TREATMENT

Medical supportive therapy consists of digoxin, diuretics, and ventilatory support; surgical treatment involves ligation; and endovascular therapy uses coil and glue embolization. Staged therapy with medical therapy initially followed by endovascular therapy and finally surgical therapy may improve survival. The overall mortality rate varies among reports in the literature and ranges between 40% and 80%. Surgical and endovascular intervention does not improve mortality rate when performed early, but may be better when performed after 1 month of age, or even after the first year.

REFERENCE

Alexander MJ, Spetzler RF, eds: *Pediatric neurovascular disease. Surgical, endovascular and medical management*, New York, Thieme, 2006.

VENOUS THROMBOSIS

CLINICAL PRESENTATION

Cerebral venous thrombosis (CVT) results in headache, seizures, and focal signs. It can occur in any age group and is more common in females.

Almost 50% of adult cases of CVT occur in pregnancy and the peripartum period. Subarachnoid hemorrhage resulting from rupture of congested veins or extension of hemorrhagic infarction, as well as papilledema, may also occur. *Superior sagittal sinus thrombosis* is the most common type and, if the parieto-occipital portion is involved, may produce elevated intracranial pressure, somnolence, and CN VI palsy.

EVALUATION

Contrast-enhanced CT scan shows a "negative delta" sign, which is characterized by opacification of the sinus wall with noninjection of the clot inside the sinus, in about 30% of cases. MRI or MR venography may be diagnostic with asymmetry. Venous phase angiography usually shows a filling defect. Other signs of parasagittal stroke or hemorrhage, or both, may be present because of propagation of the thrombus into surrounding cortical veins. Thrombosis may also involve the *cavernous sinus* (usually as a result of facial or orbital infection; involvement is characterized by facial pain, proptosis, and involvement of CN III, IV, V, and VI) and the *superior petrosal sinus* (as a result of otitis media; facial pain is prominent), *inferior petrosal sinus* (*Gradenigo's syndrome* with retro-orbital pain and CN VI palsy), *lateral petrosal sinus* (increased intracranial pressure and ear pain), or *internal jugular* vein (as a result of catheters or pacemakers, with involvement of CN IX, X, and XI). *Vein of Galen thrombosis* in neonates after trauma or infection may result in extensor posturing, fever, tachycardia, tachypnea, and death. Survivors may develop bilateral choreoathetosis. D-dimer testing is not useful to exclude CVT if negative and may be elevated in other cerebrovascular diseases, such as subacute hemorrhage and ischemic stroke.

Causes and risk factors of venous thrombosis include the following:

I. Trauma: injury, neck surgery, indwelling IV lines
II. Infection: middle ear, sinuses, meningitis
III. Endocrine: pregnancy, oral contraceptives
IV. Volume depletion: hyperosmolar coma, inflammatory bowel disease, diarrhea, postpartum, postoperative
V. Hematologic: polycythemia vera, disseminated intravascular coagulation, sickle cell disease, cryofibrinogenemia, paroxysmal nocturnal hemoglobinuria, thrombocytosis, antithrombin III deficiency, transfusion reaction
VI. Impaired cerebral circulation: arterial occlusion, congenital heart disease, congestive heart failure, anesthesia in seated position, sagittal sinus webs
VII. Neoplasm: leukemia, lymphoma, meningeal spread, meningioma
VIII. Other: Wegener's granulomatosis, polyarteritis nodosa, Behçet's syndrome, Cogan's syndrome, homocystinuria, idiopathic

Results of lumbar puncture, if not contraindicated by mass effect, are nonspecific and may reveal increased pressure and increased levels of protein, polymorphonuclear leukocytes (if infection is present), and red blood cells (if hemorrhage has occurred).

MANAGEMENT

Management involves treatment of the underlying cause and supportive care. Seizures should be aggressively treated and metabolic derangements corrected. Maintain adequate hydration and nutrition. DVT prophylaxis should be administered. Elevate the head of the bed to 30 degrees if not contraindicated by spinal injury. Infections should be treated with appropriate antimicrobial therapy for the suspected organism(s). Discontinue oral contraceptive pills. Anticoagulation therapy is usually employed if there is no major hemorrhage or bleeding disorder. Intracranial hypertension should be controlled (see also Intracranial Pressure). Standard therapy involves unfractionated heparin (although low-molecular-weight heparin may be effective, limited studies have been conducted) followed by warfarin for 3 to 6 months (or longer for underlying hypercoagulable states. *Local infusion of thrombolytics* may be considered in patients exhibiting rapid decline despite therapeutic anticoagulation, although no randomized clinical trials regarding efficacy or safety have been performed.

REFERENCES

Ameli A, Bazaar MG: *Neurol Clin* 10:87, 1992.
Lewis M: *Stroke* 30:1729, 1999.

VERTEBROPLASTY / KYPHOPLASTY

Vertebral body compression fractures are a major source of morbidity, especially in the elderly. Conservative treatment, including bed rest, bracing, and medical management, often leads to complications related to escalating narcotic and NSAID use, decreased mobility, and pulmonary compromise from bracing and progressive kyphosis. Intractable pain despite best medical management is not uncommon. Vertebroplasty and kyphoplasty offer a minimally invasive option for pain relief in this population. Both involve the percutaneous injection of polymethylmethacrylate (PMMA) into the affected vertebral body under fluoroscopic guidance. The PMMA solidifies within minutes, forming an internal cast to the fracture. Kyphoplasty differs from vertebroplasty by using an inflatable balloon to restore the vertebral body height and sagittal alignment of the spine; the balloon is removed, and the resultant space is filled with PMMA.

Indications include osteoporotic compression fractures failing medical management, painful vertebral hemangiomas, and osteolytic compression fractures from multiple myeloma and spinal metastasis. Contraindications include infection (local, spinal, or systemic), coagulopathy, neurologic deficit related to the fracture, spinal canal compromise, or fractured posterior vertebral body cortex. Treatment of "pancaked" vertebral bodies (i.e., compression fractures with >75% vertebral body height loss) is controversial, although successful treatment has been reported. The initial patient evaluation should include standard spinal imaging to identify the fracture site, as well as CT or MRI to evaluate for extent of fracture, spinal canal or neural foramen compromise by retropulsed bone or tumor, possible infections, and intactness of the posterior cortex at the involved level. Treatment timing is controversial; most defer at least 6 weeks to evaluate the effectiveness of conservative treatment, although the role of percutaneous treatment in acute fractures is being evaluated.

Significant pain relief occurs in 70% to 90% of patients, with little or no pain relief occurring in 5% or fewer. The effect is often immediate, although it may take 48 to 72 hours. Pain relief has been demonstrated to persist for at least 2 years. Slightly lower rates of pain relief are obtained from osteolytic fractures secondary to tumor.

Cement extravasation through the vertebral body cortex occurs in 20% to 40% of procedures. This is typically clinically insignificant, although rare symptomatic pulmonary embolization has occurred. Other complications include spinal cord or nerve root compression by either retropulsed bone fragments or cement extravasation; they rarely require surgical decompression.

V

VERTIGO

REFERENCES
Lieberman I, Reinhardt MK: *Clin Orthop Related Res* 415S:S176–S186, 2003.
Phillips FM: *Spine* 28(15S):S45–S53, 2003.

VERTIGO

DEFINITION
Vertigo is defined as perception of *movement* of self or surroundings or an unpleasant distortion of *orientation* with respect to gravity. Disorders causing vertigo are formulated in terms of distortion or mismatch of vestibular, visual, and somatosensory inputs. Careful questioning can better delineate the patient's perceptions and help differentiate vertigo from other forms of dizziness that result from disturbances of cardiovascular, visual, or motor function.

EXAMINATION
Evaluation of vertigo includes blood pressure measurement (lying and standing), hearing screen and otoscopy, general neurologic examination with special attention to past pointing, ophthalmoscopy, ocular motor examination, and characterization of nystagmus. Also noted are responses to specific maneuvers (if deemed safe), including tragal compression, rapid head turns, Valsalva maneuver, rotation in chair, hyperventilation, and postural testing (Dix-Hallpike). The latter is performed by abruptly moving the patient from a sitting to a lying position, with the head hanging 45 degrees over the end of the examining table and rotated 45 degrees to one side. This movement is repeated with the head rotated to the opposite side. The development of vertigo and the time of onset, duration, and direction of the fast phase of nystagmus are noted.

ETIOLOGY

I. Physiologic vertigo results from sensory distortion (e.g., change in refraction) or intersensory mismatch (such as motion sickness or height vertigo).

II. Pathologic vertigo is based on localization within vestibular pathways.

A. Labyrinths: otitis media, endolymphatic hydrops, otosclerosis, cupulolithiasis, viral infection, perilymph fistula, trauma, drug toxicity (e.g., from antibiotics)

B. Vestibular nerve and ganglia: carcinomatous meningitis, herpes zoster

C. Cerebellopontine angle: acoustic neuroma, glomus, or other tumor; demyelination, vascular compression

D. Brainstem and cerebellum: infarct, hemorrhage, tumor, viral infection, migraine, Arnold-Chiari malformation

E. Hemispheric connections: temporal or parietal dysfunction (e.g., seizure)

F. Systemic and metabolic: anemia, intoxication (such as ethanol, anticonvulsants, diuretics, and other medications), vasculitis (e.g., Cogan's syndrome of deafness, interstitial keratitis, and systemic vasculitis), metabolic derangement (e.g., thyroid disease)

III. Other causes of vertigo: Psychogenic vertigo has features of rotational or linear movement rather than isolated lightheadedness. It often begins gradually, is associated with anxiety, and terminates abruptly. Forced hyperventilation may provoke vertigo. When a patient complains of severe rotational vertigo without nausea or nystagmus, a psychogenic cause is suggested.

SPECIFIC FORMS

I. *Acute peripheral vestibulopathy* (other terms include viral labyrinthitis, vestibular neuronitis, and peripheral vestibulopathy) is associated with spontaneous vertigo, nystagmus (fast phase away from the lesion), and nausea or vomiting, or both, lasting hours to days. The environment seems to move in the direction of the fast phase (away from the lesion). There is a subjective sense of self-motion in the direction of the fast phase. The patient may fall to the side of the lesion during Romberg testing. Past pointing is to the side of the lesion. Symptoms and signs may be brought on by hurried movement ("positioning") but not necessarily by maintaining a particular position ("positional").

Hearing is usually normal. A variable residual deficit of one peripheral vestibular system (labyrinth, nerve, or both) may persist. With a unilateral fixed deficit, central compensatory mechanisms intervene and vertigo and nystagmus decrease and may resolve. Acute peripheral vestibulopathy may recur (see below). Bacterial suppurative ear infection should be excluded.

II. *Perilymph fistula* is usually due to spontaneous rupture of the inner ear membranes with resultant vertigo that may be aggravated by changes in position. It is associated with a fluctuating hearing loss. The fistula may occur during strenuous activity or Valsalva maneuver. The patient may hear a "pop" in the ear at the moment of rupture. The attacks are discrete and short-lived. The therapy is bed rest. If this fails, surgery may be required.

III. *Central vestibular vertigo* results from lesions of the vestibular nuclei or vestibulocerebellar pathways; these patients have vertigo and nystagmus, often accompanied by diplopia, dysarthria, weakness, sensory loss, involvement of cranial nerves V and VII, and pathologic reflexes. Acoustic neuromas are usually associated with hearing loss, tinnitus, and occasionally involvement of other cranial nerves, including CN VII and V.

IV. *Drug-induced vertigo* is due to effects on the peripheral end-organ or nerve and may be due to aminoglycosides, furosemide, ethacrynic acid, anticonvulsants (phenytoin, phenobarbital, carbamazepine, and primidone), some anti-inflammatory agents, salicylates, and quinine. Drugs may produce only dysequilibrium when the damage is bilateral but can produce vertigo when the damage is asymmetric. Some agents also produce hearing loss.

V. *Meniere's disease* that results from endolymph hydrops is characterized by severe episodic vertigo, vomiting, fluctuating or progressive hearing loss, distortions of sound, tinnitus, and pressure or fullness in the ears. Recovery is usually within hours to days. The interval between attacks often ranges from weeks to months. Low-salt diet and diuretics are considered most helpful. Surgical therapy (endolymphatic drainage or vestibular nerve section) may give lasting relief but should be considered only as a last resort. Newer treatments include intratympanic injections of corticosteroids or gentamicin; the latter may be a less invasive alternative to surgery.

VI. *Benign paroxysmal positional vertigo* (BPPV) is a symptom that usually indicates benign peripheral (end-organ) disease. Vertigo and nystagmus, often with systemic symptoms such as nausea and vomiting, occur when certain positions of the head are assumed, such as lying down on the back or side. Symptoms are usually transient (<60 seconds). Latency is usually several seconds but may be as long as 30 to 45 seconds. Signs and symptoms include fatigue after onset and do not recur until there is a change in position. Nystagmus is most commonly torsional toward (upper pole) the undermost ear during positional testing. With repetitive maneuvers, signs and symptoms lessen (habituate). Therapy consists of repetitive positioning exercises to stimulate central compensation or a liberatory maneuver (Brandt-Daroff maneuvers). Elderly patients compensate more slowly. Vestibular suppressant medications generally do not help in completely alleviating symptoms.

V

VERTIGO

TABLE 101

APPROACH TO PATIENT WITH VERTIGO

Do not do head maneuvers in young patient with recent trauma or possible dissection.

Do MRI and MRA in elderly patient with stroke risk factor and new vertigo.

Do the positional test and if positive for benign paroxysmal positional vertigo go on to a particle repositioning maneuver.

Do the head impulse test in the patient and if negative think of cerebellar infarction in a patient with a first-time attack of acute isolated spontaneous vertigo.

Order an audiogram and a caloric test and if they are normal think of migraine rather than Meniere's disease in a patient with recurrent vertigo.

Think of bilateral vestibular loss due to gentamicin, normal pressure hydrocephalus, early cerebellar ataxia, early progressive supranuclear palsy, sensory peripheral neuropathy, and orthostatic tremor in the patient who is off balance for no obvious reason.

LABORATORY STUDIES

Brain imaging (CT, MRI) directs attention to posterior fossa and temporal bone; MR angiography gives attention to vertebrobasilar circulation; caloric and rotational testing quantify vestibular function. Audiogram and auditory evoked potentials detect associated cochlear or brainstem dysfunction.

MANAGEMENT

Generally, management during acute vertigo (Table 101) includes bed rest, avoiding sudden head movements, clear fluids or light diet if tolerated, and reassurance. Vestibular suppressant medications such as antihistamines and benzodiazepines (Table 102) and antiemetics may be useful in acute peripheral vestibulopathy, in acute brainstem lesions near the vestibular nuclei, and for prevention of motion sickness. These agents are of no benefit in chronic vestibulopathies. After the acute phase (approximately 1 to 3 days), a graded program of exercises hastens the adaptive recalibration of the vestibular system to provide better oculomotor and postural control and reduce vertigo.

TABLE 102

MEDICATIONS USEFUL IN TREATING SYMPTOMS OF ACUTE VERTIGO

Drug	Dosage	Route
Dimenhydrinate (Dramamine)	50–100 mg q 4–6 hr	PO, IM, IV, PR
Diphenhydramine (Benadryl)	25–50 mg tid to qid	PO, IM, IV
Meclizine (Antivert)	12.5–25 mg bid to qid	PO
Promethazine (Phenergan)	25 mg bid to qid	PO, IM, IV, PR
Hydroxyzine (Atarax, Vistaril)	25–100 mg tid to qid	PO, IM

REFERENCES

Baloh RW: *J Am Geriatr Soc* 40:713–721, 1992.
Brandt T, Steddin S, Daroff RB: *Neurology* 44:796–800, 1994.
Halmagyi GM: *Clin Med* 5:159–165, 2005.
Lempert T, von Brevern M: *Curr Opin Neurol* 18:5–9, 2005.
Sharpe JA, Barber HO, eds: *The vestibulo-ocular reflex and vertigo*, New York, Raven, 1993.

VESTIBULO-OCULAR REFLEX

The vestibulo-ocular reflex (VOR) generates eye movements that compensate for head movements. Head movements are sensed by the semicircular canals and otolithic organs (utricle and saccule). Signals from the vestibular end-organs are combined with visual information in brainstem vestibular and oculomotor centers to create appropriate control signals, which are sent to the extraocular muscles. Adequate vestibular function results in eye rotations nearly equal and opposite to head movements and maintenance of a stable image on the retina, allowing high visual acuity. Overall vestibular function involves cerebral cortical centers and spinal cord relay and processing of sensory input and motor outflow. Thus, vestibular disorders (peripheral or central) can result in eye movement abnormalities or more subtle disorders of postural control and spatial orientation (Table 103).

V

VESTIBULO-OCULAR REFLEX

TABLE 103

LOCALIZATION OF VESTIBULAR DYSFUNCTION

	Peripheral	Central
History	Sudden onset; episodic; duration several days; intense vertigo; marked exacerbation with head movement; auditory symptoms (often unilateral); neurologic symptoms absent	Insidious onset; continuous; duration up to months; mild dysequilibrium; little or no exacerbation with head movement; no associated auditory symptoms; associated neurologic or vascular symptoms
Physical examination	Neurologic signs absent; *spontaneous nystagmus:* rotatory component, not vertical; *positional nystagmus:* latency before onset (≤45 sec), habituates, conjugate, uniplanar, attenuates with visual fixation	Associated neurologic or vascular signs; *spontaneous nystagmus:* horizontal or vertical, less often rotatory; *positional nystagmus:* immediate onset, no habituation, may change direction with different head positions, no change with visual fixation

VOR testing: After integrity of the neck is assured, bedside testing of the VOR is best accomplished in the following ways:

I. Rapid, passive head rotations (unpredictable, high acceleration) are applied while the patient fixates gaze on a stationary target. The examiner watches for a corrective saccadic eye movement. This occurs after the head rotation only if the VOR has not adequately maintained gaze.

II. A more continuous high-frequency, low-amplitude head oscillation is applied while the examiner views the optic disk with an ophthalmoscope. If the VOR is intact, the disk image should appear stable to the observer.

Quantitative evaluation of the VOR involves measuring eye movement responses to controlled head perturbations and calculating the "VOR gain," which is defined as eye velocity divided by head velocity.

Head rotation in comatose patients with a normal VOR results in compensatory controversive eye movements (see Caloric Testing).

VISUAL FIELDS

The visual fields can be conceptualized as an "island of vision in the sea of blindness." The peak of the island represents the point of highest acuity, the fovea. The optic disk (blind spot) is a bottomless pit in the midst of the island. Visual field testing is performed with stimuli of various sizes, colors, and intensities. There are various kinds of manual and computerized types of perimetry, but confrontation is the mainstay of clinical testing.

The characteristic features of visual field deficits have high localizing value (Fig. 51).

I. Retinal nerve fiber bundle lesions cause defects originating from the blind spot and respecting the horizontal meridian.

II. Optic disk lesions and retinal vascular occlusions often produce defects that respect the nasal horizontal meridian.

III. Optic nerve lesions produce monocular field defects that do not respect the vertical midline. Arcuate defects occur with segmental lesions of the optic nerve.

IV. Cecocentral deficits suggest an optic nerve lesion. Junctional scotoma in the contralateral field is confirmatory and is due to von Willebrand loop involvement.

V. Chiasmal lesions produce bitemporal hemianopias.

VI. All retrochiasmal lesions cause contralateral homonymous hemianopia or quadrantanopia, which increases in congruence (similarity between the eyes) as the lesions approach the occipital lobe. The visual field defects respect the vertical midline.

VII. Visual acuity is not affected by unilateral lesion posterior to the chiasm.

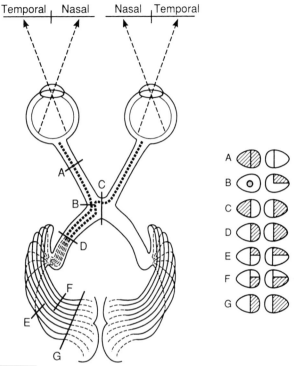

FIGURE 51

A, Complete blindness in left eye. *B*, The usual effect is a left junction scotoma in association with a right upper quadrantanopia. The latter results from interruption of right retinal nasal fibers that project into the base of the left optic nerve (Wilbrand's knee). A left nasal hemianopia could occur from a lesion at this point but is exceedingly rare. *C*, Bitemporal hemianopia. *D*, Right homonymous hemianopia. *E* and *F*, Right upper and lower quadrant hemianopia. *G*, Right homonymous hemianopia.

VIII. Parietal lobe lesions may be associated with smooth pursuit and optokinetic nystagmus asymmetry and visual field defects.

IX. Occipital lobe hemianopias are associated with macular sparing.

X. Homonymous hemianopia and alexia without agraphia are caused by dominant occipital lobe lesion extending to the splenium of corpus callosum.

REFERENCES

American Academy of Ophthalmology: *Basic and clinical science course: Neuro-ophthalmology*, 1997–1998, p 71.

Galetta SL: *Neurosurg Clin North Am* 10:563–577, 1999.

WADA TESTING

This test is named after John A. Wada, a neurologist who first described it. The WADA test is a physiologic and neuropsychological test whereby one part of the brain is chemically suppressed by injecting a short-acting anesthetic substance (such as sodium amobarbital or sodium methohexital or propofol) superselectively into a specific feeding artery. Complete neuropsychological evaluation is performed prior to and after injecting the anesthetic.

The test is usually used prior to performing epilepsy surgery for language and memory lateralization testing and to guide the surgeon regarding the potential loss of language or memory after resection. The drug is injected selectively into the internal carotid artery in this scenario. Superselective cerebral or spinal artery branch WADA testing can also be performed during arteriovenous malformation (AVM) embolization.

Occasionally the test may be performed with clinical examination for motor and sensory dysfunction prior to embolization in treating patients with AVM. Also it can be performed with EEG or evoked potential testing before and after injecting the anesthetic into the artery of interest prior to embolization.

WILSON'S DISEASE

DEFINITION AND PATHOPHYSIOLOGY

Wilson's disease, also known as hepatolenticular degeneration, is an *autosomal recessive* disorder of copper metabolism. There is a defect of hepatic copper excretion due to a mutation in the gene on chromosome 13 for a copper-transporting adenosine triphosphatase (*ATP7B*).

CLINICAL PRESENTATION

Age at onset is usually between 10 and 40 years. It presents with behavioral or personality changes, dysarthria, ataxia, and abnormal movements (chorea, athetosis, tremor, or rigidity). Hepatic dysfunction is identifiable in nearly all patients, and cirrhosis may be apparent early in the course. Other clinical features include hemolytic anemia, joint symptoms, renal stones, cardiomyopathy, pancreatic disease, and hypoparathyroidism. Kayser-Fleischer (KF) rings are present in more than 90% of patients and are virtually pathognomonic. There is brownish discoloration at the corneal limbus, consisting of copper deposits in Descemet's membrane; this may be visible only under slit lamp examination. "Sunflower" cataracts may occur.

DIAGNOSIS

The diagnosis is made by observation of the KF rings, low serum level of ceruloplasmin, elevated 24-hour urinary copper excretion, and increased level of copper in liver biopsy specimen. *Serum copper measurement is often normal.* Although the diagnosis may be relatively easy, Wilson's disease must be suspected in children and younger adults who come to medical attention with unknown hepatic or CNS syndromes.

TREATMENT

Treatment consists of chelation with D-penicillamine. Initial dosages are about 0.5 g/day in children and 1 g/day in divided doses for adults. A low-copper diet to minimize acute worsening caused by mobilization of copper store is helpful. Pyridoxine, 25 mg/day, is given to counter the antimetabolite effect of penicillamine. Acute or delayed hypersensitivity reaction to penicillamine develops in up to 20% of patients receiving treatment but may be overcome in some cases with a reduced dose and concomitant administration of corticosteroids. Trientine (a chelator) and zinc salts, which block GI penicillamine, may help. Ammonium tetrathiomolybdate has also been tried to substitute for D-penicillamine with variable results. Patients with advanced disease may require orthotropic liver transplantation. Levodopa may be of some benefit in reversing neurologic symptoms not improved by penicillamine. New drugs may be developed as studies of the underlying defects in *ATP7B* and its suspected modifiers ATOX1 and COMMD1 continue to explore the disease's genotype-phenotype correlation.

REFERENCES

Danks DM: In Scriver CR et al, eds: *The metabolic basis of inherited disease*, ed 6, New York, McGraw-Hill, 1989.

Das SK, Ray K: *Nat Clin Pract Neurol* 2(9):482–493, 2006.

Pfeil SA, Lynn DJ: *J Clin Gastroenterol* 29(1):22–31, 1999

Z

ZOSTER

Varicella-zoster virus is the infective organism in varicella (chickenpox) and herpes zoster (shingles). Varicella is usually a benign disease of childhood. Rare complications include meningoencephalitis, acute cerebellar ataxia, transverse myelitis, and Reye syndrome. Although full recovery from the first two is common, rare permanent deficits include paresis, seizures, and cognitive changes.

Herpes zoster (literally, "girdle") represents latent virus reactivation. It is most frequently seen in those with weakened cell-mediated immunity, particularly the elderly and immunocompromised. At particular risk are patients with lymphoma who have had radiation and splenectomy and patients with AIDS (who usually develop disseminated disease). Typically, zoster presents with pain in a single or several adjacent dermatomes; pain may precede the vesicular eruption by up to 3 weeks. Pain is described as sharp, lancinating, and associated with itching, dysesthesia, and allodynia (increased skin sensitivity).

Associated findings include altered sensation in the involved dermatome; fewer than 5% have segmental weakness. The CSF may show an elevated protein and a mild lymphocytic pleocytosis. *Diagnosis* is established by typical rash, Tzanck smear, direct immunofluorescence, viral culture, or comparison of acute and convalescent titers. Demonstration of the presence of varicella-zoster DNA (by polymerase chain reaction [PCR] analysis) or of antibodies in CSF to the virus is strong evidence of the infection in the appropriate clinical setting. Serum antibody analysis is of no value. Histologically, zoster is characterized by lymphocytic inflammation and vasculitis resulting in neuronal loss in ganglia. The process may spread to leptomeninges and adjacent spinal cord.

COMPLICATIONS OF THE PERIPHERAL NERVOUS SYSTEM

Varicella-zoster virus may become latent along the entire neuraxis. The most common sites of reactivation are thoracic and trigeminal dermatomes. When zoster affects the cranium (20% of cases), 90% of sites are in the trigeminal distribution and 60% of these will involve the first division— herpes zoster ophthalmicus. Complications include corneal involvement, internal or external ophthalmoplegia, iridocyclitis, and optic neuritis (rare). The prognosis for improvement of ocular motor disturbance is excellent, whereas return of lost vision is minimal. The Ramsay Hunt syndrome denotes zoster of the geniculate ganglion, presenting with painful vesicles on the tympanic membrane and external auditory canal, a peripheral seventh cranial nerve (CN VII) palsy, and variable CN VIII dysfunction. Thoracic zoster may occasionally produce arm weakness (zoster paresis), whereas lumbar reactivation may be associated with leg weakness and bowel/bladder dysfunction.

Rarely the pain occurs in the absence of any rash (zoster sine herpete), leading to considerations of carcinomatous, lymphomatous, or diabetic radiculopathies. Analysis of PCR of varicella DNA in CSF and blood mononuclear cells, and antibody titer in CSF are usually diagnostic.

Treatment: Acyclovir (800 mg five times a day), famciclovir (500 mg tid), or valacyclovir can be given. Pain management is essential but frequently difficult and there may be residual pain despite multiple medications.

Postherpetic neuralgia

Postherpetic neuralgia is characterized by persistent dysesthesias and hyperpathia persisting beyond healing of the zoster vesicles (usually beyond 2 months). The pain has three components: (1) a constant, deep burning pain; (2) paroxysms of shooting pain; (3) sharp pains after light stimulation (allodynia). Pathologically, it is associated with a localized small- and large-fiber sensory neuropathy and may result from reorganization of inputs to the second-order neurons. Postherpetic neuralgia is rare in patients younger than 50, but occurs in up to 50% of patients over 60 and in 75% of those over 70. It resolves within 1 month in 90% of patients and in half of the remainder by 2 months, but may last up to 1 year. Only about 2% of patients have persistent pain, which may last for months or years.

Treatment: Antiviral treatments tend to reduce incidence of the postherpetic neuralgia. Tricyclic antidepressants (amitriptyline/nortriptyline 25 to 75 mg PO qd); anticonvulsants, such as carbamazepine (400 to 1200 mg PO qd), phenytoin (300 to 400 mg PO qd), and gabapentin; prednisone (40 to 60 mg qd 3 to 5 days); and topical aspirin in chloroform or capsaicin 0.75% ointment five times per day for at least 4 weeks may be used. Topical lidocaine (ointment or skin patch) may also help.

Complications of the central nervous system
Occasionally, after reactivation of varicella-zoster virus in either an immunocompetent or immunocompromised patient, the virus spreads into the spinal cord and brain. CNS complications of zoster include myelitis, encephalitis, large-vessel granulomatous arteritis, small-vessel encephalitis, meningitis, and ventriculitis. Myelitis usually occurs 1 to 2 weeks after rash development and may be confirmed by CSF PCR of varicella DNA; the illness is mostly severe in immunocompromised patients. Varicella-zoster can cause encephalitis as a result of large- or small-vessel vasculopathy. Large-vessel (granulomatous) arteritis occurs predominantly in immunocompetent patients and presents with focal deficits (stroke; ischemic or hemorrhagic). Small-vessel encephalitis is the most common complication of CNS varicella-zoster and is seen in immunocompromised patients. Deep-seated ischemic or demyelinating lesions may manifest as headache, fever, vomiting, mental status changes, seizures, and focal deficits. A few cases of ventriculitis and meningitis have occurred in immunocompromised patients. The treatment for CNS complications is with IV acyclovir; steroids are used for anti-inflammatory effects.

Treatment: Oral acyclovir accelerates cutaneous healing but has no effect on acute neuritis or postherpetic neuralgia. In the immunocompromised patient, parenteral acyclovir is more effective than vidarabine in preventing dissemination and accelerating cutaneous healing. Corticosteroids may reduce acute pain and the risk of postherpetic neuralgia, but evidence of effectiveness is inconclusive.

REFERENCES
Gilden DH et al: *N Engl J Med* 342(9):635–645, 2000.
Terrence CF, Fromm GH: In Olesen J, Tfelt-Hansen P, Welch KMA, eds: *The headaches,* chapter 114, New York, Raven Press, 1993.

AAN Guideline Summaries Appendix

EVALUATION AND PROGNOSIS OF COMA
CONFOUNDING FACTORS

Some factors may confound the reliability of the clinical examination and ancillary tests. Major confounders could include the use or prior use of sedatives or neuromuscular blocking agents, induced hypothermia therapy, presence of organ failure (e.g., acute renal or liver failure), or shock (e.g., cardiogenic shock requiring isotopes). However, studies in comatose patients have not systematically addressed the role of these confounders in neurologic assessment.

COMA DECISION ALGORITHM

Exclude major confounders

No brainstem reflexes at any time
(pupil, cornea, oculocephalic, cough)
→ **Yes** Brain death testing → **No** Indeterminate outcome

-or-

Day 1: Myoclonus status epilepticus
→ **Yes** Poor outcome | FPR 0% (0–8.8) → **No** Indeterminate outcome

-or-

Day 1–3: Serum NSE >33 μg/L*
→ **Yes** Poor outcome | FPR 0% (0–3) → **No** Indeterminate outcome

-or-

Day 3: Absent pupil or corneal reflexes;
extensor or absent motor response
→ **Yes** Poor outcome | FPR 0% (0–3) → **No** Indeterminate outcome

-or-

Day 1–3: SSEP absent N20 responses*
→ **Yes** Poor outcome | FPR 0.7% (0–3.7) → **No** Indeterminate outcome

Decision algorithm for use in prognostication of comatose survivors after CPR. The numbers in parentheses are exact 95% confidence intervals. The confounding factors potentially could diminish prognostic accuracy of the algorithm.

NSE = neuron-specific enolase, SSEP = somatosensory evoked potential, FPR = false positive rate.

*These tests may not be available on a timely basis. Serum NSE testing may not be sufficiently standardized.

EVALUATION AND PROGNOSIS OF COMA

COMMUNICATION WITH FAMILY AND FURTHER DECISION MAKING

The complexity of evaluation and various options of decision making require neurologic professional expertise. More than one scheduled meeting with the family is generally required to facilitate a trusting relationship. The neurologist can explain that the prognosis is largely based on clinical examination with some help from laboratory tests. In a conversation with the family, the neurologist may further articulate that the chance of error is very small. When a poor outcome is anticipated, the need for life supportive care (mechanical ventilation, use of vasosuppressors or inotropic agents to hemodynamically stabilize the patient) must be discussed. Fully informed and more certain, the family or proxy is allowed to rethink resuscitation orders or even to adjust the level of care to comfort measures only. However, these decisions should be made after best interpretation of advance directives of the previously voiced wishes of the patient.

RECOMMENDATIONS FOR THE PROGNOSTIC VALUE OF THE CLINICAL EXAMINATION*

Strong (Level A) evidence

- Features of the neurologic examination: Glasgow coma scale (GCS) score; motor part of the GCS; brainstem reflexes (pupillary light reflexes, corneal reflexes, and eye movements)

---

*The terms "level" and "class" will be used extensively throughout this appendix. They are defined as:

Recommendation level: "Level" refers to the strength of the practice recommendation based on the reviewed literature. *Level A:* Established as effective, ineffective, or harmful or as useful/predictive or not useful/predictive; *Level B:* Probably effective, ineffective, or harmful or not useful/predictive; *Level C:* Possibly effective, ineffective, or harmful or useful/predictive or not useful/predictive; *Level U:* Data inadequate or conflicting; treatment, test, or predictor unproven.

Class of evidence for therapy: "Class" refers to the quality of research methods employed in the reviewed literature. *Class I:* Evidence provided by a prospective, randomized, controlled clinical trial with masked outcome assessment, in a representative population. The following are required: (a) primary outcome(s) is/are clearly defined; (b) exclusion/inclusion criteria are clearly defined; (c) adequate accounting for drop-outs and crossovers with numbers sufficiently low to have minimal potential for bias; and (d) relevant baseline characteristics are presented and substantially equivalent among treatment groups or there is appropriate statistical adjustment for differences. *Class II:* Evidence provided by a prospective matched group cohort study in a representative population with masked outcome assessment that meets items a to d above or a randomized control trial in a representative population that lacks one criterion in a to d. *Class III:* All other controlled trials (including well-defined natural history control subjects or patients serving as own controls) in a representative population, where outcome assessment is independent of patient treatment. *Class IV:* Evidence from uncontrolled studies, case series, case reports, or expert opinion.

- The prognosis is invariably poor in comatose patients with absent pupillary or corneal reflexes, or absent or extensor motor responses 3 days after cardiac arrest (Level A).

Good (Level B) evidence

- Presence of seizures or myoclonus status epilepticus (defined as spontaneous, repetitive, unrelenting, generalized multifocal myoclonus involving the face, limbs, and axial musculature) in comatose patients
- Patients with myoclonus status epilepticus within the first day after a primary circulatory arrest have a poor prognosis (Level B).

Good (Level B) evidence

- Circumstances surrounding CPR: anoxia time; duration of CPR; cause of the cardiac arrest (cardiac versus noncardiac); type of cardiac arrhythmia
- Prognosis cannot be based on the circumstances of CPR (Level B).

Weak (Level C) evidence

- Elevated body temperature
- Prognosis cannot be based on elevated body temperature alone (Level C).

RECOMMENDATIONS FOR THE PROGNOSTIC VALUE OF ELECTROPHYSIOLOGIC STUDIES

Good (Level B) evidence

- Somatosensory evoked potentials (SSEPs)
- The assessment of poor prognosis can be guided by the presence of bilaterally absent cortical SSEPs (N20 response) within 1 to 3 days (Level B).

Weak (Level C) evidence

- EEG and evoked/event-related potential (EP) studies
- Burst suppression or generalized epileptiform discharges on EEG predicted poor outcomes but with insufficient prognostic accuracy (Level C).

RECOMMENDATIONS FOR THE PROGNOSTIC VALUE OF BIOCHEMICAL MARKERS

Good (Level B) evidence

- Serum neuron-specific enolase (NSE)
- Serum NSE levels > 33 μg/L at days 1 to 3 after CPR accurately predict poor outcome (Level B).

Insufficient (Level U) evidence

- Serum S100: creatine kinase brain isoenzyme (CKBB)
- There are inadequate data to support or refute the prognostic value of other serum and CSF biochemical markers (Level U).

Insufficient (Level U) evidence

- Intracranial pressure; brain oxygenation
- There are inadequate data to support or refute the prognostic value of ICP monitoring (Level U).

RECOMMENDATIONS FOR THE PROGNOSTIC VALUE OF RADIOLOGIC STUDIES

Insufficient (Level U) evidence

- Neuroimaging studies: CT, MRI, PET
- There are inadequate data to support or refute whether neuroimaging is indicative of poor outcome (Level U).

DIAGNOSIS AND MANAGEMENT OF DEMENTIA

PRACTICE PARAMETER: DIAGNOSIS OF DEMENTIA

- The clinical criteria for Alzheimer's disease (AD) are reliable (DSM IIIR definition; NINCDS-ADRA and DSM IV diagnostic criteria).
- Vascular dementia, dementia with Lewy bodies (DLB), and frontotemporal dementia should be excluded, but the current diagnostic criteria for those diseases are imperfect.
- Structural neuroimaging is appropriate to detect lesions that may result in cognitive impairment.
- The CSF-14-3-3 protein is useful when Creutzfeldt-Jakob disease (CJD) is suspected and recent stroke or viral encephalitis can be excluded.
- Evidence supports the following tests in *routine evaluation of the demented patient:*
  - Complete blood cell count
  - Glucose
  - Depression screening
  - Thyroid function tests
  - Serum electrolytes
  - BUN/creatinine
  - Serum vitamin B_{12} levels
  - Liver function tests
- Evidence indicates the following tests should not be included in the routine evaluation of the demented patient:
  - Screening for syphilis (unless patient has a specific risk factor (e.g., living in a high-incidence region)
  - Linear or volumetric MRI or CT measurement strategies
  - SPECT
  - Genetic testing for DLB or CJD
  - APOE genotyping for AD
  - EEG
  - Lumbar puncture (unless presence of metastatic cancer, suspicion of CNS infection, reactive serum syphilis serology, hydrocephalus, age under 55, rapidly progressive or unusual dementia, immunosuppression, or suspicion of CNS vasculitis)
- At this time, there is not enough evidence to support or refute the use of the following tests:
  - PET
  - Genetic markers for AD not listed above
  - CSF or other biomarkers for AD
  - Tau mutations in patients with FTD
  - AD gene mutations in patients with FTD

PRACTICE PARAMETER: MANAGEMENT OF DEMENTIA

Treat cognitive symptoms of AD with cholinesterase inhibitors and vitamin E. Consider the use of cholinesterase inhibitors in patients with mild to moderate disease. Cholinesterase inhibitors may improve quality of life and cognitive functions including memory, thought and reasoning. They are proved effective for people who are mildly to moderately affected by the disease and are under evaluation in patients with MCI and severe dementia. Therefore, the early recognition and diagnosis of Alzheimer's disease is important. Consider vitamin E to slow progression of AD; selegiline is also supported, albeit by weaker evidence. Do not prescribe estrogen to treat AD.

Treat agitation, psychosis, and depression. The patient's paranoia, suspiciousness, combativeness, or resistance to maintaining personal hygiene can seem overwhelming to families and caregivers and significantly impact quality of life. Evidence indicates that several strategies can decrease problem behaviors. If environmental manipulation fails to eliminate agitation or psychosis, use antipsychotics. Selected tricyclic agents, MAO-B inhibitors, and SSRIs should be considered to treat depression.

Encourage caregivers to participate in caregiver educational programs and support groups. Short-term caregiver educational programs can improve caregiver satisfaction. Long-term caregiver educational programs can delay time to nursing home placement for the AD patient. Caregiver training programs and other support systems (computer support networks, telephone support programs, adult day care, and other respite programs) may also help delay time to nursing home placement for the AD patient.

STRATEGIES TO IMPROVE FUNCTIONAL PERFORMANCE AND REDUCE PROBLEM BEHAVIORS

Strategy	Strength of Evidence
To improve functional performance	
Behavior modification, scheduled toileting, prompted voiding to reduce urinary incontinence	Strong
Graded assistance, practice, and positive reinforcement to increase functional independence	Good
Low lighting levels, music, and simulated nature sounds to improve eating behaviors	Weak
Intensive multimodality group training may improve activities of daily living	Weak
To reduce problem behaviors	
Music, particularly during meals and bathing	Good
Walking or other forms of light exercise	Good
Simulated presence therapy, such as use of videotapes of family	Weak
Massage	Weak
Comprehensive psychosocial care programs	Weak
Pet therapy	Weak
Utilizing light, white noise	Weak
Bright light, white noise	Weak
Cognitive remediation	Weak

WOMEN WITH EPILEPSY

Recommendations: Over 90% of women with epilepsy (WWE) can expect good pregnancy outcomes. A minority of WWE will experience a worsening of seizure control during pregnancy. A coordinated approach to the care of WWE, with contributions from a primary care provider, obstetrician, geneticist, and neurologist, is ideal. Interdisciplinary communication for counseling and management is crucial.

FOR WWE DURING AND AFTER PREGNANCY
There is strong evidence (Class I) you should:
- Optimize therapy for WWE before conception.
- Complete antiepileptic drug (AED) therapy changes at least 6 months before planned conception, if possible.
- Do not change to an alternate AED during pregnancy for the sole purpose of reducing teratogenic risk.
- Offer patients being treated with carbamazepine, divalproex sodium, or valproic acid:
  - Prenatal testing with alpha-fetoprotein levels at 14 to 16 weeks' gestation.
  - Level II (structural) ultrasound at 16 to 20 weeks' gestation; and
  - If appropriate, amniocentesis for amniotic fluid alpha-fetoprotein and acetylcholinesterase levels.
  - Encourage breastfeeding for WWE; monitor the neonate for sedation or feeding difficulties.

There is evidence (Class III) you should consider:
- Monitoring non-protein-bound AED levels during pregnancy. For the stable patient, levels should be ascertained before conception, at the beginning of each trimester, and in the last month of pregnancy. Additional levels should be done when clinically indicated.
- Monitor AED levels through the eighth postpartum week. If AED dosage increases have been necessary during pregnancy, subsequent dosages can probably be reduced to prepregnancy levels safely; this may be necessary to avoid toxicity.
- Prescribe 10 mg/day of vitamin K in the last month of pregnancy for WWE taking enzyme-inducing AEDs.

FOR WWE DURING REPRODUCTIVE YEARS
There is strong evidence (Class I) you should:
- Choose the AED most appropriate for seizure type; goal should be monotherapy.
- Counsel patients entering reproductive years about the decreased effectiveness of hormonal contraception with enzyme-inducing AEDs.
- Begin folic acid supplementation with at least 0.4 mg/day; continue through pregnancy.

There is evidence (Class III) you should:

- Recommend a formulation containing 50 µg of ethinyl estradiol or mestranol if your patient's preferred method of birth control is hormonal contraception and treatment involves an enzyme-inducing AED. The risk of contraceptive failure in this setting should be discussed with the patient and discussion documented.
  - Folic acid supplementation
  - Teratogenic potential of AEDs
  - Possible change in seizure frequency during pregnancy
  - Importance of medication compliance and AED level monitoring during pregnancy
  - Inheritance risks for seizures
  - Vitamin K supplementation last month of pregnancy
  - Pros/cons of breastfeeding

NEW AED IN THE TREATMENT OF NEWLY DIAGNOSED EPILEPSY

SUMMARY OF EVIDENCE FOR AEDS IN THE TREATMENT OF NEWLY DIAGNOSED EPILEPSY

Antiepileptic Drug	Monotheraphy Partial/Mixed	Diagnosed Absence
Gabapentin	Yes**	No
Lamotrigine	Yes**	Yes**
Levetiracetam	No	No
Oxcarbazepine	Yes	No
Tiagabine	No	No
Topiramate	Yes**	No
Zonisamide	No	No

**Not FDA approved.

SUMMARY OF ADVERSE EVENTS ASSOCIATED WITH THE NEW AEDS

	Adverse Events*	
Drug	**Serious**	**Minor**
Gabapentin	None	Weight gain, peripheral edema, behavioral changes[†]
Lamotrigine	Rash, including Stevens-Johnson syndrome and toxic epidermal necrolysis (increased risk for children, also more common with concomitant valproate/divalproex use and reduced with slow titration); hypersensitivity reactions, including risk of hepatic and renal failure, DIC, and arthritis	Tics[†] and insomnia
Levetiracetam	None	Irritability/behavior change
Oxcarbazepine	Hyponatremia (more common in elderly), rash	None
Tiagebine	Stupor or spike wave stupor	Weakness
Topiramate	Nephrolithiasis, open angle glaucoma, hypohidrosis[†]	Metabolic acidosis, weight loss, language dysfunction
Zonisamide	Rash, renal caluli, hypohidrosis[†]	Irritability; photo-sensitivity, weight loss

*Psychosis and depression are associated with epilepsy and occur in open label studies with all new AEDs. Although these side effects may appear more commonly with some drugs than with others, it is difficult to ascertain whether these relationships are causal. Consequently, these side effects have been omitted from the table.

[†]Predominantly children.

Note: This is not meant to be a comprehensive list, but represents the most common adverse events, based on consensus of panel.

NEW AED IN THE TREATMENT OF REFRACTORY EPILEPSY

SUMMARY OF EVIDENCE-BASED GUIDELINE RECOMMENDATIONS FOR USE IN REFRACTORY PARTIAL EPILEPSY

AED	As Adjunctive Therapy in Adults	As Adjunctive Therapy in Children	As Monotherapy
Gabapentin	It is appropriate to use gabapentin as add-on therapy in patients with refractory epilepsy (Level A)	Gabapentin may be used as adjunctive treatment of children with refractory partial seizures (Level A)	There is insufficient evidence to recommend gabapentin as monotherapy for refractory partial epilepsy (Level U)
Lamotrigine	It is appropriate to use lamotrigine as add-on therapy in patients with refractory epilepsy (Level A)	Lamotrigine may be used as adjunctive treatment of children with refractory partial seizures (Level A)	Lamotrigine can be used as monotherapy in patients with refractory partial epilepsy (Level B, downgraded due to dropouts)
Topiramate	It is appropriate to use topiramate as add-on therapy in patients with refractory epilepsy (Level A)	Topiramate may be used as adjunctive treatment of children with refractory partial seizures (Level A)	Topiramate can be used as monotherapy in patients with refractory partial epilepsy (Level A)
Tiagabine	It is appropriate to use tiagabine as add-on therapy in patients with refractory epilepsy (Level A)		There is insufficient evidence to recommend tiagabine as monotherapy for refractory partial epilepsy (Level U)
Oxcarbazepine	It is appropriate to use oxcarbazepine as add-on therapy in patients with refractory epilepsy (Level A)	Oxcarbazepine may be used as adjunctive treatment of children with refractory partial seizures (Level A)	Oxcarbazepine can be used as monotherapy in patients with refractory partial epilepsy (Level A)
Levetiracetam	It is appropriate to use levetiracetam as add-on therapy in patients with refractory epilepsy (Level A)		There is insufficient evidence to recommend levetiracetam as monotherapy for refractory partial epilepsy (Level U)
Zonisamide	It is appropriate to use zonisamide as add-on therapy in patients with refractory epilepsy (Level A)		There is insufficient evidence to recommend zonisamide as monotherapy for refractory partial epilepsy (Level U)

NEW AED IN THE TREATMENT OF REFRACTORY EPILEPSY

SUMMARY OF EVIDENCE-BASED GUIDELINE RECOMMENDATIONS FOR USE IN REFRACTORY PRIMARY GENERALIZED EPILEPSY AND LENNOX-GASTAUT SYNDROME

AED	Refractory Primary Generalized Epilepsy	Lennox-Gastaut Syndrome
Gabapentin	There is insufficient evidence to recommend gabapentin for the treatment of refractory epilepsy in children (Level U)	
Lamotrigine	There is insufficient evidence to recommend lamotrigine for the treatment of refractory epilepsy in children (Level U)	Lamotrigine may be used to treat drop attacks associated with the Lennox-Gastaut syndrome in adults and children (Level A)
Topiramate	Topiramate may be used for the treatment of refractory generalized tonic-clonic seizures in adults and children (Level A)	Topiramate may be used to treat drop attacks associated with the Lennox-Gastaut syndrome in adults and children (Level A)
Oxcarbazepine	There is insufficient evidence to recommend oxcarbazepine for the treatment of refractory epilepsy in children (Level U)	
Levetiracetam	There is insufficient evidence to recommend levetiracetam for the treatment of refractory epilepsy in children (Level U)	
Zonisamide	There is insufficient evidence to recommend zonisamide for the treatment of refractory epilepsy in children (Level U)	

DIAGNOSIS OF PATIENTS WITH NEUROBORRELIOSIS

I. Diagnosis of definite nervous system Lyme disease requires:
   A. Possible exposure to appropriate ticks in an area where Lyme disease occurs
   B. One or more of the following:
      1. Erythema migrans or histopathologically proven *Borrelia* lymphocytoma or acrodermatitis
      2. Immunologic evidence of exposure to *B. burgdorferi*
      3. Culture, histologic, or polymerase chain reaction (PCR) proof of the presence of *B. burgdorferi*
   C. Occurrence of one or more of the neurologic disorders described below, after exclusion of other potential causes. Additional testing may be necessary. CSF analysis for cells, protein, and intrathecal

production of specific antibody is indicated if CNS infection
is suspected.
  1. Causally related neurologic disease
      a. Lymphocytic meningitis with or without cranial neuritis, painful
         radiculoneuritis, or both
      b. Encephalomyelitis
      c. Peripheral neuropathy
  2. Causally related syndrome
      a. Encephalopathy
II. Causal relationship asserted but highly unlikely
   A. Multiple sclerosis
   B. Amyotrophic lateral sclerosis
   C. Dementia
III. Based on a literature review and expert opinion, the following
     recommendations are supported as *options.*
   A. Localized disease is usually responsive to oral antimicrobial regimens
      (e.g., doxycycline or amoxicillin for 3 weeks).
   B. CNS infection probably requires parenteral antimicrobial therapy
      (e.g., ceftriaxone or cefotaxime for 2 or 4 weeks), although limited
      data suggest oral regimens may be efficacious in acute meningitis.

MIGRAINE DIAGNOSIS AND GENERAL TREATMENT CONSIDERATION

Migraine is a neurobiologic disorder that occurs in 18% of women and
6% of men, but may be undiagnosed or undertreated.
- Migraine is a genetically based disorder.
- It may be associated with altered sensitivity of the nervous system and
  activation of the trigeminal-vascular system.
- It is characterized by attacks of head pain and neurologic,
  gastrointestinal, and autonomic symptoms.
- It varies in frequency, duration, and disability among sufferers and
  between attacks.

GENERAL PRINCIPLES OF HEADACHE CARE
- Establish a diagnosis.
- Educate migraine sufferers about their condition.
- Discuss the rationale for each particular treatment, how to use it, and
  what adverse events are likely.
- Establish realistic patient expectations.
- Involve patients in managing their migraines. Encourage patients
  to use headache diaries to track triggers, frequency and severity of
  headaches, and response to treatment.
- Encourage the patient to identify and avoid triggers.
- Choose treatment based on the frequency and severity of attacks, the
  presence and degree of disability, and associated symptoms, such as
  nausea and vomiting.

- Create a formal management plan and individualize management. Consider the patient's preference, response to, and tolerance for previously administered medications. Beware of increasing frequency of acute medications. Identify coexisting conditions (such as heart disease, gastrointestinal disease, renal impairment, pregnancy, and uncontrolled hypertension), as they may limit treatment choices.

DIAGNOSIS
- Migraine is a chronic condition with episodic manifestations; attacks vary in frequency and duration among sufferers and between attacks.
- The International Headache Society criteria form the basis for migraine diagnosis.
- If atypical features are present, exclude secondary headaches.
- There is insufficient evidence to recommend any diagnostic testing other than neuroimaging. Electroencephalography is not indicated in the routine evaluation of headache.
- Neuroimaging should be considered in nonacute headache patients with:
  - Unexplained abnormal neurologic examination
  - Atypical headache, headache features, or an additional risk factor, such as immune deficiency

GOALS OF ACUTE TREATMENT
Acute care should be individualized based on the patient's symptoms and level of disability.
- Treat attacks effectively, rapidly, and consistently to minimize adverse events.
- Restore the patient's ability to function.
- Minimize the need for back-up and rescue medications.*
- Optimize self-care and reduce subsequent use of resources.

GUIDE TO ACUTE TREATMENT
- Act promptly. Failure to use an effective treatment promptly may increase pain, disability, and the impact of the headache.
- Use triptans (naratriptan, rizatriptan, sumatriptan, and zolmitriptan) and DHE in patients who have moderate or severe migraine, or whose mild-to-moderate headaches respond poorly to NSAIDs or combinations, such as aspirin plus acetaminophen plus caffeine, or other agents, such as ergotamine (see full guideline and table 1 at http://aan.com/go/practice/guidelines).
- NSAIDs (oral), combination analgesics containing caffeine, and isometheptene combinations are an option for the mild-to-moderate

---

*A rescue medication is used at home when other treatments fail. It permits the patient to achieve relief without the discomfort and expense of a visit to the physician's office or emergency department.

migraine attacks or severe attacks that have been responsive in the past to similar agents.
- Select a nonoral route of administration for patients with migraine associated with severe nausea or vomiting.
- Do not restrict antiemetics only to patients who are vomiting or likely to vomit.
- Use a self-administered rescue medication for patients whose severe migraine does not respond to (or fails) other treatments.
- Limit and carefully monitor opiate- and butalbital-containing analgesics.
- Guard against medication-overuse headache ("rebound headache"). Attempt to limit acute therapy to 2 days per week.

PREVENTIVE THERAPIES

Preventive therapies should be used when migraine has a substantial impact on a patient's life. Consider preventive therapies when any of the following are present:
- Frequent headaches (>2/week)
- Migraine that significantly interferes with patient's daily routines, despite acute treatment
- Contraindication to, failure, adverse effects, or overuse of acute therapies
- Patient preference
- Presence of uncommon migraine conditions, including hemiplegic migraine, basilar migraine, migraine with prolonged aura, or migrainous infarction

Goals of preventive therapies:
- Reduce attack frequency, severity, and duration.
- Improve responsiveness to acute treatment.
- Improve function and reduce disability.

Guide to preventive medication use:
- Use medication with best efficacy and fewest adverse events (see full guideline and table 2 at http://aan.com/go/practice/guidelines).
- Take coexisting conditions into account.
- Select a drug that will treat more than one condition, if possible.
- Be sure that the coexistent disease is not a contraindication to the migraine treatment.
- Be sure that the treatments used for coexistent conditions do not exacerbate migraine.
- Beware of drug interactions.
- Start low and increase dose slowly until benefits are achieved or limited side effects occur.
- Give the drug an adequate trial at adequate dosage (2–3 months).
- Avoid interfering medications (e.g., overuse of acute medication).
- Consider a long-acting formulation, which may improve compliance.
- Monitor the patient's headache diary.
- Re-evaluate therapy. If headache is controlled at 6 months, consider tapering or discontinuing treatment.

Nonpharmacologic therapies:

The following nonpharmacologic headache treatments may be used along or combined with preventive drug therapy to achieve additional clinical improvement:

- Relaxation training
- Thermal biofeedback with relaxation training
- EMG biofeedback
- Cognitive-behavioral therapy

ACUTE AND PREVENTIVE THERAPY OF MIGRAINE HEADACHE IN CHILDREN AND ADOLESCENTS

SUMMARY OF RECOMMENDATIONS FOR THE ACUTE TREATMENT OF MIGRAINE IN CHILDREN AND ADOLESCENTS

Strong evidence supports:

- Ibuprofen is effective and should be considered for the acute treatment of migraine in children (Class I, Level A).
- Sumatriptan nasal spray is effective and should be considered for the acute treatment of migraine in adolescents (Class I, Level A).

Good evidence supports:

- Acetaminophen is probably effective and should be considered for the acute treatment of migraine in children (Class I, Level B).

Evidence is insufficient to support or refute:

- There are no supporting data for the use of any oral "triptan" preparations in children or adolescents (Class IV, Level U).
- There are inadequate data to make a judgment on the efficacy of subcutaneous sumatriptan (Class IV, Level U).

SUMMARY OF RECOMMENDATIONS FOR PREVENTIVE THERAPY OF MIGRAINE IN CHILDREN AND ADOLESCENTS

Good evidence supports:

- Flunarizine is probably effective for preventive therapy and can be considered for this purpose, but it is not available in the United States (Class I, Level B).
- Pizotifen and nimodipine (Class I, Level B) and clonidine (Class II, Level B) did not show efficacy and are not recommended.

Evidence is insufficient to support or refute:

- There is insufficient evidence to make any recommendations concerning the use of cyproheptadine, amitriptyline, divalproex sodium, topiramate, or levetiracetam (Class IV, Level U).
- Recommendations cannot be made concerning propranolol or trazodone for preventive therapy because the evidence is conflicting (Class II, Level U).

The practice parameter closes with the statement: "Failure of an agent for either the acute or preventive treatment to demonstrate efficacy to a statistically significant degree does not imply that these medications have no role in the pediatric population and their use must be based upon good clinical judgment."

SUPPORTIVE MANAGEMENT OF PATIENTS WITH ALS

Managing the symptoms: In managing symptoms to improve the quality of life of the patient, family, and health care provider, evidence supports the following:

Nutrition: Consider PEG (percutaneous endoscopic gastrostomy) soon after symptom onset for patients who have symptomatic dysphagia (B). For optimal safety and efficacy, offer and implement PEG when the patient's vital capacity is above 50% of predicted (B). (See following treatment algorithm.)

Respiration: Deciding when to initiate noninvasive mechanical ventilation is critical because of the risk of either sudden death or ventilator dependence. Be vigilant for symptoms indicating hypoventilation (B). For best results in prolonging patient survival, initiate therapy before the patient's vital capacity falls below 50% of predicted (B). Respect the patient's right to refuse or withdraw any treatment, including mechanical ventilation. When withdrawing ventilation, use adequate opiates and anxiolytics to relieve dyspnea and anxiety (B). (See following treatment algorithm.)

Sialorrhea: Treat sialorrhea with glycopyrrolate, benziropine, transdermal hyoscine, atropine, trihexyphenidyl hydrochloride, or amitriptyline (C).

Pseudobulbar affect (emotional lability): Treat pseudobulbar affect with amitriptyline or consider fluvoxamine as an alternate choice (C).

Palliative care: As ALS progresses, the goal of the patient care changes from maximizing function to providing effective and compassionate palliative care. Two of the most prevalent and unpleasant symptoms in the terminal phase are dyspnea and anxiety. Dyspnea can be treated with opioids alone or with supplemental oxygen (B) or possibly with chlorpromazine or acupuncture (C). Anxiety can be treated with anxiolytics such as lorazepam or diazepam, opioids, or chlorpromazine. Hospice care should be considered.

Breaking the news:
- Give the diagnosis in person and never by telephone (B).
- Discuss the implications of the diagnosis, respecting the patient's cultural and social background by asking if the patient wishes to receive the information or have it communicated to a family member (B).
- Provide written reference materials about the disease and about support and advocacy organizations (B), as well as a letter or audiotape summarizing what you have discussed (B).

HOW SHOULD A PHYSICIAN BREAK BAD NEWS TO A PATIENT?*

Location:
- Quiet, comfortable, and private

Structure:
- Talk in person, face-to-face
- Choose a convenient time
- Take enough time to ensure no rushing or interruptions

*Adapted from Ptacek, Eberhardt, *JAMA* 276(6):496–502, 1996.

- Make eye contact and sit close to patient

Participants:

- Have patient's support network available

What is said:

- Find out what the patient already knows about the condition
- Ascertain how much the patient wants to know about the disease
- Give a warning comment that bad news is coming
- Acknowledge and explore patient's reaction and allow for emotional expression
- Summarize the discussion verbally, in writing, or on audiotape
- Allow for questions

Reassurance:

- Explain whether the complications of the disease are treatable
- Indicate that every attempt will be made to maintain function and that patient's decisions will be respected
- Reassure that care for the patient will continue
- Discuss opportunities to participate in research treatment protocols
- Acknowledge willingness to get a second opinion if the patient wishes

How it is said:

- Emotional manner: warm, caring, empathic, respectful
- Give news at person's pace; allow patient to dictate what he or she is told

Language:

- Simple words, yet direct; use no euphemisms or medical jargon

ALGORITHMS FOR NUTRITIONAL AND RESPIRATORY MANAGEMENT OF ALS

ALGORITHM FOR NUTRITION MANAGEMENT

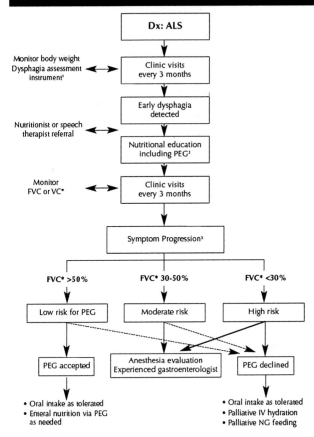

¹Rule out contraindications

²Prolonged mealtime, ending meal prematurely because of fatigue, accelerated weight loss due to poor caloric intake, family concern about feeding difficulties

*Forced vital capacity (FVC) or vital capacity (VC) can be used. VC may be more accurate in patients with bulbar dysfunction

³For example, Colorado Dysphagia Disability Inventory, bulbar questions in the ALS Functional Rating Scale, or other instrument

Dx = diagnosis   PEG = percutaneous endoscopic gastrostomy

ALGORITHMS FOR NUTRITIONAL AND RESPIRATORY MANAGEMENT OF ALS

ALGORITHM FOR RESPIRATORY MANAGEMENT

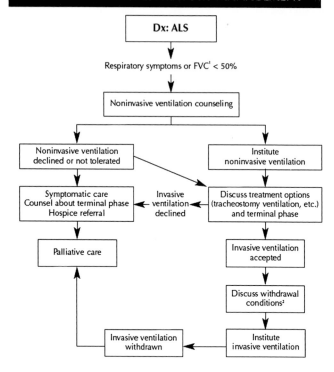

[Dx: ALS]

Respiratory symptoms or FVC[1] < 50%

Noninvasive ventilation counseling

Noninvasive ventilation declined or not tolerated

Institute noninvasive ventilation

Symptomatic care
Counsel about terminal phase
Hospice referral

Invasive ventilation declined

Discuss treatment options (tracheostomy ventilation, etc.) and terminal phase

Palliative care

Invasive ventilation accepted

Discuss withdrawal conditions[2]

Invasive ventilation withdrawn

Institute invasive ventilation

[1]*Forced vital capacity (FVC) or vital capacity (VC) can be used. VC may be more accurate in patients with bulbar dysfunction*

[2]*Agreement needed for conditions of withdrawal prior to or concurrent with instituting invasive ventilation (e.g., locked-in state, coma, etc.)*

Dx = diagnosis

Classification of management recommendations: Definitions
Standard: A principle for patient management that reflects a high degree of certainty based on Class I evidence, or very strong evidence from Class II studies when circumstances preclude randomized trials (A)
Guideline: Recommendations for patient management reflecting moderate clinical certainty (usually Class II evidence or strong consensus of Class III evidence) (B)

Option: A strategy for patient management for which the evidence (Class III) is inconclusive or when there is some conflicting evidence or opinion (C)

MRI UTILITY IN MS AND DIAGNOSTIC CONSIDERATION IN PATIENTS WITH WHITE MATTER LESIONS
EVIDENCE FOR USING MRI FOR EARLY DIAGNOSIS OF MS
Strong evidence supports:

1. On the basis of consistent Class I, II, and III evidence, in clinically isolated demyelinating (CIS) patients, the finding of three or more white matter lesions on a T_2-weighted MRI scan is a very sensitive predictor (>80%) of the subsequent development of CDMS within the next 7 to 10 years (Level A recommendation). It is possible that the presence of even a smaller number of white matter lesions (e.g., one to three) may be equally predictive of future MS, although this relationship requires better classification.
2. The appearance of new T_2 lesions or new gadolinium (Gd) enhancement 3 or more months after a clinically isolated demyelinating episode (and after a baseline MRI assessment) is highly predictive of the subsequent development of CDMS in the near term (Level A recommendation).
3. The probability of making a diagnosis other than MS in CIS patients with any of the above MRI abnormalities is quite low, once alternative diagnoses that can mimic MS or the radiographic findings of MS have been excluded.

Good evidence supports:

4. The presence of two or more Gd-enhancing lesions at baseline is highly predictive of the future development of CDMS (Level B recommendation).

Evidence is insufficient to support or refute:

5. The MRI features helpful in the diagnosis of PPMS cannot be determined from the existing evidence (Level U recommendation).

DIAGNOSTIC CONSIDERATIONS IN PATIENTS WITH SUSPECTED MS OR MRI WHITE MATTER ABNORMALITIES

- Age-related white matter changes
- Acute disseminated encephalomyelitis
- Behçet's disease
- Bacterial infections (syphilis, Lyme disease)
- Cerebral autosomal dominant arteriopathy, subcortical infarcts, and leukoencephalopathy (CADASIL)
- Cervical spondylosis or stenosis
- HIV infection
- Human T-lymphotrophic virus I/II
- Ischemic optic neuropathy (arteritic and nonarteritic)
- Leukodystrophies (e.g., adrenoleukodystrophy, metachromatic leukodystrophy)

- Neoplasms (e.g., lymphoma, glioma, meningioma)
- Migraine
- Sarcoid
- Sjögren's syndrome
- Stroke and ischemic cerebrovascular disease and spinal cord infarction
- Systemic lupus erythematosus, antiphospholipid antibody syndromes, and related collagen vascular disorders
- Unidentified bright objects
- Vascular malformations
- Vasculitis (primary CNS or other)
- Vitamin B_{12} deficiency

DISEASE-MODIFYING THERAPIES IN MULTIPLE SCLEROSIS

GLUCOCORTICOIDS

1. On the basis of several and generally consistent Class I and Class II studies, glucocorticoid treatment has been demonstrated to have a short-term benefit on the speed of functional recovery in patients with acute attacks of MS. It is appropriate, therefore, to consider for treatment with glucocorticoids any patient with an acute attack of MS (Type A recommendation).
2. There does not appear, however, to be any long-term functional benefit after the brief use of glucocorticoids in this clinical setting (Type B recommendation).
3. Currently, there is not compelling evidence to indicate that these clinical benefits are influenced by the route of glucocorticoid administration, the particular glucocorticoid prescribed, or the dosage of glucocorticoid, at least at the doses that have been studied to date (Type C recommendation).
4. On the basis of a single Class II study, it is considered possible that regular pulse glucocorticoids may be useful in the long-term management of patients with RRMS (Type C recommendation).

INTERFERON BETA

1. On the basis of several consistent Class I studies, IFN-β has been demonstrated to reduce the attack rate (whether measured clinically or by MRI) in patients with MS or with clinically isolated syndromes who are at high risk for developing MS (Type A recommendation). Treatment of MS with IFN-β produces a beneficial effect on MRI measures of disease severity such as T_2 disease burden and probably also slows sustained disability progression (Type B recommendation).
2. As a result, it is appropriate to consider IFN-β for treatment in any patient who is at high risk for developing CDMS, or who already has either RRMS or SPMS and is still experiencing relapses

(Type A recommendation). The effectiveness of IFN-β in patients with SPMS but without relapses is uncertain (Type U recommendation).

3. It is possible that certain populations of MS patients (e.g., those with more attacks or at earlier disease stages) may be better candidates for therapy than others, although, at the moment, there is insufficient evidence regarding these issues (Type U recommendation).

4. On the basis of Class I and II studies and several pieces of consistent Class III evidence, it is considered probable that there is a dose-response curve associated with the use of IFN-β for the treatment of MS (Type B recommendation). It is possible, however, that a portion of this apparent dose-effect instead may be due to differences in the frequency of IFN-β administration (rather than dose) between studies.

5. On the basis of several Class II studies, the route of administration of IFN-β is probably not of clinical importance, at least with regard to efficacy (Type B recommendation). The side effect profile, however, does differ between routes of administration. There is no known clinical difference between the different types of IFN-β, although this has not been thoroughly studied (Type U recommendation).

6. On the basis of several Class I studies, treatment of patients with MS with IFN-β is associated with the production of NAb (Type A recommendation). The rate of NAb production, however, is probably less with IFN-β-1a treatment than with IFN-β-1b treatment (Type B recommendation). The biologic effect of NAb is uncertain, although their presence may be associated with a reduction in clinical effectiveness of IFNβ treatment (Type C recommendation). Whether there is a difference in immunogenicity between subcutaneous and intramuscular routes of administration is unknown (Type U recommendation). The clinical utility of measuring NAb in an individual on IFN-β therapy is uncertain (Type U recommendation).

GLATIRAMER ACETATE

1. On the basis of Class I evidence, glatiramer acetate has been demonstrated to reduce the attack rate (whether measured clinically or by MRI) in patients with RRMS (Type A recommendation). Treatment with glatiramer acetate produces a beneficial effect on MRI measures of disease severity, such as T_2 disease burden, and possibly also slows sustained disability progression in patients with RRMS (Type C recommendation).

2. As a result, it is appropriate to consider glatiramer acetate for treatment in any patient who has RRMS (Type A recommendation). Although it may be that glatiramer acetate also is helpful in patients with progressive disease, there is no convincing evidence to support this hypothesis (Type U recommendation).

CYCLOPHOSPHAMIDE

1. Based on consistent Class I evidence, pulse cyclophosphamide treatment does not seem to alter the course of progressive MS (Type B recommendation).
2. Based on a single Class III study, it is possible that younger patients with progressive MS might derive some benefit from pulse plus booster cyclophosphamide treatment (Type U recommendation).

METHOTREXATE

1. Based on limited and somewhat ambiguous Class I evidence from a single trial, it is considered possible that methotrexate favorably alters the disease course in patients with progressive MS (Type C recommendation).

AZATHIOPRINE

1. On the basis of several, but somewhat conflicting, Class I and II studies, it is considered possible that azathioprine reduces the relapse rate in patients with MS (Type C recommendation).
2. Its effect on disability progression has not been demonstrated (Type U recommendation).

CLADRIBINE

1. On the basis of consistent Class I evidence, it is concluded that cladribine reduces Gd enhancement in patients with both relapsing and progressive forms of MS (Type A recommendation).
2. Cladribine treatment does not, however, appear to alter favorably the course of the disease, either in terms of attack rate or disease progression (Type C recommendation).

CYCLOSPORINE

1. Based on this Class I study, it is considered possible that cyclosporine provides some therapeutic benefit in progressive MS (Type C recommendation).
2. However, the frequent occurrence of adverse reactions to treatment, especially nephrotoxicity, together with the small magnitude of the potential benefit, makes the risk/benefit of this therapeutic approach unacceptable (Type B recommendation).

INTRAVENOUS IMMUNOGLOBULIN

1. The studies of intravenous immunoglobulin (IVIG), to date, have generally involved small numbers of patients, have lacked complete data on clinical and MRI outcomes, or have used methods that have been questioned. It is, therefore, only possible that IVIG reduces the attack rate in RRMS (Type C recommendation).
2. The current evidence suggests that IVIG is of little benefit with regard to slowing disease progression (Type C recommendation).

PLASMA EXCHANGE

1. On the basis of consistent Class I, II, and III studies, plasma exchange is of little or no value in the treatment of progressive MS (Type A recommendation).
2. On the basis of a single small Class I study, it is considered possible that plasma exchange may be helpful in the treatment of severe acute episodes of demyelination in previously nondisabled individuals (Type C recommendation).

SULFASALAZINE

1. Based on a single Class I study, it is concluded that treatment of MS with sulfasalazine provides no therapeutic benefit in MS (Type B recommendation).

SURGICAL THERAPY OF DIABETIC NEUROPATHY

USE OF SURGICAL DECOMPRESSION FOR TREATMENT OF DIABETIC NEUROPATHY

Insufficient Level U evidence:

There are inadequate data concerning the efficacy of decompressive surgery for the treatment of diabetic neuropathy. Given current knowledge, this treatment is unproved (Level U).

IMMUNOTHERAPY IN MANAGEMENT OF GUILLAIN-BARRÉ SYNDROME

EVIDENCE FOR IMMUNOTHERAPY IN GBS MANAGEMENT

	Plasma Exchange (PE)	IV Immunoglobulin (IVIG)	Combined Treatments	Corticosteroids
Strong evidence supports	PE recommended in nonambulant patients within 4 weeks of onset of neuropathic symptoms (Level A, Class II)	IVIG recommended in nonambulant patients within 2 weeks of onset of neuropathic symptoms (Level A, Class II)	Sequential treatment with PE followed by IVIG does not have a greater effect than either treatment given alone (Level A, Class II)	Steroids not recommended in the treatment of GBS (Level A, Class I)
	Plasma Exchange (PE)		**IV Immunoglobulin (IVIG)**	
Good evidence supports	PE recommended for ambulant patients within 2 weeks of onset of neuropathic symptoms (Level B, Class II)		IVIG recommended in nonambulant patients started within 4 weeks from the onset of neuropathic symptoms (Level B, Class II)	
	If PE started within 2 weeks of onset, there are equivalent effects of PE and IVIG in patients requiring walking aids (Level B, Class II)		If started within 2 weeks of onset, IVIG has comparable efficacy to PE in patients requiring walking aids (Level B, Class I)	
	PE is a treatment option for children with severe GBS (Level B, derived from Class II evidence in adults)		IVIG is a treatment option for children with severe GBS (Level B, derived from Class II evidence in adults)	
	Combined Treatments		**CSF Filtration**	**Immunoabsorption**
Evidence is insufficient to support	There is insufficient evidence to support or refute immunoabsorption treatment followed by IVIG (Level U, Class IV)		There is insufficient evidence to support or refute the use of CSF filtration (Level U, limited Class III)	The evidence is insufficient to support or refute immunoabsorption as an alternative to PE (Level U, Class IV)

TREATING PARKINSON'S DISEASE

RECOMMENDATIONS FOR MEDICATIONS THAT REDUCE OFF-TIME FOR PATIENTS WITH MOTOR FLUCTUATIONS

Strong Level A evidence: The following medications should be offered to reduce off-time in Parkinson's disease (PD) patients with motor fluctuations:

- Entacapone
- Rasagiline

Good Level B evidence: The following medications should be considered to reduce off-time in PD patients with motor fluctuations:

- Pramipexole
- Tolcapone (should be used with caution and requires monitoring for hepatotoxicity)
- Ropinirole
- Pergolide (should be used with caution and requires monitoring for valvular fibrosis)

Weak Level C evidence: The following medications may be considered to reduce off-time in PD patients with motor fluctuations:

- Apomorphine injected subcutaneously
- Cabergoline
- Selegiline

Weak Level C evidence:
The following medications may be disregarded to reduce off-time in PD patients with motor fluctuations:

- Sustained release carbidopa/levodopa
- Bromocriptine

RECOMMENDATIONS FOR THE RELATIVE EFFICACY OF MEDICATIONS THAT REDUCE OFF-TIME FOR PATIENTS WITH MOTOR FLUCTUATIONS

Weak Level C evidence: Ropinirole may be chosen over bromocriptine to reduce off-time in PD patients with motor fluctuations.

Insufficient Level U evidence: There is insufficient evidence to support or refute the use of any agent over another.

RECOMMENDATIONS FOR MEDICATIONS THAT REDUCE DYSKINESIA

Weak Level C evidence: Amantadine may be considered for patients with PD with motor fluctuations in reducing dyskinesia.

Insufficient Level U evidence: There is insufficient evidence to support or refute the efficacy of clozapine in reducing dyskinesia. Clozapine's potential toxicity, including agranulocytosis, seizures, myocarditis, and orthostatic hypotension with or without syncope, and required white blood cell count monitoring must be considered.

RECOMMENDATIONS FOR DEEP BRAIN STIMULATION (DBS)

Location	Recommendations for Efficacy	Factors That Predict Improvement After DBS
DBS of the subthalamic nucleus (STN)	DBS of the STN may be considered as a treatment option in PD patients to improve motor function and to reduce motor fluctuations, dyskinesia, and medication usage (Level C). Patients need to be counseled regarding the risks and benefits of this procedure.	Based upon two Class II studies, preoperative response to levodopa is probably predictive of postsurgical improvement. Preoperative response to levodopa should be considered as a factor predictive of outcome after DBS of the STN (Level B). Based on one Class II study, younger age and shorter disease duration (less than 16 years) are possibly predictive of greater improvement after DBS of the STN. Age and duration of PD may be considered as factors predictive of outcome after DBS of the STN. Younger patients with shorter disease duration may possibly have improvement greater than that of older patients with longer disease duration (Level C).
DBS of the globus pallidus interna (GPi)	There is insufficient evidence to make any recommendations about the effectiveness of DBS of the GPi in reducing motor complications or medication usage or in improving motor function in PD patients (Level U).	There is insufficient evidence to make any recommendations about factors predictive of improvement after DBS of the GPi in PD patients (Level U).
DBS of the ventral intermediate (VIM) nucleus of the thalamus	There is insufficient evidence to make any recommendations about the effectiveness of DBS of the VIM nucleus of the thalamus in reducing motor complications or medication usage or in improving motor function in PD patients (Level U).	There is insufficient evidence to make any recommendations about the effectiveness of DBS of the VIM nucleus of the thalamus in reducing motor complications or medication usage or in improving motor function in PD patients (Level U).

TREATING BEHAVIORAL CHANGES IN PARKINSON'S DISEASE

RECOMMENDATIONS FOR SCREENING FOR DEPRESSION, PSYCHOSIS, AND DEMENTIA

Depression:

- The Beck Depression Inventory (BDI-I) and Hamilton Depression Rating Scale (HDRS-17) should be considered for depression screening in PD (Level B).
- Montgomery Asberg Depression Rating Scale (MADRS) may be considered for screening for depression associated with PD (Level C).

Psychosis:

- No recommendation is made.

Dementia:

- The Mini-Mental State Examination and the Cambridge Cognitive Examination (CAMCog) should be considered as screening tools for dementia in patients with PD (Level B).

RECOMMENDATIONS FOR TREATING DEPRESSION, PSYCHOSIS, AND DEMENTIA

Depression:

- Amitriptyline may be considered in the treatment of depression associated with PD (Level C). Although the highest level of evidence is for amitriptyline, it is not necessarily the first choice for treatment of depression associated with PD.
- There is insufficient evidence to make recommendations regarding other treatments for depression in PD (Level U). Absence of literature demonstrating clear efficacy of non-tricyclic antidepressants is not the same as absence of efficacy.

Psychosis:

- Clozapine should be considered for patients with PD and psychosis (Level B). Clozapine use is associated with agranulocytosis and may be fatal. The absolute neutrophil count must be monitored.
- Olanzapine should not be routinely considered for patients with PD and psychosis (Level B).
- Quetiapine may be considered for patients with PD and psychosis (Level C).

Dementia:

- Donepezil should be considered for the treatment of dementia in PD (Level B).
- Rivastigmine should be considered for the treatment of dementia in PD or DLB (Level B).

STANDARDS OF TRANSCRANIAL DOPPLER APPLICATION

There are four standards for the application of transcranial Doppler (TCD):

I. TCD is able to provide information and clinical utility is established:

		Sensitivity %	Specificity %
Sickle cell disease	Screening of children aged 2–16 years with sickle cell disease for assessing stroke risk (Type A, Class I), although the optimal frequency of testing is unknown.	86	91
Angiographic vasospasm	Detection and monitoring of angiographic vasospasm after spontaneous subarachnoid hemorrhage (Type A, Class I-II).		
	More data are needed to show if its use affects clinical outcomes (Type U).		
	Intracranial ICA	25–30	83–91
	MCA	39–94	70–100
	ACA	13–71	65–100
	VA	44–100	42–79
	BA	77–100	42–79
	PCA	48–60	78–87

II. TCD is able to provide information, but clinical utility compared to other diagnostic tools remains to be determined:

		Sensitivity %	Specificity %
Cerebral thrombolysis	TCD is probably useful for monitoring thrombolysis of acute MCA occlusions (Type B, Class II-III). More data are needed to assess the frequency of monitoring for clot dissolution and enhanced recanalization and to influence therapy (Type U).		
	Complete occlusion	50	100
	Partial occlusion	100	76
	Recanalization	91	93
Cerebral microembolism detection	TCD monitoring is probably useful for the detection of cerebral microembolic signals in a variety of cardiovascular/ cerebrovascular disorders/procedures (Type B, Class II-IV). Data do not support the use of this TCD technique for diagnosis or monitoring response to antithrombotic therapy in ischemic cerebrovascular disease (Type U).		
Carotid endarterec-tomy	TCD monitoring is probably useful to detect hemodynamic and embolic events that may result in perioperative stroke during and after CEA in settings where monitoring is felt to be necessary (Type B, Class II-III).		
Coronary artery bypass graft (CABG) surgery	TCD monitoring is probably useful (Type B, Class II-III) during CABG for detection of cerebral microemboli. TCD is possibly useful to document changes in flow velocities and CO_2 reactivity during CABG surgery (Type C, Class III). Data are insufficient regarding the clinical impact of this information (Type U).		
Vasomotor reactivity testing	TCD is probably useful (Type B, Class II-III) for the detection of impaired cerebral hemodynamics in patients with severe (>70%) asymptomatic extracranial ICA stenosis, symptomatic or asymptomatic extracranial ICA occlusion, and cerebral small artery disease. Whether these techniques should be used to influence therapy and improve patient outcomes remains to be determined (Type U).		
Vasospasm (VSP) after traumatic subarachnoid hemorrrhage (SAH)	TCD is probably useful for the detection of VSP following traumatic SAH (Type B, Class III), but data are needed to show its accuracy and clinical impact in this setting (Type U).		
TCCS	TCCS is possibly useful (Type C, Class III) for the evaluation and monitoring of space-occupying ischemic MCA infarctions. More data are needed to show if it has greater value than CT and MRI scanning and if its use affects clinical outcomes (Type U).		

III. TCD is able to provide information, but clinical utility remains to be determined:

		Sensitivity %	Specificity %
Intracranial steno-occlusive disease	TCD is probably useful (Type B, Class II-III) for the evaluation of occlusive lesions of intracranial arteries in the basal cisterns (especially the ICA siphon and MCA). The relative value of TCD compared with MR angiography or CT angiography remains to be determined (Type U). Data are insufficient to recommend replacement of conventional angiography with TCD (Type U).		
	Anterior circulation	70–90	90–95
	Posterior circulation occlusion	50–80	80–96
	MCA	85–95	90–98
	ICA, VA, BA	55–81	96
Cerebral circulatory arrest (adjunctive test in the determination of brain death)	If needed, TCD can be used as a confirmatory test, in support of a clinical diagnosis of brain death (Type A, Class II).	91–100	97–100

IV. TCD is able to provide information, but other diagnostic tests are typically preferable:

		Sensitivity %	Specificity %
Right-to-left cardiac shunts	While TCD is useful for detection of right-to-left cardiac and extracardiac shunts (Type A, Class II), transesophageal echocardiography (TEE) is superior, as it can provide direct information regarding the anatomic site and nature of the shunt.	70–100	> 95
Extracranial ICA stenosis	TCD is possibly useful for the evaluation of severe extracranial ICA stenosis or occlusion (Type C, Class II-III), but in general, carotid duplex and MR angiography are the diagnostic tests of choice.		
	Single TCD variable	3–78	60–100
	MCA	49–95	42–100
	ACA	89	100
Contrast-enhanced TCCS	CE-TCCS may provide information in patients with ischemic cerebrovascular disease and aneurysmal SAH (Type B, Class II-IV). Its clinical utility compared to CT scanning, conventional angiography, or nonimaging TCD is unclear (Type U).		

Neurologic Emergency Appendix

ACUTE ISCHEMIC STROKE

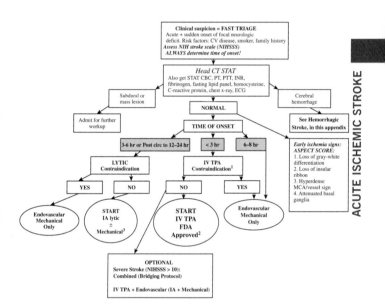

---

[1]Contraindication of IV TPA: Prior ICH, major surgery, or trauma in the past
2 months, symptoms resolving, GI bleeding in the past 3 months, MI in the past
3 months, LP in the past 7 days, stroke or brain surgery in the past 3 months,
seizures, platelets less than 100,000, INR > 1.7, elevated PTT, glucose < 50
or > 400, evidence of early infarct signs.

[2]IV TPA dose: 0.9 mg/kg (up to 90 mg); 10% over 1 min immediately, remain 60
min IV infusion with NS.

[3]Mechanical: Clot retrieval device, intra-arterial (IA) ultrasound clot disruption,
microwire clot manipulation, balloon angioplasty of clot, acute stenting

BACTERIAL MENINGITIS AND SEVERE ENCEPHALITIS

Treatment starts with the empiric antibiotics (ceftriaxone, vancomycin, ampicillin, metronidazole, acyclovir).

NEUROCRITICAL CARE

- In patients with a high risk of brain herniation, consider monitoring intracranial pressure and intermittent administration of osmotic diuretics (mannitol [25%] or hypertonic [3%] saline) to maintain an intracranial pressure below 15 mm Hg and a cerebral perfusion pressure of at least 60 mm Hg.
- Initiate repeated lumbar puncture, lumbar drain, or ventriculostomy in patients with acute hydrocephalus.
- Use EEG to monitor patients with a history of seizures and fluctuating scores on the Glasgow coma scale. Scores on the Glasgow coma scale can range from 3 to 15, with 15 indicating a normal level of consciousness.

AIRWAY AND RESPIRATORY CARE

- Intubate or provide noninvasive ventilation in patients with worsening consciousness (clinical and laboratory indicators for intubation include poor cough and pooling secretions, a respiratory rate greater than 35 breaths per minute, arterial oxygen saturation below 90% or arterial partial pressure of oxygen above 60 mm Hg, and arterial partial pressure of carbon dioxide above 60 mm Hg).
- Maintain ventilatory support with intermittent mandatory ventilation, pressure-support ventilation, or continuous positive airway pressure.

CIRCULATORY CARE

- In patients with septic shock, administer low doses of corticosteroids (if there is a poor response on corticotropin testing indicating adrenocorticoid insufficiency, corticosteroids should be continued).
- Initiate inotropic agents (dopamine or milrinone) to maintain blood pressure (mean arterial pressure, 70–100 mm Hg).
- Initiate crystalloids or albumin (5%) to maintain adequate fluid balance.
- Consider the use of a Swan-Ganz catheter to monitor hemodynamic measurements.

GASTROINTESTINAL CARE

- Initiate nasogastric tube feeding of a standard nutrition formula.
- Initiate prophylaxis with proton-pump inhibitors.

OTHER SUPPORTIVE CARE

- Administer subcutaneous heparin as prophylaxis against deep venous thrombosis.
- Maintain normoglycemic state (serum glucose level <150 mg/dL) with the use of sliding-scale regimens of insulin or continuous intravenous administration of insulin.

- In patients with a body temperature above 40°C, use cooling by conduction or antipyretic agents.

MYASTHENIA CRISIS

DIAGNOSIS
- Diagnosis begins with clinical examination, EMG/NCS (with single-fiber EMG, RNS) testing, and assessing anti-acetylcholine receptor antibodies.
- Chest imaging (CT/MRI) is used to rule out a thymoma.

TREATMENT
- Airway and respiratory support is described below.
- Consider discontinuing cholinesterase inhibitors for a short period; they cloud the clinical picture and may be causing or worsening weakness due to cholinergic crisis.
- Avoid medications that can worsen neuromuscular function: neuromuscular blockers, magnesium, aminoglycosides, beta-blockers, fluoroquinolones, D-penicillamine, quinine, quinidine, and telithromycin.
- Plasmapheresis: Usually, five exchanges is considered equivalent to intravenous immunoglobulin (IVIG) 2 g/kg, administered 0.4 g/kg/day for 5 days.

AIRWAY AND RESPIRATORY ISSUES
- Follow respiratory parameters closely (negative inspiratory force [NIF] and forced vital capacity [FVC] q 4 hr) in a *monitored setting* in nonintubated patients.
- Closely observe bulbar function with concerns for aspiration and loss of airway patency.
- Strict aspiration precautions.
- Continuous pulse oximetry with supplemental oxygen prn. CPAP or BIPAP may be used cautiously in select patients.
- Move the patient to an ICU immediately if any respiratory support is required or if the patient is fatiguing.

INTUBATION/MECHANICAL VENTILATION
Endotracheal intubation is usually indicated if NIF falls below 20 cm H_2O, FVC is less than 1 L, and $Paco_2$ is above 50 mm Hg or the patient is clinically in respiratory failure. Intubation may be performed on the spontaneously breathing patient with topical anesthesia to the oropharynx and mild sedation. Propofol and opioids should have no effect on neuromuscular transmission, although they will cause respiratory depression. Barbiturates and etomidate can be used as well without affecting NM transmission. If the situation is emergent, a *rapid sequence induction* is typically used. If neuromuscular blockade is needed, succinylcholine (1.5 mg/kg) or low-dose nondepolarizing neuromuscular blockers (0.6 mg/kg rocuronium) can be used. Succinylcholine lasts 3 to 5 minutes and rocuronium lasts 30 to 60 minutes. The duration of succinylcholine effect may be prolonged by cholinesterase inhibitors

(such as pyridostigmine). However, this is usually not clinically significant. The patient will likely be relatively resistant to succinylcholine owing to the paucity of acetylcholine receptors, necessitating the larger intubating dose (1.5 mg/kg). Nondepolarizing neuromuscular blockers may have a prolonged duration of action (up to a few hours) as a result of enhanced sensitivity to the drugs. This is usually of minimal concern clinically, as the patient will typically remain intubated for days. Infusions of neuromuscular blockers should be avoided. Endotracheal intubation facilitates maintenance of airway patency, delivery of oxygen, and pulmonary toilet. Use PEEP to reduce atelectasis and improve oxygenation. Controlled ventilatory modes can be changed to assisted modes as neuromuscular function improves.

EXTUBATION CRITERIA
Adequate bulbar function to protect airway and clear secretions, NIF at least −20 cm H_2O, and F/VT < 100 (frequency/tidal volume ratio or rapid shallow breathing index) during a spontaneous breathing trial with minimal ventilator support.

HEADACHE MANAGEMENT
APPROACH TO HEADACHE

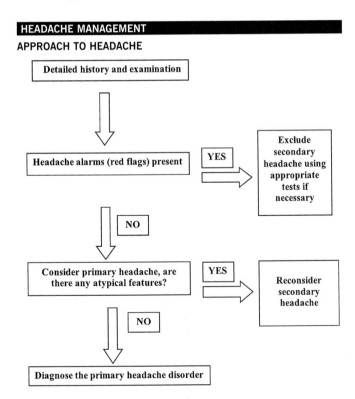

DIAGNOSIS OF HEADACHE

RED FLAGS IN THE DIAGNOSIS OF HEADACHE

Red Flag	Consider	Possible Investigation(s)
Sudden-onset headache	Subarachnoid hemorrhage, bleed into a mass or arteriovenous malformation (AVM), mass lesion (especially posterior fossa)	Neuroimaging, lumbar puncture (after neuroimaging evaluation)
Worsening-pattern headache	Mass lesion, subdural hematoma, medication overuse	Neuroimaging
Headache with systemic illness (fever, neck stiffness, cutaneous rash)	Meningitis, encephalitis, Lyme disease, systemic infection, collagen vascular disease, arteritis	Neuroimaging, lumbar puncture, biopsy, blood tests
Focal neurologic signs, or symptoms other than typical visual or sensory aura	Mass lesion, AVM, collagen vascular disease	Neuroimaging, collagen vascular evaluation
Papilledema	Mass lesion, pseudotumor, encephalitis, meningitis	Neuroimaging, lumbar puncture (after neuroimaging evaluation)
Triggered by cough, exertion, or Valsalva maneuver	Subarachnoid hemorrhage, mass lesion	Neuroimaging, consider lumbar puncture
Headache during pregnancy or post partum	Cortical vein/cranial sinus thrombosis, carotid dissection, pituitary apoplexy	Neuroimaging
New headache type in a patient with		
Cancer	Metastasis	Neuroimaging,
Lyme disease	Meningoencephalitis	lumbar puncture
HIV	Opportunistic infection, tumor	(after neuroimaging evaluation)

INTERNATIONAL HEADACHE SOCIETY CLASSIFICATION OF MIGRAINE HEADACHE

1 Migraine without aura
   1.2 Migraine with aura
        1.2.1 Migraine with typical aura
        1.2.2 Migraine with prolonged aura
        1.2.3 Familial hemiplegic migraine
        1.2.4 Basilar migraine
        1.2.5 Migraine aura without headache
        1.2.6 Migraine with acute onset aura
   1.3 Opthalmoplegic migraine
   1.4 Retinal migraine

HEMORRHAGIC STROKE

In evaluation of hemorrhagic stroke, the possibility of subarachnoid hemorrhage (SAH) must be considered.

Patient Presenting With Signs And Symptoms Suggestive of Spontaneous Hemorrhagic Stroke

STAT Head CT

Subrachonoid Hemorrhage (SAH) — Intracranial Hemorrhage (ICH)

**Admit to NEUROINTENSIVE CARE UNIT
GENERAL TREATMENT**

1. Intubate if Glasgow coma scale < 8

2. Hyperventilate, osmotic therapy, nonsurgical consult for impending herniation

3. immediate blood pressure control:
Systolic BP ~ 140 mm Hg
    a. Labetolol 10 mg IV q 10 min (hold if HR < 60), may repeat as necessary
    b. Nicardipine drip 3–5 mg/hr; titrate to goal

4. Seizure prophylaxis:
    a. For SAH: Phenytoin, valproic acid or levetiracetam IV
    b. For cortical ICH:

5. Pain control and analgesia

6. Nimodpine 60 mg p/NG q 4 hr for SAH

7. Consider factor VII 80 μg/kg IV for ICH particularly with anti coagulation

SAH EVALUATION
1. CT angiogram (CTA)
2. If CTA negative: Cerebral angiogram (DSA)
3. (See the figure on page 545.)

ICH EVALUATION
1. Consider MRI in suspicious lobar and cortical cases
2. Consider conventional angiogram in patient without history of hypertension.

1. General ICU management: DVT, GI prophylaxis, nutritional support, ventilator management, infection control

2. Neuroprotective measures:
Temperature controls
Tight glucose controls
Magnesium > 2.0
Adequate CPP

3. Cerebral edema management

4. Hydrocephalus management, if present, with external ventriculostomy drainage.

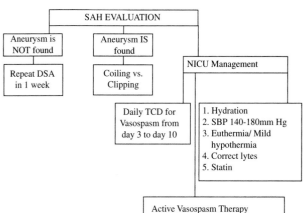

INTRACRANIAL PRESSURE MANAGEMENT

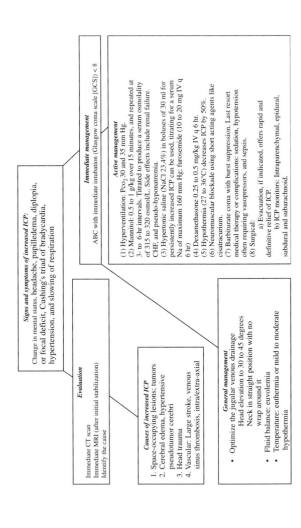

Signs and symptoms of increased ICP:
Change in mental status, headache, papilledema, diplopia, or focal deficit, Cushing's triad of bradycardia, hypertension, and slowing of respiration

Evaluation

Immediate CT scan
Immediate MRI (after initial stabilization)
Identify the cause

Causes of increased ICP
1. Space-occupying lesions; tumors
2. Cerebral edema, hypertensive pseudotumor cerebri
3. Head trauma
4. Vascular: Large stroke, venous sinus thrombosis, intra/extra-axial

General management
- Optimize the jugular venous drainage
  Head elevation to 30 to 45 degrees
  Neck in straight position with no wrap around it
- Fluid balance: euvolemia
- Temperature: euthermia or mild to moderate hypothermia

Immediate management
ABC with immediate intubation (Glasgow coma scale [GCS] < 8

Active management
(1) Hyperventilation: Pco_2 30 and 35 mm Hg.
(2) Mannitol: 0.5 to 1 g/kg over 15 minutes, and repeated at 3- to 6-hr intervals. Titrated to produce a serum osmolality of 315 to 320 osmol/L. Side effects include renal failure. CHF, and pseudo-hyponatremia.
(3) Hypertonic saline (NaCl 23.4%) in boluses of 30 ml for persistently increased ICP can be used, titrating for a serum Na of maximum 160 mm Hg; furosemide (10 to 20 mg IV q 6 hr)
(4) Dexamethasone 0.25 to 0.5 mg/kg IV q 6 hr.
(5) Hypothermia (27 to 36°C) decreases ICP by 50%.
(6) Neuromuscular blockade using short acting agents like cisatracurium.
(7) Barbiturate coma with burst suppression. Last resort medical therapy or complications: sedation, hypotension often requiring vasopressors, and sepsis.
(8) Surgical:
  a) Evacuation, if indicated, offers rapid and definitive relief of ICP.
  b) ICP monitors: Intraparenchymal, epidural, subdural and subarachnoid.

NEUROMUSCULAR DISEASES

Suggested respiratory parameters:

	Vital capacity (VC)	Negative Inspiratory Force (NIF, or MIP)	Maximum Expiratory Pressure (MEP)
Normal Values	50 to 70 mL/kg	>60 cm H_2O	>100 cm H_2O

	VC	NIF	MEP
Consider NICU Admission	25 to 30 mL/kg	-30 to -40 cm H_2O	< 50 cm H_2O

	VC	NIF	MEP
Intubation/Assisted Ventilation	10 to 15 mL/kg	<20 cm H_2O	< 40 cm H_2O

NEUROPATHIC PAIN

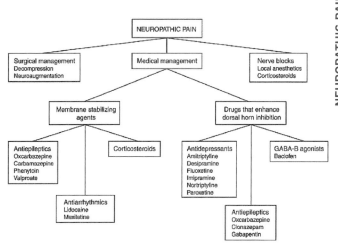

NEUROPATHIC PAIN

REFERENCE

Adapted from Chong MS, Bajwa ZH. *J Pain Symptom Manage* 25(5 Suppl):S4–S11, 2003.

NONACUTE ISCHEMIC STROKE

See the general approach suggested for acute ischemic stroke.

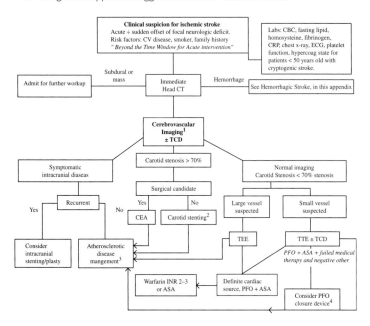

QUADRIPLEGIA

For management and further details of physical exam, workup, and differential diagnosis, see particular chapters.

A variety of conditions must be considered in patients who present with acute generalized muscle weakness including diseases of neuromuscular junction, spinal cord diseases/injuries, polyneuropathies, CNS diseases, and primary acute neuropathies.

---

[1] Cerebrovascular imaging: MRI and MRA or CTA ± carotid US.

[2] Stenting indications (SAPPHIRE study): significant cardiac or pulmonary disease, contralateral carotid occlusion, previous radical neck surgery, contralateral trigeminal nerve palsy, recurrent stenosis after CEA, >80 years old.

[3] Atherosclerotic disease management (ASA or plavix or aggrenox, lipid and metabolic syndrome control).

[4] If patient is <50 years old with cryptogenic stroke who failed medical therapy with significant PFO and atrial septal aneurysm.

DIFFERENTIAL DIAGNOSIS OF ACUTE QUADRIPLEGIA

Traumatic: Acute spinal cord injury
Autoimmune: Guillain-Barré syndrome
        Myasthenic crisis
        Transverse myelitis
Infections: (1) Tick paralysis, (2) botulism, (3) diphtheria, (4) tetanus
Toxins: Organophosphate toxicity
Vascula: Ischemic stroke/locked-in syndrome, hemorrhagic spinal cord or brain stem stroke (AVM, AVF)
Electrolyte: Hypophosphatemia/calcemia/kalemia, hypermagnesemia
Hospital acquires: Critical illness polyneuropathy and myopathy
Genetic: Acute porphyria

1. NICU admission: The common reasons for NICU admission are respiratory failure (most common), pneumonia, deep venous trombosis and/or pulmonary embolus, and autonomic dysfunction. Clinical manifestations of *respiratory failure* are increased respiratory rate and use of accessory muscles, weak shoulder shrugs and head elevation, absence of paradoxic inward movement of the abdominal wall with inspiration, complaints of air hunger, and inability to count to 20 on one breath.

2. History and physical: Trauma, ingestion of toxins, known history of myasthenia, tick bite, etc. Distinguishing true muscle weakness from functional; localizing the site of the lesion within the neuromuscular system and determining the cause of the lesion.

    Spinal cord injury: Causes to consider are traumatic, rheumatologic, neoplastic, infectious, inflammatory/immunologic, vascular, and toxic/metabolic. *Physical exam* should include inspection (spinal deformity), palpation (deformity, tenderness), motor function (including sphincter function), sensory function, and deep tendon reflexes. Goal of *imaging* is to identify the area that places the spinal cord at risk. Should be obtained in all trauma patients. When all radiographic modalities are combined (standard X-rays, CT, MRI) sensitivity is >95%. Important part of clinical approach is to determine spinal stability (combination of clinical findings and imaging). For C-spine in particular, clearing can be made by screening of clinical risk factors of neck or back pain and tenderness, sensory or motor deficits, impaired level of consciousness, alcohol or drug intoxication, painful/distracting injuries outside the spine or spinal cord region, and having normal imaging.

    Guillain-Barré syndrome (GBS), in severe cases, is a major cause of acute placid quadriplegia. Usually a preceding viral illness or immunization can be found. Diagnosis is made by through a combination of history and *physical exam*, characterized by progressive areflexic weakness. One can find a wide clinical spectrum of diseases (acute inflammatory demyelinating polyneuropathy, acute motor axonal neuropathy, acute motor sensory axonal neuropathy, Miller-Fisher syndrome). The clinical approach should focus on *predictors of mechanical ventilation*—presence of bulbar dysfunction and bilateral facial palsy, autonomic dysfunction (arrthymias, hemodynamic instability), short time to severe symptoms from the onset. It is necessary to monitor for fatigue or severe oropharyngeal weakness and respiratory function (vital capacity (VC) < 1 L, maximal inspiratory pressure < 30 cm H_2O, maximal expiratory pressure < 40 cm H_2O, reduction $> 30\%$ of baseline VC, $Po_2 < 70\%$ on room air), which would indicate the need to intubate and start mechanical ventilation.

Pearls of GBS management: (1) Do not hesitate to intubate, if needed; (2) neurologic exam does not correlate with impending respiratory failure; (3) blood gas analysis is not a good indicator of need for intubation; (4) hypoxia occurs usually late, and hypercarbia leads to decreased mental status.

Myasthenia gravis (MG) can occur at any age and is characterized by weakness and fatiguability. In the acute scenario, patients can present in *myasthenic* or *cholinergic crisis*. *Myasthenic crisis* (more frequent in patients with thymoma) is usually precipitated by infection, medications, aspiration pneumonitis, upper airway obstruction, pregnancy, or surgery. *Cholinergic crisis* (miosis, diarrhea, increased salivation, abdominal cramps, bradycardia) is typical when patients increase they intake of anticholinergic medications. It is often difficult to differentiate them, however, on *physical exam*. Pupil size should be small or pinpoint in cholinergic crisis. Tensilone test can differentiate the two crises, because symptoms improve in a myasthenic crisis. The clinical approach should focus on *predictors of mechanical ventilation,* as with GBS.

Tetanus presents typically with trismus or "lockjaw," nuchal rigidity, and dysphagia. Later, as the disease spreads, generalized muscle spasms occur. The most common source is an infection by *Clostridium tetani* through wounds, lacerations, and IV drug use, with risk factors being lack of immunization and diabetes. *Diagnosis* is solely clinical (history, clinical presentation, physical exam); however, a spatula test can be helpful (if the patient bites on a spatula inserted into the pharynx, the test is positive for tetanus; if the patient gags, the test is negative). *Therapy* should focus on controlling respiratory function (early tracheostomy), autonomic instability, muscle spasms, providing neutralizing agents (human tetanus immunoglobulin and metronidazole), and supportive care (quiet, dark room).

Botulism is caused by a neurotoxin of *Clostridium botulinum,* and most of the new cases occurr in IV drug users. *Clinical presentation* is characterized by oculobulbar muscle weakness and a descending pattern of paralysis. *Diagnosis* is based on findings of toxin (serum, stool, wound) and EMG. *Therapy* is mainly supportive and attention to respiratory status.

Periodic paralysis is a rare group of disorders, divided into two categories: *hypokalemic (HypoKPP)* or *hyperkalemic (KyperKPP)*. Patients are usually asymptomatic between episodes and have full recovery after the attacks. Both *present* usually before adulthood. In HypoKPP the attacks are often precipitated by a high-carbohydrate meal and are long in duration (many hours). In HyperKPP attacks are usually precipitated by fasting and tend to be short. *Diagnosis* is usually made by combination of clinical evaluation and measuring serum potassium levels. For *treatment* of HypoKPP, oral potassium supplementation is most effective. For HyperKPP, inhaled beta-agonists (metaproterenol nebulizers) are used. In severe cases IV calcium gluconate, insulin,   and glucose are administered.

Acute intermittent porphyria is a autosomal dominant disease of porphyrin metabolism manifested by recurrent attacks of abdominal pain and neurologic complications. The *neurologic manifestations* usually include anxiety, agitation, cranial nerve palsies, muscle paralysis, seizures, and mental status changes. The *diagnosis* is based on detection of delta amino-levulonic acid and porphobilinogen in the urine. Attacks are usually precipitated by medications or infection. The mainstay of *therapy* is avoidance of precipitating factors and supportive treatment.

Organophosphate toxicity causes irreversible inhibition of cholinesterases. Acute intoxication is most commonly the result of suicide attempts or accidental insecticide exposure. The potential use of organophosphate in chemical warfare is a concern. *Clinical presentation* is characterized by m*uscarinic symptoms* (miosis, conjunctival hyperemia, rhinorrhea, drooling, bronchospasm, increased bronchial secretion, respiratory distress, pulmonary edema, laryngeal spasms, sweating, bradycardia, hypotension, urinary and bowel incontinence) and by *nicotinic symptoms* (fasciculations, paralysis). Severe intoxication ultimately leads to ataxia, dysartria,   confusion, seizures, and coma. *Diagnosis* is made by history of exposure, clinical picture, and serum levels of organophosphates and cholinesterase activity. *Therapy* consists mainly of protecting the patient from further exposure (gastric lavage, cleaning the contaminated skin or membranes) and use of atropine and pralidoxime (cholinesterase reactivator).

Tick paralysis is caused by a paralytic toxin from the salivary glands of pregnant female ticks. Weakness begins two days post-exposure and presents with an ascending pattern with maximal evolution of symmetrical flaccid paralysis and arreflexia. The tick is commonly found in the hair of the scalp and should be removed. *Therapy* is mainly supportive.

Critical illness (polyneuropathy and myopathy) has bean found in 33% to 44% of critically ill patients and is responsible for failure to wean from mechanical ventilation in these patients. The two possible etiologic factors are severe sepsis or systemic inflammatory response syndrome and a combination of neuromuscular blocking agents or steroids. *Clinically* these patients are difficult to wean and have quadriparesis and muscle waisting. The *diagnosis* is based on EMG studies. Measurement of serum CK and muscle biopsy are helpful. *Therapy* is supportive, and most patients eventually recover despite persistent EMG abnormalities.

REFERENCES

Suarez JI: *Critical care neurology and neurosurgery,* Totowa, NJ, Humana Press, 2004.

Torbey MT: "Neuromuscular disorders," in Bhardway A, Mirski M, Ulatowski JA: *Handbook of neurocritical care,* Totowa, NJ, Humana Press, 2004.

SPINAL CORD INJURY

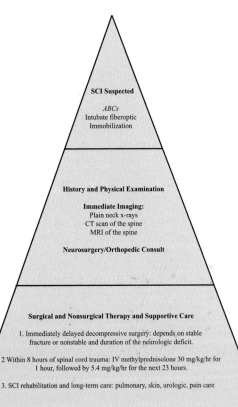

SCI Suspected

ABCs
Intubate fiberoptic
Immobilization

History and Physical Examination

Immediate Imaging:
Plain neck x-rays
CT scan of the spine
MRI of the spine

Neurosurgery/Orthopedic Consult

Surgical and Nonsurgical Therapy and Supportive Care

1. Immediately delayed decompressive surgery: depends on stable fracture or nonstable and duration of the neurologic deficit.

2. Within 8 hours of spinal cord trauma: IV methylprednisolone 30 mg/kg/hr for 1 hour, followed by 5.4 mg/kg/hr for the next 23 hours.

3. SCI rehabilitation and long-term care: pulmonary, skin, urologic, pain care

STATUS EPILEPTICUS

TREATMENT

1. ABCs, intubation basket ready (including medications and emergency airway and cardiac medical supply and ventilation in the room), two IV lines.
2. Thiamine 100 mg IV, one amp of D_{50} (if not diabetic), routine stat laboratory tests.
3. Intermittent boluses of lorazepam 2 mg IV while simultaneously asking for 20 mg/kg of fosphenytoin or phenytoin at 50 mg/minute; if status epilepticus persists; additional 10 mg/kg may be given.
4. If phenytoin intolerant; IV valproic acid 40 to 60 mg/kg or IV phenobarbital 20 mg/kg or recently levetiracetam 30 to 50 mg/kg.
5. History of progressive (PME) or juvenile (JME) myoclonus epilepsy (worsens PME and ineffective in JME); replace with IV valproic acid or IV phenobarbital.
6. Tonic status epilepticus with Lennox-Gastaut syndrome can get worse by benzodiazepines; consider IV valproic acid or IV phenobarbital.
7. Acute intermittent porphyria exacerbation with P-450 inducers, consider NG gabapentin (if possible) or IV valproic acid.
8. Focal status epilepticus without impairment of consciousness, IV treatment not indicated, load anticonvulsants orally or rectally.
9. Refractory status epilepticus: IV valproic acid, start with 40 mg/kg and, if status epilepticus persists, give an additional 20 mg/kg. Continuous intravenous infusion (CIV) usually starts with the lower dose, which is titrated to achieve seizure suppression and is increased as tolerated if tachyphylaxis develops. *Ketamine: rule out increased intracranial pressure before administration.* Other drugs include felbamate, topiramate, levetiracetam, lidocaine, inhalation anesthetics.
10. Dosage and pharmacokinetics of most anticonvulsants must be adjusted appropriately in patients with hepatic or renal failure, or with drug interactions.

STATUS EPILEPTICUS

Impending status epilepticus → Established status epilepticus → Refractory status epilepticus

5 min

30 min

Before emergency room

Diazepam rectal gel
15–20 mg

or

Intravenous lorazepam
2 mg, may repeat once

or

Intravenous diazepam
5 mg, may repeat once

Intravenous midazolam
0.2 mg/kg bolus
0.05 mg/kg/hr

or

Intravenous lorazepam
up to 0.1 mg/kg

or

Intravenous diazepam
up to 0.25–0.4 mg/kg

Emergency room

Intravenous
fosphenytoin/
phenytoin
20–30 mg/kg

Intravenous
valproic acid
40–60 mg/kg
3 mg/kg/min

Intensive care unit

Propofol loading
2–5 mg/kg
CIV 2–10 mg/kg/hr

or

Midazolam
loading 0.2 mg/kg
CIV 0.1–2 mg/kg/hr

or

Pentobarbital
loading up to 10 mg/kg
≤ 25 mg/min
CIV 0.5–2 mg/kg/hr

Ketamine
bolus 1.5 mg/kg
CIV 0.01–0.05 mg/kg/hr

and/or

Other drugs

Electroencephalographic monitoring ?

Airway, blood pressure, temperature, intravenous access, electrocardiography, CBC, glucose, electrolytes, AED levels, ABG, tox screen; central line ?

11. Supportive care: ventilator cart, tracheostomy, PEG tube placement, bowel regimen. Some patients in prolonged refractory status epilepticus will need systemic and pulmonary artery catheterization, with total parenteral nutrition, fluid, and vasopressors as indicated.

REFERENCE

Lancet Neurol 5(3):246–256, 2006.

Therapeutic Appendix

CHEMOTHERAPY: COMMON NEURO-ONCOLOGIC DRUGS

Agent	Mechanism	Dosage	Side Effects
Carboplatin (Paraplatin)	DNA alkylation	400–500 mg/m² IV every 4 weeks	Myelosuppression, nausea, altered LFTs
Carmustine (BCNU)	Nitrosourea; DNA and RNA alkylation	80 mg/m²/day for 3 days; repeat every 6 weeks	Nausea, pain at injection site, hypotension, myelosuppression, diarrhea
Carmustine wafer (Gliadel)		Wafer implanted after tumor resection	
Cisplatin	DNA alkylation	60–120 mg/m² IV every 4 weeks	Nausea, renal toxicity, ototoxicity, neuropathy, myelosuppression
Cyclophosphamide (Cytoxan)	DNA alkylation	50 mg PO qd (low-dose metronomic)	Mild nausea, stomatitis
Dexamethasone (Decadron)	Corticosteroid; decrease vasogenic edema	*Brain tumor:* 2–100 mg/day; usually started with 4 mg IV or PO every 4–6 hours *Epidural spinal cord compression:* 10–100 mg IV × 1; then 16–100 mg/day in divided doses	Immunosuppression, weight gain, myopathy, osteoporosis, cataracts, glucose intolerance/diabetes mellitus
Erlotinib (Tarceva; OSI774)	EGFR kinase inhibitor	150 mg PO qd (NEIAC) 400 mg PO qd (EIAC)	Acneiform rash, diarrhea
Erythropoietin (Epo; Procrit; Epogen)	Erythropoietin	Epo: 20,000–40,000 units SC weekly	Hypertension, allergic reaction

Darbepoietin (Aranesp)	Topoisomerase II inhibitor	Darbepoietin: 2.25 μg/kg SC or IV weekly
Etoposide (VP-16)		50 mg/m²/day PO for 21 consecutive days in 28-day cycle	Myelosuppression, nausea, stomatitis
Filgastim (Neupogen)	Granulocyte-colony stimulating factor	Filgastim: 5 μg/kg/day SC or IV	Bone pain, local reaction, mild LFT
Pegfilgastim (Neulasta)		Pegfilgastim: 6 mg SC × 1; 24 hours after chemotherapy	abnormalities
Gefitinib (Iressa; ZD1839)	EGFR kinase inhibitor	500 mg PO qd (NEIAC)	Diarrhea, acneiform rash, nausea,
		500 mg PO bid (EIAC)	altered LFTs, interstitial lung disease
Hydroxyurea (Hydrea)	Antimetabolite; inhibit nucleotide reductase	500 mg bid	Transient myelosuppression, nausea, diarrhea
Imatinib mesylate (Gleevec; STI571)	c-kit and PDGFR kinase inhibitor	500 mg PO qd (NEIAC)	Myelosuppression, edema, rash,
		500 mg PO bid (EIAC)	musculoskeletal pain
Irinotecan (Camptosar; CPT-11)	Topoisomerase I inhibitor	125 mg/m² (NEIAC); 340 mg/m² (EIAC) IV once weekly for 4 weeks in 6-week cycle	Cholinergic side effects, diarrhea, myelosuppression
Lomustine (CCNU)	Nitrosourea; DNA and RNA alkylation	110 mg/m² every 6 weeks	Nausea, vomiting, stomatitis,
		110–130 mg/m² on day 1 in 42-day cycle of PCV regimen	diarrhea, myelosuppression, lung fibrosis (in prolonged and high-dose treatment)
Methotrexate	Antimetabolite; dihydrofolate reductase inhibitor	IV: 8 g/m² every 14 days; dose adjusted by creatinine clearance	Myelosuppression, stomatitis, renal dysfunction, cortical blindness,
		Intrathecal: 10 mg twice weekly for 8 weeks	leukoencephalopathy

cont'd

CHEMOTHERAPY: COMMON NEURO-ONCOLOGIC DRUGS

CHEMOTHERAPY: COMMON NEURO-ONCOLOGIC DRUGS—cont'd

Agent	Mechanism	Dose	Side Effects
Procarbazine (Matulane)	DNA alkylation and depolymerization	125 mg/m² × 28 days; then off for 28 days or 60 mg/m² PO on days 8 to 21; in 42-day cycle of PCV regimen	Myelosuppression, nausea, flu-like symptoms, musculoskeletal pain, photosensitivity, hallucination, seizures
13-cis-Retinoic acid (Accutane)	Unknown; antiangiogenesis; inhibits protein kinase C	100 mg/m²/day for 21 consecutive days in 28-day cycle	Rash, hyperlipidemia, myelosuppression
Tamoxifen (Nolvadex)	Unknown; inhibits protein kinase C pathway	80 mg PO bid (female) 100 mg PO bid (male)	Hot flashes, nausea, fatigue, menstrual irregularities, gynecomastia, thrombogenesis
Temozolomide (Temodar)	DNA methylation	75 mg/m²/day × 42 days with radiation therapy for gliomas 150–200 mg/m²/day for 5 consecutive days every 28 days	Nausea, constipation, headache, fatigue, myelosuppression, mild LFT abnormalities
Thalidomide (Thalomid)	Antiangiogenesis	200–1200 mg PO qh	Teratogenesis, fatigue, sedation, neuropathy, constipation, skin rash, thrombogenesis
Vincristine	Inhibits RNA synthesis	1.4 mg/m² IV on days 8 and 29; in 42-day cycle of PCV regimen	Injection site reaction, neuropathy (dose-dependent), myelosuppression

EGFR, epidermal growth factor receptor; EIAC, enzyme-inducing anticonvulsants—phenytoin, carbamazepine, oxcarbazepine, primidone, and phenobarbital; LFT, liver function test; NEIAC, non-enzyme-inducing anticonvulsants—gabapentin, levetiracetam, tiagabine, valproic acid, lamotrigine, zonisamide, topiramate, and pregabalin; PCV, procarbazine, CCNU, vincristine; PDGFR, platelet-derived growth factor receptor.

CHOREA (MOVEMENT DISORDER)

Medication	Dosage	Action	Side Effects
Clozapine (Clozaril)	12.5–25 mg qh, increase by 12.5–25 mg q 3 d max 150 mg	D1 and D2 blocker, blocks serotonin type 2 (5 HT₂), alpha-adrenergic, H1, and cholinergic receptors	Sedation, diarrhea, weight gain, hypotension, dose-related seizures, agranulocytosis
Haloperidol (Haldol)	Begin 0.5–1 mg and increase by 0.5 mg qw in tid dosing max 10 mg	Blocks D1 and D2 receptors in the brain	Tardive dyskinesia, acute dystonia, akathisia, swallowing, gait difficulties, parkinsonism
Perphenazine	Begin 4 mg qd, increase by 4 mg/wk tid max 24 mg	Blocks postsynaptic mesolimbic dopaminergic receptors	Tardive dyskinesia, acute dystonia, akathisia, swallowing, gait difficulties, parkinsonism
Quetiapine (Seroquel)	25 mg qh, increase by 25 mg q 3–5 d bid max 400 mg	Proposed D2 and 5-HT2 antagonist	Parkinsonism, depression, drowsiness, hypotension
Reserpine	Begin 0.1 mg, increase by 0.1 mg q 5–7 d tid or qid max 3 mg	Depletes norepinephrine and dopamine	Parkinsonism, depression, drowsiness, hypotension
Risperdone (Risperdal)	0.5–1 mg qh, increase by 0.5 mg q 3–5 d max 6 mg	Mixed D2 and 5-HT2 antagonist	Parkinsonism, depression, drowsiness, hypotension
Tetrabenzine	Begin 12.5 mg, increase q 5–7 d tid or qid max 200 mg		Parkinsonism, depression, drowsiness, hypotension

CHOREA

DEMENTIA: PRIMARY MEDICATIONS

Characteristic	Donepezil (Aricept)	Galartamine (Reminyl)	Memantine (Namenda)	Rivastigmine (Exelon)
Indication in Alzheimer's disease	Mild to moderate	Mild to moderate	Moderate to severe	Mild to moderate
Mechanism of action	AChEI	AChB	NMDA-receptor antagonist	AChB
Absorption affected by food	No	Yes	No	Yes
Serum half-life	70–80 hr	5–7 hr	60–80 hr	2 hr
Metabolism	CYp2D6, CYP3A4	CYP2D6, CYP3A4	Nonhepatic	Nonhepatic
Dose, initial/maximum	5 mg/d, 10 mg/d	4 mg bid, 12 mg bid ER: 8 mg/d,16 mg/d, 24 mg/d	5 mg/d, 10 mg bid	1.5 mg bid, 6 mg bid
First effective dosage strength	5 mg/d	8 mg bid ER: 16 mg/d	10 mg bid	3 mg bid
Titration required	No	Yes	Yes	Yes

DEPRESSION

SELECTED ANTIDEPRESSANTS

Generic Name	Brand Name	Dosage Range (mg/d)	Sedative Effect	Anticholinergic Effect	Comments/Side Effects
Tricyclics/heterocyclics					
Amitriptyline (TCI)	Elavil	25–300	High	High	SE: Dry mouth, blurred vision,
Imipramine	Tofranil	25–300	Moderate	High	constipation, difficulty
Doxepin	Sinequan	25–150	High	High	urinating, worsening of glaucoma,
Nortriptyline	Aventyl, Pamelor	20–150	Moderate	Moderate	impaired thinking and tiredness
Desipramine	Norpramine	25–200	Low	Low	
SSRIs					
Fluoxetine	Prozac	20–60	Low	Very low	*Lexapro is effective in GAD*
Sertraline	Zoloft	25–250	Moderate	Very low	SE: Dry mouth, nausea,
					nervousness, insomnia,
Paroxetine	Paxil	20–40	Low	Very low	sexual problems,
Citalopram	Celexa	20–40	Low	Very low	and headache
Escitalopram	Lexapro	10–20	Low	Low	
SSNRIs					
Duloxetine	Cymbalta	20–60	Low	Low	*Cymbalta is efffective in diabetic*
Venlafaxine	Effexor	37.5–225	Moderate	Low	*neuropathy*
					SE: Nausea and anorexia, weight
					loss, nervousness, headache,
					insomnia and tiredness, dry
					mouth, constipation, sexual
					problems, increased heart rate,
					and increased cholesterol levels

cont'd

DEPRESSION

SELECTED ANTIDEPRESSANTS—*cont'd*

Generic Name	Brand Name	Dosage Range (mg/d)	Sedative Effect	Anticholinergic Effect	Comments/Side Effects
Reuptake inhibitors and receptor blockers					
Trazodone	Desyrel	50–600	High	Very low	SE: Dry mouth, nausea, and dizziness
Mirtazapine	Remeron	15–45	High	Low	
NDRIs					
Bupropion	Wellbutrin	200–400	Low	Very low	SE: Agitation, nausea, headache, anorexia and insomnia, increased blood pressure

NDRIs, norepinephrine and dopamine reuptake inhibitors; SE, side effects; SSNRIs, selective serotonin and norepinephrine reuptake inhibitors; SSRIs, selective serotonin reuptake inhibitors.

EPILEPSY

COMMONLY PRESCRIBED ANTIEPILEPTIC DRUGS (AEDs)

AED	Best Treated Epilepsy Type	Dosage	Comment	Adverse Reaction (Common Side Effects)*
Carbamazepine	Partial seizures, generalized seizures	400 mg PO qd, up by 200 mg/day at 1 wk intervals	(+) Cytochrome P-450 (cP450); autoinducer by active metabolite	SIADH: hyponatremia, rash, N and V, ?CBC
Ethosuximide	Absence seizures	500 mg, increase by 250 mg/day at 1 wk intervals	(−) cP450 induction or inhibition; can induce SLE-like syndrome	Anorexia, weight loss, GI: pain, N, V, D; skin: rash, hirsuitism, and gingival hyperplasia; headache, mood changes
Gabapentin (Neurontin)	Partial seizures	900 mg, increase by 300 mg/day at 24 hr intervals	No pharmacokinetic interactions; renal clearance of unmetabolized form	Weight gain, mood changes, dry mouth, periorbital edema, myalgias
Levetiracetam (Keppra)	Partial seizures	1000 mg, increase by 1000 mg/day at 2 wk intervals	Renal metabolism	Behavior changes, mood changes different in women than men
Lamotrigine (Lamictal)	Generalized and partial seizures	50 mg, increase by 50 mg/day at 2 wk intervals	Induced by phenytoin, carbamazepine; inhibited by valproate	Rash, Steven-Johnson syndrome, headache, mood changes, N, V
Oxcarbazepine (Trileptal)	Partial seizures	600 mg, increase by 600 mg/day at 1 wk intervals	(+) cP450; monohydroxy-carbamazepine Prodrug	SIADH: hyponatremia; rash, N, V
Phenobarbital	Generalized and partial seizures	90 mg, increase by 30 mg/day at 4 wk intervals	(+) cP450	Mental slowness, excessive sedative effects, physical dependence, mood changes, N, V, rash, porphyria exacerbation

EPILEPSY

cont'd

COMMONLY PRESCRIBED ANTIEPILEPTIC DRUGS (AEDs)—cont'd

AED	Best Treated Epilepsy Type	Dosage	Comment	Adverse Reaction (Common Side Effects)*
Phenytoin	Generalized and partial seizures	300 mg, increase by 100 mg/day at 4 wk intervals	(+) cP450	Coarse facies, gingival hyperplasia, hirsuitism, N, V, headache, lymphadenopathy, osteomalacia
Tiagabine (Gabatril)	Partial seizures	4 mg, increase by 4–8 mg/day at 1 wk intervals	High protein binding; no enzyme induction or inhibition; may induce spike-wave stupor	Mood changes, asthenia, N, and V
Topiramate (Topamax)	Generalized and partial seizures	25–50 mg, increase by 25–50 mg/day at 1 wk intervals	No AED enzyme induction; but may increase phenytoin levels; alters efficacy of birth control pills	Weight loss, language problems, psychomotor slowing, mood changes, paresthesia
Valproate	Generalized and partial seizures	500 mg, increase by 250 mg/day at 1 wk intervals	cP450 inhibitor; active metabolites	Weight gain, hair loss, headache, menstrual irregularities
Zonisamide (Zonegran)	Partial seizures	100 mg, increase by 100 mg/day at 2 wk intervals	Increased risk of renal stones	Headache, insomnia and mood changes, nephrolithiasis

*Common side effects to almost all AEDs: **mental status:** dizziness, drowsiness, sleepiness; **cognitive:** impaired memory, fatigue. **cerebellar/coordination:** unsteadiness, blurred vision, ataxia, tremor, nystagmus; N, nausea; V, vomiting; D, diarrhea.

ESSENTIAL TREMOR (MOVEMENT DISORDER)

Medication	Dosage	Action	Side Effects
Primidone (Mysoline)	125–250 mg tid	GABA-A agonist?	Dizziness
Propranolol (Inderal)	125–240 mg tid	Beta-adrenergic antagonist	Bradycardia
Mirtazapine (Remeron)	15 mg PO qd, may increase to 45 mg qd	SSNRIs	Somnolence, weight gain
Clonazepam (Klonopin)	0.5–2 mg qd	GABA-A agonist	Drowsiness
Thalamotomy	Surgical option		Surgery related complications, stroke, infection, failure/recurrence
Thalamic deep brain stimulation	Surgical option		Surgery related complications, stroke, infection, failure/recurrence

ESSENTIAL TREMOR

HEADACHE

TRIPTANS FOR MIGRAINE HEADACHE ABORTIVE THERAPY

Drug	Dose/Route	Other Considerations
Almotriptan (Axert)	6.25–12.5 mg PO, may repeat after 2 hours; max 2 doses/day	*Side effects:* Warm/hot sensation, tingling, chest pain/tightness, hyper/hypotension, burning, feeling of heaviness and tightness, flushing, drowsiness, malaise/fatigue, and anxiety.
Eletriptan (Relpax)	20–40 mg PO, may repeat after 2 hours; max 80 mg/day	*Precaution:* All triptans should be avoided in patients with familial hemiplegic migraine, basilar migraine, ischemic stroke, ischemic heart disease, Prinzmetal's angina, uncontrolled hypertension, and pregnancy. MAO inhibitors are contraindicated with all of the triptans other than naratriptan.
Frovatriptan (Frova)	2.5 mg, may repeat after 2 hours; max daily dose 7.5 mg	
Naratriptan (Amerge)	1–2.5 mg PO, may repeat after 4 hours; max 5 mg/day	
Rizatriptan (Maxalt)	5–10 mg PO, may repeat after 2 hours; max 30 mg/day (use 5 mg dose in patients receiving propranolol with a maximum of 15 mg in 24 hours)	Triptans should not be used within 24 hours of the use of ergotamine preparations.
Sumatriptan (Imitrex)	Oral: 50–100 mg, may repeat at 2 hours (max 200 mg/day) Intranasal: single dose of 5–20 mg SC: 6 mg; may repeat after 1 hour (max 12 mg/day)	
Zolmitriptan (Zomig)	Oral: 2.5 mg PO Nasal spray: 1 spray (5 mg) The dose may repeat after 2 hours (max 10 mg/day)	

INSOMNIA

MEDICATIONS USED TO TREAT INSOMNIA

First-line Pharmacotherapy

Drug	Dosage Range	Benefits	Side Effects
Esopiclone	1–3 mg	Short half-life provides lower risk of morning hangover effect	Rash, xerostomia, dizziness, nausea and vomiting, confusion, headache, somnolence, hallucinations, nervousness, dysmenorrhea, reduced libido
Zaleplon	5–10 mg (note: 5 mg dose is largely ineffective and not routinely recommended)	Ultra-short half-life. Used for sleep initiation and also prn for night-time awakenings when there is still a minimum of 3 to 4 hours before rising	Headache, drowsiness, nausea, and rash
Temazepam	15–30 mg	Intermediate half-life carries a low-moderate risk of morning hangover effect	Drowsiness, headache, fatigue, nervousness, lethargy, dizziness, anxiety, and confusion
Zolpidem	10 mg (12.5 extended release)	Short half-life	Nausea, vomiting, abdominal pain, caution with depressed patients

cont'd

INSOMNIA

MEDICATIONS USED TO TREAT INSOMNIA—cont'd

Drug	Dosage Range	Benefits	Side Effect
Second-line Pharmacotherapy			
Amitriptyline	10–50 mg	Longer half-life carries risk of morning hangover effect and cognitive impairment	Weight gain, bloating symptom, asthenia, constipation, xerostomia, dizziness, fatigue, headache, blurred vision, somnolence
Trazodone	25–50 mg	Shorter half-life lowers risk of morning hangover effect	Sweating, weight change, worsening depression, suicidal ideation
Variable Evidence			
L-Tryptophan	500 mg–2 g	May be preferred by patient wanting a "natural medicine"	Unknown
Melatonin	1–5 mg		
Valerian root	400–900 mg		

DRUGS NOT RECOMMENDED FOR TREATMENT OF INSOMNIA

Drug Class	Reason
Antidepressants	Lack of evidence
Antihistamines	Excessive risk of psychomotor impairment and anticholinergic side effects
Antipsychotics (conventional)	Unacceptable risk of anticholinergic and neurologic toxicity
Antipsychotics (atypical)	Lack of evidence and unacceptable risk of metabolic toxicity
Benzodiazepines (intermediate and long-acting)	Excessive risk of daytime sedation and psychomotor impairment
Benzodiazepines (short-acting)	Unacceptable risk of memory disturbances, abnormal thinking, and psychotic behaviors
Chloral agents	Risk of tolerance, dependence, and abuse, CNS and GI effects
Muscle relaxants	Excessive risk of adverse CNS effects

MULTIPLE SCLEROSIS

Generic Name	Recommended Dose	Comments	Side Effects
DISEASE-MODIFYING AGENTS			
Immune modulators:			
Interferon beta-1a (Avonex, Rebif)	30 μg (Avonex) IM qw self-injection 44 μg (Rebif) SQ 3 q tiw self-injection	RRMS, SPMS+R	Flu-like symptoms, depression, mild anemia, impaired LFT, allergy Same
Interferon beta-1b (IFNb-1b, Betaserone, Betaferone)	8 MIU or 250 μg SQ qod self-injection	RRMS, SPMS+R	Same + site reaction + reduced WBC
Glatiramer acetate (Copaxone)	20 mg SQ qd self-injection	RRMS	Local reactions, vasodilation, brief and transient panic reaction
Natalizumab (Tysabri) IgG monoclonal antibodies	300 mg IV over 1 hr q 4 weeks	RRMS only in centers with TOUCH program Approved by the FDA in June 2006	Fatal PML (? higher with other immunomodulatory and immunosuppressant drugs), infection, hypersensitivity, increased lymphocytes, and nucleated RBC
Chemotherapeutic agents:			
Mitoxantrone (Novantrone)	12 mg/m² IV over 15 min q 3 mo for 2–3 years	SPMS, worsening RRMS	Nausea (N) and vomiting (V), cytopenia, blue-green urine 24 hours later; infections, hair thinning, serious hepato- and cardiotoxicity
Azathioprine (Imuran)	50–100 mg qd or bid	Same, but not FDA approved	Cytopenia, GI symptoms, N and V, impaired LFT, rash, flu-like syndrome

Drug	Dosage	Indication	Side effects
Cyclophosphamide (Cytoxan, Neosar)	500 mg/d 8–18 days until the total WBC ≤ 4000/mm³ and booster doses at 700 mg/m² IV q 2 mo	Rapidly progressive MS, Devic's syndrome, Marburg variant MS, but not FDA approved	Cytopenia, N and V, hair loss, mouth sores, sterility, renal failure, and hemorrhagic cystitis
Cyclosporine (Sandimmune)	5–7 mg/day for 1–3 years	Same	Renal failure, hypertension, PRESS syndrome, cytopenia, hair thinning
Methotrexate (generic)	7.5 mg q w for 2–3 years	Progressive MS, but not FDA approved	Cytopenia, hair thinning, impaired LFT, N and V, stomatitis
Cladribine (Leustatin) selective lymphotoxic specificity	0.07 mg/kg/d IV for 5 days q 4 wk for 6 cycles	Progressive MS, SPMS, but not FDA approved	Bone marrow suppression and cytopenia, infection
Corticosteroids:			
Methylprednisolone (Depo-Medrol, Solu-Medrol)	250 mg IV q 6 hr × 3 d then tapered off over 1–2 wk	Acute relapses in RRMS and worsening SPMS	?AED levels, electrolyte disturbances, psychiatric effect, weight gain, osteoporosis, skin changes, and infection
Prednisone (Deltasone)	100 mg PO q d tapered off over 2 wk	Same	Same
Dexamethasone (Decadrone, Medrol)	10 mg IV or PO q 6 hr, taper slowly over 2 wk	Same	Same
SUGGESTED MEDICATION FOR SPASTICITY IN MS (SLOW TITRATION)			
Baclofen	5–20 mg PO tid	? safety in children < 12 yr, possibly teratogenic	Seizure, MS changes, hypotension, hallucination
Tizanidine (Zanaflex)	2–8 mg PO tid	Contraceptive pills reduce drug clearance, possibly teratogenic (Category C)	Dry mouth, urinary tract infection, impaired LFT (0, 1, 3, 6 mo monitoring), flu syndrome, dyskinesia, hypotension
Diazepam	2–10 mg PO tid	Possibly teratogenic	Sedation, ataxia, fatigue, urine retention

cont'd

MULTIPLE SCLEROSIS

Generic Name	Recommended Dose	Comments	Side Effects
Dantrolene	25–50 mg PO tid	Possibly teratogenic, possible photosensitivity	Impaired LFT (more in women and those > 35 years, 0, 1, 3, 6 mo monitoring), sedation, and diarrhea
Gabapentin	100–800 mg PO tid	Possibly teratogenic (Category C)	Drowsiness, ataxia, viral-like illness in children
Clonidine	0.1–0.2 mg (oral or patch)	Possibly teratogenic (Category C)	Drowsiness, hypotension, bradycardia, rebound hypertension with withdrawal
SUGGESTED MEDICATION FOR FATIGUE IN MS (SLOW TITRATION)			
Amantadine (Symmetrel)	50 or 100 PO bid	Possibly teratogenic (Category C)	Nausea, hallucination, constipation, edema, and orthostatic hypotension
Pemoline (Cylert)	18.75–75 mg PO qd	Possibly teratogenic (Category C)	Difficulty sleeping or drowsiness, dizziness, headache, nausea, anorexia
Modafinil (Provogil)	200–400 mg PO qd	Possibly teratogenic (Category C)	Headache, nervousness, rhinitis, backache, anxiety, insomnia, dizziness
Methylphenidate (Ritalin)	10–30 mg PO in 3 divided doses	Possibly teratogenic (Category C)	Seizure, nervousness, insomnia, hypersensitivity, headache, arteritis
SUGGESTED MEDICATION FOR DEPRESSION IN MS (SLOW TITRATION)			
Fluoxetine (Prozac)	20–60 mg PO qd	Anticholinergics and sedation effect—mild	Headache, anxiety, tremor, insomnia, drowsiness, fatigue, dizziness, GI complaints, excessive sweating
Bupropion (Wellbutrin)	200–300 mg daily in 2–3 divided doses	Mild anticholinergic and sedative effect	Agitation, tremor, dry mouth, insomnia, headache, N/V, constipation
Paroxetine (Paxil)	20–40 mg PO qd	Mild anticholinergic and sedative effect	N/V, insomnia, sweating, tremor, fatigue, dizziness, ejaculatory delay
Citalopram (Celexa)	20–40 mg PO qd	Mild anticholinergic and sedative effect	N/V, insomnia, somnolence, dizziness, agitation, fatigue, dry mouth

SUGGESTED MEDICATION FOR BLADDER MANAGEMENT IN MS

Oxybutynin (Ditropan XL)	5–10 mg PO qd	Anticholinergics	Dry mouth, nausea, constipation, headache, hypertension, palpitation
Tolterodine (Detrol LA)	2 mg PO qd	Anticholinergics	Dry mouth/eyes, blurred vision, headache, constipation, dizziness, drowsiness, fatigue

Suggested Management for Pain in MS (Slow Titration) (V and IX CN Neuralgia, Paroxysmal Dysesthetic Pain)

Carbamazepine	200–1600 mg in divided doses	Monitor level, slow titration	Hypersensitivity, GI side effects, SIADH
Phenytoin	300–400 mg	Monitor level, slow titration	Gingival hyperplasia, hypersensitivity, GI symptoms, SIADH
Lamotrigine	100–200 mg PO bid	Hypersensitivity reaction	Skin rash with Steven-Johnson syndrome
Topiramate	15–400 mg PO qd	Cognitive side effect	Cognitive side effects, GI tolerance
Baclofen or morphine pump, or spinal cord/deep brain stimulation		Severe pain unresponsive to conventional treatment	

RRMS, relapsing-remitting MS; SPMS+R, secondary progressive MS with relapses.

MULTIPLE SCLEROSIS

MYASTHENIA GRAVIS

ACUTE MYASTHENIA GRAVIS THERAPY (CAN BE GIVEN IN REFRACTORY CHRONIC CASES)

Generic Name	Time of Onset	Recommended Dose	Action	Indication	Side Effects
Plasmapheresis or plasma exchange	1–7 days	5 exchanges (3–5 L of plasma) over 7–10 days	Removes ACh Ab from circulation	Myasthenia crisis, bridge for immunomodulators	Catheter complications (limit chronic use), bleeding hypotension, cardiac arrhythmias
IVIG	1–2 weeks	2–4 g/kg over 2–5 days	Uncertain	MG crisis, bridge for immuno-modulators, thymoma, refractory MG if < 60 years old	Headache, chills, dizziness, aseptic meningitis, acute renal failure, thrombotic events, anaphylaxia in IgA deficiency

CHRONIC MYASTHENIA GRAVIS THERAPY

Symptomatic: Acetylcholinesterase inhibitor

Generic Name	Time of Onset	Recommended Dose	Action	Indication	Side Effects
Pyridostigmine (Mestinon)	10–15 min	30 mg tid up to 120 mg q 4 hr in crisis	AChEI	MG, myasthenia crisis, MG in children	GI: cramp/diarrhea, increased secretion, bradycardia, cholinergic crisis*
Pyridostigmine XR (Mestinon Ts)	Variable	180 mg qh	AChEI	Severe weakness upon awaking	Same
Neostigmine	10–30 min	15 mg tid, max 375 mg qd	AChEI	Less commonly used but same	Same

Symptomatic/disease-modifying?: Immunomodulators

Drug	Onset	Dose	Mechanism	Indication	Side effects
Prednisone	2–3 weeks	20 mg qd, titrate 5 mg q 3–5 d to 1 mg/kg/d Symptoms controled taper 5–10 mg q month to 5 to 10 mg qd.	Immunomodulator, T cell response	Initial therapy after ACh inhibitors	Acute: Up to 50% transient deterioration 10% respiratory failure Chronic: hypertension Diabetes mellitus Osteoporosis, fractures Gastritis Cushing syndrome
Methylprednisolone IV	1–2 weeks	500 mg IV bid × 3 days and may repeat after 2–4 weeks up to 1000 mg IV bid	Immunomodulator, T cell response	MG exacerbations	
Azathioprine (Imuran)	4–10 months	50 mg qd for 2–4 wk and increase by 50 mg q 2–4 wk up to 150–200 mg qd	Purine analogue, blocks purine synthesis in lymphocyte and (−)T and B cell proliferation	Chronic therapy ± steroids, steroid sparing	Flu-like symptoms Leukopenia. hepatotoxicity, Pancreatitis, get CBC, LFT q 1–6 mo
Mycophenolate (Cellcept)	2–4 months	500 mg bid after 2–4 wk, 1000 mg bid	Blocks purine synthesis in lymphocyte and inhibits its proliferation	Same	Nausea and diarrhea, Leukopenia, Get CBC q 6 mo, hypertension, nephrotoxic (10%)

cont'd

MYASTHENIA GRAVIS

Generic Name	Time of Onset	Recommended Dose	Action	Indication	Side Effects
Cyclosporine (CSA)	2–4 months	2.5 mg/kg/d and up to 5 mg/kg/d divided in 2 doses	Limits production of IL-2, (–) T helper cell function, (–)T lymphocyte dependent immune response	Same	Flu-like symptoms, tremors, hypertrichosis, gingival hyperplasia, cytocrome P-450 system inducer (many interactions)
Cyclophosphamide (Cytoxan)		Monthly for 6 months and then every other month for total 9 months	Alkylating agent reduces β and T cell proliferation	Refractory to previous inmunomodulators	Nausea and vomiting, hemorrhagic cystitis, bladder Ca?, alopecia, leukopenia
Tacrolimus		3–5 mg/day (level 7–8 mg/mL)	Ryanoline receptor related: sarcoplasmic calcium release	Refractory MG	Less nephrotoxicity, hypomagnesemia, tremor, paresthesias
Symptomatic/disease-modifying?: Surgery					
Thymectomy	1–10 years	NA	Affects T cell maturation	Thymoma Refractory MG if < 60 years old	Postoperative complications

Ach Ab, acetylcholine antibodies; AchEI, acetylcholinesterase inhibitor.
*AChEI side effect Rx: glycopirrolate, probantine, hyoscyamine.

Medication	Usual Dose	Class	Major Side Effects
Amphetamine	30–100 mg	Stimulant, amphetamine	Insomnia, restlessness, tachycardia, psychotic episodes, dizziness, diarrhea, constipation, hypertension, impotence
Amphetamine (sustained release)	30–100 mg	Stimulant, amphetamine	Same
Methamphetamine	40–80 mg	Stimulant, amphetamine	Same
Methylphenidate	30–100 mg	Stimulant, otherwise not defined	Nervousness, insomnia, anorexia, nausea, dizziness, hypertension, hypotension, hypersensitivity reactions, tachycardia, headaches
Modafinil	200–400 mg		Headache, nausea, eosinophilia, diarrhea, dry mouth, anorexia
Pemoline	75–150 mg	Oxazolidine	Seizures, liver failure, aplastic anemia (rare), insomnia, hallucinations, anorexia, weight loss
Selegiline	20–40 mg	MAO inhibitor (anticataplectic)	Nausea, dizziness, confusion, tremor, orthostatic hypotension, diet-induced hypertension
Fluoxetine	20–80 mg	SSRI (anticataplectic)	Asthenia, nausea, diarrhea, anorexia, insomnia, tremor, anxiety, somnolence
Protriptyline	10–60 mg	TCA (anticataplectic)	Orthostatic hypotension, hypertension, seizures, headache, anticholinergic symptoms, impotence, impaired liver function, myocardial infarction, stroke

MAO, monoamine oxidase; SSRI, selective serotonin reuptake inhibitor; TCA, tricyclic antidepressant.

OBSTRUCTIVE SLEEP APNEA–HYPOPNEA SYNDROME

Treatment	Effects	Comments
Weight loss	10% weight loss may eliminate apneic episodes by reducing the mass of the posterior airway	
Avoidance of alcohol for 4–6 hours prior to bedtime		
Sleeping on the side		
Nasal continuous positive airway pressure (CPAP)	Improves daytime sleepiness, mood, and cognitive function in people with both mild and moderate apnea. CPAP has also been shown to increase quality of life and decrease health care costs.	Side effects: dry mouth, rhinitis, and sinus congestion
	Most effective treatment of obstructive sleep apnea	Compliance: 50% of patients use prescribed CPAP on regular basis
	Sleep study recommended to titrate pressure levels	
Apnea-hypopnea index		
>15	Eligible for CPAP therapy, regardless of symptomatology	
5–14.9	Indicated only if the patient has one of the following: EDS, hypertension, or cardiovascular disease	
Oral appliances	Move tongue and mandible forward, enlarge posterior airspace, better compliance	CPAP more effective at reducing apnea hypopnea index
Surgical management		
Uvulopalatopharyngoplasty	40% effectiveness	
Craniofacial reconstruction		
Geniohyoid advancement with hyoid myotomy	70% effectiveness	Uncertain long-term prognosis
Maxillomandibular osteotomy	95% effectiveness	Uncertain long-term prognosis
Tracheostomy	Definitive treatment	

PAGET'S DISEASE

Medications	Dosage	Comments/Side Effects
Bisphosphonates:		
Alendronate (Fosamax)	40 mg PO qd x 6 months. May reinstate treatment after 6 months, if necessary.	Bisphosphonate tablets should be taken with 6 to 8 oz of tap water on an empty stomach. Do not eat or lie down for 30 minutes after taking medication. Bisphosphonates should be avoided in patients with kidney disease.
Pamidronate (Aredia)	30–60 mg IV over 4 hour period on 2–3 consecutive days. Repeat as necessary.	Pamidronate: Transient "flu-like" syndrome of fever, myalgia, and arthralgia; rarely uveitis and acute renal failure have been reported.
Tiludronate (Skelid)	400 mg PO qd for 3 months. Repeat as necessary.	
Risedronate (Actonel)	30 mg PO qd for 2 months. Repeat as necessary.	Alendronate and risedronate: the most common side effects are upper gastrointestinal symptoms.
Etidronate (Didronel)	5 mg/kg PO qd (if ineffective, 11–20 mg/kg PO qd for a maximum of 6 months). Repeat as necessary.	
Calcitonin (Miacalcin injection), calcitonin-salmon (Calcimar)	200 U/mL; 100 U SC or IM once daily for 6 to 18 months.	
Vitamin D supplement		
Calcium supplement		

PAIN (See also HEADACHE, AED, AND ANTIDEPRESSANTS IN AAN GUIDELINE SUMMARIES APPENDIX)

Medication Class	Medication	Dose/Ceiling Dose	Advantages	Comments/Caution/Side Effects
Nonopioid analgesic	Acetaminophen (APAP)	650 or 1000 mg PO/PR q 4–6 hr, not to exceed 4000 mg/day	*Mild to moderate pain*	Hepatotoxicity, usually with dose greater than 10 g/day, may occur at lower dose, within therapeutic dose in alcoholics, fasting patients, and those taking cytochrome P-450 enzyme-inducing drugs
NSAIDs	Aspirin	500–1000 mg PO q 4–6 hours, ceiling dose 1 g	*Effective in various types of pain*	All NSAIDs: sodium and water retention, NSAID-induced nephrotoxicity
	Diclofenac	start at 25 mg qid, can increase to 50 mg tid or qid	Narcotic sparing, some patients may respond to certain NSAIDs	Dose-dependent aspirin toxicity: tinnitus, emesis, encephalopathy, acidosis, increased bleeding time Misoprostol may be effective in NSAID-induced gastric erosion or peptic ulcer, contraindicated in *pregnancy*
	Ketorolac	30 mg IV or 60 mg IM in healthy adult, for multiple dosing 30 mg IV or IM q 6 hr prn, max dose 120 mg/day	Also to avoid opioid-induced respiratory depression, constipation, and nausea	*Be wary of NSAID overuse or rebound headache*
	Ibuprofen	400–800 mg qid		
	Naproxen	500 mg, then 250 mg q 6–8 hr		
Benzodiazepines	Alprazolam	0.25–0.5 mg tid	*In patient with difficulty sleeping from pain; BZD*	*Good as adjunctive therapy* Ventilatory depression and hypotension, exacerbated by opioids, worse in COPD patients,
	Chlordiazepoxide	5–10 mg tid-qid		
	Diazepam	2–10 mg bid-qid		

	Lorazepam	1 mg bid-tid	effective in treating anxiety and insomnia
Opioid analgesics			all contraindicated in first trimester of pregnancy
	Codeine	30–60 mg IM/PO q 3 hr prn, 30 mg PO is equivalent to 300 mg aspirin + acetaminophen	Opioid class with mild to severe pain control, no ceiling effect with opioids
	Propoxyphene	(Darvocet-N) 1–2 mg PO q 4–6 hr prn 50–100 mg PO	All opioids: tolerance with chronic use (1 to 2 weeks), overdose possible with respiratory depression, nausea, vomiting, ileus, impaired gastric motility, bradycardia with fentanyl, bronchospasm with morphine
	Tramadol	q 4–6 hr, max 300–400 mg/day	Tramadol is effective for neuropathic pain
	Hydrocodone	Vicodin 1tb PO q 6 hr + aspirin or + acetaminophen, also extended release	For chronic low back pain
	Oxycodone	OxyContin 10–20 mg bid	Seizure risk increases with propoxyphene, meperidine. With chronic use the IM:PO ratio falls from 1.6 to 1.3
	Hydromorphone	PO 7.5 mg, IM 1.5 mg, duration 3 hr	For phantom pain
	Morphine	PO 20–60 mg, IM 10 mg, duration 4–6 hr	For phantom pain
	Fentanyl	50–150 μg patch q 72 hr, titrate slowly	Easily titrated, naloxone for reversal
			Respiratory suppression, chest wall rigidity

cont'd

PAIN

Medication Class	Medication	Dose/Ceiling Dose	Advantages	Comments/ Caution/Side Effects
Antidepressants *(see Antidepressants, Therapeutic Appendix)*	Duloxetine (Cymbalta)	20 mg bid max 60 mg /day	Easily titrated and tolerated	Effective for diabetic neuropathy
	Tricyclic antidepressants Elavil	25–100 mg daily, qhs, titrate very slowly	For those with trouble sleeping at night	Effective in peripheral neuropathy with insomnia or chronic pain; excessive sedation or urinary retention can be a problem
Antiepileptic drugs (AEDs) (see AED, Therapeutic Appendix)	Carbamazepine	200–100 mg qd in divided doses	Trigeminal neurologic post stroke pain syndrome (thalamic Dejerine-Roussy syndrome)	Be wary of poor tolerance with rapid titration or SIADH
	Phenytoin	200–400 mg qd	Neuropathic pain	
	Gabapentin (Neurontin)	1800–3600 mg PO qd in 3 divided doses	Headaches Chronic pain	Well tolerated Variable effectiveness
	Pregabalin	600 mg PO qd, titrate slowly	Neuropathic pain Chronic headache Chronic pain	
	Topiramate	50–400 mg in 2 divided doses, titrate slowly	Chronic headache Chronic pain	Cognitive side effect, nephrolithiasis
	Valproic acid	500–2000 mg PO qd in 2 divided doses	Approved for migraine headache	Hair loss, increased appetite and weight gain, hepatotoxicity
Others	Lidocaine patch Transcutaneous electrical nerve stimulation unit PT/OT/ psychotherapy Local injection/ pump and surgery	5% patch	Postherpetic neuralgia	Post zoster/shingle infection

PARKINSON'S DISEASE (MOVEMENT DISORDER)

Medication	Dosage	Action	Side Effects
Tolcapone (Tasmar)	100–200 mg tid	Reversible COMT inhibitor	Liver failure
Amantadine (Symmetrel)	100 mg bid–tid	Dopamine-releasing, NMDA antagonist	Edema, confusion, hallucinations
Benztropine mesylate (Cogentin)	Begin 0.5–1 mg qd, increase by 0.5–1 mg q 2–3 d	Anticholinergic	Blurred vision, dry mouth, urinary retention, confusion
Entacapone (Comtan)	200 mg with each dose of Sinemet	COMT inhibitor	Discolored urine (orange)
L-Dopa, carbidopa (Sinemet)	CR 25/100–50/200 bid	Dopamine agonist	Nausea, hypotension
Pergolide (Permax)	0.05 mg bid to 6 mg/d divided	D1 and D2 receptor agonist	Dizziness, hallucinations, nausea, dyskinesia
Pramipexole (Mirapex)	0.125 mg tid to 4.5 mg/d divided	Dopamine agonist	Postural hypotension, dizziness
Ropinirole (Requip)	0.25 mg tid to 24 mg/d divided	Dopamine agonist	Dizziness, somnolence, nausea
Trihexyphenidyl hydrochloride (Artane)	Begin 1–2 mg/day, increase by 1–2 mg q 2–3 d	Anticholinergic	Blurred vision, dry mouth, urinary retention, confusion

PARKINSON'S DISEASE

RESTLESS LEGS SYNDROME

MEDICATIONS USED TO TREAT RESTLESS LEGS SYNDROME

Drug	Dosage Range	Common Side Effects
Dopaminergic Agents		
Carbidopa/levodopa		Augmentation or rebound of symptoms, dizziness upon rising, confusion, nausea, and hallucinations
Regular formulation (Sinemet)	12.5–50 mg before bed to 25–100 mg tid	
Sustained release (Sinemet CR)	25–100 mg before bed to tid	
Dopamine Agonist		Nausea, lightheadedness, drowsiness, and postural hypotension
Pergolide (Permax)	0.05–1.0 mg in 2 doses (dinner and 1 hr before bed)	
Pramipexole (Mirapex)	0.125 mg before bed to 1.0 mg tid	
Ropinirole (Requip)	0.25 mg before bed to 3 mg tid	
Benzodiazepines		Daytime drowsiness and confusion, unsteadiness and falls, and aggravation of sleep apnea
Clonazepam (Klonopin)	0.5–2.0 mg before bed	
Opioids		Risk of addiction, nausea, sleepiness, and constipation
Propoxyphene	65–130 mg tid	
Codeine	15–30 mg qid	
Oxycodone (Percocet)	5–10 mg qid	
Tramadol (Ultram)	50 mg qid	
Others		
Gabapentin (Neurontin)	100–800 mg tid	Somnolence, dizziness, ataxia, and fatigue
Clonidine (Catapres)	0.1 mg before bed to 0.3 mg bid	Dry mouth, decreased cognition, lightheadedness, sleepiness, and constipation

SEDATIVES AND PARALYTICS

Sedative Agents*	Induction Dose	Sedative Dose	Infusion Dose	Mechanism of Action	Duration	Side Effects	Contraindications/ Precautions
Propofol	2–2.5 mg/kg	Titrate	20–150 µg/kg/min	GABA-ergic	Bolus: 3–5 min	Hypotension, pain on injection	Hemodynamically unstable patients
Thiopental	3–5 mg/kg		N/A	GABA-ergic	Bolus: 3–5 min	Hypotension	Hemodynamic instability
Etomidate	0.1–0.3 mg/kg		N/A	GABA-ergic	Bolus: 3–5 min	Myoclonus, pain on injection	Adrenal suppression with continuous infusion
Dexmedetomidine			0.1–0.7 µg/kg/hr	Alpha-2 agonist	Approx. 4 hr	Hypotension	Approved only for <24 hr use
Pentobarbital			1–4 µg/kg/hr	GABA-ergic	Bolus: 5–8 min	Hypotension, immunosuppression	
Midazolam	1–4 mg		0.01–0.1 mg/kg/hr	GABA-ergic	2–6 hr	Hypotension	
Lorazepam	1–2 mg		0.01–0.1 mg/kg/hr	GABA-ergic	4–8 hr	Hypotension	Acidosis due to the solvent preparation
Fentanyl		1–2 mg/kg	0.3–10.0 µg/kg/hr	Opioid recept. agonist	60–90 min	Bradycardia	Chest wall rigidity with bolus doses
Remifentanil		1–2 µg/kg	0.05–0.3 µg/kg/min	Opioid recept. agonist	5–10 min	Hypotension, bradycardia	Chest wall rigidity with bolus doses

cont'd

SEDATIVES AND PARALYTICS

SEDATIVES AND PARALYTICS—cont'd

Paralytic Agents[†]	Intubation Dose	Maintenance Dose	Mechanism of Action	Duration	Side Effects	Contraindications/ Precautions
Succinylcholine	1–2 mg/kg	N/A	Depolarizing—Acetylcholine receptor agonist	3–5 min	Slight increase in ICP	Risk for hyperkalemia and malignant hyperthermia
Pancuronium	0.1 mg/kg	1 µg/kg/min	Non-depolarizing	90–120 min	Vagolytic (increased HR)	Renal failure
Cisatracurium	0.2 mg/kg	2.5 µg/kg/min	Non-depolarizing	45–60 min		

*Sedative infusion can be titrated to a set sedation scale (Ramsay 3) or monitoring parameter (e.g., BIS 50–60). Remember that most agents accumulate with continuous dosing with a short redistribution half-life and a much longer elimination half-life. Continuous hemodynamic and respiratory monitoring must be used.

[†]Neuromuscular blocker infusions should generally be titrated to maintain 1 out of 4 twitches on train-of-four testing. Neuromuscular blockers should only be used with concomitant sedation to avoid an awake-paralyzed state.

SPASTICITY (MOVEMENT DISORDER)

Medication	Dosage	Action	Side Effects
Tizanidine (Zanaflex)	4–8 mg q 8 hr	GABA-B agonist	Hypotension, sedation
Gabapentin (Neurontin)	300 mg tid	Unknown	Somnolence, dizziness, fatigue, ataxia
Baclofen (Lioresal)	5–40 mg tid or via baclofen pump	GABA-B agonist	Drowsiness, dizziness, weakness
Clonazepam (Klonopin)	0.5–2 mg qd	GABA-A agonist	Drowsiness
Botulinum toxin type A (Botox)	Dose varies depending on muscle size	Neuromuscular blocker	Weakness
Phenol injection	Local muscular injection under EMG guidance	Neurolytic and nerve block	Limb swelling, local pain and dysesthesia
Physical and occupational therapy			

STROKE

STROKE MEDICAL THERAPY AND RISK FACTORS MANAGEMENT

Generic Name	Trade Name	Dosage	Indications	Side Effects
Aspirin		50–325 mg/day	Reduce recurrent stroke risk Reduce risk of stroke in certain high-risk conditions (e.g., nonvalvular atrial fibrillation)	Bleeding
Alteplase	Activase	0.9 mg/kg (10% given as bolus and remainder infused over 1 hour; max dose 90 mg	Acute ischemic stroke within 3 hours of onset	Bleeding Anaphylaxis Hypotension
Clopidogrel	Plavix	75 mg/day	Reduction in atherosclerotic events in patients with stroke, coronary artery disease, and peripheral arterial disease	GI bleeding Diarrhea Rash GI symptoms
Aspirin/ extended release dipyridamole	Aggrenox	1 cap bid (25 mg aspirin/ 200 mg extended release dipyridamole per cap)	Reduce risk of stroke in patients with transient ischemic attack or completed ischemic stroke	Dizziness Headache GI effects Hypotension
Heparin		Varies	Varies	Hemorrhage Urticaria Thrombocytopenia Skin necrosis Anaphylactoid reactions Gangrene Priapism

Ticlodipine	Ticlid	250 mg PO bid with food	Reduce risk of thrombotic stroke in patients intolerant to aspirin	GI symptoms Neutropenia Purpura Abnormal liver function tests
Warfarin	Coumadin	Varies; goal PT-INR varies by indication	Prophylaxis or treatment of thromboembolic complications associated with atrial fribrillation and cardiac valve replacement	Hemorrhage from *any* tissue or organ Priapism Purple toes syndrome
Nimodipine	Nimotop	60 mg PO q 4 hr for 21 days (initiate within 96 hours)	Improvement in neurologic outcome in Hunt and Hess grades I–III subarachnoid hemorrhage	Hypotension, edema Diarrhea Rash, acne Depression Muscle pain and cramps

STROKE

MANAGEMENT OF STROKE RISK FACTORS

Risk Factor	Goal	Recommendations
Hypertension	SBP <140 mm Hg and DBP <90 mm Hg; SBP <135 mm Hg and DBP <85 mm Hg if target organ damage is present.	Lifestyle modification and antihypertensive medications.
Smoking	Cessation	Strongly encourage patient and family to stop smoking. Provide counseling, nicotine replacement, and formal programs.
Diabetes mellitus	Glucose <126 mg/dL (6.99 mmol/L)	Diet, oral hypoglycemics, insulin.
Lipids	LDL <100 mg/dL (2.59 mmol/L) HDL >35 mg/dL (0.91 mmol/L) TC <200 mg/dL (5.18 mmol/L) TG <200 mg/dL (2.26 mmol/L)	Start AHA Step II diet: ≤ 30% fat, < 7% saturated fat, < 200 mg/d cholesterol, and emphasize weight management and physical activity. If target goal not achieved with these measures, add drug therapy (e.g., statin agent) if LDL >130 mg/dL (3.37 mmol/L) and consider drug therapy if LDL 100–130 mg/dL (2.59–3.37 mmol/L).
Alcohol	Moderate consumption (≤ 2 drinks/d)	Strongly encourage patient and family to stop excessive drinking or provide formal alcohol cessation program.
Physical activity	30–60 min of activity at least 3–4 times/wk	Moderate exercise (e.g., brisk walking, jogging, cycling, or other aerobic activity). Medically supervised programs for high-risk patients (e.g., cardiac disease) and adaptive programs depending on neurological deficits are recommended.
Weight	≤ 120% of ideal body weight for height	Diet and exercise.

AHA, American Heart Association; DBP, diastolic blood pressure; HDL, high-density lipoproteins; SBP, systolic blood pressure; TC, total cholesterol; TG, triglycerides.

TICS (MOVEMENT DISORDER)

Medication	Dosage	Action	Side Effects
Clonidine (Catapres)	Begin 0.05 mg bid. Increase q 5–7 d max 0.4 mg/d	α_2-Adrenergic agonist	Drowsiness, dry mouth, itchy eyes, postural hypotension, headaches
Guanfacine (Tenex)	0.5–2 mg qd	α_2-Adrenergic agonist	Somnolence, headache, dizziness, xerostomia
Risperdone (Risperdal)	0.5 mg qh. increase by 0.5 mg q 3–5 d max 6 mg	Mixed D2 and 5-HT2 antagonist	Parkinsonism, depression, drowsiness, hypotension
Pimozide (Orap)	1–2 mg PO qd in divided doses up to 10 mg PO qd	D2+++ and D3 +++, also D1 and D4 ++2 & 5-HT2 and α_1- and α_2- antagonist	Parkinsonism, depression, drowsiness, hypotension
Clonazepam (Klonopin)	0.5 to 2 mg qd	GABA-A agonist	Drowsiness

TICS

Scales Appendix

Situation	Would never doze	Slight change of dozing	Moderate chance of dozing	High chance of dozing
1. Sitting and reading	0	1	2	3
2. Watching TV	0	1	2	3
3. Sitting and inactive in public place (theater or a meeting)	0	1	2	3
4. As a passenger in a car for an hour without a break	0	1	2	3
5. Lying down to rest in the afternoon when circumstances permit	0	1	2	3
6. Sitting and talking to someone		1	2	3
7. Sitting quietly after lunch (without alcohol)	0	1	2	3
8. In a car, while stopped for a few minutes in the traffic	0	1	2	3

Score: Add up scores for items 1 to 8 for total score (range 0 to 24)
<10 = normal awakeness
10–18 = moderately sleepy
>18 = very sleepy

FISHER SCALE

The Fisher scale assesses the amount of subarachnoid hemorrhage based on the head CT scan:
- 1: No blood, SAH diagnosed by LP
- 2: Less than 1 mm layering of SAH in the cisterns
- 3: More than 1 mm layering of SAH in the cisterns
- 4: Intraventricular or intracerebral hematoma, loculated hematoma

GLASGOW COMA SCALE

The best guide to the severity of head injury is the conscious state.
The Glasgow coma scale (GCS) allows quantitation of conscious state.
GCS 3 to 8: Severe head injury
GCS 9 to 12: Moderate head injury
GCS 13 to 15: Mild head injury

Assessment	Score	Infants	Children and Adults
Eye opening	4	Spontaneous	Spontaneous
	3	To shout	To verbal command
	2	To pain	To pain
	1	No response	No response
Best motor response	6	Norm/spontaneous movement	Follows commands
	5	Withdraws to touch	Localizes pain
	4	Withdraws to pain	Withdraws to pain
	3	Flexion to pain	Flexion to pain
	2	Extension to pain	Extension to pain
	1	No response	No response
Best verbal response	5	Coos and babbles	Orientated
	4	Irritable cry	Confused
	3	Cries to pain	Inappropriate words
	2	Moans to pain	Sounds
	1	No response	No response

Notes:
1. The GCS should be scored on the patient's best responses.
2. The GCS may be falsely low if one of the following is present – shock, hypoxia, hypothermia, intoxication, postictal state, sedative drug administration.
3. The GCS may be impossible to evaluate accurately if the patient is agitated, uncooperative, dysphasic, or intubated or has significant facial or spinal cord injuries.

GLASGOW OUTCOME RATING SCALE

The Glasgow outcome rating scale is used mainly to assess traumatic head injury but can also be used for stroke and other neurologic diseases.

Score	Description
1	**Dead**
2	**Vegetative state**
	Unable to interact with environment; unresponsive
3	**Severe disability**
	Able to follow commands/unable to live independently
4	**Moderate disability**
	Able to live independently; unable to return to work or school
5	**Good recovery**
	Able to return to work or school

HUNT HESS CLINICAL SEVERITY SCALE FOR SUBARACHNOID HEMORRHAGE

1. Asymptomatic or mild headache
2. Moderate or severe headache, nuchal rigidity, can have oculomotor palsy
3. Confusion, drowsiness, or mild focal signs

4. Stupor or hemiparesis
5. Comatose or extensor posturing

KURTZKE EXPANDED DISABILITY STATUS SCALE (EDSS)

Rating	Functional Status
0	Normal neurologic examination
1.0	No disability, minimal symptoms
1.5	No disability, minimal signs in more than one area
2.0	Slightly more disability in one area
2.5	Slightly greater disability in two areas
3.0	Moderate disability in one area but still walking independently
3.5	Walking independently but with moderate disability in one area and more than minimal disability in several others
4.0	Walking without aid, self-sufficient, up and about some 12 hours a day despite relatively severe disability; able to walk 500 meters without aid or rest
4.5	Walking without aid, up and about much of the day, able to work a full day, may have some limitation of full activity or require some help, relatively severe disability but able to walk 300 meters without aid or rest
5.0	Walking without aid or rest for about 200 meters, disability severe enough to impair full daily activities, can work a full day without special provisions
5.5	Ambulatory without aid or rest for about 100 meters; disability severe enough to prevent full daily activities
6.0	Intermittent or unilateral constant assistance (cane, crutch, brace) required to walk about 100 meters with or without resting
6.5	Needs canes, crutches, braces to walk for 20 meters without resting
7.0	Unable to walk beyond 5 meters even with aid; mostly confined to a wheelchair; wheels self in standard wheelchair and transfers alone; up and about in wheelchair some 12 hours a day
7.5	Unable to take more than a few steps; restricted to wheelchair; may need aid in transfer; wheels self but cannot carry on in standard wheelchair a full day; may require motorized wheelchair
8.0	Essentially restricted to bed, chair, or wheelchair, but may be out of bed itself much of the day; retains many self-care functions; generally has effective use of arms
8.5	Essentially restricted to bed much of day; has some effective use of arms; retains some self-care functions
9.0	Helpless bed patient; can communicate and eat
9.5	Totally helpless bed patient; unable to communicate effectively or eat/swallow
10.0	Death due to MS

REFERENCE
Kurtzke JF: *Neurology* 33:1444–1452, 1983.

KURTZKE FUNCTIONAL SYSTEMS SCORES (FSS)

- Pyramidal functions
  - 0: Normal
  - 1: Abnormal signs without disability
  - 2: Minimal disability

3: Mild to moderate paraparesis or hemiparesis (detectable weakness but most function sustained for short periods, fatigue a problem); severe monoparesis (almost no function)

4: Marked paraparesis or hemiparesis (function is difficult), moderate quadriparesis (function is decreased but can be sustained for short periods); or monoplegia

5: Paraplegia, hemiplegia, or marked quadriparesis

6: Quadriplegia

9: Unknown

- Cerebellar functions

  0: Normal

  1: Abnormal signs without disability

  2: Mild ataxia (tremor or clumsy movements easily seen, minor interference with function)

  3: Moderate truncal or limb ataxia (tremor or clumsy movements interfere with function in all spheres)

  4: Severe ataxia in all limbs (most function is very difficult)

  5: Unable to perform coordinated movements because of ataxia

  9: Unknown

  (Record #1 in small box when weakness [grade 3 or worse on pyramidal] interferes with testing.)

- Brainstem functions

  0: Normal

  1: Signs only

  2: Moderate nystagmus or other mild disability

  3: Severe nystagmus, marked extraocular weakness, or moderate disability of other cranial nerves

  4: Marked dysarthria or other marked disability

  5: Inability to swallow or speak

  9: Unknown

- Sensory function

  0: Normal

  1: Vibration or figure-writing decrease only in one or two limbs

  2: Mild decrease in touch or pain or position sense, or moderate decrease in vibration in one or two limbs; or vibratory can be substituted with decreased figure writing) decrease alone in three or four limbs

  3: Moderate decrease in touch or pain or position sense, or essentially lost vibration in one or two limbs; or mild decrease in touch or pain or moderate decrease in all proprioceptive tests in three or four limbs

  4: Marked decrease in touch or pain or loss of proprioception, alone or combined, in one or two limbs; or moderate decrease in touch or pain or severe proprioceptive decrease in more than two limbs

  5: Loss (essentially) of sensation in one or two limbs; or moderate decrease in touch or pain or loss of proprioception for most of the body below the head

  6: Sensation essentially lost below the head

9: Unknown
- Bowel and bladder function (rate on the basis of the worse function, either bowel or bladder)
  - 0: Normal
  - 1: Mild urinary hesitance, urgency, or retention
  - 2: Moderate hesitance, urgency, retention of bowel or bladder, or rare urinary incontinence (intermittent self-catheterization, manual compression to evacuate bladder, or finger evacuation of stool)
  - 3: Frequent urinary incontinence
  - 4: In need of almost constant catheterization (and constant use of measures to evacuate stool)
  - 5: Loss of bladder function
  - 6: Loss of bowel and bladder function
  - 9: Unknown
- Visual function
  - 0: Normal
  - 1: Scotoma with visual acuity (corrected) better than 20/30
  - 2: Worse eye with scotoma with maximal visual acuity (corrected) of 20/30 to 20/59
  - 3: Worse eye with large scotoma, or moderate decrease in fields, but with maximal visual acuity (corrected) of 20/60 to 20/99
  - 4: Worse eye with marked decrease of fields and maximal visual acuity (corrected) of 20/100 to 20/200; grade 3 plus maximal acuity of better eye of 20/60 or less
  - 5: Worse eye with maximal visual acuity (corrected) less than 20/200; grade 4 plus maximal acuity of better eye of 20/60 or less
  - 6: Grade 5 plus maximal visual acuity of better eye of 20/60 or less
  - 9: Unknown
  - (Record #1 in small box for presence of temporal pallor.)
- Cerebral (or mental) functions
  - 0: Normal
  - 1: Mood alteration only (does not affect EDSS)
  - 2: Mild decrease in mentation
  - 3: Moderate decrease in mentation
  - 4: Marked decrease in mentation (chronic brain syndrome, moderate)
  - 5: Dementia or chronic brain syndrome, severe or incompetent
  - 9: Unknown

REFERENCE

Kurtzke JF: *Neurology* 33:1444–1452, 1983.

MODIFIED RANKIN CLINICAL DISABILITY SCALE

- 0: No symptoms at all (Used often in stroke patients)
- 1: No significant disability despite symptoms; able to carry out all usual duties and activities

2: Slight disability; unable to carry out all previous activities but able to look after own affairs without assistance

3: Moderate disability requiring some help, but able to walk without assistance

4: Moderate-severe disability; unable to walk without assistance and unable to attend to own bodily needs without assistance

5: Severe disability; bedridden, incontinent, and requiring constant nursing care and attention

6: Death

NIH STROKE SEVERITY SCALE (NIHSSS)

Level of consciousness

- Alert, keenly responsive (0 points)
- Obeys, answers, or responds to minor stimulation (1 point)
- Responds only to repeated stimulation or painful stimulation (excludes reflex response) (2 points)
- Responds only with reflex motor or totally unresponsive (3 points)

Ask the month and patient's age; answer must be exactly right

- Answers both correctly (0 points)
- Answers one correctly or patient unable to speak because of any reason other than aphasia or coma (1 point)
- Answers neither correctly, or too stuporous or aphasic (2 points)

Ask patient to open and close eyes and then grip and release nonparetic hand

- Performs both tasks correctly (0 points)
- Performs 1 task correctly (1 point)
- Performs neither task correctly (2 points)

Best gaze: only horizontal movements tested; oculocephalic reflex use is ok, but not calorics

- Normal (0 points)
- Partial gaze palsy (1 point)
- Forced deviation or total gaze paresis not overcome by oculocephalic maneuver (2 points)

Visual fields tested by confrontation

- No visual loss (0 points)
- Partial hemianopia (1 point)
- Complete hemianopia (2 points)
- Bilateral hemianopia (blind from any cause including cortical blindness) (3 points)

Facial palsy: encourage patient to smile and close eyes or grimace; check symmetry

- Normal symmetrical movement (0 points)
- Minor paralysis (flattened nasolabial fold, asymmetry on smiling) (1 point)
- Partial paralysis (total or near total lower face paralysis) (2 points)

- Complete paralysis (absence of facial movement upper/lower face) (3 points)

Right arm motor: extend right arm palm down at 90 degrees (sitting) or 45 degrees (supine)

- No drift, holds for full 10 seconds (0 points)
- Drifts down before 10 seconds but does not hit bed/support (1 point)
- Some effort against gravity, but cannot get up to 90 (or 45 if supine) degrees (2 points)
- No effort against gravity, limb falls (3 points)
- No movement (4 points)

Left arm motor: extend left arm palm down at 90 degrees (sitting) or 45 degrees (supine)

- No drift, holds for full 10 seconds (0 points)
- Drifts down before 10 seconds but does not hit bed/support (1 point)
- Some effort against gravity, but cannot get up to 90 (or 45 if supine) degrees (2 points)
- No effort against gravity, limb falls (3 points)
- No movement (4 points)

Right leg motor: extend right leg and flex at hip to 30 degrees

- No drift, holds for full 5 seconds (0 points)
- Drifts down before 5 seconds but does not hit bed/support (1 point)
- Some effort against gravity (2 points)
- No effort against gravity, limb falls (3 points)
- No movement (4 points)

Left leg motor: extend left leg and flex at hip to 30 degrees

- No drift, holds for full 5 seconds (0 points)
- Drifts down before 5 seconds but does not hit bed/support (1 point)
- Some effort against gravity (2 points)
- No effort against gravity, limb falls (3 points)
- No movement (4 points)

Limb ataxia: finger/nose and heel/shin done on both sides (Not ataxia if hemiplegic or unable to comprehend. Ataxia must be out of proportion to any weakness present.)

- Absent (0 points)
- Present in 1 limb (1 point)
- Present in two limbs (2 points)

Sensory to pinprick

- Normal (0 points)
- Pinprick less sharp or dull on affected side (1 point)
- Severe to total sensory loss; patient unaware of being touched (2 points)

Best language using pictures, naming items, and reading short sentences

- No aphasia (0 points)
- Some loss of fluency or comprehension (1 point)

- Severe aphasia—fragmentary communication, listener carries burden of communication (2 points)
- Mute, global aphasia, no usable speech or auditory comprehension (3 points)

Dysarthria: if not obviously present, have patient read
- Normal (0 points)
- Slurs some words (1 point)
- So slurred as to be unintelligible, or mute (2 points)

Extinction/inattention
- No abnormality (0 points)
- Inattention to any sensory modality or extinction to bilateral simultaneous stimulation in one sensory modality (1 point)
- Profound hemi-inattention or hemi-inattention to more than one modality; does not recognize own hand (2 points)

PARKINSON'S DISEASE RATING SCALES

HOEHN AND YAHR STAGING OF PARKINSON'S DISEASE

1. Stage One
   1. Signs and symptoms on one side only
   2. Symptoms mild
   3. Symptoms inconvenient but not disabling
   4. Usually presents with tremor of one limb
   5. Friends have noticed changes in posture, locomotion, and facial expression
2. Stage Two
   1. Symptoms are bilateral
   2. Minimal disability
   3. Posture and gait affected
3. Stage Three
   1. Significant slowing of body movements
   2. Early impairment of equilibrium on walking or standing
   3. Generalized dysfunction that is moderately severe
4. Stage Four
   1. Severe symptoms
   2. Can still walk to a limited extent
   3. Rigidity and bradykinesia
   4. No longer able to live alone
   5. Tremor may be less than earlier stages
5. Stage Five
   1. Cachectic stage
   2. Invalidism complete
   3. Cannot stand or walk
   4. Requires constant nursing care

UNIFIED PARKINSON DISEASE RATING SCALE (UPDRS)

The UPDRS is a rating tool to follow the longitudinal course of Parkinson's disease. It is made up of the (1) Mentation, Behavior, and Mood, (2) ADL, and (3) Motor sections. These are evaluated by interview. Some sections require multiple grades assigned to each extremity. A total of 199 points are possible, with 199 representing the worst (total) disability, and 0 representing no disability.

I. Mentation, Behavior, Mood
- Intellectual Impairment
  - 0: None
  - 1: Mild (consistent forgetfulness with partial recollection of events with no other difficulties)
  - 2: Moderate memory loss with disorientation and moderate difficulty handling complex problems
  - 3: Severe memory loss with disorientation to time and often place, severe impairment with problems
  - 4: Severe memory loss with orientation only to person, unable to make judgments or solve problems
- Thought Disorder
  - 0: None
  - 1: Vivid dreaming
  - 2: "Benign" hallucination with insight retained
  - 3: Occasional to frequent hallucination or delusions without insight, could interfere with daily activities
  - 4: Persistent hallucination, delusions, or florid psychosis.
- Depression
  - 0: Not present
  - 1: Periods of sadness or guilt greater than normal, never sustained for more than a few days or a week
  - 2: Sustained depression for >1 week
  - 3: Vegetative symptoms (insomnia, anorexia, abulia, weight loss)
  - 4: Vegetative symptoms with suicidality
- Motivation/Initiative
  - 0: Normal
  - 1: Less of assertive, more passive
  - 2: Loss of initiative or disinterest in elective activities
  - 3: Loss of initiative or disinterest in day to day (routine) activities
  - 4: Withdrawn, complete loss of motivation

II. Activities of Daily Living
- Speech
  - 0: Normal
  - 1: Mildly affected, no difficulty being understood
  - 2: Moderately affected, may be asked to repeat
  - 3: Severely affected, frequently asked to repeat
  - 4: Unintelligible most of time

- Salivation
  - 0: Normal
  - 1: Slight but noticeable increase, may have nighttime drooling
  - 2: Moderately excessive saliva, minimal drooling
  - 3: Marked drooling
- Swallowing
  - 0: Normal
  - 1: Rare choking
  - 2: Occasional choking
  - 3: Requires soft food
  - 4: Requires NG tube or G tube
- Handwriting
  - 0: Normal
  - 1: Slightly small or slow
  - 2: All words small but legible
  - 3: Severely affected, not all words legible
  - 4: Majority illegible
- Cutting Food/Handing Utensils
  - 0: Normal
  - 1: Somewhat slow and clumsy but no help needed
  - 2: Can cut most foods, some help needed
  - 3: Food must be cut, but can feed self
  - 4: Needs to be fed
- Dressing
  - 0: Normal
  - 1: Somewhat slow, no help needed
  - 2: Occasional help with buttons or arms in sleeves
  - 3: Considerable help required but can do some things alone
  - 4: Helpless
- Hygiene
  - 0: Normal
  - 1: Somewhat slow but no help needed
  - 2: Needs help with shower or bath or very slow in hygienic care
  - 3: Requires assistance for washing, brushing teeth, going to bathroom
  - 4: Helpless
- Turning in Bed/Adjusting Bed Clothes
  - 0: Normal
  - 1: Somewhat slow, no help needed
  - 2: Can turn alone or adjust sheets but with great difficulty
  - 3: Can initiate but not turn or adjust alone
  - 4: Helpless
- Falling Unrelated to Freezing
  - 0: None
  - 1: Rare falls
  - 2: Occasional, less than one per day

    3: Average of once per day

    4: >1 per day

- Freezing When Walking

    0: Normal

    1: Rare, may have start hesitation

    2: Occasional falls from freezing

    3: Frequent freezing, occasional falls

    4: Frequent falls from freezing

- Walking

    0: Normal

    1: Mild difficulty, may drag legs or decrease arm swing

    2: Moderate difficultly requires no assist

    3: Severe disturbance requires assistance

    4: Cannot walk at all even with assist

- Tremor

    0: Absent

    1: Slight and infrequent, not bothersome to patient

    2: Moderate, bothersome to patient

    3: Severe, interferes with many activities

    4: Marked, interferes with many activities

- Sensory Complaints Related to Parkinsonism

    0: None

    1: Occasionally has numbness, tingling, and mild aching

    2: Frequent, but not distressing

    3: Frequent painful sensation

    4: Excruciating pain

III. Motor Exam

- Speech

    0: Normal

    1: Slight loss of expression, diction, volume

    2: Monotone, slurred but understandable, moderately impaired

    3: Marked impairment, difficult to understand

    4: Unintelligible

- Facial Expression

    0: Normal

    1: Slight hypomimia, could be poker face

    2: Slight but definite abnormal diminution in expression

    3: Moderate hypomimia, lips parted some of time

    4: Masked or fixed face, lips parted 1/4 inch or more with complete loss of expression

- Tremor at Rest

    A. Face

        0: Absent

        1: Alight and infrequent

        2: Mild and present most of time

    3: Moderate and present most of time

    4: Marked and present most of time

B. Right Upper Extremity (RUE)

    0: Absent

    1: Slight and infrequent

    2: Mild and present most of time

    3: Moderate and present most of time

    4: Marked and present most of time

C. Left Upper Extremity (LUE)

    0: Absent

    1: Slight and infrequent

    2: Mild and present most of time

    3: Moderate and present most of time

    4: Marked and present most of time

D. Right Lower Extremity (RLE)

    0: Absent

    1: Slight and infrequent

    2: Mild and present most of time

    3: Moderate and present most of time

    4: Marked and present most of time

E. Left Lower Extremity (LLE)

    0: Absent

    1: Slight and infrequent

    2: Mild and present most of time

    3: Moderate and present most of time

    4: Marked and present most of time

- Action or Postural Tremor

  A. RUE

    0: Absent

    1: Slight, present with action

    2: Moderate, present with action

    3: Moderate present with action and posture holding

    4: Marked, interferes with feeding

  B. LUE

    0: Absent

    1: Slight, present with action

    2: Moderate, present with action

    3: Moderate present with action and posture holding

    4: Marked, interferes with feeding

- Rigidity

  A. Neck

    0: Absent

    1: Slight or only with activation

    2: Mild/moderate

    3: Marked, full range of motion

    4: Severe

B. RUE
- 0: Absent
- 1: Slight or only with activation
- 2: Mild/moderate
- 3: Marked, full range of motion
- 4: Severe

C. LUE
- 0: Absent
- 1: Slight or only with activation
- 2: Mild/moderate
- 3: Marked, full range of motion
- 4: Severe

D. RLE
- 0: Absent
- 1: Slight or only with activation
- 2: Mild/moderate
- 3: Marked, full range of motion
- 4: Severe

E. LLE
- 0: Absent
- 1: Slight or only with activation
- 2: Mild/moderate
- 3: Marked, full range of motion
- 4: Severe

- Finger Taps
  A. Right
  - 0: Normal
  - 1: Mild slowing and/or reduction in amplitude
  - 2: Moderately impaired, definite and early fatiguing, may have occasional arrests
  - 3: Severely impaired, frequent hesitations and arrests
  - 4: Can barely perform

  B. Left
  - 0: Normal
  - 1: mild slowing, and/or reduction in amp.
  - 2: Moderately impaired, definite and early fatiguing, may have occasional arrests
  - 3: Severely impaired, frequent hesitations and arrests
  - 4: Can barely perform

- Hand Movements (open and close hands in rapid succession)
  A. Right
  - 0: Normal
  - 1: Mild slowing and/or reduction in amplitude
  - 2: Moderately impaired, definite and early fatiguing, may have occasional arrests

      3: Severely impaired, frequent hesitations and arrests

      4: Can barely perform

  B. Left

     0: Normal

     1: Mild slowing and/or reduction in amplitude

     2: Moderately impaired, definite and early fatiguing, may have occasional arrests

     3: Severely impaired, frequent hesitations and arrests

     4: Can barely perform

- Rapid Alternating Movements (pronate and supinate hands)
  A. Right
     0: Normal
     1: Mild slowing and/or reduction in amplitude
     2: Moderately impaired, definite and early fatiguing, may have occasional arrests
     3: Severely impaired, frequent hesitations and arrests
     4: Can barely perform
  B. Left
     0: Normal
     1: Mild slowing and/or reduction in amplitude
     2: Moderately impaired, definite and early fatiguing, may have occasional arrests
     3: Severely impaired, frequent hesitations and arrests
     4: Can barely perform

- Leg Agility (tap heel on ground, amplitude should be 3 inches)
  A. Right
     0: Normal
     1: Mild slowing and/or reduction in amplitude
     2: Moderately impaired, definite and early fatiguing, may have occasional arrests
     3: Severely impaired, frequent hesitations and arrests
     4: Can barely perform
  B. Left
     0: Normal
     1: Mild slowing and/or reduction in amplitude
     2: Moderately impaired, definite and early fatiguing, may have occasional arrests
     3: Severely impaired, frequent hesitations and arrests
     4: Can barely perform

- Arising from Chair (patient arises with arms folded across chest)
  0: Normal
  1: Slow, may need more than one attempt
  2: Pushes self up from arms or seat
  3: Tends to fall back, may need multiple tries but can arise without assistance
  4: Unable to arise without help

- Posture
  - 0: Normal erect
  - 1: Slightly stooped, could be normal for older person
  - 2: Definitely abnormal, moderately stooped, may lean to one side
  - 3: Severely stooped with kyphosis
  - 4: Marked flexion with extreme abnormality of posture
- Gait
  - 0: Normal
  - 1: Walks slowly, may shuffle with short steps, no festination or propulsion
  - 2: Walks with difficulty, little or no assistance, some festination, short steps or propulsion
  - 3: Severe disturbance, frequent assistance
  - 4: Cannot walk
- Postural Stability (retropulsion test)
  - 0: Normal
  - 1: Recovers unaided
  - 2: Would fall if not caught
  - 3: Falls spontaneously
  - 4: Unable to stand
- Body Bradykinesia/Hypokinesia
  - 0: None
  - 1: Minimal slowness, could be normal, deliberate character
  - 2: Mild slowness and poverty of movement, definitely abnormal, or decreased amplitude of movement
  - 3: Moderate slowness, poverty, or small amplitude
  - 4: Marked slowness, poverty, or amplitude

SCHWAB AND ENGLAND ACTIVITIES OF DAILY LIVING

Rating can be assigned by rater or by patient.

- 100%: Completely independent. Able to do all chores without slowness, difficulty, or impairment.
- 90%: Completely independent. Able to do all chores with some slowness, difficulty, or impairment. May take twice as long.
- 80%: Independent in most chores. Takes twice as long. Conscious of difficulty and slowing
- 70%: Not completely independent. More difficulty with chores. 3 to 4 times along on chores for some. May take large part of day for chores.
- 60%: Some dependency. Can do most chores, but very slowly and with much effort. Errors, some impossible
- 50%: More dependant. Needs help with half of chores. Difficulty with everything.
- 40%: Very dependent. Can assist with all chores but few alone.
- 30%: With effort, now and then does a few chores alone or begins alone. Much help needed.

- 20%: Nothing alone. Can do some slight help with some chores. Severe invalid.
- 10%: Totally dependent, helpless.
- 0%: Vegetative functions such as swallowing, bladder, and bowel function are not functioning. Bedridden

SPETZLER-MARTIN SCALE FOR ARTERIOVENOUS MALFORMATION

	Score
Size of AVM	
Small (<3 cm)	1
Medium (3–6 cm)	2
Large (>6 cm)	3
Eloquence of Adjacent Brain	
Noneloquent	0
Eloquent	1
Pattern of Venous Drainage	
Superficial only	0
Deep	1

Score: Grade the AVM by adding the scores on each feature (range 1 to 5).

Common Abbreviations

AIDS—acquired immunodeficiency syndrome
bid—twice a day
BP—blood pressure
BUN—blood urea nitrogen
CBC—complete blood count
CN—cranial nerve
CNS—central nervous system
CPR—cardiopulmonary resuscitation
CT—computed tomography
CVP—central venous pressure
DBP—diastolic blood pressure
ECG—electrocardiogram
EEG—electroencephalogram
ELISA—enzyme-linked immunosorbent assay
EMG—electromyelogram
fMRI—functional magnetic resonance imaging
HIV—human immunodeficiency virus
ICH—intracranial hemorrhage
ICP—intracranial pressure
IVIG—intravenous immunoglobulin
LP—lumbar puncture
MAP—mean arterial pressure
MRI—magnetic resonance imaging
MRS—magnetic resonance spectroscopy
PCR—polymerase chain reaction
PT—prothrombin time
PTT—partial thromboplastin time
qid—four times a day
RBC—red blood cell
REM—rapid eye movement
SBP—systolic blood pressure
tid—three times a day
TSH—thyroid-stimulating hormone
WBC—white blood cell

Index

Note: Page numbers followed by f refer to figures; page numbers followed by t refer to tables.